Table of Contents

Contributors

The following list contains the location and practice for each contributor at the time of their article submission.

Patricia Martin Arcari, PhD(C), RN
Codirector
Behavioral Medicine General Programs
Division of Behavioral Medicine
Deaconess Hospital
Boston, Massachusetts

Carol Ann Baer, PhD, RN
Nurse Researcher
Wellness Division
VNA Care Plus
Danvers, Massachusetts

Julia W. Balzer, MN, RN
Independent Consultant
Staff Educator
Training and Development
Baptist Medical Center
Jacksonville, Florida

Sharon E. Beck, DNSc, RN
Assistant Hospital Director
Nursing Education and Quality Improvement
Temple University Hospital
Philadelphia, Pennsylvania

Patricia Hentz Becker, EdD, RN
Associate Professor
School of Nursing
La Salle University
Philadelphia, Pennsylvania

Joyceen S. Boyle, RN, PhD, FAAN
Department of Community Nursing
School of Nursing
Medical College of Georgia
Augusta, Georgia

Harriette L.K. Buchanan, MS, Ed, MS Counseling
Former Full-Time Volunteer
Trauma Unit
Codeveloper and Former Coordinator
Allegheny General Hospital Trauma
   Bereavement Program
Allegheny General Hospital
Pittsburgh, Pennsylvania

Pamela Buckalew, RN, CNS, C
Coordinator
New Jersey Sudden Infant Death Syndrome
   Resource Center
Department of Neonatology
St. Peter's Medical Center
New Brunswick, New Jersey

Margaret A. Burkhardt, PhD, RNCS
Associate Professor of Nursing
West Virginia University School of Nursing,
   Charleston Division
Charleston, West Virginia

Patricia E. Camp, DSN, RN
Assistant Professor
Ida V. Moffett School of Nursing
Samford University
Birmingham, Alabama

Susan K. Chase, EdD, RN
Assistant Professor
Boston College
Graduate School of Nursing
Chestnut Hill, Massachusetts

Tabiri Chukunta, BA, MA
Manager of Safety and Coordinator of Diversity
New Jersey Sudden Infant Death Syndrome
    Resource Center
Department of Neonatology
St. Peter's Medical Center
New Brunswick, New Jersey

Carolie J. Coates, PhD
Assistant Professor
School of Nursing
University of Colorado Health Sciences Center
Denver, Colorado

Teresa P. Cooper, MSN, RN, CPNP, CTN
Coordinator
Community Health Outreach with the
    Department of Pediatrics
Division of Community Pediatrics
University of California San Diego
San Diego, California

Nina M. Coppens, PhD, RN
Professor
Department of Nursing
University of Massachusetts Lowell
Lowell, Massachusetts

Alice D. Domar, PhD
Staff Psychologist
Division of Behavioral Medicine
Deaconess Hospital
Senior Scientist
Mind/Body Medical Institute
Assistant Professor in Medicine
Harvard Medical School
Boston, Massachusetts

Marge Drugay, MS, RN, C
Consultant
Drugay & Associates
Glenview, Illinois
Associate Faculty
Rush University
Department of Gerontological Nursing
Chicago, Illinois

Katie Eriksson, RN, PhD
Professor
Department of Caring Science
Åbo Akademi University
Vasa, Finland

Linda M. Esposito, RN, MPH
Assistant Coordinator
New Jersey Sudden Infant Death Syndrome
    Resource Center
Department of Neonatology
St. Peter's Medical Center
New Brunswick, New Jersey

Marie D. Geubtner, RN, CCRN
Staff Nurse
Trauma Unit
Coordinator
Allegheny General Hospital Trauma
    Bereavement Program
Allegheny General Hospital
Pittsburgh, Pennsylvania

Evelyn K. Goldberg, MS, RN
Community Health Educator
Tru Care Home Health Agency, Inc.
Philadelphia, Pennsylvania

Barbara W. Girardin, PhD, RN
Graduate Lecturer
Division of Nursing
California State University
Carson, California

Joyce P. Griffin, PhD, RN, OCN
Director
Clinical Nursing Research
Naval Hospital
Portsmouth, Virginia

Joanne M. Hall, RN, PhD
Assistant Professor
University of Wisconsin
Madison School of Nursing
Madison, Wisconsin

Betty Halpern, RN, CPAN
Postanesthesia Care Unit Staff Nurse
Shore Memorial Hospital
Somers Point, New Jersey

Cathy S. Heriot, RN, PhD
Assistant Professor
College of Nursing
Medical University of South Carolina
Charleston, South Carolina

Sue C. Jacobs, PhD
Associate Professor and Director of PhD
    Counseling Psychology Training Program
Department of Counseling
University of North Dakota
Grand Forks, North Dakota

Jennifer Jenkins, MBA, RN, CNAA
Principal
Jenkins and Associates
Senior Consultant
Healthcare Concepts, Inc.
Memphis, Tennessee

Kelly Johnston, MSN, RN, CCRN
Staff Nurse
Department of Nursing
Ann Arbor Veterans Administration Hospital
Ann Arbor, Michigan

Rauni Prittinen King, RN, BSN, CCRN
Staff Nurse
Intensive Care Unit
Scripps Memorial Hospital
La Jolla, California

Lori L. Kondora, RN, CS, MS
Doctoral Candidate
University of Wisconsin
Madison School of Nursing
Madison, Wisconsin

Janet Wessel Krejci, MS, RN, PhD
Assistant Professor
College of Nursing
Marquette University
Milwaukee, Wisconsin

Patricia LaCarrubba, RN
Pediatric Sedation Nurse
Shore Memorial Hospital
Somers Point, New Jersey

Sarah Steen Lauterbach, EdD, RN
Associate Professor
School of Nursing
La Salle University
Philadelphia, Pennsylvania

Carol Lynn Mandle, RN, PhD
Associate Professor
Boston College School of Nursing
Associate for Research and Consultation
Beth Israel Hospital
Codirector
Behavioral Medicine General Programs
Division of Behavioral Medicine
Deaconess Hospital
Scientist
Mind/Body Medical Institute
Harvard Medical School
Boston, Massachusetts

Evelyn Martin-Lewis, MSN, RN
Data Coordinator
Cardiac Data Bank
Crawford Long Hospital of Emory University
Atlanta, Georgia

Susan McCue, MSN, RN, PNP
Former Graduate Student
College of Nursing
University of Tennessee
Knoxville, Tennessee

Cynthia Jean Medich, PhD, RN
Clinical Director
Affiliate Programs
Faculty and Scientist
The Mind/Body Medical Institute
Beth Israel Deaconess Medical Center and
    Harvard Medical School
Boston, Massachusetts

Joni Miller, RN
Clinical Nurse
Cardiology
Emory Clinic
Atlanta, Georgia

Mary Anne Modrcin-McCarthy, PhD, RN
Director and Associate Professor
Undergraduate Program
College of Nursing
University of Tennessee
Knoxville, Tennessee

Carol Leppanen Montgomery, RN, PhD
Assistant Professor
School of Nursing
University of Colorado Health Sciences Center
Denver, Colorado

Rita I. Morris, PhD, RN
Associate Professor
School of Nursing of San Diego State
    University
Adjunct Faculty Member
University of Phoenix
San Diego, California

Rachel Beaty Muller, RN, MSN
Doctoral Student
School of Nursing
Medical College of Georgia
Augusta, Georgia

Steffanie S. Mulloney, MS, RN
Brigham and Women's Hospital
Newborn Intensive Care Unit
Boston, Massachusetts

Judy G. Ozbolt, PhD, RN, FAAN
Professor and Director
Doctoral Program
School of Nursing
University of Virginia
Charlottesville, Virginia

Belinda Utley Peebles, MN, RN, CCRN
Nurse Coordinator
Crawford Long Hospital of Emory University
Atlanta, Georgia

Janet F. Quinn, PhD, RN, FAAN
Associate Professor and Senior Scholar
Center for Human Caring
University of Colorado School of Nursing
Denver, Colorado

Roberta Reed, BSN, RN
Clinical Nurse
Cardiology
Emory Clinic
Atlanta, Georgia

Sherry Rodriquez, BBA/BHA, RN
Technical Director
Cardiac Catheterization Laboratory
Crawford Long Hospital of Emory University
Atlanta, Georgia

Jacqueline Rohaly-Davis, MS, RN, OCN
Staff Nurse
Edward J. Hines Jr. Veterans Administration
    Hospital
Hines, Illinois

Marion E. Rudek, MSN, RN, CRNP
Maternal Child Health Nurse Practitioner
Shore Memorial Hospital
Somers Point, New Jersey

**Albert A. Rundio, Jr., PhD, MSN, RN,
    CNAA**
Vice President for Nursing Services
Shore Memorial Hospital
Somers Point, New Jersey

Susan D. Ruppert, PhD, RN, CCRN, FNP
Associate Professor
Division of Critical Care and Transplantation
The University of Texas-Houston Health
    Science Center
School of Nursing
Houston, Texas

**Elaine Fogel Schneider, PhD, CCC-SLP,
    ADTR, CIMI**
Founder and Executive Director
Baby Steps/Antelope Valley Infant
    Development
First Touch
Lancaster, California

Julie Anderson Schorr, PhD
Associate Professor
Department of Nursing
Northern Michigan University
Marquette, Michigan

Victoria E. Slater, MSN, RN
Doctoral Student
University of Tennessee
Knoxville, Tennessee

Carolyn Kay Snyder, MSW, LSW
Clinical Social Worker
Trauma Unit
Codeveloper and Supervisor
Allegheny General Hospital Trauma
    Bereavement Program
Allegheny General Hospital
Pittsburgh, Pennsylvania

Maria Spear, BS
Child Life Specialist
Shore Memorial Hospital
Somers Point, New Jersey

Cynthia M. Steckel, RN, MSN, CCRN
Director
ICU/SDU/Telemetry
Scripps Memorial Hospital-La Jolla and Green
Hospital of Scripps Clinic
La Jolla, California

Anthony J. Strelkauskas, PhD
Associate Professor
Microbiology and Immunobiology
Medical University of South Carolina
Charleston, South Carolina

Eileen Stuart, MS, RN, C
Project Director
CAD Reversal Project
The Mind/Body Medical Institute
Beth Israel Deaconess Medical Center and
    Harvard Medical School
Boston, Massachusetts

Maureen Bryan Thompson, MS, RN-C
Family Nurse Practitioner
Newburyport, Massachusetts

Julie Walker, MSN, RN, PNP
Former Graduate Student
College of Nursing
University of Tennessee
Knoxville, Tennessee

Christi Deaton Warner, MN, RN, CCRN
Clinical Nurse Coordinator
Crawford Long Hospital of Emory
    University
Atlanta, Georgia

Carol L. Wells-Federman, MEd, RN
Nurse Specialist
Division of Behavioral Medicine
Director of Clinical Training
Mind/Body Medical Institute
Deaconess Hospital
Adjunct Clinical Instructor in Nursing
Graduate School for Health Studies
Simmons College
Adjunct Instructor in Public Health
School of Medicine
Boston University School of Public Health
Boston, Massachusetts

Susan Ann Williams, DNS, RN
Assistant Professor
Department of Adult Health
School of Nursing
East Carolina University
Greenville, North Carolina

Patty Wooten, BSN, RN, CCRN
Founder and President
Jest for the Health of It Services
Davis, California

Preface

If we could entertain the notion of "weaving a tapestry of holism and healing," the imagery would include the complexity of the task and the multifaceted composition of its many foundational threads. Several of those threads have been gathered for *Essential Readings in Holistic Nursing* to provide a clearer, more vivid understanding about the frequently elusive nature of holistic nursing.

PURPOSE

The purpose of *Essential Readings in Holistic Nursing* is to provide information to supplement the content found in the *American Holistic Nurses' Association Core Curriculum for Holistic Nursing* (Dossey, 1997), and *Holistic Nursing: A Handbook for Practice* (Dossey et al., 1995). The book focuses on clients/families and their nurse caregivers. It is intended for all students, practitioners, educators, and researchers who are interested in exploring the real-world issues of holistic nursing. Forty articles have been selected for this book culled from 10 Aspen nursing journals over the past five years. The articles were chosen because of their relevance, insight, clarification, and alternative perspectives on holism and healing in clinical practice.

ORGANIZATION

The articles include a variety of current subjects (although taken only from Aspen journals because of copyright and permission issues) ranging from practice-based clinical and "how-to" reports (17 articles), research investigations (14 articles), clinical reviews (four articles), and theory-based topics (five articles).

I was awestruck when I realized how the articles selected for this book exposed decisive, changing trends that are emerging from nursing practice—trends reflecting care of the body-mind-spirit of clients, families, and caregivers. Some of these trends, justified by the sheer number of articles that have been published on specific topics over the past five years, have been captured in the six units of this book. Unit I, for example, reflects the soul of holism and healing by covering some of its foundational threads, including caring, spirituality, synchronicity, and expanded consciousness. Unit II reflects the heightened awareness across the profession that nurses must first take care of themselves before they are able to deliver transformational care to their clients. Units III and IV uncover a renewed emphasis on intervention for those problems that we know affect client outcomes but are too often ignored (e.g., culturally sensitive health care issues and unhealthy environmental variables), as well as some problems that often tend to be hidden from view (i.e., unrecognized lifestyle alterations and abuse). The literature chosen for Unit V also clearly confirms that nurses, across all types of practice settings, are becoming more committed to meeting the client's body-mind-spirit needs by implementing alternative/complementary therapies, including relaxation techniques, imagery, music therapy, therapeutic touch, and massage for a multitude of bio-psycho-social-spiritual problems (e.g., stress, anxiety, fear, denial, depression, pain, and sleep pattern disturbance). Unit VI unveils several exemplars of holistic nursing practice demonstrating the translation of theory into practice. These exemplars provide practical details about implementing holistic programs for a variety of clients ranging from those children and adults who are chronically or critically ill, undergoing surgery, recovering from a cardiac crisis, dealing with the traumatic loss of a loved one, or placing a relative in a long-term care setting.

The research articles selected for this book also reveal changing trends that are driving investigational designs. We are seeing, for example, emphasis placed on measuring the effects of holistic programs and nursing interventions based on valued consumer outcomes such as functional status, health-related quality of life, perceived effectiveness of therapy, and satisfaction with care rather than exclusively on the traditional, biomedical outcome measures that have been heavily used so much in the past (i.e., clinical endpoints such as vital signs and laboratory measurements, morbidity, and mortality). In addition, we are observing a tendency to investigate multidimensional measures of health status and the bio-psycho-social-spiritual outcomes of health and illness rather than only studying the absence of disease.

FEATURES

There are several valuable features of *Essential Readings in Holistic Nursing*. As a companion text to the *Core Curriculum* and *Holistic Nursing, Essential Readings* provides supplemental articles that can serve as a basis for studying and group discussions in preparing for the certification examination in holistic nursing (HNC). The book also is useful as a teaching tool in both the clinical and academic settings. For nurses who have neither the time, energy, nor access to a nursing library to search for updated literature, this book provides a ready-made compilation of topical articles that can be used to stay current in the field, maintain professional standards of practice, guarantee professional advancement, and evaluate the strength of evidence supporting the interventions we deliver.

Essential Readings in Holistic Nursing reveals the sights and sounds of changing times. These sights and sounds validate that holistic nursing is no longer on the fringe, no longer confined to theoretical abstractions, and no longer endorsed by only a few. These sights and sounds disclose the stories of clinicians and researchers throughout the country who are successfully integrating and investigating the effects of holism and healing in clinical practice.

Tapestries are created by an intermeshing, intertwining, and interconnecting of carefully selected individual threads configured by the weavers' consciousness and spirit. As each of us creates our own tapestry of holism and healing, I believe we will find that the insights and wisdom of our expert colleagues will help us to unravel some of the mysterious, theoretical threads to transform such concepts into concrete implications for nursing practice.

Cathie E. Guzzetta, RN, PhD, FAAN
Editor

Foundations of Holism and Healing

Some of the foundational threads of holism and healing, including caring, spirituality, synchronicity, and expanded consciousness, have been selected for this unit to provide a more discerning, real-world understanding about the frequently theoretical nature of holistic nursing.

CARING

Caring has been delineated as the core or soul of nursing. As a framework to understand this core, a clinical caring science paradigm is proposed (Eriksson) for integrating caring into clinical practice. Caring also is explored in terms of its emotional (both positive and negative) demand on nurses (Montgomery) and its presumed incompatibility with technology (Ozbolt). The message here is that caring experiences can become transformational events producing healing and growth toward wholeness even in the midst of technology, devastating crisis, and death.

If caring is the soul of nursing, it is imperative that we determine whether such caring practices make a difference in the lives of our clients and families. To that end, the Caring Efficacy Scale (CES) was developed (Coates) to assess belief in one's ability to care and develop caring relationships with clients. Likewise, in an outcome study of caring (Williams), a positive relationship between patients' perceptions of nurse caring and satisfaction with nursing care is presented. The Holistic Caring Inventory (HCI), which was used in this study, is published as part

of the article. Nurse researchers might explore using the CES and the HCI for future clinical and educational caring studies.

SPIRITUALITY

The three articles on spirituality provide rich descriptions of the human spiritual dimension as the core of the individual's existence. Two of the articles document the findings from qualitative research studies to provide us with a fuller understanding of spirituality in women (Burkhardt) and for clients in crisis (Camp). The third article on spiritual aging (Heriot) contains a thorough review of findings from religious and spiritual research and practical suggestions for assessing spirit titre and intervening with the spirit.

SYNCHRONICITY

Synchronicity and synchronous connections are concepts that have not been well documented or researched, yet appear to have enormous implications for holistic nursing practice. Synchronicity is described by Slater (via a concept analysis) in terms of its definition, attributes, and types with intuition selected as an example of a synchronous event. Krejci propels this concept into the clinical sphere by documenting (via qualitative clinical research) how the synchronous connections between client and nurse have major impact on client outcomes. Recommendations are offered for documenting, teaching, and incorporating synchrony in practice as well as for ideas on researching outcomes associated with facilitating client synchrony.

EXPANDED CONSCIOUSNESS

The potential healing effects associated with the intentional use of expanded consciousness are proposed by Quinn and supported by the findings from her pilot study using therapeutic touch. In this seminal article, Quinn views *the nurse as* the healing environment of the client.

Such a healing environment facilitates the synergistic, multidimensional response of clients in the direction of healing and wholeness. Although no one and no thing can heal another human being, nurses can remove the barriers and create environments that support healing. The suggestion that nurses can intentionally use expanded consciousness to facilitate the healing process in themselves and others, and that such a process has the potential to be measured by research, catapults the role of the nurse healer to an unparalleled new level. It is imperative that this line of research be supported and fostered.

Understanding the World of the Patient, the Suffering Human Being: The New Clinical Paradigm from Nursing to Caring

Katie Eriksson, RN, PhD
Professor, Department of Caring Science
Åbo Akademi University
Vasa, Finland

Caring science is now entering a new paradigmatic phase. Thus the world of the patient and the caring reality can be molded in a new way (Eriksson, 1993; Eriksson et al., 1996). A clinical caring and nursing science paradigm implies that nursing work has an ontological basis. This basis includes a new conceptual model and central fundamental presumptions about the human being, the patient, health, suffering, caring, and the values that form the basis of patient care. The clinical caring paradigm also includes a new methodological and epistemological basis. A change of paradigm implies a change of the core of theory (Törnebohm, 1985). The new core presupposes a return to the original concept of patient—the suffering human being—and to the original historical conditions of caring.

Watson (1995) follows the same reasoning in her discussion about the necessity for a change of paradigm, which may require a redefinition of the nursing discipline as a whole. According to Watson, this development can already be seen in epistemological shifting, which is a development from "analytic, descriptive—toward critical, interpretative hermeneutics, con-constructed meaning . . . ontic [fixed] categories, entities—toward the ontologically authentic" (Watson, 1995, p. 63).

The author acknowledges the patients, relatives, and nurses who participated in this study and made it possible. The author thanks Inger Myllymäki, MNSc, for analyzing the results of the study and Marina Aittamäki for compiling the article.

Source: Reprinted from K. Eriksson, *Advanced Practice Nursing Quarterly,* Vol. 3, No. 1, pp. 8–13, © 1997, Aspen Publishers, Inc.

The discussion about a "new" paradigm, a more authentic, autonomous, and clinically practical form of nursing, has been going on for the last few years (Fawcett, 1993; Newman, 1992; Parse, 1987, 1992; Watson, 1988). Cody (1990), in discussing all paradigms, says that many paradigms exist throughout the universe but there are only two in nursing: the old and the new. The old paradigm is reductional and scientific. The new is a more total paradigm.

The discussion about paradigms may sometimes seem diffuse, moving on different levels, ontologically, epistemologically, methodologically, and so forth. In spite of this fact, there is a trend toward developing a clinical paradigm based on an ontology where the human being, the patient, and true caring comprise the essence. True caring is not a form of behavior, not a feeling or state. It is an ontology, a way of living. It is not enough to "be there"—it is the way, the "spirit" in which it is done; and this spirit is caritative (Eriksson, 1992). During the years to come it will be important to discuss how the new paradigm can be integrated into a complex world that is, in many respects, foreign to caring in a deep sense. The purpose of this article is to discuss different paradigms and perspectives of interpretation, as well as the consequences they might have with respect to gaining knowledge about the patient's world. In order to enlight the new clinical paradigm, an example of ongoing research is used (Eriksson et al., 1996).

Do the ideals of caring exist in the patient's world today? The basic ontological questions are: What is the nurse's view of the patient? and What do nurses regard as the basic motive for caring? (Eriksson et al., 1996; Lindholm & Eriksson, 1993). The fundamental epistemological questions are: How do we search for knowledge? What do we want to know? and How do we make it knowable or understandable?

THE CLINICAL PARADIGMS—THE PATIENT'S WORLD AS AN IDEAL AND AS A REALITY

The clinical caring science paradigm can, as its starting point, choose a field of science or a field of research. The primary question is whether caring science is viewed as an autonomous or an applied science. When choosing a field of science as a starting point, an ideal model is also chosen as a starting point for empirical research (see Figure 1). Research is then guided by this ideal model, and reality is viewed from this special point of view (Alvesson & Sköldberg, 1994). The ideal model represents a special form of abductive hypothesis (i.e., the idea of what reality could be like), which helps in the identification of the meaningful, deep structures in one's field of research.

If a field of research is chosen as the starting point, there is no explicit model guiding research. This absence of a model often leads to diffuseness in the development of science, because research and interpretation of the results are guided by concepts and models from different sciences and perspectives. It also means that the development of knowledge takes place on a superficial level.

The integration of a clinical caring science paradigm into nursing practice also means that nurses become more aware of caring science. When caring science and practice are integrated, the unique identity of the nurses develops, which in turn makes the nurses feel that they are part of the scientific community. It also becomes natural for them to take part in research work, to

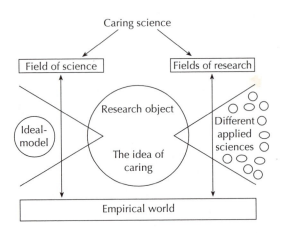

Figure 1. Epistemological perspectives in caring and nursing science.

implement research findings, and to develop the care of patients.

THREE PERSPECTIVES OF NURSING

During the last few years, the ongoing discussion within caring science has increasingly focused on the question of what the innermost core of caring is (Eriksson, 1987; Leininger, 1988; Roach, 1987). The discussion can be characterized as a question about the concepts of "caring" and "nursing." Lately, the concept has often been referred to simply as caring. *Caring* relates to the innermost core of nursing. *Nursing* relates to the actual work of the nurses. Nursing does not necessarily involve caring. When talking about nursing and caring, different nursing and caring cultures exist. For example, it is possible to distinguish between different nursing traditions, which are identified here as nursing perspectives and are referred to as nursing I, II, and III (see Figure 2).

Nursing I (caring nursing) describes the innermost core of caring. It represents a kind of caring without prejudice that emphasizes the patient and his or her suffering and needs. Such care may seem unstructured and chaotic from the outside, but its inner structure reflects good, individual patient care. The caring relation is a communion, and the caring profile is caritas (Eriksson, 1992).

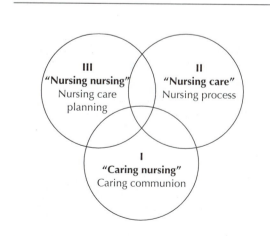

Figure 2. Caring and nursing perspectives.

Nursing II (nursing care) is based on the nursing process. It aims to meet the patient's needs systematically. It is based on illness and diagnosis. Nursing II represents good care when it is controlled by the innermost core of caring. However, if the innermost part is not taken into consideration, nursing may be technically good, but it is still not caring.

Nursing III (nursing nursing) is based on the structures of nursing care planning. Its aim is systematic planning of patient care. Unless it is based on the nursing process and the essence of nursing, there is a risk that nursing could become an administrative structure without caring substance. Good nursing care must include all three perspectives.

These three nursing traditions imply that there are three different worlds and cultures in the clinical nursing reality. They also mean that there are three different traditions of science and research. Each tradition is based on different ontologies and conceptual models.

THE HERMENEUTICAL IDEA IN CLINICAL CARING RESEARCH

Hermeneutical, abductive or reflective research makes a deeper understanding possible and allows the context of meaning to be maintained (Gadamer, 1988). When one wants to explore the patient's world in order to understand it in a deeper sense, the difficulty of being able to describe it without reducing its context of meaning is problematic. Referring to Aristotle, von Wright (1995) points out that a distorted picture of reality occurs if one tries to achieve greater exactitude than the nature of the phenomenon allows. A complex and nuanced world cannot be explained in exact terms. It can only be understood broadly.

The hermeneutical, abductive research approach includes three phases that constantly alternate between theory and empiricism toward deeper levels of understanding. Reality is penetrated through explorative reflection and earlier interpretations are revisited through reflective seeing (Alvesson & Sköldberg, 1994; Føllesdal, Walloe, & Elster, 1992; Peirce, 1990). When analyzing and interpreting, one moves from a whole to its parts and then back to the whole. First, the meaning of the whole has to be captured and then the nuances of the whole must be deepened by interpreting its different parts. Through interpretation new patterns that are presented as caricatures or metaphors are sought (Nygren, 1972). The interpretation also involves pendulating between empirical theory and theoretical empiricism through which the meaning emerges (Alvesson & Sköldberg, 1994). The dynamic process pendulating between theory and empiricism leads to inductive, deductive, and abductive conclusions.

THE STUDY APPROACH

In order to find basic patterns in different caring cultures, the study employed a hermeneutical research approach using notes from diaries. Patients, relatives, and nurses at a number of Finnish hospitals were asked to keep a diary regarding their experiences of caring and the caring culture. Through these notes, different stories about or descriptions of the context of meaning in caring were obtained.

The "story" makes a deeper understanding of the patient's world possible. According to Carter (1993), a story should always have a living main character who is involved in a struggle where there is clear insight and a story should always describe a course of events. The idea is to set "captive" knowledge free. Stories clearly emerge when there is discrepancy between the ideals and the reality (Parker, 1990; Riessman, 1994); that is, stories emerge when patients, relatives, and nurses reflect on the question of the care experienced and their idea of how care could be.

Keeping a diary made it possible for the informants to reflect more freely on their experiences and to describe them more or less immediately. There was, however, a threshold that the informants had to cross in order to be able to express themselves. One disadvantage was that some patients had to be excluded from the study because they could not write things down for one reason or another. The collection of data was supplemented by observation.

THE CARING WORLD

The study showed that there is a caring world. This world looks different from the perspectives of the patient, the nurse, and the relative. The patient's world stands out as a world of suffering. This theme emerges from the diaries of patients, nurses, and relatives, even though they also include joy and many positive experiences. Patients described different kinds of suffering. The first, suffering related to illness, involved pain, worry, waiting for different treatments and operations, and an uncertain future. The most profound suffering related to care involved the patient's perception of having been deprived of his or her dignity, of not being understood, of not being taken seriously, and of being reduced from being a human being to being a physical body.

Relatives suffer too when they see the patient's situation. The patient's total life situation is seen as a suffering, as evidenced by relatives' diaries. They write about uncertainty, loneliness, and feelings of estrangement in an unknown world. It is interesting to note that research indicates that nurses pay more attention to suffering related to illness (Lindström, 1995).

A caring perspective of the patient's world can only be understood from a perspective of suffering. Only when the suffering that the patient goes through is understood can the patient's total situation with all its different nuances be understood. A patient who suffers is not open to teaching or information, nor does he or she think about self-care. Such pursuits feel like a violation and cause further suffering.

The nurse is important in the patient's world. A close relationship with one single nurse may be of crucial importance. The patient longs for true communion with a nurse. This true communion is the essence of the caring world. In an article written almost 40 years ago, van Kaam (1959) emphasized the importance of communion between patient and nurse. Real communion implies an understanding that reaches beyond mere understanding to truly sharing the patient's world with all its experiences. In order to alleviate suffering and offer comfort, nurses must see the patient's suffering in a deep sense from the patient's perspective as a unique human being (Eriksson, 1992).

The caring world is characterized by the paradigm that Watson (1995) refers to as the postmodern paradigm, where the seeking of knowledge is based on the seeking of one's own unique core and historical roots. Caring is based on the original view of the patient as a suffering human being, and caring means communion between patient and nurse.

THE IDEAL—A GOOD CARING CULTURE

A good caring culture is a culture that reflects the good as well as the evil. Jonas (1994) points out that it is only through being aware of evil and the things that are at stake that an awareness of good can emerge. Evil is the suffering related to care that emerges in the different cultures. Awareness of this suffering is, however, most clearly seen in the caring cultures.

Despite the progress that has taken place and the high-quality care available today, many factors still threaten good care. Current research shows that there is a trend toward increased suffering in care (Lindström, 1995; Lindholm & Eriksson, 1993). In addition to suffering caused by illness and its treatment, there is suffering caused by nursing. Florence Nightingale (1859) indicated this phenomenon nearly 140 years ago:

> In watching disease, both in private houses and in public hospitals, the thing which strikes the experienced observer most forcibly is this, that the symptoms or the sufferings generally considered to be inevitable and incident to the disease are very often not symptoms of the disease at all, but of something quite different—of the

> want of fresh air, or of light, or of warmth, or of quiet, or of cleanliness, or of punctuality and care in the administration of diet, of each of all of these. . . . The reparative process which nature has instituted and which we call disease has been hindered by some want of knowledge or attention, in one or in all of these things, and pain, suffering, or interruption of the whole process sets in. . . . If a patient is cold, if a patient is feverish, if a patient is faint, if he is sick after taking food, if he has a bed-sore, it is generally the fault not of the disease, but of the nursing. (pp. 5–6)

Thus, one problem is the violation of human dignity. There is an abuse of power that limits the patient's ability to participate in decisions about his or her care. Another central problem is poor patient information. Other problems are connected with nurses' ability to reflect and see—their "clinical eye." Basically, it is all a question of whether the necessary concept resources are available to shape this reality.

Alleviating the suffering related to care calls for a deeper understanding of the patient's world, of the inner side of caring and how care is experienced and perceived by the patient. From a human and a financial point of view, it is increasingly urgent to find ways to alleviate patient suffering and eliminate the suffering caused by nursing.

Nurses have to take a stand on the integrated clinical caring science paradigm and its starting points. They must reflect on and critically consider how the results of nursing research can lead to a development of patient care. There must also be reflection on the things about which little or nothing is known, what central fields within clinical nursing have not yet been researched and how these central fields should be researched.

From a caring science perspective the patient-nurse relationship is the essence of clinical nursing as well as the basis for the caring community. The significance of clinical caring science should primarily be evaluated from the patient's perspective. To return to the patient means a return to the suffering human being. The patient's experiences of his or her own suffering, poor health, or illness is the starting point of the clinical paradigm. Clinical nursing and clinical decisions cannot be based merely on scientific knowledge. It is necessary but not sufficient. Values are needed (i.e., decisions must be made on what is good for the patient in a deep sense).

A caring culture must be developed that upholds the cultural values that research related to the history of ideas has emphasized as the essence of caring. This culture must be open to change when it comes to integrating and innovating based on the results of science and research.

A caring culture where the context of meaning has been elucidated is protected against atomism, fragmentation, and death. It makes it possible to base arguments on a given tradition and on given values. In the culture-scientific paradigm "content" is the ontological (fundamental) meaning, the firm basis, in much the same way as causality is the basis for the natural science paradigm. Because understanding the unique and the individual is central, it imposes greater demands on research than those in a natural science paradigm. In a reality where a number of different scientific and occupational paradigms meet, it is the scientific dialogue that is a prerequisite to cooperation and the striving for an entity. This entity must take advantage of all possibilities concerning the care of the individual patient.

MacIntyre (1981) said that "A practice that fails to develop by realizing possibilities is dead." In order to achieve the "good," nurses must aim at providing good care and at developing nursing practice in accordance with the results of caring and nursing research. Science has to develop ideal models that make improvement of patient care possible. Nurses must create new goals for their work and realize the possibilities science offers. The nursing reality and patient care are not simple. A complex reality implies the need for a complex model of reality in order to understand the uniqueness of the patient's world and to offer good patient care. The essence of ethical codes in nursing obliges nurses to view their responsibility and make use of the possibilities that science, research, and practice offer.

REFERENCES

Alvesson, M., & Sköldberg, K. (1994). *Tolkning och reflektion. Vetenskapsfilosofi och kvalitativ metod* [Interpretation and reflection. Philosophy of science and qualitative method]. Lund, Sweden: Studentlitteratur.

Carter, K. (1993). The place of story in the study of teaching and teaching education. *Educational Researcher, 22*(1), 5–12.

Cody, W.K. (1990). Norms and nursing science. A question of values. *Nursing Science Quarterly, 6*(3), 110–112.

Eriksson, K. (1987). *Vårdandets idé* [The idea of caring]. Stockholm, Sweden: Almqvist & Wiksell.

Eriksson, K. (1992). Nursing: The caring practice "being there," caring communion. In D. Gaut (Ed.), *The presence of caring in nursing* (pp. 201–210). New York, NY: National League for Nursing.

Eriksson, K. (Ed.). (1993). *Möten med lidanden* [Encounters with suffering]. Reports from the Department of Caring Science. Vasa, Finland: Åbo Akademi University.

Eriksson, K. (Ed). (1996). Research programme for the project "In the patient's world—A study of health, suffering and caring." Vasa, Finland: Department of Caring Science, Åbo Akademi University.

Fawcett, J. (1993). From a plethora of paradigms to parsimony in worldviews. *Nursing Science Quarterly, 6,* 56–58.

Føllesdal, D., Walloe, L., & Elster, J. (1992). *Argumentationsteori, språk og vitenskapsfilosofi* [Theory of argumentation, language and philosophy of science]. Oslo, Norway: Universitetsförlaget AS.

Gadamer, H-G. (1988). *Truth and method.* London, England: Sheed and Ward Stagenbooks.

Jonas, H. (1994). *Ansvarets princip. Utkast till en etik för den teknologiska civilisationen* [The principle of responsibility. A draft to an ethics for the technological civilization]. Gothenburg, Sweden: Daidalos.

Leininger, M.M. (1988). *Caring—An essential human need.* Detroit, MI: Wayne State University Press.

Lindholm, L., & Eriksson, K. (1993). To understand and alleviate suffering in a caring culture. *Journal of Advanced Nursing, 18,* 1354–1361.

Lindström, U. (1995). *Ensamhetskänslan sviker inte* [The feeling of loneliness still remains]. Reports from the Department of Caring Science. Vasa, Finland: Åbo Akademi.

MacIntyre, A. (1981). *After virtue.* Notre Dame, IN: University of Notre Dame Press.

Newman, M.A. (1992). Prevailing paradigms in nursing. *Nursing Outlook, 40*(1), 10–13.

Nightingale, F. (1859). *Notes on nursing: What it is and what it is not.* London, England: Harrison.

Nygren, A. (1972). *Meaning and method.* London, England: Epworth Press.

Parker, S.R. (1990). Nurses stories: The search for a relational ethic of care. *Advanced Nursing Science, 13*(1), 31–40.

Parse, R.R. (1987). *Nursing science: Major paradigms, theories and critiques.* Philadelphia, PA: W.B. Saunders.

Parse, R.R. (1992). Human becoming: Parse's theory of nursing. *Nursing Science Quarterly, 5,* 35–42.

Peirce, C. (1990). *Pragmatism och kosmologi* [Pragmatism and cosmology]. Gothenburg, Sweden: Daidalos.

Riessman, C.K. (1994). *Narrative Analysis* (Qualitative Research Methods Series 30). Newbury Park, CA: Sage Publications.

Roach, M.S. (1987). *The human act of caring—A blueprint for the health professions.* Ottawa, Canada: Canadian Hospital Association.

Törnebohm, H. (1985). *Vad betyder vetenskapsteori?* (Rapport nr. 149) [What does the theory of science mean, (report nr.149)]. Institutionen för vetenskapsteori, Department of theory of science, University of Gothenburg, Sweden.

Watson, J. (1988). *Nursing: Human science and human care. A theory of nursing.* New York, NY: National League for Nursing.

Watson, J. (1995). Postmodernism and knowledge development in nursing. *Nursing Science Quarterly, 8*(2), 60–64.

van Kaam, A.L. (1959). The nurse in the patient's world. *American Journal of Nursing, 59*(12), 1708–1710.

von Wright, G.H. (1995). Om behov [About needs]. In K. Klockars & B. Österman (Eds.), *Begrepp om hälsa. Filosofiska och etiska perspektiv på livskvalitet* [Concepts about health. Philosophical and ethical perspectives on quality of life] (pp. 43–59). Stockholm, Sweden: Liber Utbildning.

Coping with the
Emotional Demands of Caring

Carol Leppanen Montgomery, RN, PhD
Assistant Professor
School of Nursing
University of Colorado Health Sciences Center
Denver, Colorado

Karen (all names are fictitious), an oncology nurse, became deeply involved with a patient with acquired immunodeficiency syndrome (AIDS) during the long ordeal of his dying. His death was felt as a personal loss, and she still grieves for him; however, she describes his death as "the most powerful, the most uplifting, the most complete experience. . . . I felt exhausted and depleted, but with a sense of peace and accomplishment. . . . This to me is the greatest thing in nursing. It's the greatest reward."

Debra, a medical-surgical nurse, also was involved with a difficult death. Two days after the incident in which the patient died, she returned to work, but found herself in the staffing office because she was unable to stop crying. She hadn't slept or eaten in the 2 days following the incident. She was referred to a therapist and diagnosed with severe posttraumatic stress disorder.

Nurses are continually exposed to human breakdown, suffering, violence, and the utter unpredictability of life-altering events. Those who take the risk to get involved with patients and to care, even in such difficult circumstances, experience a profound sense of fulfillment expressed so eloquently by the first nurse, Karen. However, caring is not without risks, as the second nurse, Debra, reminds us. A grounded-theory investigation studied the experience of exemplar caregivers and resulted in a descriptive theory of caring (Montgomery, 1991a, 1991b, 1992, 1993) and a model for how caregivers are affected by the experience of caring (Montgom-

Source: Reprinted from C.L. Montgomery, *Advanced Practice Nursing Quarterly,* Vol. 3, No. 1, pp. 76–84, © 1997, Aspen Publishers, Inc.

ery, 1993). The purpose of this article is to use this model to explain the differences in the experiences of nurses such as Karen and Debra and to offer suggestions for the resources necessary for nurses to thrive as caregivers.

Ultimately, whether nurses had a positive or negative experience with caring depended on the meanings they were able to create or the way they made sense of the experience. These meanings were drawn from inner personal resources, as well as the resources from each unique context in which caring occurs.

THE EMOTIONAL RISKS OF CARING

It is important to recognize that getting involved carries some risk, for the very nature of caring implies that caregivers open themselves up to the experience of vulnerability. Gadow (1985) explains that in order to overcome the objectification to which patients are often reduced in health care, the caregiver must approach patients not from the patronizing position of one who is whole to one who is not whole, but from the caregiver's awareness of his or her own vulnerability. It is impossible to expect caregivers to be involved with patients in this way when their own dignity or personhood is at risk. Those who experience this type of distress may feel no choice but to disengage and try to nurse without caring. The emotional risks of caring fall within two general areas. The first is the experience of personal loss, and the second is emotional overload.

Experience of personal loss

As one nurse explained, "Every time you get involved with somebody you risk a lot. You stand to lose something." Many of the caregivers interviewed for this study recalled an experience with a patient that involved a death. As one commented, "The things that I remember that are memorable have to do with dying; maybe that's because those things stand out in your mind, life and death." All of these caregivers felt the personal loss and emotional pain that go with grief;

however, as we saw with Karen, it was also seen as a personally enriching experience. Marsha, a perioperative nurse, began to cry when talking about a patient she had become close to who had died, but she explained that she was not crying because she was sad, but "sometimes I think tears are a sign of fullness, and when you overflow, you overflow." As this nurse saw it, grief did not leave her feeling empty. It made her so full that she literally spilled over with feeling.

However, as Debra illustrated, grief can be devastating. Meagan, a pediatric intensive care nurse, also felt devastated after a patient's death. She now keeps an emotional distance between herself and her patients and tries to avoid getting involved:

> Each time I let someone like that come into my heart, when they die, it's just like I close off even more, it's just like, okay, I'm going to do what I have to do. I can feel sorry for you but that's it, you know, when you die you are gone. I won't even remember your name.

The emotional risks involved in losing a patient are increased on units that are set up to save lives. Death on these units is viewed as defeat and failure. A nurse describes how he lost "that spark" after one of his patient died unexpectedly in the intensive care unit (ICU):

> You do all this neat work and put all this energy into it and what happens is the patient dies. . . . It's a big letdown. . . . After she died I just, it felt different. . . . There is something there that is not there anymore . . . boy you talk about a letdown. . . . Maybe we look at ourselves like uh oh, we failed, we failed them, we failed ourselves. They come in the hospital to beat death.

Emotional overload

Emotional overload can lead to emotional depletion, disillusionment, and what is commonly known as burnout. Emotional overload is created when a nurse's human sensibilities are over-whelmed with exposure to trauma, loss, and suf-fering. Meagan, the nurse who disengaged from caring following a child's death, described being just emotionally and physically exhausted:

> It's like I can see [the families] want-ing to feel like somebody cares but they just don't understand. We see this three or four times a month and when you see something like this three or four times a month for 10 years you, you don't have it to care. I mean—I don't mean that you don't care, but . . . it's kind of like you close off a certain part of yourself. You have nothing else to give these people other than you try to be nice.

Emotional overload occurs when caregivers are stretched beyond their capacities to reconcile these assaults within their human sensibilities. Only time, space, and caring will allow them to make sense of these experiences so that they can come to some type of resolution, some meaning that will allow them once again to risk involvement.

RESOURCES THAT SUSTAIN CARING

As we have begun to see, the meanings that caregivers create to make sense out of their ex-periences with caring determine whether they experience the positive transformative effects of caring, or whether they suffer the emotional depletion and trauma that lead to disengagement from caring. But these meanings do not arise from a vacuum. They are derived from both in-ner personal and contextual resources.

PERSONAL RESOURCES

The inner personal resources that sustain car-ing include both spiritual and philosophical re-sources and the personal characteristics of flex-ibility, depth (or soulfulness), and balance.

Spiritual and philosophical resources

As we saw earlier, nurses are constantly chal-lenged to make sense of the insensible when they are confronted with inhumanity, violence, suffering, and trauma. One nurse tried to make sense of why a "very, very nice" 32-year-old woman died, when "you see some old codger on 14th and Colfax with his emphysema machine going and smoking away with his oxygen, and you are just like, where are the variables here; It just doesn't make sense." He called this "philo-sophical doo doo." One nurse commented, "I feel like in 6 years I've probably aged 20 or 30 years, and I probably have seen more in 6 years as far as human nature and the basics of human life, more than most people will ever see in a lifetime." This exposure has the potential to lead to philosophical or spiritual growth, or it may result in a gradual wearing down of the spirit. In order to grow from this kind of exposure, nurses are challenged to develop a transcendent view of life that lends itself to a deeper acceptance of what may appear to others as senseless, mean-ingless tragedy.

The caring relationship itself facilitates this growth by allowing nurses to become part of a larger consciousness that lends itself to accep-tance and understanding. It occurs through the process of spiritual transcendence, found in this study to be the essence of a caring-centered in-volvement. *Spiritual transcendence* is experi-encing oneself, during an encounter with a pa-tient, as part of something greater than oneself. It involves stepping outside one's own ego to be-come immersed in a larger source of energy or meaning. Watson described this phenomenon as a common humanity, shared phenomenological fields, or a universal psychic energy (Watson, 1985, 1988a, 1988b); however, one nurse de-scribed it more personally when she remarked that when she cares, she has the opportunity to "experience a thousand different lifetimes through someone else's eyes" (Montgomery, 1993, p. 93).

While connection at this level constitutes a transpersonal experience, nurses also need to de-velop their own specific spiritual and philo-sophical beliefs that provide a higher order schema, one that can absorb and assimilate these assaults to human sensibilities within a universal and enduring set of meanings (Tedeschi & Calhoun, 1995).

As we saw earlier, nurses are also challenged with a significant personal experience of loss every time they let themselves become close to someone who will die. How they cope with this loss is greatly influenced by their philosophical and spiritual understanding of death. A spiritual understanding that allows for a sense of connection and continuity within the cycle of life and death helps nurses to transcend their personal experience of loss.

Karen, the nurse who felt fulfilled in spite of her grief over the patient who died of AIDS, illustrates how her spiritual values allowed her to find positive meaning in his death:

> I have many images of patients I've lost. They're real for me, they're spirits. . . . They pass life on to me. I am instructed to live because they are not able to. . . . I have a responsibility to them who died so young—to live life [more fully] to really be aware of what life is.

This ongoing sense of connection is expressed in a different way by a nurse who had changed specialties from obstetrics to oncology: "They feel the same in some ways because I almost cry at a birth the same way I cry at a death. It's so poignant at the beginning and at the end . . . it's very alike."

In contrast, the nurse who lost "that spark" after the death of a patient does not express any sense of connection or peace with death:

> Well Kubler-Ross's theory is that death is just basically one of the most wonderful advancements in life and you go through all these neat little channels and changes. How can it possibly be neat? You know. It's like, let's get real. You die, you die. . . . How can you possibly be at peace with the end of your life?

The lack of meaning makes it impossible for this nurse to move beyond the feeling of loss and devastation.

Personal qualities

Flexibility and depth (or soulfulness)

While caring has certain attributes, such as authenticity, receptivity, commitment, and so on (Montgomery, 1993), caring cannot be defined by its attributes because each attribute associated with caring is a dialectic rather than a fixed trait. In other words, every quality of caring is defined by its opposite dimension, and there will be times when the opposite dimension will need to be called forth. In fact, caring itself requires the ability to choose not to care, and to have the wisdom to know what to care about. Nurses have the potential to be exploited by others who expect that they will always care indiscriminately and at all costs to themselves. Nurses may also be exploited by their own need to maintain an ego-identity consistent with a stereotype of caring as being "nice," or of always pleasing others. Nurses in this study who were successful at caring showed a more expanded repertoire of personal responses, beyond those stereotypically associated with caring. One nurse who was known for her acceptance and gentleness with patients did not hesitate to show another side of her personality when she filed a letter of intent to sue a physician for slander after he berated her work in front of her patients. ICU nurses criticized "caring" for its seemingly "passive" qualities, pointing out that they showed caring more often by their ability to take control on behalf of the patient.

Shrinking resources, combined with the enormity of needs in the health care environment, demand that nurses balance a tendency to want to be able to respond with caring to all that needs caring. A perfectionistic, idealized view of caring creates an overly expansive view of one's own obligation and abilities to meet all unmet human needs. This idealistic over-expansiveness must be balanced with realism and humility. Furthermore, a perfectionistic approach that overemphasizes ideal outcomes and standards does not contribute to the ability to cope with complex patient conditions and circumstances that do not lend themselves to control, resolution, or easy answers. In fact, this perfectionism may lead to anger and victim blaming as caregivers experience disappointment when they are unable to meet these idealistic standards (Benner & Wrubel, 1989). The phrase "make a difference" was used frequently by successful caregivers in this study, and it seemed to reflect how they coped with overwhelming demands or seemingly hopeless patients. Having an intent to make a difference in a situation rather than to solve all of the problems or meet all of the needs seemed to help caregivers focus on discovering possibilities rather than on becoming immobilized by all of the deficits. One nurse explained, "I don't think it makes any difference how big the case is or how little the case is because there are always those little pockets of where you can make a difference." Sometimes making a difference can mean deriving satisfaction from providing comfort or even simply providing a moment of meaningful human interaction in the face of deterioration.

Perhaps another way to understand the depth and breadth of human responses that caring demands is as "soulfulness." A soulful nature, according to Moore (1992), is characterized by genuineness and depth. Soulfulness is grounded in the nature of human foibles and imperfections. While the quest for perfection seeks an identity exclusive of these traits, soulfulness implies a wholeness that is achieved through acceptance of one's imperfections. Some of the more powerful stories of caring heard during this study occurred as a result of a nurse's mistake, or when nurses forgot their professional persona and allowed the "unprofessional" expression of their own vulnerability and humanness. A nurse who has experienced his or her own human failings or one who has honestly admitted his or her potential for these failings will be more capable of generating an authentic concerned response to a patient who, because of his or her failings, may be shunned by society. An example of an authentic response might be concerned anger.

A student in the author's class once shared a story that she had been reluctant to reveal. While she was working in an inner-city emergency de-partment, a patient came in with a gunshot wound to his stomach as a result of a drug deal that had turned sour. In spite of his injuries he was combative and threatening to kill the staff. They all maintained their "professional" dispassionate composure while they tied him down with leather restraints. After they all left, he continued to thrash, curse, and threaten them, endangering his own condition and making it very hard for this nurse to "work on him." Having lived in a similar inner-city culture herself, this nurse felt she knew how to "handle" him. After making sure no one was around, she went and got the biggest syringe she could find, held it in front of his face, and said in her fiercest tone, "Look, I can be your best friend, or your worst enemy. Now I suggest you cooperate with me, and maybe I can help save your life." He immediately shrunk away, and said "Hey that's cool, I'll be cool." He then settled down and let her do what she needed to do. She then went out into the hallway and ran into his cousin who got "in her face" and threatened to kill her if his cousin died. Once again, in the fiercest tone she could muster, she looked him in the eye and said "Don't ever threaten me. Your cousin is in good hands and we will do everything we can for him, but we won't tolerate threats from you or anyone else." The cousin also backed off and said "Hey, he's like my brother." She said she understood, and the cousin left, apparently feeling the situation was under control.

While this exchange would not typically be thought of as a caring nurse-patient encounter, she managed to engage with him out of concern. Her response was real and it was soulful, an alternative to the dispassionate professionalism of the others, an obviously inauthentic response that, not surprisingly, resulted in mistrust and a resulting sense of panic. In fact, based on the outcome, I would put forth that her response was the "ideal" caring response for this particular situation.

Balance

The intense exposure to suffering requires that caregivers seek a balance in their life so that they can remain whole and intact. A hospice nurse found solace in spending time with her infant grandson. A psychiatric nurse balanced the mental intensity of her work with "mindless" physical exercise. The nurse who worked with the deterioration of AIDS sought out beauty by going to art museums. Grim and depressing treatment settings produced gallows humor, an important outlet that helped to counteract despair.

CONTEXTUAL RESOURCES

While personal resources are important, to expect caregivers to handle such challenging demands through individual coping skills alone is unrealistic and victimizing (Benner & Wrubel, 1989). Involvement, especially under such intense circumstances, always involves risk, and anyone, no matter how skillful he or she is at coping, has the potential to be psychologically wounded by exposure to trauma (Tedeschi & Calhoun, 1995). The context needed to sustain involvement under such intense circumstances needs to include patient-centered support and caregiver-centered support, as well as the reciprocity within the caring relationship.

Patient-centered support

Caring is not a heroic, independent act; instead it arises from within a context of a community or a team. Successful caregivers always perceive themselves as part of a network, and mobilizing this network is an important way in which they express caring (Montgomery, 1993). Therefore, caring is at risk unless this type of support is available. The contrast between the experiences of Karen and Debra, mentioned at the beginning of this article, best illustrates the differences this support can make.

For Debra, the lack of support resulted in her extreme reaction, later diagnosed as posttraumatic stress disorder, following a patient's death. Her experience involved what she perceived as a preventable death that resulted from a physician who ignored her assessment and coworkers who did not follow through with her

concerns by monitoring the patient's condition and calling the physician after she left for the day. When she returned the following day she was left "holding the bag" as she had to deal with this patient's rapidly deteriorating condition, along with his frantic family. Finally she had to perform the procedure that, while medically necessary, triggered the violent physical reaction that supposedly caused his death. Those team members who had neglected the patient were not on the scene to assist her, so she was left with the existential experience of having to be with this patient, whom she cared about, look him in the eye and see his terror, knowing that they had failed him. And, as often happens with nurses who are "at the scene of the crime," she became the target of the family's anger. When tragic and violent situations like this one are not assuaged with caring they are reduced to stark horror, and that is how she experienced this scene over and over again in her mind.

In contrast, Karen had to deal with some painful and gruesome aspects during her care of the young man who died of complications from AIDS. Yet when it was all over she could feel, "We lost, but we all won. . . . My commitment to nursing, knowing that I do make a difference. . . . It was a win for everyone. I felt proud that the institution had supported me." She described how the chaplain, the physician, the psychiatric liaison nurse, and others who were involved in his care made such an experience possible. These caregivers saw themselves as part of a team that included his family and his lover. They all became bonded with one another out of common love for this patient, and they were left with the sweet feeling of knowing that he had received the best care that everyone could give.

Caregiver-centered support

These contrasting cases also illustrate the devastating impact that isolation and alienation from the team can have on the caregiver. Debra did not have a strong connection with the team because she floated between units. "No one would listen to me!" After the death, she felt that people were staring at her or avoiding her. No one offered to take over her assignment or suggest that she go home. People did ask her how she was feeling, but she could not talk about it because she would start crying so violently that she could not function, and her perception was that she was expected to continue to function. Karen, on the other hand, felt very comfortable with her team and was well respected. Team members were concerned about the intensity of her involvement with this patient and often "checked in" with her. They trusted that she could feel deeply and continue to do her work, but at certain times they also "cut her some slack" and gave her the time and space to cry and just be with the patient and his family. If there were any doubts about the use of her time these were relieved by the kudos the hospital received from the family following the death. This case illustrates the kind of support that allows nurses to risk the personal sense of loss that may result from a caring involvement.

The environment must also provide resources to manage the risk of emotional overload described earlier. This exposure to suffering and death needs to be balanced with exposure to life-affirming events, the whole picture of a patient recovery, resolution of grief, or transcending disability. Hospitals that are organized around a mechanistic industrial model of efficiency caused staff to feel that they were in, as one ICU nurse described it, "packaging and processing." Successful caregivers sought out this balance by visiting patients on other units after the initial trauma, or by attending funerals. Their caring relationships resulted in patients coming back to the unit to show off their recovery, or sending postcards relating their successes and triumphs. The environment, however, needs to allow for and encourage these kinds of opportunities so that nurses can be involved with the "whole story" rather than just being left with the images of the patient's worst moments. Neonatal intensive care units that sponsor parties for their "graduates" are an example of this holistic approach.

RECIPROCITY OF THE CARING RELATIONSHIP

Because caring is an intersubjective experience that is characterized by mutual participation, the patient will shape not only the communication of caring, but also the experience of the caregiver. Theories of caring that do not acknowledge a patient's participation risk dehumanizing patients by reducing them to "objects" of our caring.

This is not to say that caring depends on the interpersonal abilities of patients to engage their caregivers, for the spiritual transcendence characteristic of caring is not motivated by the individual egos or personalities, but by some greater source of meaning. In caring, one goes beyond the superficial manifestations of self to connect with that that is universal: the person's humanity, his or her center or inner spirit. Therefore, the impulse to care does not necessarily depend on the participation of the patient, but the unfolding of the relationship does. Two general areas emerged from nurses' narratives of their experiences with patients. The first is the patient's ability to respond, and the second is the ability to find meaning or to transcend.

Ability to respond

The impulse to care is often elicited by a patient's vulnerability and by presenting the nurse with an opportunity to make a difference. As one nurse noted, "You tend to get involved with the ones that . . . need you more." On the other hand, patients who do not respond, who alienate, or who exploit their caregivers make caring difficult. As one nurse explained, "You feel alienated because you try, you give of yourself, and they don't want it." On the other hand, other nurses saw this situation as a challenge. They loved working with the "troublemakers," explaining "There are people who just want you to leave them alone, but 99% of the time you can get around that."

In any case, vulnerability in the caring relationship does not rest solely with the patient; instead, it shifts back and forth between the participants. When caregivers are willing to go beyond the professional-role persona and allow themselves to interact at a human level, they risk being hurt. Developing their capacities for self-awareness, authenticity, and depth allows them to manage their own vulnerability so that they are not forced to retreat or disengage from involvement.

Ability to find meaning

Patients who have the ability to participate in a caring relationship and are able to transcend despair by finding meaning are a source of inspiration to caregivers. These are often the patients whom nurses remember when asked to talk about their most significant experiences with caring. These patients serve as an important resource for the broader perspective nurses have to find in order to sustain themselves and to mobilize hope in other patients who are struggling to find meaning. Being involved with these patients is not as much of an emotional risk because they teach caregivers to transcend the pain.

On the other hand, caring for patients who are caught in despair is difficult to sustain emotionally, because nurses who are willing to participate in the client's world will experience, on some level, the same challenges as the patient. It helps if they both bring resources to the experience so that they can learn together. These patients challenge nurses to continue to expand their perspective so that they can reconcile or make peace with the patient's condition, at least in their own mind.

SUMMARY

To summarize, this article has presented a grounded theory of how nurses create meanings that sustain them and allow them to continue to risk caring by entering into the world of another, during what is most often an intense and perilous time. Nurses draw from both personal inner resources as well as contextual resources, includ-

ing the patient, in order to make sense of their experiences. These meanings will determine the nature of their experience with caring. Positive meanings result in positive fulfillment, personal growth, and the alchemical effects described as a "peak experience." These feelings reinforce commitment and the desire to engage further. Negative meanings result in feelings of emotional depletion and possible trauma. As a result, these nurses may feel no choice but to disengage and withdraw from caring involvements (Figure 1).

IMPLICATIONS

Nurses face unique existential challenges that are rarely addressed in educational or practice settings. In educational settings studies of philosophy, humanities, and religions can help nurses arrive in practice settings with a broader repertoire of ways to understand the existential

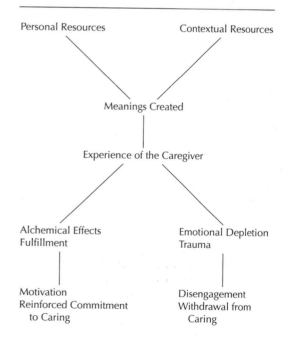

Figure 1. Coping with the emotional demands of caring. *Source:* C. Montgomery, *Healing through Communication: The Practice of Caring,* © 1993, by Sage Publications, Inc. Reprinted by permission of Sage Publications, Inc.

questions raised by exposure to human suffering (Bevis & Watson, 1989). Both education and practice settings can introduce health care workers to a variety of practices such as meditation, contemplation, and other spiritual methods that encourage ego-transcendence and compassion (Cooper, 1992; Novak, 1990). Of course these activities should reflect as much diversity as possible, and participants should not feel coerced to take part.

The healthy personal growth and development of the nurse are important as well. However, activities toward this end should keep in mind the greater sense of purpose that we share as caregivers, and avoid being promoted in a way that is individualistic or solipsistic, the focus being on the nurse for the nurse's sake. Health care settings exist for the care of patients, and in the healthiest teams support and love flow with abundance, but always toward a common sense of purpose and focus. One caregiver described her work setting as being characterized by "healthy human exchange." Everyone felt that they were safe and would be taken care of, so they were all able to settle into their own cycles in a way that worked for everyone. Humor, play, spontaneity, and diversity were the qualities that stood out for her. As a result "people were able to reveal their basic kindness." Self-development activities that focus on individual stress management risk losing that focus.

Sharing stories is a way to develop a common culture and to keep caring soulfully grounded in what Street (1990) has called the "messy swamps" of nursing practice, where nurses learn to find their way expertly amidst the messy realm of subjective involvement. Guidelines are also available to help nurses understand the difference between caring-centered involvements and destructive "over-involvements" (Montgomery, 1993).

When extreme situations occur, hospitals need to take advantage of the many resources available for helping individuals and teams cope with trauma. One nurse described feeling very burned out after a plane disaster and lamented the fact that trauma teams had worked with the rescue workers and others in the community that had been involved in the disaster, but no one had thought to provide any support for the ICU nurses who worked with four or five "horrifyingly incredible patients at one time" and could not get away from their "deep sad stories." These traumas act as a threat to our frame of reference or a challenge to our sense of order and coherence (Antonovsky, 1987; McCann & Pearlman, 1990). Again, the cultivation of a transcendent view serves a protective function by providing the enduring universal meanings that help to maintain coherence; however, as we have seen contextual factors can be so severe, that even the most seasoned professionals may need professional debriefing within the context of a concerned and caring team to help reconcile the event.

Health care systems need to allow for consistent personal involvement with patients, and the time and space to prioritize workloads based on caring rather than task completion. If such allowances are not made, increasing numbers of nurses will withdraw emotionally or leave the profession altogether because they find it impossible to care. Hospital administration should not feel intimidated by the "burden" of supporting caregivers. Caring is a natural state that has been a part of human culture far longer than curing. Those nurses who are given the autonomy to organize their work and their team based on their natural desires to care, tend to care for one another in the process and enjoy tremendous satisfaction as they reap the shared joy of being able to express themselves in this way.

REFERENCES

Antonovsky, A. (1987). *Unraveling the mystery of health: How people manage stress and stay well.* San Francisco, CA: Jossey-Bass.

Benner, P., & Wrubel, J. (1989). *The primacy of caring: Stress and coping in health and illness.* Menlo Park, CA: Addison-Wesley.

Bevis, E., & Watson, J. (1989). *Toward a caring curriculum: A new pedagogy for nursing.* New York, NY: National League for Nursing.

Cooper, D.A. (1992). *Silence, simplicity and solitude.* New York, NY: Bell Tower.

Gadow, S.A. (1985). Nurse and patient: The caring relationship. In A.H. Bishop & J.R. Scudder (Eds.), *Caring, curing, coping: Nurse, physician, patient relationships* (pp. 31–43). Tuscaloosa, AL: University of Alabama Press.

McCann, I.L., & Pearlman, L.A. (1990). *Psychological trauma and the adult survivor: Theory, therapy, and transformation.* New York, NY: Brunner/Mazel.

Montgomery, C. (1991a). Caring v. curing. *Common Boundary, 9*(6), 37–40.

Montgomery, C. (1991b). The care-giving relationship: Paradoxical and transcendent aspects. *Journal of Transpersonal Psychology, 23*(2), 91–104.

Montgomery, C. (1992). The spiritual connection: Nurses' perceptions of the experience of caring. In D. Gaut (Ed.), *The presence of caring in nursing* (pp. 39–52). New York, NY: National League for Nursing.

Montgomery, C. (1993). *Healing through communication: The practice of caring.* Thousand Oaks, CA: Sage Publications.

Moore, T. (1992). *Care of the soul: A guide for cultivating depth and sacredness in everyday life.* New York, NY: HarperCollins.

Novak, P. (1990). The practice of attention. *Parabola, 15*(2), 4–13.

Street, A. (1990). *Nursing practice: High, hard ground, messy swamps and the pathways in between.* Geelong, Australia: Deakin.

Tedeschi, R.G., & Calhoun, L.G. (1995). *Trauma and transformation: Growing in the aftermath of suffering.* Thousand Oaks, CA: Sage Publications.

Watson, J. (1985). *Nursing: Human science and human care.* Norwalk, CT: Appleton-Century-Crofts.

Watson, J. (1988a). *Nursing: Human science and human care—A theory of nursing.* New York, NY: National League for Nursing.

Watson, J. (1988b). New dimensions of human caring theory. *Nursing Science Quarterly, 1*(4), 175–181.

Nursing and Technology: A Dialectic

Judy G. Ozbolt, PhD, RN, FAAN
Professor and Director
Doctoral Program
School of Nursing
University of Virginia
Charlottesville, Virginia

NURSING: THE PRIMACY OF CARING

Nurses care. Those two words contain the essence of nursing practice. Caring, as Benner and Wrubel define it, "means that persons, events, projects, and things matter to people."[1(p1)] In nursing, caring also means doing for, supporting, supplementing, teaching, and helping those for whose welfare nurses take responsibility. Both aspects are critical. Without involvement, the techniques of care are likely to be less effective, or even counterproductive. Without knowledge of and skill in how to help, concern, good wishes, and good intentions will rarely be enough to restore patients to health or to promote their development and well-being.

Benner and Wrubel[1] assert that, in late 20th century industrialized society, the primacy of caring is rarely recognized. Indeed, they say, "Nursing and other caring practices have become paradoxical in a highly technical culture that seeks sweeping technological breakthroughs to provide liberation and disburdenment"[1(pxv)] of the individual. Such liberation, however, is costly. Benner and Wrubel continue: "Embracing this version of negative freedom, in which one finally loses all bonds and is free from every care, deprives one of the positive freedom to choose and to act. Of course, such utter disconnectedness is a practical impossibility, and the quest for negative freedom frustrates as it impoverishes."[1(p2)]

In a world where the acuity of illness and the complexity of care demand technologic assis-

Source: Reprinted from J. Ozbolt, *Holistic Nursing Practice,* Vol. 11, No. 1, pp. 1–5, © 1996, Aspen Publishers, Inc.

tance for the nurse, and the technology often seems designed to free the nurse from caring, how can nurses maintain the primacy of caring? How can we change the negative freedom to a positive one and use the technology to free ourselves for caring? Before answering these questions, it is necessary to examine other dimensions of nursing, nurses, and technology.

NURSING: THE DEVELOPMENT OF EXPERTISE

If caring is the soul of nursing, expertise is its mind and body. Expertise includes both *knowing that*, or theoretical knowledge, and *knowing how*, or experiential knowledge involving intuition and insight.[2–5] Moving from novice to expert in nursing means moving from a minimum of experiential knowledge and a maximum reliance on theoretical knowledge to a high degree of experiential knowledge with a minimum need to rely on theoretical knowledge expressed as rules or maxims. Evans, analyzing Henderson and Nite's text *Principles and Practice of Nursing*,[6] likened the development of expertise in the caring nurse to the conduct of scientific research:

> The habits of mind that inform the everyday tasks of the nurse are exactly the same as those that undergird the very finest published research; in this way Everynurse ought not just to *do* simple research tasks as part of her work, but she ought also *always* to *be* a researcher, whether or not she writes or speaks a word in print or public. Nurses are given lots of token encouragement to participate in research or to be aware of the need for research-based nursing care, but not enough emphasis has been placed on those qualities of mind that essentially make the publishing scholar *identical*, in a way, to Everynurse, when she is truly being a nurse as she should.[7(pp338–339)]

In this view, nursing as it should be practiced involves entering into a relationship with a pa-

tient for whose particular benefit the nurse raises questions, draws on stores of experiential and theoretical knowledge, formulates hypotheses, tests them, and remains open to the richness of the situation and all it has to teach. From such experiences with a variety of patients, the nurse is always drawing new knowledge to add to and to transform what was previously known.

The best nursing, then, occurs in the union of caring and expertise. Anything that alienates the nurse from caring or thwarts the growth of expertise is inimical to nursing and to patient welfare. Technology, if it is to enhance nursing, must support the primacy of caring and the development of expertise.

TECHNOLOGY: ALIENATION OR ENHANCEMENT?

Examples of the dehumanizing effects of technology abound: the nurse who pays more attention to the fetal monitor than to the woman in labor, the computer monitor that becomes a wall between nurse and patient, the erroneous bill blamed on "computer error" that cannot be corrected because no one can seem to find or solve the problem, the patient care information system that forces the clinician to scroll through unwanted screens to reach the desired data. The technologies in these examples are alienating because they impede human interactions or block orderly or creative thought.

But what of the cardiac monitor that sounds an alarm to alert the nurse to a dangerous dysrhythmia? How about the community-based information system that allows widely dispersed providers to communicate their perspectives and to plan together for the comprehensive, coherent care of an elderly woman with multiple chronic illnesses? What of the workstation that enables the clinician to review the patient record, check federal guidelines, consult the most recent literature, and develop a plan of care, all in the presence of the patient, who participates in evaluating options and makes sure that his or her preferences are known and respected? How about support groups that depend on computer networks to communicate with one another and with health professionals whenever they feel the need? These technologies put people in touch with one another and provide the information needed for effective care and learning.

Why do some technologies block caring and learning whereas others support good nursing? The answer lies in the function that the technology was designed to serve, the quality of the execution, and the technology's flexibility in adapting to the needs of different users.

Function

Intended function is fundamental. Nurses do not need technology to tell them what they already know or to perform functions that humans do better than machines. Nurses are excellent at collecting, analyzing, and interpreting data from multiple sensory channels to determine the patient's status and at creating a holistic perception of the patient's situation. To try to replace this human function with a computer system would be futile. On the other hand, information technologies exist for continuous monitoring of multiple channels of physiologic data and for signaling dangerous values or trends. Such technologies are helpful because they are untiringly attentive to the evolving data, they can rapidly calculate complex interactions, and they can remember all the rules about normal and abnormal parameters. Their function is not to replace the nurse but to enhance and extend the nurse's performance. By putting the data from the monitoring system into the context of the patient's total situation, the nurse can make better judgments about the patient's overall needs and response to care—better than the nurse without the monitor, and certainly better than the monitor without the nurse.

Quality

Even if a technology is intended to serve a useful and needed function, it can succeed only if the design is well executed. A network system intended to improve communications among caregivers cannot work if the interface is so awkward that users find it difficult to send or retrieve information. Nurses are already sufficiently challenged by trying to identify and meet their patients' needs in a work environment that does not always seem to support that objective. They must be able to focus more on the clinical problem than on the mechanics of using the technology. Thus systems that are intuitively obvious, that minimize keystrokes and mouse manipulation, that take advantage of patient data already in the record, and that respond quickly have a greater probability of being used. To be useful, the technology not only must fulfill its intended function but must do so without interfering with the nurse's primary concern: patient care.

Flexibility

Because nurses have different levels of expertise, the same pathway from data to decision will not be appropriate for every nurse or for every decision problem. The nurse needs to be able to start from his or her current level of knowledge and understanding of the situation and work through to a decision by a process that neither skips so many steps that the nurse cannot follow it nor plods through so many obvious steps that the nurse loses patience and interest.

For students or other novices planning care for a patient, for example, a good information system might request assessment data, indicate hypotheses for which there are not yet sufficient data for diagnoses and request additional data, generate diagnoses, explain their basis in the data, and work through care planning and evaluation in a similar manner.

Such a process would quickly exasperate an expert. It would be desirable for the same system to be able to operate in an "express" mode, requesting from the nurse the diagnoses that he or she had already determined together with the supporting data. The system might also offer the expert the option of simply entering objectives and interventions or viewing a set of alternatives that the knowledge base suggested might be appropriate to the situation, with actual data on the effectiveness of the interventions in achieving the objectives in similar situations. Once the expert had sketched in the essentials of a care plan, the system could use its files and its "help" functions to fill in the details or, for example, to instruct a novice in carrying out the plan that the expert had developed. With the flexibility to accommodate different levels of expertise, appropriate, well-designed information technology can become tightly integrated into the thinking, planning, evaluating, and caring that drive nursing actions.

SYNTHESIS: THE UNION OF CARING, EXPERTISE, AND TECHNOLOGY

But what will ensure that appropriate, well-designed, flexible technology will be available to nurses? To get information technology that supports nursing, nurses must pursue education, research, and development in the discipline of nursing informatics. By studying nursing practice from the perspective of information science, nurses will learn which information processing functions they do well and which functions can be done better by computers. They will articulate priorities for the development of applications and participate in the design of technologies that will serve nurses and patients well. Through studies of judgment, expertise, and nurse performance, nurses will specify the kinds of assistance that

technology will provide for nurses at different levels of expertise. When deep knowledge of nursing and profound commitment to patients unite in the mind of the nurse informatician with thorough understanding of information science and technology, the spark of creation ignites, and better technologies are born.

If the technology is right for nursing in function, quality, and flexibility, it will neither alienate the nurse from caring nor block the development and use of expertise. On the contrary, it will provide more information and knowledge for the caring nurse to bring to bear on the patient's situation and promote the growth of both individual expertise and nursing knowledge. If Everynurse, to use Evans'[7] image, is considering each patient's situation in the light of available knowledge and learning from each encounter, then the best information technology can provide more of the relevant information and knowledge, offer options for actions, describe their probable consequences, and then store, aggregate, and analyze the results of the encounter to give better advice next time. This way of incorporating information technology into nursing will enrich the expertise of the individual nurse and add to the general store of nursing knowledge. When the nurse unites technology with expertise and caring, both the art and the science of nursing will flourish, and patients will receive better care.

REFERENCES

1. Benner P, Wrubel J. *The Primacy of Caring: Stress and Coping in Health and Illness.* Menlo Park, Calif: Addison-Wesley; 1989.
2. Benner P. From novice to expert. *Am J Nurs.* 1982;82: 402–407.
3. Benner P. *From Novice to Expert: Excellence and Power in Clinical Nursing Practice.* Menlo Park, Calif: Addison-Wesley; 1984.
4. Benner P, Wrubel J. Skilled clinical knowledge: The value of perceptual awareness. *Nurse Educ.* 1982;7:11–17.
5. Benner P, Tanner C. Clinical judgment: How expert nurses use intuition. *Am J Nurs.* 1987;87:23–31.
6. Henderson V, Nite G. *Principles and Practice of Nursing.* New York, NY: Macmillan; 1978.
7. Evans D. Everynurse as researcher: An argumentative critique of principles and practice of nursing. *Nurs Forum.* 1980;19:337–349.

The Caring Efficacy Scale: Nurses' Self-Reports of Caring in Practice Settings

Carolie J. Coates, PhD
Assistant Professor
School of Nursing
University of Colorado Health Sciences Center
Denver, Colorado

Source: Reprinted from C.J. Coates, *Advanced Practice Nursing Quarterly,* Vol. 3, No. 1, pp. 53–59, © 1997, Aspen Publishers, Inc.

Today's rapidly changing health care environments are increasingly calling upon nurses to conduct patient outcome and cost studies as part of a current emphasis on accountability of health care programs (Lorig, Stewart, Ritter, Gonzales, Laurent, & Lynch, 1996). While recognizing and valuing the importance of the trend toward more outcome and cost accountability studies, nurses have a tradition of valuing the process and quality of care as well as the outcomes. Fitzpatrick (1995) reminds us that although the current focus on cost has seemingly relegated care and quality to a secondary position, nursing research should be a force to restore the balance. The construct of caring in nursing has proved an elusive one to conceptualize, define, and assess. Despite the difficulties nursing needs to continue to explore and assess the nature of caring and to pursue the implications of the research for nursing practice and education.

The Caring Efficacy Scale (CES) was developed to assess conviction or belief in one's ability to express a caring orientation and to develop caring relationships with clients or patients. The caring efficacy belief implies that one has the underlying cognitions and attitudes, as well as the behavioral repertoire, to produce results in the desired direction. Development of the CES was based on Watson's (1979, 1985, 1988, 1996) theory of transpersonal caring and on Bandura's (1977, 1986) concept of efficacy as explained later. The approach is unique in that it is theoretically grounded and does not exclusively focus on caring behaviors.

This article outlines initial reliability and validity testing of the self-report CES scale. Coates (1996) provides more detailed information including description of a companion supervisor version to assess supervisor perceptions of a nurse's caring efficacy.

REVIEW OF QUANTITATIVE APPROACHES TO CARING ASSESSMENT

Most existing caring instruments are designed to assess caring behaviors or, in a few cases, caring attributes or abilities. For the most part content validity has been established, and the scale reliabilities are acceptable. The studies are methodologically limited by small sample sizes and fledgling attempts at validity testing, as is often the case with new measures. Most of the studies appear to be atheoretical; a few are linked to Watson's caring theory (Watson, 1979, 1985, 1988, 1996).

Behaviorally oriented measures

Many caring assessment scale originators view the measurement challenge as one of assessing nursing behaviors. Larson's development of the Caring Assessment Report Evaluation-Q Sort (CARE-Q) (Larson 1984, 1986, 1987; Mayer, 1987) and more recently the CARE/SAT (Larson & Ferketich, 1993) is one of the more well-known behavioral approaches to nurse and patient perceptions of caring behaviors. Von Essen and Sjoden (1991a, 1991b, 1993, 1995) report on development of a Swedish version of the CARE-Q. Further use of the CARE-Q is documented by Komorita, Doehring, and Hirchert (1991); Mangold (1991); and Rosenthal (1992). McDaniel (1990) describes less well known behaviorally oriented caring scales and Nkongho (1990) explains the development of an inventory to assess ability to care.

Measurement approaches

Several measurement approaches have been influenced by Watson's (1979, 1985, 1988, 1996) theory. Wolf (1986) reports on the development of the Caring Behavior Inventory (CBI) in which respondents rank caring words or phrases. The revised CBI (Wolf, Giardino, Osborne, & Ambrose, 1994) contains factors representing Watson's caring theory.

Cronin and Harrison (1988) report on the development of the Caring Behaviors Assessment (CBA), comprised of subscales congruent with Watson's carative factors. Parsons, Kee, and Gray (1993) and Huggins, Gandy, and Kohut (1993) report further modifications and use of the CBA. Nyberg (1990) developed the Nyberg Caring Assessment Scale based on concepts from a variety of nursing theorists including Watson. Duffy (1992) developed the Caring Assessment Tool (CAT), using Watson's theory as a theoretical framework. The CAT was modified to assess nurses' perceptions of nurse managers. This tool is known as the CAT-A (Duffy, 1993).

CONCEPTUAL FRAMEWORKS

Caring theory

Watson's transpersonal caring theory (1979, 1985, 1988, 1996) was selected as the nursing theoretical framework for development of the CES because of its emphasis on the caring relationship. The development of the CES was informed by Watson's theory, although separate items were not systematically written for each of Watson's carative factors. The CES attempts to reflect the spirit of Watson's approach by emphasizing the caring relationship and the experience of caring as a whole, enriching process and not a sum of discrete behaviors.

Efficacy theory

The social learning theory of Bandura (1977, 1986) was selected as a framework because it offers a perspective that bridges human beliefs and behaviors in environmental contexts and thus informs the definition and assessment of caring. According to Bandura (in press), "Perceived self-efficacy refers to beliefs in one's capabilities to organize and execute courses of action required to meet given situational demands." Hurley (1990) paraphrases self-efficacy as a sense of "I can do."

Cervone and Peake (1986) explain that efficacy beliefs are not generalized feelings of confidence or success, but judgments of how well one can perform in specified domains. The specific efficacy domain under consideration in this study is nurses' beliefs in their abilities to express caring orientations, attitudes, and behaviors and to establish caring relationships with clients or patients.

PHASE 1: CES DEVELOPMENT

Description and sample

The original CES contained 46 items, and subjects responded on a 6-point Likert-type scale, strongly disagree (–3) to strongly agree (+3). Positively worded items were converted to a 1 to 6 scale for scoring purposes, and negatively worded items were reversed. Items were reviewed for content validity by nursing faculty members in the United States and Canada. The first version of the CES contained 39 positively worded and 7 negatively worded items. The initial sample was a convenience sample of 47 novice nurses.

Initial findings

Inter-item correlations and a factor analysis (performed for descriptive purposes despite the small number of subjects) were used in guiding decisions to drop 16 items that failed to exhibit a pattern of significant relationships with other items. The reduced 30-item scale, CES Self-Report Form A, contains 23 positively worded and 7 negatively worded items. The mean student novice nurse scale score for Form A was 3.97, with a standard deviation of .55. Cronbach's al-

pha, a measure of internal consistency, was very favorable (.92).

PHASE 2: RELIABILITY AND VALIDITY TESTING

Samples and administration

Data were collected as part of an evaluation plan to assess the student outcome of caring for an accreditation review. All of the samples were convenience samples because of the need to sample graduating students, their preceptors, alumni, and their employers from three academic programs: baccalaureate (BS), nursing doctorate (ND), and master's (MS).

New graduates

Questionnaire packets were distributed near the end of students' final semester to 83 BS students, 10 ND students, and 51 MS students. The response rates for the graduating student samples were defensible, ranging from 61% to 90%.

Almost all of the students' clinical preceptors were mailed an assessment packet to rate students in their final semester of study. The preceptor response rates were slightly lower than for the students.

All responses were confidential. The three samples of graduating students were very similar in demographic characteristics, except that the MS sample was slightly older. The majority of graduating students were female and Caucasian.

Experienced nurse alumni

A second sample consisted of alumni who had graduated at least 1 year prior. For the BS and MS programs, current mailing addresses were obtained (when possible) for alumni cohorts for the past 5 years. The ND alumni sample was an exception, in that only one cohort had graduated at the time of the study. All responses were confidential.

The potential alumni population as defined included 453 from the BS program (22% response rate), 10 from the ND program (90% response rate), and 387 from the MS program (35% response rate). Because alumni identified their employers on a voluntary basis, responses were completed by only 11% of the BS employers, 80% of the ND employers, and 18% of the MS employers; however, these response rates are typical for alumni who have graduated some years ago. Almost all of the responding alumni reported current employment in nursing or a related health field. The alumni characteristics, except for age (slightly older), were similar to those reported by the graduating students.

Instrument descriptions, internal consistency, and findings

CES

The response format was the same as the 6-point Likert-type format described earlier. CES Self-Report Form A was used for the ND graduating students so a comparison could be made with their scores 2 years previous; however, no significant mean difference was found. Form A was also used for half of the BS students.

CES Self-Report Form B (content the same as Form A but balanced for positive and negative items) was used for half of the BS students and all of the MS students. Cronbach's alpha was .85 and .88 for Form A and Form B, respectively. Internal consistency thus appears to be relatively high for both 30-item self-report forms.

A reduction in the length of the CES had to be made for purposes of mailing evaluation packets to alumni. A 12-item self-report Form B version (7 positively worded and 5 negatively worded items) was developed based on items with the highest factor loadings obtained in the initial study. The Cronbach alpha obtained for the short CES alumni self-report form, .84, indicates a relatively high level of internal consistency.

Table 1 contains the CES means and standard deviations obtained from the graduating and alumni students. Despite the different forms of the 30-item CES (Forms A and B), the means for graduating students are identical for all programs. As shown in Table 1 the means for CES alumni ratings are also relatively high, ranging from 5.3 to 5.5. (Note the CES was only mailed to half of the BS alumni and the MS alumni to conserve space in the questionnaire for another measure.) No statistical tests of difference were performed due to the unequal sample sizes.

Validation instrument

The CES and a validating measure, the Clinical Evaluation Tool (CET), should be positively correlated, if one supports the proposition that caring and competence are positively related in nursing practice. Graduating students and alumni completed CET self-ratings, while preceptors rated graduating students and employers rated alumni using the CET.

Table 1. Caring efficacy scale score descriptive statistics for graduating student and alumni ratings

Sample	Form	n	Mean	Standard deviation
Graduating students				
BS	Self-report A	38	5.3	.38
BS	Self-report B	25	5.3	.37
ND	Self-report A	8	5.3	.38
MS	Self-report B	39	5.3	.42
Alumni				
BS	Self-report short	47	5.3	.62
ND	Self-report short	9	5.3	.47
MS	Self-report short	63	5.5	.36

BS = baccalaureate; ND = nursing doctorate; MS = master's.

Building on Bondy's (1983, 1984) work on five criterion-referenced performance standards, University of Minnesota School of Nursing faculty members developed the CET. It consists of 10 clinical practice dimensions for baccalaureate students and has adequate psychometric properties (Laura Duckett, personal communication, April 7, 1993). Because the CET was used to evaluate ND and MS students in the current study, as well as experienced alumni from all programs, a sixth performance level was added. It is an "expert" level, adapted from Benner (1984) and Hester and Foster (1991). This modification resulted in a revised CET scale with six levels of performance, with expert being the highest and dependent the lowest. Graduating student and alumni self-rating samples were combined to determine a Cronbach's alpha of .85, supporting the contention that the ten scale items were consistently measuring a single concept. The Cronbach's alpha for the CET supervisor version (preceptors of graduating students and alumni employers) was also high (.95).

Surprisingly, the mean CET graduating student self-ratings and preceptor ratings for the three different academic programs are very similar (Table 2). This finding may be, in part, because the scale is not designed to assess nuances of advanced practice nursing. As shown in Table 2, while there is an order effect for mean CET scores from low to high for alumni and alumni employer ratings for the BS, ND, and MS programs, respectively, the means are all very positive. No statistical tests of difference were conducted because of the unequal sample sizes.

Table 2. Clinical evaluation tool descriptive statistics for graduating student and preceptor ratings, and alumni and employer ratings

Sample	n	Mean	Standard deviation
Graduating student			
BS	63	4.8	.38
ND	9	5.1	.29
MS	38	5.1	.39
Preceptor			
BS	43	4.5	.89
ND	6	4.5	.44
MS	14	4.8	.50
Alumni			
BS	94	5.0	.52
ND	9	5.3	.40
MS	123	5.4	.41
Employer			
BS	44	4.8	.77
ND	8	5.1	.75
MS	61	5.5	.48

BS = baccalaureate; ND = nursing doctorate; MS = master's.

Initial validity testing of CES

Content validity

Faculty associates at the University of Colorado Center for Human Caring rated each of the 30 items in CES Self-Report Form B for the Watson carative factor or factors the item appeared to represent. The findings revealed that 3 items represented one carative factor, 11 items were scored as representing two factors, 13 were rated as representing three factors, and 3 items were rated as representing four factors. All of the carative factors were assigned in the rating process, except number ten. The CES therefore appears to be congruent with Watson's carative factors.

Concurrent validity

Concurrent validity was assessed by testing the relationships between the measure of caring, CES, and the measure of clinical competence, CET. First, correlations (two-tailed tests) were examined among the two types of measures for program graduates and their preceptors.

Graduates' ratings of caring, CES, are positively correlated with graduates' ratings of their clinical competence, CET (Form A: $r = .34$, n = 47, $p = .05$; Form B: $r = .37$, n = 63, $p = .01$). However, there are no significant correlations (two-tailed tests) between graduates' CES self-ratings and preceptors' ratings of graduates on the CET. Interestingly, there is no significant correlation between graduates' and preceptors' ratings on the CET.

Alumni self-ratings on the caring measure, CES, are positively correlated with alumni self-ratings of clinical competence, CET ($r = .63$, n = 110, $p = .01$) and perhaps most important with the independent employer CET ratings ($r = .30$, n = 50, $p = .05$). Employer and alumni CET ratings are positively correlated ($r = .46$, n = 107, $p = .01$).

DISCUSSION

While development of the CES is still in its early stages, the scale has some promising features. The reliabilities for the various forms suggest high levels of internal consistency. Expert nurse judges validated the content validity of the scale early in its development, and Center for Human Caring faculty associates have concurred that the scale assesses the majority of Watson's carative factors. In addition, the scale is positively correlated with an independent measure of clinical competence.

The study has a number of significant limitations. The practical purpose of the study, its role as part of an accreditation review, may have induced bias toward socially desirable responses. The extent of a socially desirable response bias in the CES needs to be explored. In the case of alumni, it is possible that the more confident and satisfied responded to the questionnaires. Future studies need larger samples, either randomly selected from diverse populations or selected using a known groups strategy. Future studies need to use the longer 30-item form with large samples so that a factor analysis can be conducted. More diverse samples need to be employed to investigate if the restricted ranges found in this study, high means and low variance, remain psychometric problems. The CES needs to be administered concurrently with other instruments that assess personal control variables such as coping style, general self-efficacy, locus of control, and social desirability. In addition the relationship of the CES to other important nursing process variables in the realm of clinical competence needs to be explored.

As von Essen and Sjoden (1995) point out, the correspondence between nursing perceptions and actual behavior is far from clear. Social psychology has documented the often weak linkages between self-report belief measures and actual behaviors. For example, Triandis (1982) identified 40 factors that complicate the relationship between attitudes and behaviors. Multiple sources and measures are needed to triangulate the CES self-report and the newly developed CES preceptor/supervisor versions of the scale (Coates, 1996). Additional sources of data for triangulation could be explored in the form of independent patient ratings of caring and observations of caring behaviors. Caring efficacy needs to be studied as an aspect of the nursing process in relationship to patient outcome measures.

In conclusion, while most of the quantitative measurement tools designed to assess caring report reasonable internal consistency with modest sample sizes and good content validity, concurrent and predictive validity testing with large samples of diverse populations of nurses and patients remains a research challenge for the future for the caring efficacy scale as well as other measures of caring. The assessment of caring has an important role to play in specifying the nature of caregiver processes and interventions that result in desired patient outcomes.

REFERENCES

Bandura, A. (1977). Self-efficacy: Toward a unified theory of behavioral change. *Psychological Review, 84,* 191–215.

Bandura, A. (1986). *Social foundations of thought and action: A social cognitive theory.* Englewood Cliffs, NJ: Prentice Hall.

Bandura, A. (in press). Self-efficacy mechanism in physiological activation and health-promoting behavior. In J. Madden IV, S. Mattyhss, & J. Barchas (Eds.), *Adaptation.* New York, NY: Raven Press.

Benner, P. (1984). *From novice to expert.* Menlo Park, CA: Addison-Wesley.

Bondy, K.N. (1983). Criterion-referenced definitions for rating scales in clinical evaluation. *Journal of Nursing Education, 23,* 376–382.

Bondy, K.N. (1984). Clinical evaluation of student performance: The effects of criteria on accuracy and reliability. *Research in Nursing and Health, 7,* 25–33.

Cervone, D., & Peake, P.K. (1986). Anchoring, efficacy, and action: The influence of judgmental heuristics on self-efficacy judgments and behavior. *Journal of Personality and Social Psychology, 50,* 492–501.

Coates, C.J. (1996). *Development of the caring efficacy scale: Self-report and supervisor versions.* Unpublished manuscript, University of Colorado Health Sciences Center, Denver, CO.

Cronin, S.N., & Harrison, B. (1988). Importance of nurse caring behaviors as perceived by patients after myocardial infarction. *Heart and Lung, 17*(4), 374–380.

Duffy, J.R. (1992). The impact of nurse caring on patient outcomes. In D.A. Gaut (Ed.), *The presence of caring in nursing* (pp. 113–136). New York, NY: National League for Nursing.

Duffy, J.R. (1993). Caring behaviors of nurse managers: Relationships to staff nurse satisfaction and retention. In D.A. Gaut (Ed.), *A global agenda for caring* (pp. 365–378). New York, NY: National League for Nursing.

Fitzpatrick, J.J. (1995). Editorial: Where has all the caring gone? *Applied Nursing Research, 8*(4), 155.

Hester, N., & Foster, R. (1991). *Nurses' clinical decision-making: Pain in children* (Research grant funded by NIH NCNR, RO1NR01964). Denver, CO: School of Nursing, University of Colorado Health Sciences Center.

Huggins, K.N., Gandy, W.M., & Kohut, C.D. (1993). Emergency department patients' perception of nurse caring behaviors. *Heart and Lung, 22*(4), 356–364.

Hurley, A.C. (1990). Measuring self-care ability in patients with diabetes: The Insulin Management Diabetes Self-Efficacy Scale. In C.F. Waltz & O.L. Strickland (Eds.), *Measurement of nursing outcomes: Measuring client self-care and coping skills* (Vol. 4, pp. 289–294). New York, NY: Springer.

Komorita, N., Doehring, K., & Hirchert, P. (1991). Perceptions of caring by nurse educators. *Journal of Nursing Education, 30*(1), 23–29.

Larson, P.J. (1984). Important nurse caring behaviors perceived by patients with cancer. *Oncology Nursing Forum, 11,* 46–50.

Larson, P.J. (1986). Cancer nurses' perceptions of caring. *Cancer Nursing, 9,* 86–91.

Larson, P. (1987). Comparison of cancer patients' and professional nurses' perceptions of important nurse caring behaviors. *Heart and Lung, 16*(2), 187–193.

Larson, P.J., & Ferketich, S.L. (1993). Patients' satisfaction with nurses' caring during hospitalization. *Western Journal of Nursing Research, 15,* 690–707.

Lorig, K., Stewart, A., Ritter, P., Gonzales, V., Laurent, D., & Lynch, L. (1996). *Outcome measures for health education and other health care interventions.* Thousand Oaks, CA: Sage Publications.

Mangold, A.M. (1991). Senior nursing students' and professional nurses' perceptions of effective caring behaviors: A comparative study. *Journal of Nursing Education, 30*(3), 134–139.

Mayer, D.K. (1987). Oncology nurses' versus cancer patients' perceptions of nurse caring behaviors: A replication study. *Oncology Nursing Forum, 14*(3), 48–52.

McDaniel, A.M. (1990). The caring process in nursing: Two instruments for measuring caring behaviors. In C.F. Waltz & O.L. Strickland (Eds.), *Measurement of nursing outcomes: Measuring client self-care and coping skills* (Vol. 4, pp. 17–27). New York, NY: Springer.

Nkongho, N.O. (1990). The caring ability inventory. In C.F. Waltz & O.L. Strickland (Eds.), *Measurement of nursing outcomes: Measuring client self-care and coping skills* (Vol. 4, pp. 3–16). New York, NY: Springer.

Nyberg, J. (1990). The effects of care and economics on nursing practice. *Journal of Nursing Administration, 20*(5), 13–18.

Parsons, E.C., Kee, C.C., & Gray, D.P. (1993). Perioperative nursing care behaviors. *AORN Journal, 57*(5), 1106–1114.

Rosenthal, K.A. (1992). Coronary care patients' and nurses' perceptions of important nurse caring behaviors. *Heart and Lung, 21*(6), 536–539.

Triandis, H.C. (1982, August 25). *Incongruence between intentions and behavior: A review.* Paper presented at the American Psychological Convention, Washington, D.C.

von Essen, L., & Sjoden, P-O. (1991a). The importance of nurse caring behaviours as perceived by Swedish hospital patients and nursing staff. *International Journal of Nursing Studies, 28,* 267–281.

von Essen, L., & Sjoden, P-O. (1991b). Patient and staff perceptions of caring: Review and replication. *Journal of Advanced Nursing, 16,* 1363–1374.

von Essen, L., & Sjoden, P-O. (1993). Perceived importance of caring behaviors to Swedish psychiatric inpatients, patients with somatic illness, and staff. *Research in Nursing and Health, 16,* 293–303.

von Essen, L., & Sjoden, P-O. (1995). Perceived occurrence and importance of caring behaviours among patients and staff in psychiatric, medical and surgical care. *Journal of Advanced Nursing, 21,* 266–276.

Watson, J. (1979). *Nursing: The philosophy and science of caring.* Boston, MA: Little, Brown and Company.

Watson, J. (1985). *Nursing: Human science and human care.* Norwalk, CT: Appleton-Century-Crofts.

Watson, J. (1988). New dimensions of human caring theory. *Nursing Science Quarterly, 1,* 175–181.

Watson, J. (1996). Watson's theory of transpersonal caring. In P.H. Walker & B. Neuman (Eds.), *Blueprint for use of nursing models: Education, research, practice, and administration* (pp. 141–184). New York: National League for Nursing.

Wolf, Z.R. (1986). The caring concept and nurse identified caring behaviors. *Topics in Clinical Nursing, 8*(2), 84–93.

Wolf, Z.R., Giardino, E.R., Osborne, P.A., & Ambrose, M.S. (1994). Dimensions of nurse caring. *Image: The Journal of Nursing Scholarship, 26*(2), 107–111.

The Relationship of Patients' Perceptions of Holistic Nurse Caring to Satisfaction with Nursing Care

Susan Ann Williams, DNS, RN
Assistant Professor
Department of Adult Health
School of Nursing
East Carolina University
Greenville, North Carolina

The profession of nursing has only recently begun to look at what the term *care* means.[1] In the current health care environment, the measurement of patient satisfaction, defined by some investigators as patients' perceptions of quality care, has become important as hospitals compete for patients and struggle to control costs.[2,3] Although nursing care has been found to be the most significant variable influencing patient satisfaction, few efforts have been made to link nursing care and patient outcomes.[4,5]

REVIEW OF LITERATURE

Historically, the term *caring* denoted the task of giving physical care to another person. Florence Nightingale used the term *nursing care* primarily to indicate environmental and physical care.[6] In the 20th century, however, the idea evolved that nursing care has both affective and task dimensions, incorporates a humanistic approach, and includes the concepts of existentialism and humanism.[7–13]

In part, this evolution of the view of nursing may be related to the incorporation of information from other disciplines into the realm of nursing. Social scientists recognize care and caring as essential for human growth and healing. Freud considered care an essential component of survival of the species.[14] Maslow defined care as a biological phenomenon that requires awareness of the need of humans for caring.[15] Erikson, Jourard, and Rogers each identified caring or

Source: Reprinted from S.A. Williams, *Journal of Nursing Care Quality,* Vol. 11, No. 5, pp. 15–29, © 1997, Aspen Publishers, Inc.

concern as essential in a helping or loving relationship.[16–18]

Over the last 20 years, a number of nursing theorists have discussed the phenomenon of caring from different perspectives. Gaut, Leininger, and Watson all recognized caring as essential for growth and healing of the patient.[1,7,10] These theorists viewed caring somewhat differently from earlier writers. Gaut saw caring as a therapeutic action, Leininger viewed caring as the essence of nursing and as a basic human trait, and Watson believed caring to be the moral core of nursing.

Caring is now viewed as a central component of nursing. Indeed, caring has been identified as central to most nursing interventions, necessary for cure to take place, the moral and ethical basis of nursing, and the essence of nursing.[1,10,19–23] Caring interactions are seen as beneficial not only to the patient but also to the nurse.[8,10,19,24,25]

In the last two decades, research has attempted to determine what constitutes care. A number of qualitative studies have identified what care means to patients and nurses.[26–37] The majority of studies show that patients place more emphasis on the task dimension than the affective dimension of nursing care. Patients value the affective dimension, however, and want nurses to be kind, friendly, considerate, careful, and gentle as well as to provide proficient and timely technical skills. Nurses view the affective component as more important than the physical tasks and value listening, showing respect, communicating, helping, and giving of self. Few quantitative studies have been conducted, and all but two of these sought only to identify perceptions of caring.[9,38–40] Only Duffy and Latham linked patients' perceptions of nurse caring to selected patient outcomes.[41,42] Duffy found a positive relationship between nurse caring and patient satisfaction.

Investigators have found that several patient characteristics influence perceptions of caring. These include age, gender, and degree of pain. Brown and Latham both reported that the younger patients in their studies (under 47 years old) valued affective dimensions of care significantly more than the older patients.[27,42] Reimen and Weiss reported that the male patients in their samples focused more on the physical aspects of nursing care, whereas the female patients focused more on the emotional aspects of nursing care.[36,40] Latham found that patients who had higher levels of pain desired and received more supportive nursing care.[42] Baer and Lowery found that pain influenced nursing students' desires to care for patients.[26] The results of both these studies may be indicative of a circular process in the patient–nurse interaction. Patients in pain need more caring, and nurses feel good about being able to provide more caring, which influences patients' perceptions of the caring received.

There are gaps and biases in the research on caring. Questions have been raised about the utility of caring to nursing, the uniqueness of caring to nursing, the difficulty in identifying and measuring the concept of caring, and the need to develop a view of caring that combines its physical and emotional aspects.[43–45] In addition, caring has been examined as if it were an outcome rather than a process with resulting outcomes.[46]

The connections between caring and patient outcomes remain poorly understood because few efforts have been made to link nursing care and patient outcomes. Although it is important to ensure that the concept of care is clearly understood from the perspective of the caregiver and the care receiver, it is equally important to identify patient outcomes of nursing care.

Although there are problems with the measurement of patient satisfaction, the fact remains that researchers assess patient satisfaction as a means of monitoring quality of care and evaluating the effectiveness of nursing interventions, as an indicator of patient outcomes, as a therapeutic nursing activity, and as a predictor of overall satisfaction with hospital care.[47] In the current competitive environment of health care, researchers are studying patient satisfaction to identify what patients expect in health care and what they like about health care providers. Studies have consistently shown that patients' satisfaction with hospital care is influenced by their satisfaction with nursing care. Patients are more discriminating about nursing care than about other service areas, and their satisfaction with nursing care is the most important factor in their decision to return to a hospital.[2,4,5,48–52]

Patients value the humanistic quality of the nurse–patient interaction and the opportunity to be active participants in their own care.[41,48,49,51–56] Furthermore, patients generally see nursing care as an important factor in their satisfaction with overall care and in their decision to return to a hospital. Nurses' technical abilities and the quality of nurse–patient interactions are considered important variables in patient satisfaction. The research to date, however, has assessed satisfaction with overall health care. Essentially no studies have examined the relationship of patients' perceptions of holistic nurse caring to their satisfaction with nursing care.

PURPOSE

The purpose of this study, therefore, was to assess patients' perceptions of the extent to which holistic care was received. The study was also designed to assess the relationship between patients' perceptions of the dimensions of holistic caring and their satisfaction with nursing care and to determine whether the patient variables of age, gender, and pain influenced perceptions of caring and satisfaction with care among patients in the sample.

SAMPLE

Two rural hospitals in the southeastern United States were used for data collection. The sample consisted of 94 hospitalized medical patients older than 18 years of age who were able to read and write English. Patients being prepared for, or recovering from, an extremely invasive procedure and patients under the influence of pain medications were excluded from the sample. All subjects were hospitalized for 2 days to 2 weeks. Patients who were potential subjects were approached by the researcher. After the study was explained and patients agreed to participate, written informed consent was obtained. Patients

were given a packet with the demographic data form, the Holistic Caring Inventory (HCI), the Pain Thermometer (PT), and the Patient Satisfaction Inventory (PSI) to complete. Completion of the instruments took approximately 20 to 30 minutes.

INSTRUMENTS

The HCI, developed by Latham, was used to measure patients' perceptions of nurse caring[42] (see Appendix). The HCI is designed to measure the holistic, humanistic, caring component of the health care provider–patient interaction. Holistic nurse caring incorporates the principle that the patient is a person with social, physical, mental, and spiritual components. The nurse addresses each of these components in planning and implementing nursing care for the patient. Humanistic nursing care incorporates the principle that the patient is a unique individual with inherent worth, is free to make decisions and act on those decisions, and is recognized as equal in status. Both concepts were measured with the HCI. The 40-item Likert scale is scored from 1 (the patient does not feel cared for) to 4 (caring is evident to the patient). Two expert judges established a content validity index of 1.00. Item clarity of the HCI was confirmed through a pilot study, and the reading level of the inventory was estimated at the sixth to seventh grade level.[42] Discriminant validity of the instrument was established using the Impact Message Inventory (IMI).[42]

Four dimensions of nurse caring were identified through factor analysis of the inventory: physical caring, which addresses patients' physical well-being (10 items); interpretive caring, which assists patients in discussing and interpreting the meaning of their feelings (11 items); spiritual caring, which focuses on the spiritual needs of the patient (9 items); and sensitive caring, which is sensitivity to individual feelings and needs (9 items).

The PT, developed by Johnson and colleagues, was used to quantify the intensity of pain from each patient's perspective.[57] The PT measures pain on a simple scale from 0 to 100.

Validity of the PT was reported by Johnson and colleagues and Latham.[42,57]

The PSI, originally developed by Risser and revised for inpatient use by Hinshaw and Atwood, is a 25-item Likert scale that includes three dimensions of satisfaction with nurses and nursing care.[52,58] These include technical-professional activities (involving nurses' knowledge and technical abilities), trust (characteristics that enhance trust and comfortable nurse–patient interactions), and educational activities (involving nurses providing information to patients). Items are scored from 1 (high satisfaction) to 5 (low satisfaction). Reliability and validity estimates were reported by Hinshaw and Atwood in five studies, and acceptable levels of validity and reliability were demonstrated through successive estimates.[58]

Coefficient αs for the HCI and PSI demonstrated a high degree of internal consistency. Coefficient αs for the HCI global, physical, interpretive, sensitive, and spiritual subscales ranged from 0.87 (spiritual) to 0.97 (HCI global). Coefficient αs for the PSI global, education, trust, and technical-professional subscales ranged from 0.86 to 0.96.

RESULTS

The mean age of the subjects who reported their age was 50.5 years (standard deviation [SD], 14.5 years; range, 20 to 82 years; median, 49.5 years). The sample consisted of 45 men and 49 women. Subjects' mean pain rating on a 100-point scale (<50, minimal; >50, moderate to severe) was 24 (SD, 31; range, 0 to 100; median, 8). Eighty percent of the patients rated their pain at less than 50 on the PT, with 34 percent of those rating their pain at 0. Only 20 percent of the patients rated their pain greater than 50 on the PT.

The mean number of years of education was 11.8 years (SD, 3.5; range, 1 to 20 years; median, 12 years). Of the subjects indicating educational level, a small percentage had a seventh grade education or less (9.6 percent), 37.2 percent had completed high school, 12.8 percent had earned college degrees, and an additional 3

percent had completed graduate studies. Of the subjects indicating marital status, 50.5 percent were married, with the remainder of the sample being divided among divorced (8.6 percent), widowed (10.8 percent), single (15.0 percent), and separated from spouse (15.1 percent).

Sample means for the perception of holistic caring ranged from a low of 2.53 (SD, 0.5) for interpretive caring to a high of 2.95 (SD, 0.5) for sensitive caring. The sample means for patient satisfaction ranged from a low of 3.58 (SD, 0.83) for the educational subscale to a high of 3.92 (SD, 0.71) for the professional subscale.

As identified in Table 1, the global HCI score and each of the subscales scores correlated significantly with the global PSI as well as the PSI subscale scores. Fisher's R to Z transformations were applied to determine whether the simple correlations between the global PSI score and each of the HCI dimensions differed significantly.[59] The correlation between spiritual caring and the PSI score ($r = .43$, $p < .0001$) was significantly weaker than the correlations between physical ($r = .68$, $p < .0001$), interpretive ($r = .60$, $p < .0001$), and sensitive caring and the PSI score ($r = .75$, $p < .0001$; all $z = 1.96$, $p < .05$). The correlation between sensitive caring and PSI was significantly stronger than the correlation between interpretive caring and PSI ($Z = 2.09$, $p < .05$).

Multiple regression analyses assessed the relationships between the combined holistic caring subscale variables (physical, interpretive, spiritual, and sensitive) and each of the satisfaction with nursing variables. The correlations (R) between the four subscale scores and each of the satisfaction with nursing variables ranged from .73 to .77 ($p < .0001$; Table 2).

A stepwise multiple regression analysis using the four holistic subscale variables as predictor variables indicated that the perception of sensitive caring accounted for the greatest proportion of the variance in each dimension of satisfaction. Physical caring explained a relatively small (from .02 to .03) but significant (all $p < .05$) increment in variance in global PSI, the educational subscale, and the trust subscale.

Table 1. Pearson's correlations between perception of holistic caring and satisfaction with nursing care

Satisfaction variable	Perception of holistic caring				
	Global caring (n = 82)	Physical caring (n = 86)	Interpretive caring (n = 83)	Spiritual caring (n = 84)	Sensitive caring (n = 84)
Global satisfaction	.71***	.68***	.60***	.43***	.75***
Educational subscale	.72***	.67***	.61***	.47***	.73***
Trust subscale	.66***	.66***	.55***	.36*	.72***
Professional subscale	.67***	.63***	.58***	.40**	.73***

*$p < .001$.
**$p < .0005$.
***$p < .0001$.

There were significant positive correlations between patient age and perceptions of global HCI ($r = .28$, $p < .05$), interpretive caring ($r = .29$, $p < .01$), and spiritual caring ($r = .25$, $p < .05$). There was a significant negative relationship between pain and the global HCI score ($r = -.25$, $p < .05$). No patient variables correlated significantly with the PSI global score or the three PSI subscale scores. Multiple regression analysis demonstrated that the predictor variables of age, gender, and level of pain did not account for a significant proportion of the variance in global PSI ($R^2 = .05$, $F(4,69) < 1.0$).

The relationship between perceptions of holistic caring and global satisfaction with nursing care was assessed while controlling for subject variables. The global HCI score and the physical, interpretive, spiritual, and sensitive subscales each produced a significant increment in the variance accounted for (R^2) in the PSI global score (Table 3). Sensitive caring accounted for the largest amount of variance, and spiritual caring accounted for the smallest amount.

DISCUSSION

These patients did not report a high level of satisfaction with their nursing care. The finding of low patient satisfaction levels raises questions about communication and trust between nurses

Table 2. Variability in satisfaction with nursing care accounted for by the combination of holistic care subscale scores*

Satisfaction with nursing variable	n	R^2	p
Global satisfaction score	82	.59	< .0001
Educational subscale	82	.57	< .0001
Trust subscale	82	.55	< .0001
Professional subscale	82	.54	< .0001

*Combined holistic care subscales of perceived physical caring, interpretive caring, spiritual caring, and sensitive caring.

Table 3. Variability in satisfaction with nursing care (global PSI) accounted for by dimensions of caring

		R^2	
Holistic caring variable	n	increment*	p
Global caring	67	.46	< .0001
Physical caring	71	.43	< .0001
Interpretive caring	68	.31	< .0001
Spiritual caring	69	.20	< .0001
Sensitive caring	69	.49	< .0001

*Variability accounted for (r^1) after statistically controlling for predictor variables of age, gender, and level of pain.

and patients. Also, it conflicts with the widely held view that patients are reluctant to relate negative feelings about caregivers and contradicts previous reports that hospitalized patients are highly satisfied with their care.[4,41,60–63]

This study does support the view that holistic nurse caring is a significant factor in selected patient outcomes. Patients in the study indicated that caring was evident and that they were more satisfied when they perceived nurses to be caring. Patients rated interpretive and spiritual caring lowest and sensitive and physical caring highest. Sensitive caring was the best predictor of patient satisfaction.

The finding that patients valued sensitive, physical, and interpretive caring is consistent with other studies of patient satisfaction.[5,48,49,52,64] The fact that sensitive caring was the strongest predictor of patients' satisfaction supports the view that patients value the affective aspect of nursing care over physical care.[27,31,36,49] The fact that physical care was the only HCI subscale that added any predictive value to sensitive caring, however, also lends support to studies that found that patients value technical skills, competency, and timely physical care.[9,27,28,34,36,38,65]

There were significant positive relationships between age and patients' perceptions of global caring, interpretive caring, and spiritual caring but no relationship between age and satisfaction with care. As in the studies by Brown and by Cronin and Harrison, gender made no difference in perceptions of caring or in patients' satisfac-

tion with care.[27,28] The finding that pain was negatively related to perceptions of holistic caring did not support Latham's finding that patients with high levels of pain desire and receive more supportive nursing care.[42] Neither does it support the view that there is a circular process in the nurse–patient interaction whereby patients with more pain elicit more positive feelings and actions of caring from the nurse. In fact, the more pain the patients in this study experienced, the less they felt cared for. Pain was also not related to satisfaction with nursing care. Thus, although the research literature suggests that patient variables may confound the relationship between nurse caring and patient satisfaction, in the present sample no patient variable was significantly related to either global satisfaction with nursing care or any of the three satisfaction subscales.

To control for the subject variables, the proportion of variability in patient satisfaction uniquely accounted for by holistic care was assessed after entry of the subject variables into the regression equation. The result was that the significant relationships between global HCI score and the HCI physical, interpretive, spiritual, and sensitivity subscales on one hand and patient satisfaction on the other were independent of subject variables. Thus this study indicates that holistic nurse caring was evident to the subjects, that nurse caring was significantly related to the subjects' satisfaction, and that the predictor variables of subject age, gender, and magnitude of pain were not significant predictors of the relationship between caring and satisfaction.

IMPLICATIONS

The current approach to the delivery of nursing care focuses on the tasks of nursing rather than on the interpersonal relationship between nurse and patient. Time and resources are allocated based on the physical care needs of the patients and rarely, if ever, on the subjective, interpersonal, or caring needs of patients.[66] Clearly, nurse caring behaviors are important to patient perceptions of quality care (patient satisfaction) regardless of patient age, gender, and level of pain. Therefore, greater emphasis should be placed on nurse caring behaviors. This necessitates defining and standardizing nurse caring in the institution, considering nurses' caring behaviors a nursing resource, increasing nurses' knowledge of what caring behaviors are through educational programs, providing support from peers and supervisors for those nurses who provide a caring environment for their patients, including caring standards in performance evaluations, and including the concept of caring in documents that guide nursing care, such as policies and procedures, standards of practice, and the philosophy of the nursing service. What patients consider caring should also be given greater emphasis in nursing education. At present, many curricula do include information about caring, but increased emphasis on this aspect of nursing would help ensure its inclusion in practice.

Maintaining caring in today's health care institutions is difficult, especially with the rapid changes in health care delivery systems that are challenging nurses. Given the strong association between patients' perceptions of nurse caring and their perceptions of quality care (satisfaction with nursing care), it is important to find ways to enhance institutions' caring environment. Without providing for caring time, there is likely to be a negative effect on patients' experiences of care, nurses' perceptions of their ability to deliver good nursing care, and institutions' ability to attract patients.

REFERENCES

1. Leininger, M. "The Phenomenon of Caring: Importance, Research Questions and Theoretical Considerations." In *Caring: An Essential Human Need*, edited by M.M. Leininger. Detroit: Wayne State University Press, 1981.

2. McDaniel, C., and Nash, J. "Compendium of Instruments Measuring Patient Satisfaction with Nursing Care." *Quality Review Bulletin* 16 (1990): 182–188.

3. Joiner, G.A. "Caring in Action: The Key to Nursing Service Excellence." *Journal of Nursing Care Quality* 11 (1996): 38–43.

4. Abramowitz, S., et al. "Analyzing Patient Satisfaction: A Multianalytic Approach." *Quality Review Bulletin* 13 (1987): 122–130.

5. Valentine, K.L. "Comprehensive Assessment of Caring and Its Relationship to Outcome Measures." *Journal of Nursing Quality Assurance* 5 (1991): 59–68.

6. Nightingale, F. "Notes on Nursing: What It Is and What It Is Not." New York: Dover, 1969.

7. Gaut, D.A. "Development of a Theoretically Adequate Description of Caring." *Western Journal of Nursing Research* 5 (1983): 313–323.

8. Griffin, A.P. "A Philosophical Analysis of Caring in Nursing." *Journal of Advanced Nursing* 8 (1983): 289–295.

9. Larson, P. "Oncology Patients' and Professional Nurses' Perceptions of Important Nurse Caring Behaviors." University Microfilms No. 81-16511, 1981.

10. Watson, J. *Nursing: Human Science and Human Care. A Theory of Nursing.* New York: National League for Nursing Press, 1988.

11. Patterson, J.G., and Zderad, L.T. *Humanistic Nursing.* New York: John Wiley & Sons, 1976.

12. Peplau, H.E. *Interpersonal Relationship in Nursing.* New York: G.P. Putnam's Sons, 1952.

13. Howard, J. "Humanization and Dehumanization of Health Care: A Conceptual View." In *Humanizing Health Care*, edited by J. Howard and A. Strauss. New York: John Wiley & Sons, 1975.

14. Freud, S. *Inhibitions, Symptoms, Anxiety.* London: Hogarth Press, 1966.

15. Maslow, A. "Love in Healthy People." In *The Practice of Love*, edited by A. Montagu. Englewood Cliffs, NJ: Prentice-Hall, 1975.

16. Erikson, E. *Identity, Youth, and Crisis.* New York: W.W. Norton, 1968.

17. Jourard, S.M. *The Transparent Self.* New York: Van Nostrand Reinhold, 1971.

18. Rogers, C. "The Therapeutic Relationship: Recent Theory and Research." *Australian Journal of Psychology* 17 (1965): 96–99.

19. Benner, P., and Wrubel, J. *The Primacy of Caring: Stress and Coping in Health and Illness.* Menlo Park, CA: Addison-Wesley, 1989.

20. Carper, B.A. "The Ethics of Caring." *Advances in Nursing Science* 1 (1979): 11–19.

21. Condon, E.H. "Reflections on Caring and the Moral Culture of Nursing." *Virginia Nurse* 56 (1988): 23–27.

22. Fry, S.T. "The Ethic of Caring: Can It Survive in Nursing?" *Nursing Outlook* 36 (1988): 48.

23. Noddings, N. *Caring: A Feminine Approach to Ethics and Moral Education.* Berkeley: University of California Press, 1984.

24. Minick, P. "The Power of Human Caring: Early Recognition of Patient Problems." *Scholarly Inquiry for Nursing Practice: An International Journal* 9 (1995): 303–315.

25. Montgomery, C.L. "The Spiritual Connection: Nurses' Perceptions of the Experience of Caring." In *The Presence of Caring in Nursing*, edited by D.A. Gaut. New York: National League for Nursing Press, 1992.

26. Baer, E.D., and Lowery, B.J. "Patient and Situational Factors That Affect Nursing Students' Like or Dislike of Caring for Patients." *Nursing Research* 36 (1987): 298–302.

27. Brown, L.J. "Behaviors of Nurses Perceived by Hospitalized Patients as Indicators of Care." *Dissertation Abstracts International* 42 (1981): 43–61B.

28. Cronin, S.N., and Harrison, B. "Importance of Nurse Caring Behaviors as Perceived by Patients after Myocardial Infarction." *Heart & Lung* 17 (1988): 374–380.

29. Ford, M. "Nurse Professionals and the Caring Process." *Dissertations Abstracts International* 43 (1981): 967–968B.

30. Forrest, D. "The Experience of Caring." *Journal of Advanced Nursing* 14 (1989): 815–823.

31. Warren, L.D. "Review and Synthesis of Nine Nursing Studies on Care and Caring." *Journal of the New York State Nurses Association* 19 (1988): 10–16.

32. Miller, B.K., et al. "The Experience of Caring in the Acute Care Setting: Patient and Nurse Perspectives." In *The Presence of Caring in Nursing*, edited by D.A. Gaut. New York: National League for Nursing Press, 1992.

33. Mullins, I.R. "Nurse Caring Behaviors for Persons with Acquired Immunodeficiency Syndrome/Human Immunodeficiency Virus." *Applied Nursing Research* 9 (1996): 18–23.

34. Paternoster, J. "How Patients Know That Nurses Care about Them." *Journal of the New York State Nurses Association* 19 (1988): 17–21.

35. Ray, M.S. "The Development of a Classification System of Institutional Caring." In *Care: The Essence of Nursing and Health*, edited by M.M. Leininger. Detroit: Wayne State University Press, 1984.

36. Reimen, D.J. "The Essential Structure of a Caring Interaction: Doing Phenomenology." In *Nursing Research: A Qualitative Perspective*, edited by P. Munhall and C. Oiler. Norwalk, CT: Appleton-Century-Crofts, 1986.

37. Reimen, D.J. "Noncaring and Caring in the Clinical Setting: Patients' Descriptions." *Topics in Clinical Nursing* 8 (1986): 30–36.

38. Gardner, K.G., and Wheeler, E. "Patients' and Staff Nurses' Perceptions of Supportive Nursing Behaviors: A Preliminary Analysis." In *Caring: An Essential Human Need*, edited by M.M. Leininger. Detroit: Wayne State University Press, 1988.

39. Mayer, D.K. "Oncology Nurses' versus Cancer Patients' Perceptions of Nurse Caring Behaviors: A Replication Study." *Oncology Nursing Forum* 14 (1987): 48–52.

40. Weiss, C. "Gender-Related Perceptions of Caring in the Nurse–Patient Relationship." In *Care: The Essence of Nursing and Health*, edited by M.M. Leininger. Detroit: Wayne State University Press, 1984.

41. Duffy, J.R. "The Impact of Nurse Caring on Patient Outcomes." In *The Presence of Caring in Nursing*, edited by D.A. Gaut. New York: National League for Nursing Press, 1992.

42. Latham, C.L. "Humanistic Caring: Personal Influences, Coping Processes, Psychological Outcomes and Coping Effectiveness." Dissertation Abstracts International No. 9030761, 1990.

43. Ben-Sira, Z. "The Primacy of Caring: Stress and Coping in Health and Illness." *Social Science and Medicine* 30 (1990): 517–519.

44. Lundh, U., et al. "Nursing Theories: A Critical View." *Image* 20 (1988): 36–40.

45. Bottoroff, J.L. "Nursing: A Practical Science of Caring." *Advances in Nursing Science* 14 (1991): 26–39.

46. Shiber, S., and Larson, E. "Evaluating the Quality of Caring: Structure, Process, and Outcome." *Holistic Nursing Practice* 5 (1991): 57–66.

47. Lin, C.C. "Patient Satisfaction with Nursing Care as an Outcome Variable: Dilemmas for Nursing Evaluations Researchers." *Journal of Professional Nursing* 12 (1966): 207–216.

48. Lemke, R.W. "Identifying Consumer Satisfaction through Patient Surveys." *Health Progress*, March 1987: 56–58.

49. Bader, M.M. "Nursing Care Behaviors That Predict Patient Satisfaction." *Journal of Nursing Quality Assurance* 2 (1988): 11–17.

50. Cleary, P.D., et al. "Patient Assessment of Hospital Care." *Quality Review Bulletin* 15 (1989): 172–179.

51. Petersen, M.B. "Using Patient Satisfaction Data: An Ongoing Dialogue To Solicit Feedback." *Quality Review Bulletin* 15 (1989): 168–171.

52. Risser, N.L. "Development of an Instrument To Measure Patient Satisfaction with Nurses and Nursing Care in Primary Care Settings." *Nursing Research* 24 (1975): 45–52.

53. Taylor, A.G., and Haussmann, G.M. "Meaning and Measurement of Quality Nursing Care." *Applied Nursing Research* 1 (1988): 84–88.

54. Guzman, P.M., et al. "Tapping Patient Satisfaction: A Strategy for Quality Assessment." *Patient Education and Counseling* 12 (1988): 225–233.

55. Heffring, M.P., et al. "High Tech, High Touch: Common Denominators in Patient Satisfaction." *Hospital and Health Services Administration* 31 (1986): 81–93.

56. Vuori, H. "Patient Satisfaction: An Attribute or Indicator of the Quality of Care?" *Quality Review Bulletin* 13 (1987): 106–108.

57. Johnson, J.E., et al. "Psychosocial Factors in the Welfare of Surgical Patients." *Nursing Research* 19 (1970): 18–29.

58. Hinshaw, A.S., and Atwood, J.R. "A Patient Satisfaction Instrument: Precision by Replication." *Nursing Research* 31 (1982): 170–175.

59. Hays, W.L. *Statistics.* New York: Holt, Rinehart & Winston, 1988.

60. Oberst, M.T. "Patients' Perceptions of Care: Measurement of Quality and Satisfaction." *Cancer* 53 (1984): 2366–2373.

61. Pascoe, G.C., and Attkisson, C.C. "The Evaluation Ranking Scale: A New Methodology for Assessing Satisfaction." *Evaluation and Program Planning* 6 (1983): 335–347.

62. Steptoe, A., et al. "Satisfaction with Communication, Medical Knowledge, and Coping Style in Patients with Metastatic Cancer." *Social Science Medicine* 32 (1991): 627–632.

63. Ventura, M.R., et al. "A Patient Satisfaction Measure as a Criterion To Evaluate Primary Nursing." *Nursing Research* 3 (1982): 226–230.

64. Taylor, A.G., et al. "Quality Nursing Care: The Consumers' Perspective Revisited." *Journal of Nursing Quality Assurance* 1 (1991): 23–31.

65. Mayer, D.K. "Cancer Patients' and Families' Perceptions of Nurse Caring Behaviors." *Topics in Clinical Nursing* 8 (1986): 63–69.

66. Milne, H.A., and McWilliams, C.L. "Considering Nursing Resource as 'Caring Time.'" *Journal of Advanced Nursing* 23 (1996): 810–819.

APPENDIX

Instruments

Instructions: Place a circle around the appropriate number to the right of each statement. Keep a specific registered nurse in mind who has taken care of you during your current hospitalization.

Example: The following statement is an example of how to answer this survey:

	STRONGLY DISAGREE	DISAGREE	AGREE	STRONGLY AGREE
I am able to get information from the nurse to help me deal with my condition.	1	(2)	3	4

This answer indicates that the person did not always get information from the registered nurse about his or her condition.

The following 10 statements refer to getting physical help from a nurse:

	STRONGLY DISAGREE	DISAGREE	AGREE	STRONGLY AGREE
1. I am able to discuss my physical problems with the nurse.	1	2	3	4
2. The nurse is sensitive to the possible effect that information may have on my recovery.	1	2	3	4
3. The information given by the nurse about my physical problems helps me to adjust to my condition.	1	2	3	4
4. The nurse considers my feelings when giving me information about my physical condition.	1	2	3	4
5. The nurse shows concern about how my physical condition will affect other areas of my life.	1	2	3	4
6. The nurse allows time for me to think over my physical problems.	1	2	3	4
7. The nurse shares his/her view of my physical condition with me.	1	2	3	4

	STRONGLY DISAGREE	DISAGREE	AGREE	STRONGLY AGREE
8. The nurse helps me with my feelings about changes happening to my body.	1	2	3	4
9. The nurse understands my condition, and this helps me to deal with physical problems.	1	2	3	4
10. The nurse knows when I need help in dealing with physical problems.	1	2	3	4

The following 10 statements refer to the way the nurse deals with your feelings:

	STRONGLY DISAGREE	DISAGREE	AGREE	STRONGLY AGREE
11. When I am depressed, the nurse leaves me alone.	1	2	3	4
12. The nurse listens to my feelings when taking care of me.	1	2	3	4
13. The nurse helps me to interpret the meaning of my feelings.	1	2	3	4
14. The nurse shares his/her feelings about my situation to help me to understand my condition.	1	2	3	4
15. The nurse helps me to discuss my feelings when I need to make changes in the way I live.	1	2	3	4
16. The nurse is sensitive to my feelings when I am trying to understand my condition.	1	2	3	4
17. The nurse shows concern for my feelings.	1	2	3	4
18. The nurse openly discusses my feelings to help me to adjust to being ill.	1	2	3	4
19. The nurse tells me how he/she sees my feelings affecting others who are close to me.	1	2	3	4
20. The nurse reacts to my feelings in a way that helps me to adjust to a new situation.	1	2	3	4

The following 10 statements refer to how nurses handle other important areas of your life:

	STRONGLY DISAGREE	DISAGREE	AGREE	STRONGLY AGREE
21. The nurse gives information about how my condition will affect other areas of my life.	1	2	3	4
22. The nurse allows me time to reflect on how my condition will affect my family, friends, etc.	1	2	3	4
23. The nurse talks about my condition to family, friends, or other people who I go to for help.	1	2	3	4
24. When I have a new condition, I find that the nurse is easy to talk to.	1	2	3	4
25. The nurse helps me with my feelings about my relationships with others.	1	2	3	4
26. The nurse discusses how my condition will affect the sexual aspects of my life.	1	2	3	4

	STRONGLY DISAGREE	DISAGREE	AGREE	STRONGLY AGREE
27. The nurse shows concern about how my condition will affect the work or job that I am normally involved with.	1	2	3	4
28. The nurse shares his/her view of how my family or friends are reacting to my situation.	1	2	3	4
29. I find the nurse is interested in knowing what I have done, or would like to do during my lifetime.	1	2	3	4
30. The nurse is aware of my idiosyncrasies and other things important to my care.	1	2	3	4

The following 10 statements refer to how the nurse handles your need for hope and spiritual needs:

	STRONGLY DISAGREE	DISAGREE	AGREE	STRONGLY AGREE
31. While ill, I feel the nurse has shown concern for my spiritual needs.	1	2	3	4
32. The nurse considers my need for some hope when telling me about my condition.	1	2	3	4
33. I find that the nurse encourages me to reflect on my spiritual needs.	1	2	3	4
34. The nurse recognizes that my spiritual beliefs may help me to adjust to new situations in my life.	1	2	3	4
35. The nurse openly discusses how this situation fits into the rest of my life.	1	2	3	4
36. The nurse helps me obtain spiritual guidance when I am dealing with difficult feelings.	1	2	3	4
37. The nurse accepts my need to sometimes feel like the situation is out of my hands.	1	2	3	4
38. The nurse is able to sense times when I need help from a higher power.	1	2	3	4
39. The nurse assists me in obtaining religious or spiritual advice to help me to deal with health-related situations.	1	2	3	4
40. The nurse does not get involved with my spiritual needs.	1	2	3	4

Source: C.L. Latham, *Humanistic Caring: Personal Influences, Coping Processes, Psychological Outcomes and Coping Effectiveness* (University Microfilms No. DAO 64793, 1990).

PSI

Directions: The researcher is interested in your opinion of the care you have received. Please give your honest opinion for each statement on this list by circling one of the five answers to describe the nurse(s) caring for you:

1. The nurse should be more attentive than he/she is.

   STRONGLY AGREE   AGREE   UNCERTAIN   DISAGREE   STRONGLY DISAGREE

2. Too often the nurse thinks you can't understand the medical explanation of your illness, so he/she just doesn't bother to explain.

   STRONGLY AGREE   AGREE   UNCERTAIN   DISAGREE   STRONGLY DISAGREE

3. The nurse is pleasant to be around.

   STRONGLY AGREE   AGREE   UNCERTAIN   DISAGREE   STRONGLY DISAGREE

4. A person feels free to ask the nurse questions.

   STRONGLY AGREE   AGREE   UNCERTAIN   DISAGREE   STRONGLY DISAGREE

5. The nurse should be more friendly than he/she is.

   STRONGLY AGREE   AGREE   UNCERTAIN   DISAGREE   STRONGLY DISAGREE

6. The nurse is a person who can understand how I feel.

   STRONGLY AGREE   AGREE   UNCERTAIN   DISAGREE   STRONGLY DISAGREE

7. The nurse explains things in simple language.

   STRONGLY AGREE   AGREE   UNCERTAIN   DISAGREE   STRONGLY DISAGREE

8. The nurse asks a lot of questions, but once he/she finds the answers, he/she doesn't seem to do anything.

   STRONGLY AGREE   AGREE   UNCERTAIN   DISAGREE   STRONGLY DISAGREE

9. When I need to talk to someone, I can go to the nurse with my problems.

   STRONGLY AGREE   AGREE   UNCERTAIN   DISAGREE   STRONGLY DISAGREE

10. The nurse is too busy at the desk to spend time talking with me.

    STRONGLY AGREE   AGREE   UNCERTAIN   DISAGREE   STRONGLY DISAGREE

11. I wish the nurse would tell me about the results of my tests more than he/she does.

    STRONGLY AGREE   AGREE   UNCERTAIN   DISAGREE   STRONGLY DISAGREE

12. The nurse makes it a point to show me how to carry out the doctor's orders.

    STRONGLY AGREE   AGREE   UNCERTAIN   DISAGREE   STRONGLY DISAGREE

13. The nurse is often too disorganized to appear calm.

STRONGLY AGREE   AGREE   UNCERTAIN   DISAGREE   STRONGLY DISAGREE

14. The nurse is understanding in listening to a patient's problems.

STRONGLY AGREE   AGREE   UNCERTAIN   DISAGREE   STRONGLY DISAGREE

15. The nurse gives good advice.

STRONGLY AGREE   AGREE   UNCERTAIN   DISAGREE   STRONGLY DISAGREE

16. The nurse really knows what he/she is talking about.

STRONGLY AGREE   AGREE   UNCERTAIN   DISAGREE   STRONGLY DISAGREE

17. It is always easy to understand what the nurse is talking about.

STRONGLY AGREE   AGREE   UNCERTAIN   DISAGREE   STRONGLY DISAGREE

18. The nurse is too slow to do things for me.

STRONGLY AGREE   AGREE   UNCERTAIN   DISAGREE   STRONGLY DISAGREE

19. The nurse is just not patient enough.

STRONGLY AGREE   AGREE   UNCERTAIN   DISAGREE   STRONGLY DISAGREE

20. The nurse is not precise in doing his/her work.

STRONGLY AGREE   AGREE   UNCERTAIN   DISAGREE   STRONGLY DISAGREE

21. The nurse gives directions at just the right speed.

STRONGLY AGREE   AGREE   UNCERTAIN   DISAGREE   STRONGLY DISAGREE

22. I'm tired of the nurse talking down to me.

STRONGLY AGREE   AGREE   UNCERTAIN   DISAGREE   STRONGLY DISAGREE

23. Just talking to the nurse makes me feel better.

STRONGLY AGREE   AGREE   UNCERTAIN   DISAGREE   STRONGLY DISAGREE

24. The nurse always gives complete enough explanations of why tests are ordered.

STRONGLY AGREE   AGREE   UNCERTAIN   DISAGREE   STRONGLY DISAGREE

25. The nurse is skillful in assisting the doctor with procedures.

STRONGLY AGREE   AGREE   UNCERTAIN   DISAGREE   STRONGLY DISAGREE

Becoming and Connecting: Elements of Spirituality for Women

Margaret A. Burkhardt, PhD, RNCS
Associate Professor of Nursing
West Virginia University School of Nursing,
   Charleston Division
Charleston, West Virginia

Nursing has acknowledged that spirituality is an essential component of the human condition and an important factor in health, yet nursing research in the area of spirituality has been limited. Authors have discussed the need for nurses to be attentive to the spiritual needs of clients, offering a few guidelines for the process.[1–17] Since no consistent definition of the concept of spirituality has been found in the literature,[18] this study aimed at developing a fuller understanding of the concept of spirituality in order to better appreciate how spirituality can be incorporated into nursing and health care.

Women writers and theologians have suggested that spirituality may be experienced and expressed differently by women than by men.[19–26] Attempting to redress the limited documentation of women's experiences in the literature, this study focused on women's expressions and understandings relative to spirituality. Appreciating these experiences may provide insight into dealing with women's health concerns.

The purpose of this investigation was to expand nursing's knowledgebase relative to spirituality from the perspective of women. The researcher's experiences within Appalachia led to seeking participants from this region. The study question asked how women in Appalachia view their spirituality.

LITERATURE REVIEW

Terms found in the literature in reference to the concept of spirituality are spirit, spirituality, spiritual well-being, spiritual dimension and spiritual

Source: Reprinted from M.A. Burkhardt, *Holistic Nursing Practice,* Vol. 8, No. 4, pp. 12–21, © 1994, Aspen Publishers, Inc.

needs,[18] and spiritual perspective.[27] The elderly, terminally ill, and chronically ill have frequently been the target of research on spirituality reported in nursing literature. Studies have focused on nurses' attitudes, conceptions, and practice regarding spirituality and spiritual care[6,9,28,29]; perceptions and practices of patients concerning spiritual needs or care[30–32]; and examination of the relationship between spiritual well-being and factors such as anxiety, loneliness, hope, or quality of life.[8,33–35] In most of these studies the main indicators of spirituality included religious beliefs or practices reflective of a deistic orientation, primarily from a Judeo-Christian perspective, which might suggest that someone who does not believe in a Judeo-Christian God is not spiritual.

Some studies have focused on determining characteristics of the spiritual dimension and describing the experience of spiritual well-being. Research by Banks, Poehler, and Russell[36] suggested that the spiritual dimension is characterized by a unifying force, meaning and purpose in life, relating to God, a common bond between individuals, and individual beliefs and perceptions that guide behavior. The investigation of spiritual well-being with older adults conducted by Hungelmann and associates[37] described major themes of harmonious interconnectedness of time and relationships. In Trice's study[38] of meaningful experiences of the elderly, major themes were reported to be concern for others, helpfulness, action, and positiveness. A study conducted by Burkhardt[39] suggested that characteristics of spirituality among women in rural Appalachia included belief in God or Greater Source, prayer and meditation, a sense of inner strength, and relationship with others and nature. Barker's[40] investigation with women who described themselves as having spiritual well-being noted that the essential structure of spiritual well-being incorporated the themes of relationships and self within the metatheme of being whole.

DESIGN AND ASSUMPTIONS

The nature of the information sought through this study indicated the need for a qualitative approach. In-depth, face-to-face interviews were conducted with women. Data analysis was guided by the constant comparison process described by Lincoln and Guba[41] and Glaser and Strauss.[42] The researcher made the assumption that spirituality is an essential component of each person, thus all persons can contribute to a fuller explication of the concept.

PARTICIPANTS

Participants were selected from among adult women living in southern West Virginia. Data from early interviews guided the selection of later participants. The unfolding selection process included choosing participants from various racial, ethnic, and religious orientations found in the Appalachian region. Women who had religious affiliations and those who claimed no religious affiliation were sought for the study. In order to participate in the study, women had to be 18 years of age or older, not hospitalized or a resident of an institution, and have been raised in Appalachia or have chosen this region as home. Participants were identified with assistance from staff at primary health care centers where the researcher was known and through personal contacts in the community. The researcher contacted potential participants by phone to describe the study and schedule interviews.

The 12 women who agreed to participate in the study ranged in age from 30 to 80 years with half being in their 40s. Eight of the participants had lived in the Appalachian region all of their lives. The other four had chosen to live in the region and had been there between 15 and 32 years. All except one of the participants had children. All except two of the participants completed high school, five completed college, and one completed graduate studies. Three of the participants were retired and one was taking some time between jobs to reassess her life and career goals. All of the other participants were employed outside of the home. In addition to one woman who was single and two who were divorced, one other participant was the primary income earner in her family. Self-described ethnic backgrounds of participants included Scotch-Irish, Pennsylvania Dutch, German Dutch, Polish, Jewish, Norwegian, native American, African American, and Eastern European. Racially, two of the participants described themselves as Black or African American, the others as White or Caucasian. Five participants listed affiliation with a Protestant church denomination, five listed no affiliation, one listed Jewish, and one listed Unitarian/Quaker.

DATA COLLECTION AND ANALYSIS

Data was collected through face-to-face interviews, lasting about 1 hour, conducted at the participant's convenience and choice of location. At the initial meeting the researcher described the study, addressed any questions, reviewed the informed consent, and obtained the person's written permission to participate in the study and to have the interview audiotaped. The initial interview was then conducted. The opening question, which asked the participant to describe her understanding of the term spirituality, was the same for each participant. Subsequent probing questioning, which was aimed at gaining further insight and clarity into the participant's understanding of spirituality, was guided by the participant's responses. At the end of the initial interview, demographic data were obtained. After the tapes were transcribed, a second meeting was arranged with each participant to review the transcript and to clarify and further explore the participant's views.

PROCEDURES IN THE ANALYSIS PROCESS

In order to assure a full elaboration of the concept and to minimize potential presupposition on the part of the researcher, the following procedures were utilized in the analysis process. Each audiotaped interview was transcribed by a professional transcriptionist. The researcher reviewed each tape with the transcription, using field notes to supply missing data and to indicate areas needing further exploration. The transcrip-

tion of each interview was reviewed with the participant so that she could clarify, expand upon, or modify anything she had said.

Transcripts were reviewed line by line to identify and code units of information. Data that appeared to relate to the same content were sorted into categories. Categories were clustered or connected in order to identify and fill in the patterns. This process led to a collapsing of categories and forming of more inclusive categories with related dimensions. Member check was done by taking the synthesis of a participant's responses, based on the analysis process, back to the individual participant for validation.

This process was repeated for each participant. Through the process of comparison, categories and dimensions common among the participants began to emerge. During this process, four intensive days were spent with a peer debriefer knowledgeable in the area of spirituality. These sessions were for the purpose of reflecting on and discussing the emerging categories in order to assure that the researcher's interpretations were remaining true to the meaning and feeling tones of the participants' descriptions. This process led to further clarification of the categories. At a final meeting with each participant a description of spirituality, which was synthesized from all data, was presented to each participant and was validated by all.

FINDINGS

A common pattern was discovered in the interview process. In describing their understandings of spirituality, participants tended to respond initially with statements such as "connectedness to all things," "relationship with and dependency on God," "underpinnings of life, reliable guide," "religion, going to church, doing what is right." They then expanded their descriptions by recounting life experiences related to "the beyond" and to their connections with family, friends, acquaintances, nature, self, and God or Higher Power. They illustrated their understandings of spirituality by telling personal stories that described their own journeys, awarenesses of self that have come along the way, things that have affected, shaped, and given meaning to their lives. In the telling of their stories, they enfleshed an otherwise abstract concept.

The core category reflects that spirituality is a unity or wholeness permeating all of one's life, and manifested through one's becoming and connecting. Neither becoming nor connecting can occur in isolation, as will be evident in this discussion. Although it is artificial to divide spirituality into elements, for the purpose of clarity, the various categories that have been identified will be discussed separately. The elements will then be synthesized into a description of the concept of spirituality as understood by the participants. Participants are identified by coded initials.

Becoming

In describing spirituality, all of the women spoke of things that mattered in their lives (meaning), and how they have changed over time (journeying). Spirituality was described in terms of important relationships and sense of connection with oneself, which included the essence of who one is (one's being), what and how one knows (one's knowing), and what one does and how one acts (one's doing). Participants indicated that spirituality was both a reflection of and a source of their inner strength.

Being

The experience of being was expressed in many ways. Women spoke of "going inward" and of the importance of taking time to be in touch with themselves. BB described "going inside and trying to allow that part of myself to be, and to develop more . . . just paying attention to the quiet place inside." A sense of communion with others, with God, and the world was a source of nourishment for the women. IH talked about spirituality in terms of "being at peace with yourself," suggesting that "unity with other people gives you that sense of being more than yourself." For HC, "just being at the ocean" was soothing. Being was reflected in attitudes toward

life, and was experienced alone, with others, and through ritual. Participants described being "open to new things," and reflected that when they were in "the right place," there was a feeling of inner synchrony and harmony.

Knowing

Knowing incorporated an evolving understanding of the processes and events of life. Awarenesses about self, connections, and the process of life journeys were described. EG talked about "knowing what was important and figuring out about what I wanted to do, what my mission was." One participant noted "I know what I should be praying for, but I can't ask for that because at this point in my life that's not what I want." GK described a "consolidating moment" that occurred after a process that "was real painful. It happened in the night and I realized I had to allow myself to have faith in something about being alive and about myself as a living piece of it. I had to take a different base that would give me courage to move out into life." A sense of inner knowing or trust in God was described by several women, expressing the awareness of "a force that looks over the whole universe, sort of oversees what's happening."

The process of coming to know involved both a receptive openness to life and an active seeking, discovering, and figuring out. Trusting in one's own experiences was illustrated by LR's saying: "You go up the road and you look back and you know why it happened. Not only does it fall into place, but somewhere up the road it will be explained to you why. If you just ride it out and keep an open mind, you'll know why it happened." Knowing included "a more intuitive sense," which was linked to the spiritual self, as well as a physical component. In describing how she knew that an important decision was right, GK stated, "It was very clear when it happened and I had physical clear reaction of absolute relief."

Doing

The active component of spirituality was described by BB in stating that "spirituality isn't being in a cave somewhere for 3 years alone doing meditating, but it needs to be expressed in the world, and you need to do or develop in relation to others." What participants did for others, the earth, and themselves was related to connection with something bigger than themselves. Activities such as prayer, going to church, meditation, doing ritual, raising children, taking care of parents, and assisting friends were described. Noting one's connectedness with the earth led to activities such as gardening, recycling, and composting. DP illustrated this when she said, "because of that realization that you are connected and like other things, you tend to want to preserve those things and not bring any harm to them, to protect them."

Strength

Participants described experiencing a sense of inner strength, derived through nature, other people, and God, which grounded their lives. EG talked about finding "strength from either looking outside or being there." BB described a group in which she felt safe in pursuing the spiritual side of herself as "a sustaining community for being able to go out into the world."

Inner strength was evident in choices like moving on with life after a divorce and drawing on inner resources to be supportive to friends and family. Inner resources were often discovered within life events in which they initially felt limited in their abilities to deal with the situation. AJ illustrated this when she described having to relay news of her best friend's mother's death to the friend, saying: "I just begged God to help. I don't know, it's just like an inner something that takes over, that you know you have to do it. I mean, I love her, she's the very best friend I've ever had in my life, and to see her hurt was agonizing. I don't know, it's just like an inner strength. It sort of comes over me when I feel that need."

Meaning

The women described what gave purpose to their lives. For all of the participants, the "why"

of living was expressed and experienced in the context of caring relationships. Meaning was discovered and demonstrated through choices and actions. For IH meaning was found in being "part of a group of people who had the same ideals that you do, that can accomplish some great good." CV found meaning in caring for others, noting "I look back on my life, I guess I feel all my good deeds have helped some." Meaning was found in relationships with God, and in how one lived life. HC stated that "you might be the only God someone sees. How your actions affect other people are more important than what you can tell them." Meaning was connected to values, which may or may not be related to religious beliefs. EG talked about "discovering more about things that I thought were important and what my values were. It didn't really have much to do with religion."

Having a sense of place or of how one fit in the world was another way in which meaning was addressed. DP spoke of people being "confident of who they are and where they fit in, a sense of some purpose, that their life is not just passing." The meaning of life events was not always clear in the midst of the experience; rather, it was in looking back that the women discovered a pattern unfolding in their lives. When reflecting on her life FE noted, "you see how the threads, how one little thing leads, and if somewhere along the way you leaned this way instead of this way your life might have been entirely different." The women reflected that they could deal with the unexpected because of a basic trust that there is a reason for what happens within one's life, and that they had or would receive the resources needed to deal with all life events.

Journeying

All participants expressed a sense of changing over time. Changing involved learning through experiences of both harmony and disharmony, and developing new awarenesses through the process. One woman noted becoming more aware of spirituality "since my later years and since I got older." For BB and EG this meant coming to honor parts of themselves that had been denied. Changing sometimes meant struggling to reconcile new experiences with values that had guided their lives. Women were aware that their lives were shaped through daily experiences. AJ noted that "the things that happen in your life make you become the person that you are. Every experience makes you stronger or weaker, you just have to try to make it the best you can." One woman summed up the sense of journey in saying, "I've found things in my life that helped me to become that spiritual person I want to be. It's all about becoming and I figure I'll be becoming until I die."

CONNECTING

Connections with the past and future, as well as those significant relationships of the present, were seen as a part of the greater unity that is important for one's becoming. These connections were marked by care, and involved an intentional commitment, embracing the difficult, painful, and mysterious as well as the supportive, loving, and known. Connectedness with God or Higher Power was frequently mentioned first by the participants as they shared understandings of spirituality; however, connectedness with self, others, and nature tended to receive more focus as each interview progressed.

Connecting with Ultimate Other

Relationship with an Ultimate Other incorporated both mystery and trust, and a sense of being connected with something greater than, and a part of oneself. Those who named the Ultimate Other God, Maker, or Lord tended to speak of a relationship with a person. Those who used terms such as Higher Power, Inner Light, Goddess, Force, and Ultimate Energy reflected a sense of being aligned with or in harmony with this Force. For DP "it means a connectedness to the universe and a sense that you have purpose here, a feeling that all of it is one substance." God was not limited to the context of church or religion. Going to church was described in terms of connecting with communities in which one felt safe and experienced caring relationships more than in terms of beliefs and expectations about God. Women described meditation, prayer, being in nature, ritual, and talking with other people as ways of connecting with the Higher Power.

Connecting with nature

Women frequently spoke of spirituality in terms of being outside, connecting with the earth, and deriving strength from nature. For some, being in the mountains was special, some described experiences of the ocean, and some spoke of activities related to gardening, recycling, and appreciating flowers. Goddess worship was described by one woman as a part of her spirituality that helped her to appreciate the earth energy and become grounded. Another woman noted that "the times that I feel most spiritual are when I am alone and when I'm outside and walking or sitting. It happens outside usually in connection to the earth or the sun." EG stated that "trying to respect the earth, since it's so important to me, may be a way that I express spirituality."

Connecting with others

Spirituality was enfleshed through relationships with family, friends, communities, coworkers, and acquaintances, whether loving or painful, supportive or difficult. Love, honesty, acceptance, support, and reconciliation were valued within these relationships. The sense of connection across the generations was evident in the life stories of these women. JS described trying "to use my spirituality in raising my children, pretty much the way I was brought up, knowing the importance of it." AJ talked about her grandmother "who was really strong. I guess maybe those things are passed down, traits, or strengths and character." It was KA's will to be with her children that kept her from dying when she was in the hospital after her accident. She described the experience this way:

I was so bad that they didn't know if I was going to live or die . . . and I went to sleep one night, and I just kept dreaming, you know, I know it was dreaming that I was going through that tunnel, and the wind was real strong and was blowing me to the other side. And the voices kept saying, 'Don't let yourself go through the tunnel. If you do you'll never see your children again.' . . . And I was fighting so hard to keep from going . . . and I thought, I can't let myself go through it, they won't know where I am.

The women's stories included many situations in which they were caring for others, both when it was easy and when difficult. Sometimes giving felt rewarding as seen in FE's experiences of "making life simpler for my kids" by going through things and getting her finances in order. Sometimes it left a sense of emptiness, such as JS's "having to be there for everybody else; sometimes it feels like there's nobody there for me."

Their stories reflected the many-faceted importance of relationships. GK noted that she had "always had people that I could be absolutely honest with in life. Always it's women. There's something in the dynamic process, it just opens up a lot of places for me." CV described the caring relationship she has with her neighbor who "takes me to church; and he's the one that sees that I have a little garden." FE stated that "this is what I appreciate, the little things that people do, call it spirituality, call it whatever."

DESCRIPTION OF SPIRITUALITY

The description of spirituality synthesized from the data presented above is: the unifying force that shapes and gives meaning to the pattern of one's self-becoming. This force is expressed in one's being, in one's knowing, and in one's doing, and is experienced in caring connections with Self, Others, Nature, and God or Higher Power.

DISCUSSION AND IMPLICATIONS

The findings of this study support a unitary view of the human person in that the various categories reflect an interrelating pattern of different manifestations of the same phenomenon. The unity described by the women includes paradox and unfolding, incorporating joy and pain, struggle and peace, stillness and action, sometimes as different aspects of the same experience. Their stories illustrate that as "we come to identify with more and more of our world by knowing through being, we become more and more related to all of reality."[25(p141)]

Elements of becoming and connecting identified through this study give insight relative to important considerations for women's health. Nursing assessments need to incorporate information about a woman's sense of fit in her world, the meaning of events in her life, where she has experienced peace and struggle, how she connects with her inner knowing, and what activities, places, and rituals provide nurturance and a sense of connection. Assessments with women need to include exploration of sources of strength and of relationships that are important. Assessment processes that facilitate a woman's giving voice to her story, and focus more on being with and coming to know the woman than on completing a checklist, are suggested. Encouraging women to take time for self-reflection, honoring their own experiences, and promoting opportunities for making important connections are appropriate nursing actions.

The need for integrating women's views into nursing theory is supported by this study. The importance of including women's perspectives is expressed by Belenky and associates in stating, "When the woman's voice is included in the study of human development, women's lives and qualities are revealed and we can observe the unfolding of these qualities in the lives of men as well."[43(p7)] Appreciating women's experiences may give insight into the affect on health of valuing and understanding oneself and one's authentic connection. Further clarification of the relationship between spirituality and health among those who are healthy and among those experiencing various degrees of alterations in health is needed. Ongoing exploration of the value of narrative, of telling one's story, as an approach to assessment and intervention is recommended. Data from this study demonstrate the variety and richness of the language used by women to speak about the spiritual manifestation of self. A challenge for nursing is to communicate appreciation for the spirituality of each client in language that can be understood.

REFERENCES

1. Brallier L. *Successfully Managing Stress.* Los Altos, Calif: National Nursing Review; 1982.

2. Burkhardt MA, Nagai-Jacobson MG. Dealing with spiritual concerns of clients in the community. *J Community Health Nurs.* 1985;2(4):191–198.

3. Byrne M. A zest for life. *J Gerontol Nurs.* 1985;11(4): 30–33.

4. Clark CC, Cross JR, Deane DM, Lowry LW. Spirituality: integral to quality care. *Holistic Nurs Pract.* 1991;5(3):67–76.

5. Dennis PM. Components of spiritual nursing care from the nurse's perspective. *J Holistic Nurs.* 1991;9(1):27–42.

6. Dettmore D. Spiritual care: remembering your patients' forgotten needs. *Nursing 84.* 1984;14(10):46.

7. Ellis D. Whatever happened to the spiritual dimension? *The Canadian Nurse.* 1980;76(8):42–43.

8. Granstrom SL. Spiritual nursing care for oncology patients. *Topics in Clinical Nursing.* 1985;7(1):39–45.

9. Highfield MF, Cason C. Spiritual needs of patients: are they recognized? *Cancer Nursing.* 1983;6(3):187–192.

10. Lane JA. The care of the human spirit. *Journal of Professional Nursing.* 1987;3(6):332–337.

11. Nagai-Jacobson MG, Burkhardt MA. Spirituality: cornerstone of holistic nursing practice. *Holistic Nurs Pract.* 1989;3(3):18–26.

12. Ruffing-Rahal MA. The spiritual dimension of well-being: implications for the elderly. *Home Healthcare Nurse.* 1984;2(12):12–14.

13. Stiles MK. The shining stranger: Nurse-family spiritual relationship. *Cancer Nurs.* 1990;13(4):235–245.

14. Stoll RI. Guidelines for spiritual assessment. *Am J Nurs.* 1979;79(9):1574–1577.

15. Stoll RI. The essence of spirituality. In: Carson VB, ed. *Spiritual Dimensions of Nursing Practice.* Philadelphia, Pa: WB Saunders; 1989.

16. Stuart EM, Deckro JP, Mandle CL. Spirituality in health and healing: a clinical program. *Holistic Nurs Pract.* 1989;3(3):35–46.

17. Thomas SA. Spirituality: an essential dimension in the treatment of hypertension. *Holistic Nurs Pract.* 1989;3(3):47–55.

18. Burkhardt MA. Spirituality: an analysis of the concept. *Holistic Nurs Pract.* 1989;3(3):69–77.

19. Anderson SR, Hopkins P. *The Feminine Face of God.* New York, NY: Bantam Books; 1991.

20. Christ CP, Plaskow J, eds. *Womanspirit Rising.* San Francisco, Calif: Harper & Row; 1979.

21. Christ CP. *Diving Deep and Surfacing: Women Writers on Spiritual Quest.* 2nd ed. Boston, Mass: Beacon Press; 1980.

22. Collins S. *A Different Heaven and Earth.* Valley Forge, Pa: Judson Press; 1974.

23. Gilligan C. *In a Different Voice.* Cambridge, Mass: Harvard University Press; 1982.

24. Gray ED. *Sacred Dimensions of Women's Experience.* Wellesley, Mass: Roundtable Press; 1988.

25. Ochs C. *Women and Spirituality.* Totowa, NJ: Rowman & Allenheld; 1983.

26. Reuther RR. Motherearth and the megamachine. In: Christ CP, Plaskow J, eds. *Womanspirit Rising.* San Francisco, Calif: Harper & Row; 1979.

27. Haase JE, Britt T, Coward DD, Leidy NK, Penn PE. Simultaneous concept analysis of spiritual perspective, hope, acceptance, and self-transcendence. *Image.* 1992;24(2):141–148.

28. Carson VB, Winkelstein M, Soeken K, Brunins M. The effect of didactic teaching on spiritual attitudes. *Image.* 1986;18(4):161–164.

29. Soeken KL, Carson VJ. Study measures nurses' attitudes about providing spiritual care. *Health Prog.* 1986;67(3):52–55.

30. Sodestrom K, Martinson I. Patients' spiritual coping strategies: a study of nurse and patient perspectives. *Oncol Nurs Forum.* 1987;14(2):41–46.

31. Reed PG. Religiousness among terminally ill and healthy adults. *Res Nurs Health.* 1986;9:35–41.

32. Reed PG. Spirituality and well-being in terminally ill hospitalized adults. *Res Nurs Health.* 1987;10(5):335–344.

33. Kaczorowski JM. Spiritual well-being and anxiety in adults diagnosed with cancer. *Hospice J.* 1989;5(3/4):105–116.

34. Mickley JR, Soeken K, Belcher A. Spiritual well-being,

religiousness, and hope among women with breast cancer. *Image.* 1992;24(4):267–272.

35. Miller JF. Assessment of loneliness and spiritual well-being in chronically ill and healthy adults. *J Prof Nurs.* 1985;1(2):79–85.

36. Banks R, Poehler D, Russell R. Spirit and human–spiritual interaction as a factor in health and in health education. *Health Educ.* 1984;15(5):16–18.

37. Hungelmann J, Kenkel-Rossi E, Klassen L, Stollenwerk RM. Spiritual well-being in older adults: harmonious interconnectedness. *J Relig Health.* 1985;24(2):147–153.

38. Trice LB. Meaningful life experience to the elderly. *Image.* 1990;22(4):248–251.

39. Burkhardt MA. Characteristics of spirituality in the lives of women in a rural Appalachian community. *J Transcult Nurs.* 1993;4(2):19–23.

40. Barker ER. *Spiritual Well-Being in Appalachian Women.* Austin, Tex: University of Texas; 1989. Dissertation.

41. Lincoln YS, Guba EG. *Naturalistic Inquiry.* Beverly Hills, Calif: Sage Publications; 1985.

42. Glaser BG, Strauss AL. *Discovery of Grounded Theory: Strategies for Qualitative Research.* Hawthorne, NY: Aldine Publishing; 1967.

43. Belenky MF, Clinchy BM, Goldberger NR, Tarule JM. *Women's Ways of Knowing.* New York, NY: Basic Books; 1986.

Having Faith: Experiencing Coronary Artery Bypass Grafting

Patricia E. Camp, DSN, RN
Assistant Professor
Ida V. Moffett School of Nursing
Samford University
Birmingham, Alabama

A few years ago the author worked on a cardiac unit that admits clients the day before open heart surgery and was responsible for the preoperative teaching of clients and families regarding open heart surgery. Even with the rather brief time spent with them, a bonding or connecting occurred. After the teaching, the author would frequently comment to clients and their families that she would be praying for them the next day as they went for surgery. Clients and families responded to this statement in myriad ways. Some would say nothing, some would say "thank you," and others were eager to talk of their anxieties and fears about the surgery and possible outcomes. They expressed their hopes and faith in God. Others wanted reassurance they would make it through surgery. These clients were expressing a need for hope, faith, and encouragement that would be a source of strength and support for them as they faced this unprecedented life event. Hearing their concerns led the author to realize that clients have needs that transcend the physical, emotional, or sociocultural realm and are spiritual in nature. Nurses may not address spiritual concerns of clients until they are directly confronted with spiritual needs that cannot be ignored.[1]

Historically, nursing has been concerned with physical, emotional, and spiritual needs of humans; meeting such needs is the essence of nursing.[2–5] Looking at nursing's history, one finds that religious and spiritual considerations have had a great influence on nursing practice and

Source: Reprinted from P. Camp, *Journal of Cardiovascular Nursing,* Vol. 10, No. 3, pp. 55–64, © 1996, Aspen Publishers, Inc.

nursing education. Donahue,[6] in a discussion of the history of nursing, describes how religion has been at the forefront of many of the first nursing schools. With the advent of modern technology and the movement of schools of nursing from the hospital setting to the university campus in the 1960s, the spiritual aspect of care in nursing curricula has dwindled. Spiritual factors profoundly affect responses to health, illness, crisis, and death[1,7–9] and nurses must be prepared to address the spiritual concerns of their clients.[10] Research findings indicate clients who are faced with life-threatening situations such as illness, disease, and perhaps death focus on spiritual concerns.[11–13] Persons admitted to the hospital for coronary artery bypass grafting (CABG) are no different. They are apprehensive and fearful, and they understand that the surgery is serious and perhaps life threatening. Clients typically seek ways to cope with the stress surrounding the event. If nurses are aware of the client's spiritual needs, then appropriate spiritual care can be offered that can help meet client needs[14] and reduce the stress, apprehension, fear, and anxiety experienced.

LITERATURE REVIEW

Prior nursing studies have focused on spiritual coping,[15–16] spiritual well-being,[7,12] spirituality,[17–21] spiritual care,[14,22–25] and spiritual needs.[26–31] Although there is no single definition for spirituality, terms such as spirit,[32] spirituality,[10,20,33,34] religion,[32,35,36] spiritual dimension,[37] spiritual well-being,[12,17] spiritual distress,[38] spiritual needs,[26–28] and spiritual care[11,14,22,24] have been used in reference to spirituality.[21,39,40] The words "spirit" and "spiritual" are used most often. According to Lane, spirit is "that which gives life, the animator of existence"[32(p332)] and is characterized by transcending, connecting or belonging, giving life, and being free. Stoll defines spiritual as a "vertical dimension of a forgiving, loving, trusting relationship with God (as defined by that person) and meaningfully lived out in love, forgiveness, hope, and trust of oneself and others."[33(p4)] Carson states evidence of

growth in spirituality is seen when one becomes "increasingly aware of the meaning, purpose, and values in life."[41 (p26)] Spirituality is a dimension of all humans and involves a belief in someone or something greater than self and provides a source of faith for the individual.[20,32,42] Emblen defines religion as "faith, beliefs, and practices that nurture a relationship with a superior being, force, or power."[39(p43)]

Religion is often viewed as synonymous with a group of persons who hold similar beliefs, ideas, and values. Spiritual dimension[37] refers to that part of a person that gives meaning and purpose to life, a set of principles or ethics to live by, a sense of selflessness and a feeling for others, a commitment to God, and recognition of powers beyond the natural and rational. The National Interfaith Coalition on Aging defines spiritual well-being as "an affirmation of life in a relationship with God, self, community and environment that nurtures and celebrates wholeness."[43(p1)] Spiritual well-being may refer to a sense of inner peace that occurs even in the midst of unpleasant circumstances because one is in harmony with self, others, and God (as defined by individual), and it is a source that strengthens faith and hope in the individual.

Spiritual distress is defined by the North American Nursing Diagnosis Association[38] as a disruption in the belief system and values that integrate and transcend the physical and psychosocial dimension. Spiritual needs refer to "involving any essential variables required for the support and viability of that element which inspires in man the desire to transcend the realm of the material."[42(p85)] In a study by Conrad[44] spiritual needs were categorized as a search for meaning and purpose, a sense of forgiveness, and the need for love and hope. Taylor, Amenta, and Highfield defined spiritual care as "the health-promoting attendance to responses to stress that affect the spiritual perspective of an individual or group."[24(p31)]

In examining these definitions, relationship appears as a common thread in most of them. It is relationship with self, God (as defined by individual), and with others that is woven together by communication (verbal and nonverbal) and helps to bring about wholeness of the individual. Spirituality is maintained through relationships, and nurses should work toward maintaining open lines of communication to enhance the spirituality of clients. However, research is needed to better delineate what spiritual needs are and what nursing interventions would be worthwhile to clients in meeting those spiritual needs. Clark and colleagues[45] suggest that nursing should give priority to conducting research that focuses on spiritual care as defined and needed by the patients themselves. Therefore, the purposes of this research were to discover what cardiovascular clients say their spiritual needs are and how these needs are met during hospitalization for CABG.

METHOD

To discover what spiritual needs are for CABG clients and how these needs are met during hospitalization, the researcher used grounded theory methodology. Grounded theory is an inductive method of inquiry used for the purpose of discovering patterns of life experiences of individuals and relating these patterns for the development of constructs or variables for theory development.[46–48] This methodology allows the theory to emerge from the data in an inductive process. The investigator seeks to discover human experience as it is lived and defined by the person having the experience. Glaser and Strauss[46] and Glaser,[47] the founders of grounded theory, suggest using the following five steps: (1) Open-ended data gathering guided by a general conceptual perspective; (2) concurrent coding and analysis to identify basic categories; (3) literature review to suggest additional categories; (4) concurrent hypothesis formulation; and (5) final review of data for refinement of categories, properties, and hypothesis. A continuous process of data collection and data analysis occurs.

Data collection took place in a large medical center in the South. Tape recorded interviews were conducted in each participant's room 4 to 7 days post-CABG. The criteria for sample selection required that this be the first time participants had experienced CABG surgery. Participation in the study was voluntary and subjects were told they could withdraw from the study any time before data analysis. Each participant was told the purposes of the interview and signed a consent form before taking part in the study. Data were systematically obtained through the process of theoretical sampling rather than statistical sampling. That is, rather than choosing a sample to represent the population, the subjects were considered to be experts about CABG and were chosen because these persons are believed to maximize the possibilities of obtaining the best data about spiritual needs of CABG clients. After each interview, the data from the taped sessions were transcribed by a professional transcriptionist. Tapes were then erased by the researcher in order to ensure confidentiality and anonymity of the subjects. Of the 17 study participants, 11 were males and 6 were females, ranging from 34 to 83 years of age. Participants included nine Protestants, one Catholic, and seven people who had no religious or denominational preference.

Before the taped interview was begun, demographic data were collected. Even though the interview was taped, the researcher took notes as subjects talked and as thoughts or impressions came to mind. These thoughts, feelings, and ideas served to enhance the credibility of the data. Initial questions were open ended, such as, "Tell me what led to your having this surgery" and "When thinking about your hospitalization, what is there about it that led you to think about spiritual things?" The interviews were tape recorded and transcribed as soon as possible after each interview.

Data analysis began with the first transcribed interview and continued throughout the last interview. As the data were collected, analysis began with open coding of each line of the data before putting the data into categories. The coded words were frequently the participants' own words such as "believe," "count on," "trust," and "God." Each piece of data was compared with data obtained from each of the earlier interviews to determine similarities or differences of content before the data bits were placed into categories. As data were analyzed, a pattern began to emerge that led the researcher to ask more focused questions related to the emerging concepts such as "Tell me about your decision to have surgery," "What was uppermost in your mind?" "Did you recognize this as having any spiritual relevance?" and "Did faith have any part in your spiritual needs?" These questions allowed the investigator to be able to guide the development of the theory by asking questions that fit the needs of the emerging theory.[46,47] The categories obtained from the data were developed into concepts (depend, trust, rely, believe) that formed a pattern. From theoretical sampling of participants, there was continuous confirmation and verification of the concept characteristics as the defined category continued to emerge from the data. Throughout this process, the researcher wrote memos about the codes and their relationships. This process continued until the data were saturated and no new categories emerged, allowing the researcher to conclude the sampling.

The computer program ETHNOGRAPH was used to prepare data files by setting margins and numbering the data line by line. Codes were entered in segments with overlapping and nesting of code words, allowing easy access to codes. Patterns emerged as the memos were sorted according to similarities, connections, and conceptual orders, giving an outline or conceptual map that guided the researcher in developing the theoretical concepts. To establish credibility, the researcher consulted a nurse researcher who has considerable experience using grounded theory and two nurse colleagues to verify the codes to determine whether the emerging codes and categories were congruent with those of the researcher.[49] Telephone calls were made to six local participants after they were discharged from the hospital to ask whether they agreed with the core category and the subconcepts that emerged from the data. They gave responses such as "yes," "most definitely," and "sure was."

FINDINGS

A common pattern was discovered from the interview data of the participants. In describing what their spiritual needs were and how these needs were met during hospitalization, participants believed their greatest spiritual need centered around having faith. The spiritual need of having faith was expressed within the subconcepts of *trusting in self, depending on God,* and *relying on hospital staff. Trusting in self* involved transcending or rising above or beyond the current materialistic situation in order to "make the right decision" about one's health. Knowing the risk involved with the surgery, these participants were willing to be risk takers, to "step out in faith," and they "believed they were making the right choice" to have surgery. Most of the participants expressed fear when they realized they had to decide about surgery and some "had to make a quick decision." They had to consider the benefits and hazards and evaluate their options before they "knew what I had to do." At this point in the hospital experience, faith was experienced as letting go when they wanted to hold on and saying "yes" when they wanted to say "no," while realizing what was most important at this time in their life and doing it.

After confirming their "right choice," the subjects' faith was turned in another direction, to someone, to God, who they believed "would get them through" surgery. One participant stated, "I have to depend on someone greater than myself to meet my (spiritual) needs." *Depending on God* was the most commonly expressed spiritual need of the participants and was alluded to in statements such as "...the Lord would see me through it," "I just had faith in Him, and He got me through it," "I did a lot of praying and asking God to protect me," and "I knew I was in God's hands." It was a process of letting go, of depending on a higher being to be in control because they "felt like I had lost control." "I felt I was ready to go if it was my time." One man stated he believed God was in control and that he did not need to worry. Once they believed they were "in God's hands," the patients felt as if they would "get through it (surgery)."

From depending on God, the participants began to consider *relying on hospital staff* to "take care of me and see that nothing went wrong." They were reaching out to others whom they believed to be more capable, knowledgeable, and willing to care for them when they were unable to care for themselves. Previous positive experiences with hospital staff led to believing "I'd get good care this time." Others reflected on the good reputation of the hospital which led to their "having a lot of confidence in them (hospital staff)." Some stated "they (doctors and nurses) knew what they were doing," "I felt like I'd be all right," and "I trusted them." The faith in themselves, in God, and in the hospital staff was a developing process that occurred in stages. The progression from deciding to have surgery, to seeking help beyond self from someone they believed "was in control," to questioning and then relying on the abilities of the hospital staff to care for them shows the process of a mental journey participants traveled in their quest for inner peace, security, and a feeling that "all was well." Participants indicated their spiritual needs were met through the caring behaviors shown to them by others. They believed their spiritual needs were met by friends and family, hospital staff, and God.

Family and friends were significant in meeting the participants' spiritual needs. As one man said, "I had quite a few (friends) come over here . . . and we have prayer . . . it helps." Others stated, "We had prayers (of friends and family), prayed in two or three different towns . . . we knew we was gonna be all right," or "I got cards from a bunch today." Others believed the presence and prayers of their minister or priest helped to meet their spiritual need. As one man said, "He (pastor) stayed with me, prayed with me, and helped me . . . The Priest was the first one I called . . . He helps me spiritually."

Hospital staff (particularly nurses) were instrumental in meeting spiritual needs by "giving words of encouragement." One woman stated the nurse told her, "You are going to be all right. You are doing fine. You are recuperating like you should. . . ." Another said, "It was just kind words (by the nurse) that helped me spiritually." One man mentioned that when he could "walk a little better . . . if that's not reaching some spiritual need, what is it?" When the nurses were "being efficient . . . watching . . . asking if you need anything" met a spiritual need for one man. Some of the routine nursing activities that were carried out in a caring, professional, and knowledgeable manner were perceived as meeting a spiritual need for these participants. Three of the participants whose family and friends did not come to visit very often stated they would have welcomed a nurse sitting down to talk with them. One woman said she would have welcomed prayer but would like for the nurse to offer to pray "because I don't know how to word a prayer." Others stated the hospital chaplain who came by and prayed with them helped meet their spiritual need because, "I need every bit of prayer." The majority (13 of 17) of the participants stated that God had met their spiritual needs. They believed "God had been with them through it all" and "He got me through it." One man said, "I prayed the Lord would get me through it. I just had faith in Him . . . He cares about His children."

Dependence on God gave the participants peace of mind to make it through the surgical experience. They believed through prayer they would be in touch with God and would know that He cared for them and would not leave them alone.

DISCUSSION

According to Carson, faith "represents a way of being, of living, of imagining; it implies a way of acting and responding."[50(p27)] Fowler[51] views faith as a developmental process, occurring in stages throughout one's life span with the stages many times overlapping, making it difficult to recognize when faith has changed from one form to another. Dykstra and Parks[49] wrote that Fowler's concept of faith includes the idea that faith is a human activity that occurs through relationships with the most significant aspects being trust and loyalty to someone or some group or to superordinate centers of value and power (ie, the gods), which provides meaning to life and gives shape and order to one's world to provide comfort, security, and a sense of harmony within. Faith implies trust, reliance, and dependence on another and does not necessarily have a religious meaning, suggesting the universality of faith. Faith is a way of behaving,[52] and is seen as trust, assent, obedience, and self-surrender.[53]

Faith has an intrinsic and extrinsic component. It is not only a belief, an internal process, but also a way of acting, an external process. One believes in self and then acts on that belief. The process of faith is not static, but continually evolves to different forms as one matures and encounters various life events. Gooden[54] stated that crisis can bring about faith development. As one encounters life-changing situations, the organization, structure, and meaning of life are threatened or disrupted. One's self-concept and identity are no longer sources of support; there is a need to find a new way to bring meaning out of the chaotic present. The crisis becomes a "central theme in the development of faith, and as faith encounters new crisis and works through them, it may develop."[54(p105)] However, crisis can sometimes threaten or destroy faith and leave the person with feelings of doubt and dismay. As one participant stated, "I wondered what I had done to deserve all this."

Faith can be described as a dimension of spirituality. It is a way of getting through a present situation because of the fulfilling relationship one has with self, God (as defined by individual), and others. Horizontal and vertical dimensions of spirituality can be seen in faith. It is having a relationship horizontally with others and a vertical relationship with God that empowers the person to transcend the present in hopes of future rewards. Having faith in themselves, in God, and in the hospital staff enabled the participants to bond or connect with others who could help in restoring some semblance of order and structure to life, which

provided peace and security. Their relationship with themselves, others, and God brought about integrity of their spirit. Highfield and Cason support this description by stating that man's "deepest relationship with others, himself, and with God are the center of his spiritual dimension."[27(187)] The findings of Gooden's study[54] may be transferable and used with other clients.

Persons having CABG surgery need additional support to cope with the swift, continual changes taking place. They need to believe they can depend on support from others during these times of change. Because nurses are present with these clients on a consistent basis, they are in a position to offer support and hope. These interventions may have a significant impact on the person's recovery and future health. Most of the participants in this study believed the spiritual support they received made a difference in their hospital experience of having bypass surgery.

Because the pendulum is once again swinging toward spiritual concerns of clients, schools of nursing should be ready to include spiritual care in their nursing curricula. As the students graduate and begin to practice nursing, they will be better prepared to meet not only the physical and emotional needs of their clients, but also the spiritual needs. Nurses are taught the therapeutic use of self in their basic nursing education but often fail to realize how broad this use of self can become in the nurse–client relationship. Using one's self to establish sound therapeutic relationships with clients demonstrates to clients that nurses care, trust, and support them as individuals. Participants of this study described some of the caring behaviors by nurses and how these behaviors and words gave them confidence, encouragement, and hope. Some of the actions by the nurse may not have been interpreted by the nurse as spiritual care, but for the client it met a spiritual need. Soeken and Carson[30] support the idea that use of self may be the most effective means the nurse has to support the person.

Leininger[55] stated that an understanding of the client's religious system is an essential component in meeting the client's health needs. Through religion and religious practices one may demonstrate faith to God (as defined by the individual) and to others. Encouraging clients to elaborate on aspects of their faith increases their faith as they talk and discuss meaningful experiences within their religion. Nurses who are sensitive to the client's religious beliefs and support faith can nurture that faith by striving to gain the client's trust. By demonstrating a caring attitude, knowledge, competence, and skill nurses show clients faith in themselves and in their abilities, which boosts the faith of the patients.

The strength of one's faith may be an important factor in the healing process. If a patient notices that the nurse lacks faith in his or her skills and abilities or lacks faith in other health care providers, it can threaten the patient's own faith in the hospital staff. Encouraging patients in even the small accomplishments made in daily care or recovery increases their faith in self and in the nurse.

●   ●   ●

Responding to the spiritual needs of patients does not require the nurse to share the patients' beliefs, nor does it require the nurse to be an expert in matters of spiritual care. It does necessitate that the nurse be alert for spiritual needs and open to those needs. Responding involves listening, taking patients' concerns seriously, talking with them, and being alert to others who may help in meeting their spiritual needs. When spiritual needs are identified, nurses can then try specific nursing interventions designed to assist in meeting those needs.[14]

Spirituality, spiritual needs, and spiritual care remain virtually uncharted in nursing research, and there is a need for research that further addresses these concepts. Some of the following are recommendations for further research: (1) Exploring the concept of faith more fully to delineate its components of trust and dependability, (2) exploring the nurse's perspective about faith and its impact on client wellness and healing, and (3) further exploration of components of spirituality in nursing.

REFERENCES

1. Beakman LA. Spiritual care. *Nursing.* 1981;81:14–15.
2. Brittain JN, Boozer J. Spiritual care: integration into a collegiate nursing curriculum. *J Nurs Educ.* 1987;26: 155–160.
3. Ellerhorst-Ryan J. Selecting an instrument that measures spiritual distress. *J Psychol Theol.* 1985;12:93–99.
4. Ruffing-Rahal MA. The spiritual dimension of well-being, implications for the elderly. *Home Health Nurse.* 1984;2:12–14.
5. Whitmire VM, Utz SW. Teaching the art of holistic nursing care. *Nurs Health Care.* 1985;3:147–150.
6. Donahue MP. *Nursing: The Finest Art.* St. Louis, Mo: Mosby; 1985.
7. Mickley JR, Soeken K, Belcher A. Spiritual well-being, religiousness and hope among women with breast cancer. *Image.* 1992;24:267–272.
8. Quesenberry L, Rittman MR. When other words fail. *Am J Nurs.* 1993;93:120.
9. Shelly JA, Fish S, eds. *Spiritual Care: The Nurse's Role.* Downers Grove, Ill: Intervarsity Press; 1988.
10. Robinson A. Spirituality and risk: toward an understanding. *Holist Nurs Pract.* 1994;8(2):1–7.
11. Davis MC. The rehabilitation nurse's role in spiritual care. *Rehabil Nurs.* 1994;19:298–301.
12. Miller JF. Assessment of loneliness and spiritual well-being in chronically ill and healthy adults. *J Prof Nurs.* 1985;1:79–85.
13. Reed PG. Religiousness among terminally ill and healthy adults. *Res Nurs Health.* 1986;9:35–41.
14. Clark C, Heidenreich T. Spiritual care for the critically ill. *Am J Crit Care.* 1995;4:77–81.
15. Simen B. The spiritual dimension. *Nurs Times.* 1986;82: 41–42.
16. Sodestrom KE, Martinson IM. Patient's spiritual coping strategies: a study of nurse and patient perspectives. *Oncol Nurs Forum.* 1987;14:41–46.
17. Burkhardt MA. Becoming and connecting: elements of spirituality for women. *Holist Nurs Pract.* 1994;8(4): 12–21.
18. Burkhardt MA. Spirituality: an analysis of the concept. *Holist Nurs Pract.* 1989;3(3):69–77.
19. Forbes EJ. Spirituality, aging, and the community dwelling caregiver and care recipient. *Geriatr Nurs.* 1994;15:297–302.
20. Miller MA. Culture, spirituality, and women's health. *J Obstet Gynecol Neonatal Nurs.* 1995;24:257–263.

21. Burkhardt MA, Nagai-Jacobson MG. Dealing with the spiritual concerns of clients in the community. *J Commun Health Nurs*. 1985;2:191–198.

22. Conco D. Christian patient's views of spiritual care. *West J Nurs Res*. 1995;17:266–276.

23. Granstrom SL. Spiritual nursing care for oncology patients. *Top Clin Nurs*. 1985;7:39–45.

24. Taylor EJ, Amenta M, Highfield M. Spiritual care practices of oncology nurses. *Oncol Nurs Forum*. 1995;22:31–39.

25. Taylor EJ, Highfield M, Amenta M. Attitudes and beliefs regarding spiritual care. *Cancer Nurs*. 1994;17:479–487.

26. Chadwick R. Awareness and preparedness of nurses to meet spiritual needs. In: Fish S, Shelly JA, eds. *Spiritual Care: The Nurses' Role*. Downers Grove, Ill: Intervarsity Press; 1988.

27. Highfield MF, Cason C. Spiritual needs of patients: are they recognized? *Cancer Nurs*. 1983;6:187–192.

28. Martin S, Burrows C, Pomilio. Spiritual needs of patients study. In: Fish S, Shelly JA, eds. *Spiritual Care: The Nurses' Role*. Downers Grove, Ill: Intervarsity Press; 1988.

29. Narayanasamy A. Nurses' awareness and educational preparation in meeting their patients' spiritual needs. *Nurse Educator Today*. 1993;13:196–201.

30. Soeken KL, Carson VB. Responding to the spiritual needs of the chronically ill. *Nurs Clin North Am*. 1987;22:603–611.

31. Stallwood-Hess J. Spiritual needs survey. In: Fish S, Shelly JA, eds. *Spiritual Care: The Nurses' Role*. Downers Grove, Ill: Intervarsity Press; 1988.

32. Lane JA. The care of the human spirit. *J Prof Nurs*. 1987;3:332–337.

33. Stoll RI. Guidelines for spiritual assessment. *Am J Nurs*. 1979;79:1,574–1,577.

34. Peri TC. Promoting spirituality in persons with acquired immunodeficiency syndrome: a nursing intervention. *Holist Nurs Prac*. 1995;10(1):68–76.

35. Lilliston L, Brown PM. Perceived effectiveness of religious solutions to personal problems. *J Clin Psychol*. 1981;37:118–122.

36. Lilliston L, Brown PM, Schliebe HP. Perceptions of religious solutions to personal problems of women. *J Clin Psychol*. 1982;38:546–549.

37. Banks RL, Poehler DL, Russell RD. Spirit and human-spiritual interaction as a factor in health and in health education. *Health Educ*. 1984;4:16–19.

38. North American Nursing Diagnosis Association. *NANDA Nursing Diagnosis: Definitions and Characteristics*. Philadelphia, Pa: NANDA; 1992.

39. Emblen JD. Religion and spirituality defined according to current use in nursing literature. *J Prof Nurs*. 1992;8:41–47.

40. Reed P. An emerging paradigm for the investigation of spirituality in nursing. Res Nurs Health. 1992;15:349–357.

41. Carson VB. *Spiritual Dimensions of Nursing Practice*. Philadelphia, Pa: WB Saunders; 1989.

42. O'Brien ME. The need for spiritual integrity. In: Yura H, Walsh MB, eds. *Human Needs and Nursing Process*. Norwalk, Conn: Appleton-Century-Crofts; 1982.

43. National Interfaith Coalition on Aging. *Spiritual Well-being: A Definition*. Athens, Ga: National Interfaith Coalition on Aging; 1975.

44. Conrad NL. Spiritual support for the dying. *Nurs Clin North Am*. 1985;20:415–425.

45. Clark C, Cross J, Deane D, Lowry L. Spirituality: integral to quality care. *Holist Nurs Pract*. 1991;5(3):67–76.

46. Glaser BG, Strauss AL. *The Discovery of Grounded Theory, Strategies for Qualitative Research*. Chicago, Ill: Aldine; 1967.

47. Glaser BG. *Theoretical Sensitivity*. Mill Valley, Calif: Sociology Press; 1978.

48. Atwood J, Hinds P. Heuristic heresy: application of reliability and validity criteria to products of grounded theory. *West J Nurs Res*. 1988;8:135–147.

49. Dykstra C, Parks S. *Faith Development and Fowler*. Birmingham, Ala: Religious Education Press; 1986.

50. Carson VB. Meeting the spiritual needs of hospitalized psychiatric patients. *Perspect Psychiatr Care*. 1980;18:17–20.

51. Fowler JW. *Stages of Faith*. San Francisco, Calif: Harper & Row; 1981.

52. Westerhoff J. *Will Our Children Have Faith?* New York, NY: Seabury Press; 1976.

53. Aden L. Faith and the developmental cycle. *Pastoral Psychol*. 1976;24:215–230.

54. Gooden W. Responses from adult development perspectives. In: Stokes K, ed. *Faith Development in the Adult Life Cycle*. Minneapolis, Minn: Adult Faith Resources; 1983.

55. Leininger MM. *Transcultural Nursing: Concepts, Theories, and Practice*. New York, NY: Wiley; 1978.

Spirituality and Aging

Cathy S. Heriot, RN, PhD
Assistant Professor
College of Nursing
Medical University of South Carolina
Charleston, South Carolina

Come hell or high water
Hang on to the basics of being human!![1(p83)]*

With these words, Snyder exhorts older adults not to give in to the decrements and changes that may come with increasing age. He urges them instead to continue to ground their spirits in the people and things of the world.

The body, mind, and spirit are the basics of being human. According to Frankl,[2] the spirit is what separates humans from animals, so the spirit may be the most fundamental unit of being human, of being a person. Just as people choose to either nurture or neglect their bodies and minds, so too can they elect to nurture or neglect their spirits. Nurturance of any aspect of the person supports health and well-being, whereas neglect results in decreased function or illness. Aging changes are known to affect the body and mind. There is no evidence, however, that the spirit succumbs to the aging process, even in the presence of debilitating physical and mental illness. Rather, Philibert[3] has proposed that aging is a spiritual rather than a biologic process. This proposition should inspire gerontological health care professionals to target the spirit in the pro-

---

*Reprinted with permission from Snyder R. In the Aging Years: Spirit. In: LeFevre C, LeFevre P, eds. *Aging and the Human Spirit: A Reader in Religion and Gerontology.* 2nd ed. Chicago, Ill: Exploration Press; 1981. © 1981 Martha Snyder.

Source: Reprinted from C.S. Heriot, *Holistic Nursing Practice,* Vol. 7, No. 1, pp. 22–31, © 1992, Aspen Publishers, Inc.

vision of health care. Through a review of concepts associated with the spirit and related research, the reader may become better prepared to implement the interventions discussed herein.

SPIRITUALITY

In its broadest sense spirituality is the manifestation of the spirit, just as physiology is one manifestation of the body, and emotions are one manifestation of the mind. Landrum and associates claim "spirituality is at the core of the individual's existence, integrating and transcending the physical, emotional, intellectual, and social dimensions."[4(p303)] Spirituality is a broader notion than religion. In fact, spirituality may be conceived as the umbrella concept under which one finds religion and the needs of the human spirit. Religion and spirituality, therefore, are not synonymous. Religion refers to an external, formal system of beliefs, whereas spirituality is concerned more with a personal interpretation of life and the inner resources of people.

The needs of the spirit include the development of a sense of meaning and purpose of life, including finding meaning in suffering; a means of forgiveness; a source of love and relatedness, including the ability to both give and receive love; a sense of transcendence; a sense of awe or wonder about life; and a deep experience of trustful relatedness to God, a Supreme Being, or a universal power or force.[4-7] Thus, a notion of deity is not essential to spirituality.

In proposing that aging is a spiritual process, Philibert[3] was not suggesting that continued growth in creativity and wisdom, with their concomitant final fulfillment, is a universal feature of people's lives. Rather, he believed creativity and wisdom represented compensation for a lifelong dedication to education of the self. Philibert further asserted that, like choosing to commit to self-growth in general, "aging as spiritual growth is an opportunity that may either be enjoyed or neglected."[3(p189)] If one espouses a perspective of aging as a continuing, life-span developmental process, then aging will be viewed as a time of opportunities—opportunities for inner growth and continued spiritual development.

SPIRITUAL AGING AND DEVELOPMENT

Spiritual aging pertains to changes of self and self-perceptions, relationships of self to others, the place of self in the world, and the self's world view.[8] The spiritual self is defined partly through interaction with others and partly, in the later years, through introspection and contemplation. In older adults interpersonal relationships tend to take priority over concerns with such matters as status in the working world and acquisition of material objects. Thus, the older adult receives the impetus for redevelopment of the spiritual self in keeping with changes in interpersonal relationships.

According to Gress and Bahr,[8] spiritual aging develops across the life span in concert with continuing evolvement of one's philosophy of life. It involves "getting to know the interpersonal relationships defining *self* in give-and-take situations,"[8(p48)] as well as attaining an appreciation of one's relationship to the universe. Acceptance of the fullness of one's experiences, both pleasant and unpleasant, is part of spiritual development. "Sharing experiences with others helps to develop inner strength and establishes the human bond, love, which is a source of support. If aging is seen as the unfolding of human potential, the development and use of inner resources comprise the spiritual growth and development of older persons."[8(p48)]

Development of personal identity precedes discovery of the meaning of life.[7] Children begin "the quest for identity by raising such questions as *Who am I?* and later *Why am I?*"[8(p85)] The pursuit of answers to these questions is the first step in attaining personhood and is indicative of spiritual development. As people age, the emphasis shifts to *Why am I?* and *What is the meaning of my life?* Searching for answers to these questions can result in a greater sense of being and self-identity. The older person frequently achieves identity, only to be forced into a struggle with the possibility of "becoming a nobody in a world that has placed high value on productivity and materialism."[8(p85)] This situation brings into sharp focus the question of the purpose of life.

Development of the spirit is less clearly defined in the literature than is development of the body and mind. This, however, should not be construed as meaning that the spiritual dimension of the person is less important than the other facets of the person. Older people often emphasize the spiritual aspects of life,[8] making the development of knowledge about the spirit imperative for those who work with the older adult.

RESEARCH WITH AGED ADULTS

Religious research

Researchers in gerontology and psychology have limited their efforts to descriptions of religious practices,[9,10] their effects on suicide rates[11] and well-being,[12–16] relationships between religious practices and coping,[17–20] and attempts to measure spiritual well-being.[21–23] The problem these studies share is that regardless of whether the terminology refers to spirituality or religion, the researchers have all used either religiosity (religious behavior), as measured by church attendance or other organized religious activity, or a Judeo-Christian framework to conceptualize the variable for tool development.

Critique of these studies reveals two major gaps in the research on religion and the aged. First, there is a need to conduct research with older adults from more diverse philosophical and religious orientations using tools with a broader framework than Judeo-Christianity. Second, it would be useful to employ random-sampling techniques in order to be able to generalize the findings to populations other than those under immediate review.

Spiritual research

Most spiritual research has used phenomenological approaches. Trice[24] studied older adults to determine a description of the essential structure of a single experience of the meaning of life. Common themes resulting in Trice's development of the essential structure of a meaningful experience were concern for others, helpfulness, action, and positiveness.

Heriot[25] built on Trice's research by studying older adults' experiences of the personal meaning of life across their life spans. Three concepts emerged from the data

- sources of personal meaning,
- meanings associated with the sources, and
- outcomes of the presence of personal meaning of life

In yet another phenomenological study, Prodoehl[26] found that the informants' ideas about spirituality had to do with "their beliefs and questions concerned with self and their orientation to the universe." The major themes that emerged from the data were world view, spiritual process, spiritual feelings and behaviors, religion and church, and spirituality and health.

In a study of residents of four nursing homes and retirement units, Uhlman and Steinke[27] found that whereas the majority felt that general communication or interaction with their source of spiritual help gave them the most pleasure and comfort, most stated they had no current source of spiritual help. This study clearly indicated that spiritual needs were recognized but not met.

From the preponderance of qualitative studies regarding matters of the spirit, it is evident that further research into this global concept is needed to develop measures of spirituality. It will then be possible to test hypotheses about relationships between health and the human spirit.

NURTURING THE AGED SPIRIT

Assessment

In his compelling poem, Snyder[1] pleaded,

Still to be Spirit!
though dimly, and at times murky
Still to be *lived* moments
which light up with significances!
even though I am in process of disappearing.

Still to be a meaningful story
since soon that will be all.
I have a story
and I have a song

And the song will be sung
till my day is done.[1(p85)]*

With these words Snyder advanced several ideas about where nurses can start to meet their clients spirit-to-spirit. When combined with the information from the literature and research reviews, these words indicate areas nurses need to address to nurture the spirits of aging adults.

The first step to nurturing the spirit is to assess what Jourard[28] referred to as spirit-titre. Noting that "hard-headed empiricists banish the spirit to limbo from time to time,"[28(p80)] he attempted to look at what is observable and describable when a person is said to be *spirited* or *broken in spirit* as a means of developing an operational definition for spirit. Rather than looking specifically at spiritual development, Jourard developed the concept of spirit-titre as a means of facilitating the assessment of a person's level of wellness. Spirit-titre reflects the person's sense of hope, of having something for which to live. Jourard contended that when this spirit-titre falls below some wellness-sustaining level, the individual can be characterized subjectively by depression, boredom, or diffuse anxiety. At the same time he stated, the "elegance, precision, and zeal of the person's behavioral output"[28(p82)] diminishes. Jourard went so far as to suggest that in time, the low spirit-titre "permits illness to take root; microbes or viruses multiply, stress by-products proliferate, latent illnesses become manifest."[28(p82)] Furthermore, he proposed that identity may be the psychological counterpart of spirit. He maintained that when identity is rooted in the occupational role, the loss of the role can result in loss of spirit (ie, it de-spirits the individual).

In the past, nursing assessment of the spiritual dimension has usually been limited to noting the client's religious preference and desire to see a member of the clergy. Richards,[29] however, suggested that it is not sufficient to know the church, synagogue, or fellowship group a person attended. Although these may be indicators of religious involvement, she believed they are not necessarily the only manifestations of the spiritual orientation of one's life.

In addition to religious preference, the client's spiritual history should include questions about clients' ideas about the meaning of life, how they express love for others, whether they feel loved, what gives them a sense of wonderment about life, their experiences with transcendence, and their sources of forgiveness.

Intervening with the spirit

Holistic health is based on the supposition that the body, mind, and spirit are interdependent. This belief suggests that an imbalance in any one of these facets of the person can affect the remaining two. Neglect of the spirit may contribute to physical and/or emotional disease, and nurturance of the spirit can generate physical and/or emotional well-being. As Mattson noted, "spiritual integration is necessarily concomitant with all healing and well-being, and no amount of body healing will work if the spirit is not healed also."[30(p12)] A less extreme view is that well-being is enhanced when the spirit is incorporated in a holistic approach.

According to Ross, "the spiritual resources of aging are . . . the strengths and learnings gleaned from a lifetime of experiences."[31(p346)] People who have survived more than 65 years of life, coping with myriad disappointments, losses, and tragedies, will have cultivated some know-how that will serve them in the last years of life. Nurses need to listen to their older clients to ascertain these strengths and strategies.

Most interventions to aid older adults to nurture their spirits involve them in reflecting on their lives. Reflective interventions usually entail eliciting older adults' life stories through a variety of methods. Reflective techniques include life review, guided autobiographies, and eliciting stories in an unstructured way.[32–34] Stimulation of life memories provides older

---

*Reprinted with permission from Snyder R. In the Aging Years: Spirit. In: LeFevre C, LeFevre P, eds. *Aging and the Human Spirit: A Reader in Religion and Gerontology.* 2nd ed. Chicago, Ill: Exploration Press; 1981. © 1981 Martha Snyder.

adults with an opportunity to work through their losses and maintain self-esteem, to come to grips with guilt and regrets, and to emerge feeling good about themselves.

Haight[35] developed a comprehensive list of questions designed to prompt memories related to childhood, adolescence, family and home, and adulthood. Haight's Life Review and Experiencing Form (LREF) also includes summary questions aimed at eliciting the older person's perceptions of life. The guide has been used extensively by the author's undergraduate nursing students. At most, the students require only a two-paragraph explanation and 10-minute discussion to be able to use the form.

Wysocki[36] provided nurses with a detailed guide to performing life reviews with elderly patients. She provided specific suggestions for initiating the process; handling each visit; managing specific difficulties, such as the apathetic and withdrawn client; ending the interview; and terminating the sessions. With the LREF and Wysocki's instructions, nurses should find it easy to incorporate reflective interventions into spiritual care of older adults.

Birren[32] found that autobiography is a helpful way of giving meaning to one's present life. He stated that "writing an autobiography puts the contradictions, paradoxes and ambivalence of life into perspective."[32(p91)] The autobiographical technique can be used with both institutionalized and noninstitutionalized older adults. Birren noted that guided autobiographies are the most useful. Nurses might assign topics such as the roles of money, health, exercise, food, and humor in the older adults' lives. After a week of remembering and writing, or tape-recording their life experiences, the older adults would then be asked to share those experiences with others in the group.

Kopp believed that each person "must work at telling his own story if he is to be able to reclaim his personal identity."[34(p21)] He insisted that everything depends on the telling of one's personal story. According to Kopp, the "principle of explanation consists of getting the story told—somehow, anyhow—in order to discover how it

begins,"[34(p22)] with a basic presumption that the telling of the story will itself yield good counsel. He further believed that this second look at one's personal history can transform a person "from a creature trapped in his past to one who is freed by it."[34(p22)]

In his work with older adults and their autobiographies, Birren[32] noted that something happens when people go beyond the mere recollection and writing of their experiences to sharing those life experiences with others. The interaction that occurs when individuals divulge their deeply personal selves with those in their social environment reveals new dimensions of the self.

Kopp[34] also concluded that merely relating one's tale is not enough. He claimed there must be a caring person available to listen to the story. The listener attempts to learn about each person's unique journey through life. Payne believed that the caring listener "confirms"[37(p13)] others rather than directing them. The caring person needs also to be present to the storyteller; that is, "for genuine dialogue to occur there must be a certain openness, a receptivity, readiness, or availability."[38(p30)]

Heriot[25] found that sharing their life stories offered older adults a rare moment of reflection. This moment of reflection provided for stimulation of memories, categorization and organization of thoughts that resulted, an opportunity to reflect on their lives, and an occasion for verbal catharsis to an empathic listener. The telling of this story allowed the participants to bring thoughts and ideas they had not considered in years, or ever, to awareness. The opportunity to categorize and organize thoughts, ideas, beliefs, and emotions related to the idea that people are not always aware of their thoughts until they say them out loud. This organization of thoughts led in turn to establishment of relationships in thinking in such a way that insights were gained. Sharing meaning-of-life experiences also enabled elderly individuals to analyze their lives and to get better acquainted with themselves. This often enabled them to experience themselves in a more positive light than normally. Another benefit of this evaluative time was that it permitted the participants to reassess their life goals. Participants noted they are not often provided with opportunities for unburdening themselves, and they found just talking to someone who cared was helpful.

Sharing one's life experiences can be a way of developing inner strengths. Since the spirit, in its broadest sense, pertains to the inner resources of the person, it is likely that sharing the story of one's life experiences will support development of one's spirit.

Since sharing of human experiences is so important, Ross[31] suggested that people who work with the elderly must fine-tune their listening skills. She believed this started with developing the ability to "suspend our own viewpoint long enough to receive the report of another."[31(p349)]

According to Paterson and Zderad,[38] humanistic nurses approach nursing as an existential experience. They view an existential experience as an intersubjective transaction, a lived dialogue. Paterson and Zderad stated that "nursing is an experience lived between human beings."[38(p3)] Therefore, instead of asking the nurse, *What did you do in the nurse–patient situation?* (they believed) one ought to ask, *What happened between you?*[38(p14)] In her study, Heriot[25] found the intersubjective dialogue enabled participants to share with the interviewer their meaning-of-life experiences. Intersubjective dialogue entails both indications of awareness of the older adult as a person outside the role as a client and selective sharing of the nurse's experiences with clients.

Bianchi[39] wrote a how-to guide on enhancing spirituality from midlife through elderhood. In this book he suggested that "spiritual becoming in elderhood consists of a 'lifelong growth in creativity and wisdom.' "[39(p190)] He further proposed that those who have attained elderhood are "summoned to fuller participation in the great concerns of humanity."[39(p2)] Nurses can help their older clients to find ways to participate in humanitarian concerns, from writing letters to politicians to serving as volunteers.

Bianchi[39] also suggested that healthy interiority in old age leads to reidentifications. He proposed the following guidelines to the development of *beneficial* new identities: (1) get in touch with one's true inner voices (inner exploration); and (2) turn to a life of services. As Beck noted, "this stage in the life cycle often provides time to think about spiritual matters; issues such as mortality and immortality, love relationships, and transcendence take on new meaning as death approaches."[40(p1264)] Health care professionals can facilitate such inner exploration by fostering the older adult's internal mechanisms of dreaming, visualization, and meditation. Nurses can further assist older adults by encouraging them to serve in volunteer capacities and to share their expertise with the younger generations. Mother Teresa[41] once said that the fruit of faith is love; the fruit of love is service; and the fruit of service is peace. Older adults can be the harbingers of peace on earth if only they believe in themselves and their continuing abilities.

SPIRITUALITY AND THE COGNITIVELY IMPAIRED OLDER ADULT

Richards[29] provided a succinct and practical guide to encouraging, fostering, and maintaining a sense of spiritual connectedness in clients with cognitive impairments. She claimed that even those clients with the most severe mental limitations have moments of lucidity. Nurses need to learn to capitalize on those precious few flashes of clearheadedness, to recognize and use them constructively.

Richards[29] spoke to four areas of client need: relatedness, caring, memory (identity), and grief. She claimed that cognitively impaired clients can experience relatedness to a Higher Force through the love of people who reach out to them. "Persons with dementia can understand the kindness and love of caregivers."[29(p3)] Nouwen and Gaffney characterized caring as "to be always present to each other."[42(p111)] Nurses can be present to clients by taking them seriously, by truly listening to their words and their nonverbal communication, even when they do not make sense to the listener at first. Often a tender touch or gentle tone of voice will transcend the curtain between the cognitively intact and the cognitively impaired. The most fundamental principle nurses must employ in their work with cognitively impaired clients is to see them as unique and special people. To view them merely as dementia patients denies them their personhood.

Nurses frequently see memory impairments as obstacles, and excuses, to providing spiritual care to cognitively impaired clients. However, Richards[29] reminds nurses that the earliest long-term memories are the last to leave a person. Even clients with dementia may have spiritual memories that go back to a much earlier time. Nurses can unlock some of those memories and the feelings that accompany them through the use of rituals and symbols. Music, pictures, and religious symbols (crosses, rosaries, menorahs) may be the keys to accessing the person's memory.

Accessing the memory is important because memory helps people to hold onto their identities. As Richards notes, "an older person may recite words of the 23rd Psalm and gain comfort and a sense of peace from the rhythm of the words even when there is no awareness of where he or she is living. Something deep in memory unlocks a connection to the spirit."[29(p7)]

Richards also noted that the grief of past losses may be experienced with the original intensity due to an altered sense of time. Nursing staffs of nursing homes sometimes become callous toward dementia patients who cry incessantly. They need to remember that memories of the death of a spouse, child, or parent may be as fresh as they were years earlier.

Richards[29] also addressed the need for nurses to share their knowledge with family members, visitors, and members of the clergy. Visitors may ignore the cognitively impaired client because they fail to elicit traditional responses. Nurses can provide these people with the tools to facilitate visits. They can tell them to bring in church programs, tapes of church services, taped music, and poetry and spiritual readings.

• • •

Nurturing the human spirit can prove a valuable resource when working with elderly clients. Herein the reader has found a brief literature review and a guide to assessing and intervening with the aging spirit. Terminological confusion abounds and is responsible in part for nurses' reluctance to address their clients' spiritual needs. Nurses must be encouraged to accept the proposition that the human spirit can be addressed both within and outside of the context of religion. If nurses adopt this idea, they will recognize that it is not imperative they share their clients' beliefs in order to assist them in clarifying and strengthening those beliefs.

It should be clear to the reader that more research is needed in this area. A crucial part of conducting such research will be to conceptualize the concepts clearly. More distinct conceptualizations will help to clear up the terminological problems and free nurses and other health care professionals from the biases associated with them.

Varying levels of consciousness need not prevent nurses from addressing their clients' spiritual needs. It is possible to meet clients spirit-to-spirit through noncognitive means. The author urges nurses to free themselves from their preconceptions and be creative. Not only will the older client benefit, but the nurse will, too.

Older adults will benefit from a holistic approach to health care. As Moberg noted, the one human domain "that stands out as providing the most opportunity for continued growth in the later years is the spiritual."[43(p8)] Nurses can take advantage of this opportunity and facilitate well-being throughout the life span if only they have the courage to do so.

REFERENCES

1. Snyder R. In the aging years: spirit. In: LeFevre C, LeFevre P, eds. *Aging and the Human Spirit: A Reader in Religion and Gerontology.* 2nd ed. Chicago, Ill: Exploration Press; 1981.

2. Frankl VE. *The Unheard Cry for Meaning; Psychotherapy and Humanism.* New York, NY: Simon & Schuster; 1978.

3. Philibert M. The phenomenological approach to images of aging. In: LeFevre C, LeFevre P, eds. *Aging and the Human Spirit: A Reader in Religion and Gerontology.* 2nd ed. Chicago, Ill: Exploration Press; 1981.

4. Landrum PA, Beck CM, Rawlins RP, Williams SR, Culpan FM. The person as a client. In: Beck CM, Rawlins RP, Williams SR, eds. *Mental Health-Psychiatric Nursing: A Holistic Life-Cycle Approach.* St. Louis, Mo: Mosby; 1984.

5. Clinebell HJ. *Basic Types of Pastoral Counseling: New Resources for Ministering to the Troubled.* New York, NY: Abingdon; 1966.

6. Fish S, Shelly JA. *Spiritual Care: The Nurse's Role.* 2nd ed. Downers Grove, Ill: InterVarsity Press; 1983.

7. Travelbee J. *Intervention in Psychiatric Nursing: Process in the One-to-One Relationship.* Philadelphia, Penn: F.A. Davis; 1969.

8. Gress LD, Bahr RT Sr. *The Aging Person: A Holistic Perspective.* St. Louis, Mo: Mosby; 1984.

9. Ainley SC, Smith DR. Aging and religious participation. *Journal of Gerontology.* 1984;39(3):357–363.

10. Heisel MA, Faulkner AO. Religiosity in an older black population. *The Gerontologist.* 1982;22(4):354–358.

11. Martin WT. Religiosity and United States suicide rates, 1972–1978. *Journal of Clinical Psychology.* 1984; 40(5):1,166–1,169.

12. Koenig HG. Religion as a coping resource in later life. In: *Psychogeriatrics: Selected Abstracts from the Third Congress of the International Psychogeriatric Association.* Ridgefield, Conn: Altier & Maynard; 1988.

13. Koenig HG, Kvale JN, Ferrel C. Religion and well-being in later life. *The Gerontologist.* 1988;28(1):18–28.

14. Reed PG. Religiousness among terminally ill and healthy adults. *Research in Nursing and Health.* 1986;9:35–41.

15. Reed PG. Spirituality and well-being in terminally ill hospitalized adults. *Research in Nursing and Health.* 1987;10:335–344.

16. Tellis-Nayak V. The transcendant standard: the religious ethos of the rural elderly. *The Gerontologist.* 1982;22(4):359–363.

17. Bearon LB, Koenig HG. Religious cognitions and use of prayer in health and illness. *The Gerontologist.* 1990;30(2):249–253.

18. Lilliston L, Brown PM. Perceived effectiveness of religious solutions to personal problems. *Journal of Clinical Psychology.* 1981;37(1):118–122.

19. Lilliston L, Brown PM, Schliebe HP. Perceptions of religious solutions to personal problems of women. *Journal of Clinical Psychology.* 1982;38(3):546–549.

20. Nelson PB. Intrinsic/extrinsic religious orientation of the elderly: relationship to depression and self-esteem. *Journal of Gerontological Nursing.* 1990;16(5):29–35.

21. Fehring RJ, Brennan PF, Keller ML. Psychological and spiritual well-being in college students. *Research in Nursing and Health.* 1987;10:391–398.

22. Moberg DO. Spirituality and science: the progress, problems, and promise of scientific research on spiritual well-being. *Journal of the American Scientific Affiliation.* 1986;38(3):186–194.

23. Paloutzian RF, Ellison CW. Loneliness, spiritual well-being, and the quality of life. In: Peplau LA, Perlman D, eds. *Loneliness: A Sourcebook of Current Theory, Research and Therapy.* New York, NY: Wiley; 1982.

24. Trice L. *Human Spirit as a Meaningful Experience to the Elderly: A Phenomenological Study.* [microfilm] Ann Arbor, Mich: University Microfilms International (Catalog No. 8608503 02800); 1986.

25. Heriot CS. *A Descriptive Analysis of Experiences of Personal Meaning of Life Among Older Adults.* Thesis. University of Utah; 1991.

26. Prodoehl T. *The Spiritual Dimension of Health as Perceived and Experienced by Older Adults: A Qualitative Investigation.* Abstract from a poster presentation based on an unpublished dissertation. Carbondale, Ill: Southern Illinois University; 1991.

27. Uhlman J, Steinke RD. Pastoral care for the institutionalized elderly: determining and responding to their need. *The Journal of Pastoral Care.* 1985;39:22–30.

28. Jourard SM. *The Transparent Self,* rev. New York, NY: Van Nostrand Reinhold Company; 1971.

29. Richards M. *The Institutionalized Dementia-Affected Person: The Spiritual Challenge for Connectedness.* Paper presented at the Spiritual Maturity and the Older Adult Conference. April 23–24, 1987; Claremont, California.

30. Mattson PH. *Holistic Health in Perspective.* Palo Alto, Calif: Mayfield; 1980.

31. Ross P. Discovering the spiritual resources in aging. In: LeFevre C, LeFevre P, eds. *Aging and the Human Spirit: A Reader in Religion and Gerontology.* 2nd ed. Chicago, Ill: Exploration Press; 1981.

32. Birren J. The best of all stories. *Psychology Today.* 1987;21(5):91–92.

33. Butler R. Successful aging and the role of the life review. *Journal of the American Geriatrics Society.* 1974;22(12):529–535.

34. Kopp, SB. *If You Meet the Buddha on the Road, Kill Him.* Toronto, Canada: Bantam Books; 1972.

35. Haight, BK. Life review: a method for pastoral counseling: Part I. *Journal of Religion and Aging.* 1989;5(3): 17–29.

36. Wysocki MR. Life review for the elderly patient. *Nursing '83.* 1983;83(2):46–49.

37. Payne B. *Spiritual Maturity and Meaning-Filled Relationships.* Paper presented at the Spiritual Maturity and the Older Adult Conference. April 23–24, 1987; Claremont, California.

38. Paterson JG, Zderad LT. *Humanistic Nursing.* New York, NY: Wiley; 1976.

39. Bianchi EC. *Aging as a Spiritual Journey.* New York, NY: Crossroad; 1986.

40. Beck CM. The Aged Adult. In: Beck CM, Rawlins RP, Williams SR, eds. *Mental Health-Psychiatric Nursing: A Holistic Life-Cycle Approach.* St. Louis: Mosby; 1984.

41. Mother Teresa of Calcutta. *Love of Fruit Always in Season.* San Francisco, Calif: Ignatius Press, 1987.

42. Nouwen HJM, Gaffney WJ. *Aging.* New York, NY: Doubleday; 1974.

43. Moberg DO. 1987. Spiritual maturity and holistic religion in the later years. Paper presented at the Spiritual Maturity and the Older Adult Conference. April 23–24, 1987; Claremont, California.

Modern Physics, Synchronicity, and Intuition

Victoria E. Slater, MSN, RN
Doctoral Student
University of Tennessee
Knoxville, Tennessee

Synchronicity, a term and concept introduced by Jung in 1951, is a difficult concept to understand or accept as valid. The purpose of this article is to present a description of Jung's original explanation, link it to current understanding in physics, and show its similarity to intuition. The concept will be analyzed according to the strategy described by Walker and Avant.[1]

Concept analysis is a tool used to clarify the attributes of a concept; the analysis clearly depicts what a concept entails and what it does not. Walker and Avant include the following four steps in analyzing a concept:

1. Identify all uses of the concept that you can discover.
2. Determine the defining attributes.
3. Construct a model case, and
4. Identify antecedents and consequences.

USES OF THE CONCEPT OF SYNCHRONICITY

Jung first proposed the existence of synchronicity in a lecture in 1951 and defined it at that time as, "a meaningful coincidence of two or more events, where something other than the probability of chance is involved."[2(p520)] The next year, in a longer treatise, he defined it as, "the simultaneous occurrence of a certain psychic state with one or more external events which appear as meaningful parallels to the momentary subjective state—and, in certain cases, vice versa."[2(p441)] He added,

Source: Reprinted from V.E. Slater, *Holistic Nursing Practice,* Vol. 6, No. 4, pp. 20–25, © 1992, Aspen Publishers, Inc.

I chose this term because the simultaneous occurrence of two meaningfully but not causally connected events seemed to me an essential criterion. I am therefore using the general concept of synchronicity in the special sense of a coincidence in time of two or more causally unrelated events which have the same or a similar meaning, in contrast to "synchronism," which simply means the simultaneous occurrence of two events.[2(p441)]

The three significant terms in his definition are *coincidence in time, causally unrelated events*, and *same or similar meaning*. Two examples will help to illustrate his meaning. Craven[3] has written a charming book, *I Heard the Owl Call My Name*, in which she builds her story around an Indian belief that when you hear the owl call your name, you will die. Your dying and the owl calling your name are unrelated. The coincidence is that the person who hears the owl call his name dies shortly thereafter. The meaning is attached by the listener, in this case, that one's death will follow soon after the owl's call. The owl's call and the person's dying are a synchronistic phenomenon.

A second example is psychic knowledge. Jung considered descriptions of future events synchronistic. The prediction did not cause the event; its accuracy was validated only when the event occurred. The meaning (ie, that someone accurately predicted the future) was imposed at the time of the prediction but verified perhaps years later. The two events, the prediction and the event, are unrelated except in meaning.

Synchronicity, then, has two predominant characteristics: a timelessness and a "coincidence." Many people have experienced coincidences that fit the description of synchronicity. For example, one might dream about something, see the subject of the dream several times during the next day, and hear someone else mention the subject of that dream. There is no cause involved, and the coincidence is the close relationship in time of the events. The awareness of the coincidence is up to the person, and any meaning to the events is attached by that person.

However, the aspect of synchronicity involving timelessness is the part having the most significance. How does someone foretell an event that will occur, sometimes years in the future? Why does someone sit next to a stranger on the airplane and that stranger has just the answer the person needed? What, if anything, put them together at just that time, at just the right time? Those types of synchronistic events go beyond mere coincidence.

PHYSICS AND A HOLOGRAPHIC WORLD

Most nonphysicists understand reality in terms of Newtonian physics. According to that understanding, nature and people act as machines. A surgeon, for example, can be seen as a bioplumber, one who skillfully removes or repairs a broken part and reconnects the system so that the body functions normally again.[4] The approaches designed to treat the body from a mechanical, Newtonian perspective work at the macromolecular level, but not at the subatomic level.[5]

The study of the subatomic level is quantum mechanics. A quantum is an amount, a quantity; mechanics is the study of motion. Quantum mechanics, then, "is the study of the motion of quantities. Quantum theory says that nature comes in bits and pieces (quanta), and quantum mechanics is the study of this phenomenon."[5(p45)]

From the study of the bits and pieces of the universe has come an understanding of the effects waves have upon each other when they meet. They will interfere with each other, mixing and interacting. The result of laser light waves that have interfered with each other is a three-dimensional projection. It is a hologram.[4]

One of the properties of holograms is that each small piece of the photographed image contains an entire three-dimensional image of the whole. If you were to tear that image into the tiniest pieces, each piece would contain a complete and intact, three-dimensional image of the thing you photographed with your laser.[4]

WHERE IS THE MIND?

Dossey[6] has taken on the question of the location of the mind. Is it in the brain? He argues that it is not, that it "permeates the entire body—and, indeed, that it reaches beyond the body into the world beyond."[6(p19)] He reaches his conclusions from studies of "body-wide chemicals" such as endorphins, which affect our mental life and moods.

He also cites the Sprindrift studies.[7] This research on prayer indicates that, at least in those studies, patients who are prayed for recover faster. So where, he asks, is the mind—in the brain, in the entire body, or beyond the body?

Dossey also reports studies in which average students have been identified to their teachers as superior. At the end of the year, those students had above-average increases in their results on their annual achievement tests. The difference between the students identified as "superior" and their classmates "existed only in the minds of the teachers."[6(p3)] Similar studies have been done by psychology students using rats and worms. The results were similar. The animals identified as "gifted" performed the learning experiments far better than the animals labeled as genetically poor learners. The only difference, in fact, was in the minds of the students.[6]

Dossey asks, "Did the psychology students escape their own brains to interfere with the 'world outside?' Could they have interacted with the minds of the students, rats, and worms to shape their performances?"[8(p3)] He recognizes that the easiest answer is "No." He then proposes that "if minds are non-local—if they are not bounded in space and time—this means that they are not fundamentally separated from each other. And if not separate, there cannot be then, five billion single minds inhabiting this earth today, but *only one Mind*."[8(p4)]

If Dossey is correct, one may ask if that mind is a hologram and if each of the five billion single minds inhabiting the world today is not a tiny piece of the larger whole. If so, each of us has in our mind a complete, intact image of the larger mind.

Pribram[9] has also looked at the mind and has come to the conclusion that our minds are made up of holographic patches. "Information about the environment is . . . converted into simple waves and these waves are transmitted and stored as interference patterns."[8(p259)] Those patterns, those holograms, are an exact image of what the person sees, hears, smells, tastes, and feels. He concludes, like Dossey, that the mind is a hologram.

In addition, he asks, "What is the hologram the hologram of?"[10(p46)] Another physicist, Bohm, who was writing at the same time as Pribram, proposed that the universe, itself, is a hologram.[10]

So now we have a hologram mind that is proposed to have within it a complete, intact, picture of the larger hologram it reflects, that is, the universe. If, as Bohm and Pribram suggest, the universe is a hologram and our minds are holograms, then perhaps Dossey is correct. We are all part of one mind.

If these physicists are correct, then synchronicity, those meaningful coincidences that cannot be explained by cause and effect, can be explained by holography. If our minds are intact images of a larger mind, of which all minds are a part, it is reasonable to expect that one mind will know what another mind does. And if, as Einstein proposed, time is elastic, then a holographic universe enmeshed in elastic time requires synchronicity.

AN ANALYSIS OF SYNCHRONICITY AND INTUITION

Definition and attributes

Because Jung defined synchronicity so specifically, the word has no other uses. When it is used by other authors, they return to Jung's original work and quote or paraphrase his definition.[11,12] Jung, however, described three types of synchronicity. Bolen lists them as, first, "a coincidence between mental content (which could be a thought or feeling) and outer event,"[11(p16)] such as the owl calling your name. The second is when "a person has a dream or vision, which coincides with an event that is taking place (at that time and) at a distance (and is later verified)."[11(p16)] Such events might be a friend's or relative's death or a catastrophic event such as an earthquake or fire. The third type of synchronistic event is when "a person has an image (as a dream, vision, or premonition) about something that will happen in the future, which then does occur."[11(p16)]

Defining attributes

The defining attributes of synchronicity are a *connection* between two events that had *no discernable cause*, but the person involved gives the connection *meaning*. Jung, in fact, titled his original monograph, *Synchronicity: an Acausal Connecting Principle*.[2] It is the meaning given the connection that distinguishes synchronicity from a synchronous event.

Intuition, as defined by Rew[13] and Benner and Tanner[14] echoes the defining attributes of synchronicity. Rew lists three attributes of intuition: "Knowledge as a whole, immediate awareness of the knowledge, and knowledge that does not result from linear analysis."[13(p32)] Benner and Tanner define it as "understanding without a rationale."[14(p23)]

The defining attributes of both synchronicity and intuition require a connection between two events that have no discernable cause but for which a person attributes meaning. For the remainder of this article, intuition will be discussed as a synchronous event.

A model case

Model cases of intuition have been described by Rew in several articles[13,15,16] and by Benner and Tanner.[14] Rew gives the example of a nurse discussing her intuition about a patient.

"His neuro signs were the same (as the day before) but it was that gut feeling that he was changing . . . and later that evening he had to be put back on the respirator."[13(p32)]

In this case, the nurse experienced the third type of synchronicity, a premonition. There was no discernable cause, but the nurse gave her sense meaning and called it a "gut feeling."

Antecedents and consequences

By definition, there are no antecedents to synchronistic events. However, Benner and Tanner[14] and Rew[13] discuss the difference between the novice nurse, whom Benner describes as one who relies on rules, checklists, and procedures, and the expert, who "no longer relies on an analytical principle (rule, guideline, maxim) to connect an understanding of the situation to an appropriate action. The expert nurse . . . has an intuitive grasp of the situation and zeros in. . . ."[14(p28)]

Rew, and Benner and Tanner, present intuitive events as ones that occur more often with expert nurses and less with novices. An antecedent event may be that the nurses giving meaning to the events must have had enough experience to be able to free themselves from reliance upon the rules and checklists, and be open to a synchronistic, intuitive event.

The consequence of any synchronistic event is a function of the meaning given to that event by the person involved. It may be no more than recognition that such an event has occurred. Or it may be, as with expert nurses, that the nurse acts. A nurse may call a doctor because "the patient does not look right." Benner and Tanner relate just such a situation:

> I was on nights. The patient was not my patient but I went into the room. I knew that the patient was going sour at that point, and I elected to call a code. The patient had not stopped breathing, his pulses were still there, but as I told a nurse colleague on the way home, "I could have bet my last paycheck that he was going to arrest."[14(p29)]

Intuition as a synchronistic event

Jung[2] defined and described synchronicity as a meaningful coincidence that has no discernable cause. Rew[13] and Benner and Tanner[14] define intuition with similar overtones, such as Benner and Tanner's definition of intuition as "understanding without a rationale." Standing alone, neither synchronicity nor intuition makes sense, and they are greeted with suspicion. As Benner and Tanner point out, "a mistrust of knowledge other than formal logic and mathematics has been handed down in the Western tradition since Plato."[14(p30)]

Both synchronicity and intuition, however, can be understood through the current theories of the universe proposed by physicists. According to one modern physics theory, as opposed to the theories of Newtonian physics, the universe is a hologram. Each part reflects a three-dimensional portrait of the whole. Humans and their minds are holograms. They reflect, if they are not actually a part of, the whole universe. If that is the case, and data suggest that it is, the meaningful coincidences (ie, synchronistic events and intuitive awareness) do not need causes. They simply are a recognition by a small piece of the universal hologram (one person's mind) of another piece of the same hologram.

Further development of both concepts within nursing must begin with the intriguing views of the universe being proposed by physicists. Only through an appreciation of the universe as a hologram made up of constantly moving waves and quantities (quanta) of subatomic particles can synchronicity and intuition be explained and understood. Once one puts these phenomena into the context of modern physics, one must rationally conclude that they frequently occur.

• • •

As Rew is doing, nursing needs to continue to explore its intuitive experiences and synchronistic events. Physics provides a theoretical explanation for a phenomenon that is more than a "gut feeling." It is the tuning in of the nurse into the larger holographic universe in which both he or she and the patient exist. The nurse is less able to tune into this level of understanding when bound by rules and lack of experience. But expert nurses who learn to trust their intuition and the synchronistic events that surround them know, as Benner and Tanner state, that "intuitive knowledge and analytic reasoning are not in an either/or opposition; they can—and often do—work together."[14(p31)] One might even say that one is an expert nurse only when one is appreciative of the holographic universe and the synchronistic events that surround us, and when intuitive knowledge and analytic reasoning are blended.

REFERENCES

1. Walker L, Avant K. *Strategies for Theory Construction in Nursing.* 2nd ed. Norwalk, Conn: Appleton & Lange; 1988.
2. Jung CG. *The Structure and Dynamics of the Psyche.* 2nd ed. Princeton, NJ: Princeton University Press; 1969.
3. Craven M. *I Heard the Owl Call My Name.* New York, NY: Dell; 1973.
4. Gerber R. *Vibrational Medicine.* Santa Fe, NM: Bear & Co.; 1988.
5. Zukav G. *The Dancing Wu Li Masters: An Overview of the New Physics.* New York, NY: William Morrow; 1979.
6. Dossey L. *Recovering the Soul: A Scientific and Spiritual Search.* New York, NY: Bantam; 1989.
7. Owen, R. *Qualitative Research: The Early Years.* Salem, Ore: Greyhaven Books; 1988.
8. Dossey L. Where in the world is the mind? *Advances.* 1989;6(3):38–47.
9. Briggs J, Peat F. *Looking Glass Universe: The Emerging Science of Wholeness.* New York, NY: Simon & Schuster; 1983.
10. Weber R. The enfolding–unfolding universe: A conversation with David Bohm. In: Wilkes K, ed. *The Holographic Paradigm and Other Paradoxes.* Boston, Mass: Shambhala; 1982.
11. Bolen JS. *The Tao of Psychology: Synchronicity and the Self.* San Francisco, Calif: Harper & Row; 1979.
12. Dyer WW. *You'll See It When You Believe It.* New York, NY: William Morrow; 1989.
13. Rew L. Intuition in critical care nursing practice. *Dimensions of Critical Care.* 1990;9(1):30–37.
14. Benner P, Tanner C. Clinical judgment: How expert nurses use intuition. *American Journal of Nursing.* 1987;87(1):23–31.
15. Rew L. Intuition: Concept analysis of a group phenomenon. *Advances in Nursing Science.* 1986;8(2):21–28.
16. Rew L, Barrow EM. Intuition: A neglected hallmark of nursing knowledge. *Advances in Nursing Science.* 1987;10(1):49–62.

Synchronous Connections:
Nursing's Little Secret

Janet Wessel Krejci, MS, PhD, RN
Assistant Professor
College of Nursing
Marquette University
Milwaukee, Wisconsin

. . . helping people get in synch totally, totally affects their ability to become whole . . . their recovery . . . their rehabilitation . . . and I don't think we document that . . . ever! . . . We don't talk about the magic moment!

Nurses have the potential to move to the forefront of the evolving health care system. Nurses could prove themselves as effective and cost-efficient primary health care providers as well as managers of care within the acute, long-term, community, and home health care settings. There is a detour on this road to quality nursing care for recipients of our health care system, however. The detour is mechanistic care provided by technicians who do not understand the complexity of human response. To avoid this detour nurses must bring their contribution to the forefront and begin to articulate clearly and value the art as well as the science of nursing.

Intuitively and rationally, the public seems to be aware that nurses are important health care providers. Recipients of health care want what most call (for lack of a better term), good nurses, and they know that their personal health care seems to go better when they have these good nurses. Because the nursing profession has not always communicated nurses' value to society in ways that are clearly understood, however, the outcomes of competent professional nursing care are often subsumed under the more general rubric of medical care. Thus nurses lose visibil-

Source: Reprinted from J.W. Krejci, *Journal of Nursing Care Quarterly,* Vol. 9, No. 4, pp. 24–30, © 1995, Aspen Publishers, Inc.

ity in important policy and economic discussions and decisions. Even so, nurses are now becoming more comfortable articulating their contribution within the case management and care coordination frameworks because these frameworks are congruent with the cost-effective mind-set of the health care system.[1–3] This progress, albeit exciting, stops short of where the profession needs to go.

Although many nurses are moving forward in various dimensions of a more independent practice (e.g., nurse practitioners and care managers), some of the most unique and powerful nursing contributions continue to go unacknowledged, unarticulated, and invisible. These contributions are often based on connections nurses make with their patients. These connections and subsequent interventions that nurses make are often too complex and intangible for our present language because they go beyond the objective descriptions that are almost exclusively used in health care today.

In quality programs, nurses spend time identifying quality measures from the tangible and technical aspects of practice. This may suggest to others that nurses see these pieces as the most significant to quality outcomes. In reality, nurses may focus on these pieces as they are most easily identifiable and congruent with the dominant health care paradigm. This practice, however, continues to render powerful nursing interventions focused on complex human responses and based on holistic connections with patients partially or completely invisible. These connections and interventions have defied measurement in traditional quality programs, although recipients of health care will surely identify outcomes associated with such connections.[4]

These connections make a powerful contribution to the person's overall health but are almost never charted, discussed, or valued, although they are always remembered by nurses and patients. Connections have often been discussed by nurses and patients as something that happens between the nurse and the patient whereby healing is optimized and access to knowing is maximized.

The care providers of the traditional health care system (more aptly called a disease treatment system), being influenced by the medical paradigm, have primarily attended to health with a unidimensional focus on pathophysiology and high-technology treatments. Nurses have adapted to this paradigm while continuing to struggle for a more holistic perspective that focuses not only on pathophysiology but also on human response.[5]

Throughout the years, nurses have been almost exclusively reinforced and rewarded for congruence with the traditional medical model.[6,7] At the same time nurses have been devalued for focusing on a more holistic perspective that, although not necessarily adversarial to the medical model, is not definitive of it. As Reverby has stated, nurses have been expected to care without having the right to care or the support to organize systems that support both caring and curing.[8]

Nurses, like the women studied by Belenky and colleagues, have often kept their voices silent because their contribution is rarely valued and sometimes belittled.[9] The nursing contribution is not easily or directly measured in the financial paradigm that drives health care today. As a result, nurses themselves often value the traditional medical paradigm, which negates their own unique contributions.[7]

Thus if one reviews medical or patient care records, one finds evidence of nursing tasks (e.g., performing dressings changes, starting intravenous lines, monitoring, and administering medications). One does not usually find articulation of interventions focused on the human response, other than those sanctioned by the traditional medical model.

NURSE EXPERTS ON SYNCHRONY AND CONNECTIONS WITH CLIENTS

A recent study of nurse experts exemplifies and challenges this problem.[10] The study focused on synchrony (a movement of harmonious intraaction and interaction) and synchronicity (meaningful events unexplained by causal reality) experienced in nursing practice by nurse experts (nurses with at least 5 years of experience nominated by their peers on the basis of Benner's model[11]). In-depth initial and follow-up interviews were conducted with 15 nurse experts from a variety of settings.

Although several nurse theorists included the concept of synchrony directly or indirectly, a clear articulation of synchrony in practice had not been presented.[12,13] A phenomenon noted by the author when witnessing nurse experts seemed to resemble synchrony. An analysis of synchrony and synchronicity was completed and then investigated with nurse experts.[14]

One of the unexpected findings of the study included the communication, or actually the lack of communication, by nurse experts about synchronous connections they had made with their clients. Nurse experts detailed complex interventions and assessment approaches that they used with their clients related to these connections. The experts had difficulty articulating these interventions and approaches because they were not traditional approaches congruent with the objective, technical world of present day health care. They were extremely confident however, that these interventions and approaches had major impact on the outcomes of their clients/patients. The experts delineated outcomes including accessing important information that would have been missed with traditional approaches, helping people die with dignity, and preventing major crises.

DISSEMINATION OF EXPERTISE?

When asked how they communicated these findings to fellow nurses and other health care professionals, the experts were almost unanimous in their response. Some nurse experts related that one could rarely find such information in the patient records, and then only if one could read between the lines. Several nurse experts laughed at the thought of communicating the nontraditional approaches that related more to caring connections than to curing. An example from their responses is as follows:

> . . . very little [would she ever document]. . . . I mean we're talking about . . . it's a sort of quality. . . . I don't think we document that . . . ever!

> I mean we talk about what the patient does . . . and the movement that occurs . . . and our intervention modes . . . maybe . . . but we don't talk about the magic moment. . . .

The reasons nurse experts gave for not documenting the interventions that were more nontraditional and influenced by caring connections rather than curing were twofold. The first related to a lack of language that captures the process. The language available that is accepted and encouraged is more closely related to the high-technology approach. One expert struggled with even articulating the dilemma of language:

> I mean you know there's always other information . . . the tip of the iceberg, to see the whole you have to go get rid of the water . . . you know . . . I mean . . . if you could . . . [explain it] you could write a book . . . you'd make a fortune . . . I don't know how else to be more. . . . It doesn't satisfy me to not be able to verbalize or quantify. . . .

The second reason given was that the health care system specifically, and society in general, is perceived to value and thus reinforce the objective, tangible, medical model almost exclusively. The price of clashing with the authority structure that controls the setting is perceived as potentially too high for both patient and nurse.

Nurse experts who did not work in acute care settings (but rather in home care, hospice, long term care, or more autonomous settings) believed that it might be possible to document some of these more intangible, complex, and holistic interventions. The traditional, medical, high-technology approach is not so overwhelming in these settings, so that obstacles to capturing the caring and the connections might be overcome. Nurse experts were still doubtful, however. As one nurse expert explained,

> . . . some of the stuff I do is so bizarre [to help clients in home care], how do you chart it . . . how do you? . . . they told me . . . "don't chart it."

Another reacted in response to documentation of synchrony and synchronistic events:

> Ha! You probably couldn't find a thing, and that is real sad . . . we are so into the objective data . . . probably sometimes the connection piece would get written down . . . [after a pause] . . . but I don't think it happens. . . .

One nurse expert stated that the lack of documentation of these interventions that are beneficial to patients are a disservice not only to nurses but to patients as well. Excluding powerful interventions from research data (collected from patient records) skews knowledge generation about patient outcomes. One could draw erroneous conclusions about outcomes. As one nurse expert explained:

> I don't think a lot of it [nursing interventions of a more caring or connecting nature] gets on the chart . . . the results may be there, but I think how those results got there, was not described too well . . . it is not documented.

NURSING'S "LITTLE SECRET"

Not only did nurse experts not document interventions associated with the connections they make with patients, they also admitted that they rarely spoke with anyone about them. Many of the nurse experts believed that their experiences were not necessarily shared by other nurses and that they might feel odd talking about them. Interestingly, interventions based on connections with clients were unanimously experienced and experienced as powerful and influential. Yet nurses believed that they might be alone in their experiences and were not sharing these experiences, or their thoughts about them, with many people, if anyone at all. Three separate nurse experts used the same phrase when told that other nurse experts experienced the same thing: that maybe it was nursing's "little secret."

One nurse expert said that it might have something to do with power. She shared:

> . . . if it has to do with power . . . it is really hard for me to talk about . . . it is real hard . . . it's like it has to do with, a sense of healing or doing something real important . . . like making something happen. . . . I don't think nurses are used to feeling that kind of power . . . you know? . . . or maybe we're all good girls and we're not supposed to talk about that?

One nurse expert even cautioned about exposing nursing's "little secret." She said that it was possible that nurses keep it to themselves because they believe it might be distorted. She said with sadness:

> . . . you can't let this out of the bag too quick because it will be quickly bumped off. Someone will come along and attempt to put a lid on it because it is very threatening . . . you can't be too free and easy with this kind of stuff . . . we're under cover agents. . . .

This was not a nurse of questionable stability or one with paranoid delusions; rather, this was a strong nurse expert with a clear track record of being a practice leader.

Other nurse experts wondered whether peer pressure from other nurses or other health care providers prevents the sharing of these experiences. The nurse experts interviewed were all respected by their peers as experienced, seasoned nurses with wisdom, compassion, and competence. Because competence is often associated with the ability to manage highly technical care in an efficient manner, dialog about connections with clients as powerful could be construed as a weakening of their high-technology, cognitive, and competent judgment. One might begin to question whether these nurse experts had become distorted in their perceptions. These experiences, as articulated, do not (at least at first) appear congruent with the traditional high-technology competence that is a hallmark of the present day health care system.

RECOMMENDATIONS FOR CHANGE

If seasoned, respected nurse experts all agree to the power of their ability to facilitate synchrony by connecting with their clients, what can be done to expose nursing's "little secret" in a way that is beneficial to patients, nurses, and the entire health care system? If nurses do not attend to these powerful contributions, it is possible that a health care system could be created that is technician driven, without consideration for the importance of the human spirit or the need for human synchrony to restore, maintain, and promote health.

Education is one place to begin. Nurse experts agreed that, although the nurse–patient relationship was identified as important in their education, it was always framed within a traditional paradigm of carrying out the medical, technical regime. In other words, the nurse–patient relationship was emphasized in nursing education, but only within the framework of collecting empirical data or facilitating the traditional interventions and tasks. Only in psychiatric clinical settings did the nurse–patient relationship take on a slightly more important dimension in the nurses' education. Even in the mental health settings, the nurse–patient relationship was emphasized as a prelude to establishing trust, not necessarily as having outcomes in and of itself.

Although nurse theorists have written about healing and caring related to energy fields, expanding consciousness, and other nontraditional approaches that represent the core of caring in nursing, this focus is rarely explored and encouraged in undergraduate programs.[12,13,15–17] This content is often seen as too esoteric for generic students and is saved for graduate programs in nursing. Yet almost half the nurse experts (most did not have graduate degrees) described their experiences by discussing energy, energy fields, and other nontraditional concepts. Few of these

nurse experts were aware that nurse theorists have proposed that nursing's impact may not always be observable.

Nurses and nursing students could be exposed to the traditional health care paradigm as well as to the potential for outcomes based on, and/or influenced by, the connections that nurses make with clients (even though these connections cannot always be captured with traditional health care language). Courses or continuing education offerings might be titled "Connection as Core: Experiences with Nurse Experts" or "Outcomes Associated with Facilitation of Patient Synchrony."

Inservice quality programs could begin to identify differential outcomes when patients perceive that they receive high-quality nursing care. Although this approach could be criticized for being too subjective, it is a beginning approach to sorting out and discerning differences between care provided by a nurse expert and care that could be defined as technical care. With the work of Benner and others, we are beginning to develop a systematic process to identify nurse experts.[11] Care provided by those identified as nurse experts could be compared with care given by those not identified as experts. Patient perceptions could also help discern differences in care. Outcomes such as length of stay, lost work days, recidivism, perceptions of health, family functioning, use of medications, and other concrete outcomes would begin to identify the results of synchronous connections between patients and nurse experts.

●　　●　　●

Because we live in a paradigm that is focused on an empirical, reductionist reality, it is no surprise that our educational programs have followed suit.[13,17] Educators and practicing nurses need to stop the exclusive focus on objective data and begin to stress multiple ways of knowing. We need to stress expert judgment and how to articulate logically our expert judgment even when it is not completely within the empirical paradigm.

Psychologists, ministers, and social workers are not always expected to document each and every conclusion with empirical data. They use empirical data, their relationships with their clients, and their expertise to form a judgment. If they are well-respected experts in their field, their expert judgments are assumed to have validity. Nurses need to be encouraged to document their expert judgments like other professionals. Benner and Tanner, like Pyles and Stern, have written on expert judgments and different ways of knowing; although accepted at a professional level, these different ways of knowing have yet to make major impact on the process of nursing in organizations.[18,19]

As new structures are created for information systems to capture the Nursing Minimum Data Set, and as quality programs become more sophisticated, nurses and health care leaders must not exclude documentation of assessments, interventions, and outcomes that may fall outside the traditional, technical paradigm and may be more closely aligned with the caring paradigm.[20] In this age of cost-effective care, we cannot afford to exclude expertise that may bring beneficial outcomes.

Nurse experts must be encouraged to forward their perceptions and experiences to individuals working on classification systems, such as the *Nursing Intervention Classification Manual* group and the North American Nursing Diagnosis Association (NANDA).[21-23] Diagnoses such as "alteration in synchrony" could be forwarded to NANDA for further testing. There needs to be a better communication loop among theorists, researchers, and practitioners. There is often much common ground, as shown in this study, although communication may be lacking.

People receiving health care need both caring and curing, both high technology and high touch. It would be a grave mistake to negate either. As Kuhn has documented, we will remain prisoners of a limited view if we judge all new ideas within the present popular paradigm.[24] Nurse experts have a wisdom that cannot remain a "little secret." This evolving health care system needs to tap into the art as well as the science of nursing. Nurses who are practicing as well as those in traditional leadership positions need to nurture nursing expertise by celebrating it and valuing it, not by hiding it.

REFERENCES

1. Etheridge, P., and Lamb, G. "Professional Nursing Case Management Improves Quality, Access, and Costs." *Nursing Management* 20 (1989): 30–35.

2. Sinnen, M., and Schifalacqua, M. "Coordinated Care in a Community Hospital." *Nursing Management* 22 (1991): 38–42.

3. Zanders, K. "Focusing on Patient Outcomes: Case Management in the 90's." *Dimensions of Critical Care Nursing* 11 (1992): 127–129.

4. Krejci, J. Synchrony: A Pilot Study. Typescript.

5. American Nurses Association (ANA). *Nursing: A Social Policy Statement*. Kansas City, Mo.: ANA, 1980.

6. Ashley, J. *Hospitals, Paternalism, and the Nurse*. New York, N.Y.: Teachers College, 1979.

7. Roberts, S. "Oppressed Group Behaviors: Implications for Nurses." *Advances in Nursing Science* 5 (1983): 21–30.

8. Reverby, S. "A Caring Dilemma: Womanhood and Nursing in Historical Perspective." *Nursing Research* 36 (1987): 3–15.

9. Belenky, M.F., et al. *Women's Ways of Knowing: The Development of Self, Voice, and Mind*. New York, N.Y.: Basic, 1986.

10. Krejci, J. "Synchrony: Nurse Experts Perspectives." Ph.D. diss., University of Wisconsin–Milwaukee, 1992.

11. Benner, P. *From Novice to Expert*. Menlo Park, Calif.: Addison-Wesley, 1984.

12. Rogers, M. *An Introduction to the Theoretical Basis of Nursing*. Philadelphia, Pa.: Davis, 1970.

13. Newman, M.A. *Health as Expanding Consciousness*. St. Louis, Mo.: Mosby, 1986.

14. Krejci, J. Synchrony: A Concept Analysis. Typescript.

15. Watson, J. *Nursing: Human Science and Human Care*. New York, N.Y.: National League for Nursing, 1989.

16. Barrett, E.M. *Visions of a Roger-Based Science*. New York, N.Y.: National League for Nursing, 1990.

17. Parse, R.P. *Nursing Science: Major Paradigms, Theories, and Critiques*. Philadelphia, Pa.: Saunders, 1987.

18. Benner, P., and Tanner, C. "How Expert Nurses Use Intuition." *American Journal of Nursing* 87 (1987): 23–31.

19. Pyles, S.H., and Stern, P.N. "Discovery of Nursing Gestalt in Critical Care Nursing: The Importance of the Gray Gorilla Syndrome." *Image* 15 (1983): 51–57.

20. Werley, H.H., et al. "Why the Nursing Minimum Data Set (NMDS)?" In *Current Issues in Nursing*, 4th ed., edited by J. McCloskey and H.K. Grace. St. Louis, Mo.: Mosby, 1994.

21. McCloskey, J., and Bulachek, G. *Nursing Intervention Classification Manual*. Philadelphia, Pa.: Saunders, 1992.

22. Carrol-Johnson, R.M., and Paquette, M. *Classification of Nursing Diagnosis Association: Proceedings of the Tenth Conference*. Philadelphia, Pa.: Lippincott, 1994.

23. Clark, J., and Lang, N. "Nursing's Next Advance: An International Classification for Nursing Practice. *International Nursing Review* 39 (1992): 109–112.

24. Kuhn, T. *The Structure of Scientific Revolutions*. Chicago, Ill.: University of Chicago Press, 1970.

Holding Sacred Space:
The Nurse as Healing Environment

Janet F. Quinn, PhD, RN, FAAN
Associate Professor and Senior Scholar
Center for Human Caring
University of Colorado Health Sciences Center
School of Nursing
University of Colorado
Boulder, Colorado

While the concept of environment has been considered central to nursing's paradigm since Florence Nightingale, along with person, health, and nursing, there has been little emphasis on this concept in the nursing literature or in nursing curricula. The focus of this article is the client-environment process as a special case of the human-environment relationship.

There are at least two ways of conceptualizing the nurse's place in the client-environment process. The first, which is most common, is to think of the nurse as being *in* the environment of the client. In this view, nurse and client are looking out, if you will, from the same vantage point into the same environment. "Nursing care in this [Rogers'] system is concerned with patterning the environmental field. The nurse, together with the client, patterns the environment to promote healing and comfort."[1(p108)] Questions we might ask if this is the focus would be, "What can the nurse *do* to create (pattern) an environment that is more healing for the client? What changes could be made in this environment? What could be deleted and what could be added?" Issues of color, light, sound, activity, temperature—in essence, many of the issues with which Nightingale[2] was so concerned—would call for our attention. Following appraisal and alteration of the physical environment, the holistic nurse *in* the environment might then turn

Source: Reprinted from J.F. Quinn, *Holistic Nursing Practice,* Vol. 6, No. 4, pp. 24–36, © 1992, Aspen Publishers, Inc.

The study reported herein was funded by the Institute of Noetic Sciences.

attention to the use of particular healing modalities to assist in patterning a more healing environment for the client. Barrett said, "Regardless of the practice modality being used, the nurse's objective is to pattern the client's environment to promote health and well being."[3(p35)] Imagery, visualization, relaxation, and music therapy might all be used to alter the environment with which the client is interacting at that moment such that a more harmonious, healing process is possible. The nurse, while theoretically integral with the client's environment, continues to act from the position of a separate self *in* the environment, shaping and sculpting it in efforts to facilitate client healing.

Consider now another view of the nurse's place in the client-environment process. In addition to thinking of the nurse *in* the environment of the client, think of the nurse *as* the environment of the client. In this perspective, the nurse turns toward her or his understanding of the "nurse-self" as an energetic, vibrational field, integral with the client's environment. Questions we might ask if this is the focus might be, "If I *am* the environment for this client, how can I *be* a more healing environment? How can I become a safe space, a sacred healing vessel for this client in this moment? In what ways can I look at, into this person to draw out healing? How can I use my consciousness, my being, my voice, my touch, my face, for healing?"

This later perspective provides the focus for the remainder of this article. In a 1982 study, I raised the question, "What are the limits of influence if the means of influence is an energy field?"[4(p107)] I have considered the question from many viewpoints, and this article is an attempt at response based on 17 years of clinical and theoretical work with the use of nonordinary states of consciousness for healing, including Therapeutic Touch and, more recently, transpersonal psychology[5] and holotropic breathwork.[6–8]

CONCEPTUAL FRAMEWORK

The conceptual framework within which this article has been developed incorporates theoretical perspectives originated in nursing by Rogers,[9–11] expanded by Newman,[12–15] and tested by Quinn[4,16,17] and others. The framework is supported and further expanded by the works of Bentov,[18] Bohm,[19,20] Grof,[6–8] Pribram,[21,22] Watson,[23] and others. In the early 1970s, Rogers introduced into nursing the concept that the fundamental unit of the living system was an energy field, coextensive with the environmental energy field.[9] At the time, this was a revolutionary idea in nursing, and an unacceptable conjecture of little or no interest to Western medicine. Today, one cannot approach the cutting edge of essentially any modern scientific discipline, nor the tradition of any major spiritual culture, and not see that same idea proposed. No longer merely conjecture, the interconnectedness of all of life seems clear. Scholars, artists, and futurists alike are writing about this phenomenon in fields as diverse and different from each other as quantum physics,[18–20] biology,[24] Western medicine,[25–29] Ayurveda,[30,31] psychology,[6–8,32,33] psychoneuroimmunology,[34] philosophy,[35,36] theology and spirituality,[37–40] and nursing.[23,41–43] The emerging view of our world includes the concepts that the human being is a nonmaterial, multidimensional field integral with the environment/universal field; that consciousness is nonlocal, unbounded by physical structure and function; and that separateness of the individual from all other individuals is an illusion. Western mystics like Hildegard of Bingen[37] and contemporary artists like Alex Grey[44] provide us with insight into this same phenomenon through exquisite paintings, poetry, and prose depicting contact with the energetic nature and underlying unity of all of life.

What are the implications of these ancient/emerging views of the nature of person and environment? How do our conceptions of harmony in the human-environment relationship shift when we are talking fundamentally about an energetic resonance, a vibrational phenomenon, patterning? Most importantly for this article, how can nursing utilize these views to maximize healing—for ourselves, our clients, our communities, and our planet?

PURPOSE

Taking these ideas as basic assumptions, the purpose of this article is to explore the potentials of this model of reality for creating healing environments. A healing environment is one that facilitates the emergence of the Haelan effect, the synergistic, organismic, multidimensional response of whole persons in the direction of healing and wholeness.[45] Healing, the emergence of right relationship at, between, and among all the levels of human being, is always accomplished by the one healing. No one and no thing can heal another human being. All healing is creative emergence, new birth, the manifestation of the powerful inner longing, at every level, to be whole. Yet there is a role for nurses. We can remove barriers to the healing process. We can participate in creating environments that will support healing. We can become midwives to this process of healing, creating and being safe, sacred space into which the healing might emerge. We can, literally, become the healing environment.

THE NURSE AS HEALING ENVIRONMENT

Given that we are interconnected to all of life, our consciousness is not separate and apart but integral with all consciousness. We can knowingly participate in this web of interconnectedness toward repatterning and healing for ourselves and for others through the intentional use of our own consciousness. The clinical practice of Therapeutic Touch is an exemplar of this premise because its modus operandi is a shift in the consciousness of the practitioner (centering) through which, clinical experience and empirical study[16,46,47] demonstrate, there can also be a shift in consciousness of the recipient. Cowling suggests that "the nurse could knowingly participate in human field patterning through his/her interconnectedness to the client, possible in a four-dimensional universe of open fields. For instance, it has been suggested that a human to human field process operates in Therapeutic Touch through the mode of . . . intentionality on the part of the nurse."[48(p51)]

At the start of a Therapeutic Touch session, the nurse centers, that is, turns attention first inward, reaching a calm, relaxed, and open state of consciousness akin to a meditative state. In this meditative state of consciousness, the Therapeutic Touch practitioner then formulates the intent to help or to heal and focuses outwardly on wholeness and balance in the recipient, which, it is hypothesized, has the potential to accelerate the recipient's innate inner healing process. Please note that the terms "inner" and "outer" are, of course, incongruent with a world view of unity and must be understood as metaphors or heuristic devices to describe in a three-dimensional language a nonlinear, multidimensional phenomenon.

In the context of the present discussion, this process on the part of the Therapeutic Touch practitioner may be thought of as a repatterning of her or his own energy field in the direction of expanded consciousness, a consciousness experienced as unified, harmonious, peaceful, ordered, and so forth, and understood to be a "healing meditation."[46] It is proposed here that being in process with a nurse in such a meditative state of consciousness may provide a template of sorts upon which the client may repattern. Using the metaphor of sound, the pattern, or vibration of the nurse's consciousness becomes a tuning fork, resonating at a healing frequency, while the client has the opportunity within the mutual person-environment process to tune, to resonate, to that frequency. Bentov approximates this perspective in the following words:

> the real reality—the microreality, that which underlies . . . our solid reality—is a rapidly pulsating matrix of fields of energy, an interference pattern of waves filling the vast vacuum of our bodies and continuing beyond them in a more diluted fashion . . . we may look at a disease as an out-of-tune behavior . . . When a strong harmonizing rhythm is applied to it, the interference pattern of waves, may start

beating in tune again. This may be the principle of psychic healing.[18(p47)]

This may also be the principle or mechanism of Therapeutic Touch. This perspective involves a shift in previous descriptions of the phenomenon of Therapeutic Touch. Previously, Therapeutic Touch has been described as an "energy exchange," requiring a model that includes at least theoretically a here and a there: a source of energy and a recipient of energy. However, in a model of interconnectedness, there is no here or there. The understanding of Therapeutic Touch as presented herein is, I believe, more consistent with the evolution in Rogers' own thinking.[11]

Thus, it is postulated that the nurse, centered in a meditative state of consciousness, an expanded consciousness in Newman's terms,[12–15] may knowingly participate in the repatterning of the client's consciousness such that the client's consciousness may also expand. In this sense, the nurse and the client share consciousness. In Newman's framework, expansion of consciousness is equivalent to health/healing. Thus, the repatterning of consciousness that can occur during Therapeutic Touch may be viewed as movement toward health.

TIME EXPERIENCE DURING THERAPEUTIC TOUCH

One of the indices of expanded consciousness is postulated to be an alteration in time perception.[13–15,18] To begin exploration of the idea that an expanded consciousness may be shared during Therapeutic Touch, data about time perception during Therapeutic Touch treatment were collected during a larger research project.[49] This descriptive pilot study explored the effects of Therapeutic Touch on selected psychoimmunologic parameters in both practitioners and recipients. Participants were two very experienced Therapeutic Touch practitioners and four recently bereaved Therapeutic Touch recipients. All participants completed informed consent forms prior to entry into the data collection for

the study. Only the information relevant to time perception shall be presented here.

Treatment consisted of the practitioner administering Therapeutic Touch in the manner in which it has been taught, that is, using the sequential steps developed by Krieger[50] and Kunz and described elsewhere.[16] Beyond this general guideline, the practitioner was permitted to perform Therapeutic Touch as she usually does and for the length of time that she deemed appropriate. Both practitioners and recipients were asked to estimate the amount of time that had elapsed since the Therapeutic Touch treatment had begun. Actual clock time for the length of treatment was also recorded by means of a stopwatch that was kept face down in the treatment room after being started by the practitioner. The practitioner stopped the stopwatch at the end of the treatment without turning it over, and a research assistant recorded the actual elapsed time. Time estimates were obtained for three sessions for recipient CB, and six for the remaining recipients, MG, VD, and GS.

RESULTS

Table 1 presents the amount and direction of time distortion, the difference between actual time elapsed and subject's report of elapsed time, in both practitioners and recipients. A (−) sign indicates that the estimated elapsed time was under, or less than, the actual elapsed time. No sign indicates that the estimate was over, or more than, the actual elapsed time. Each practitioner-recipient pair of estimates has also been graphed (see Figures 1–4).

It can be observed that there is no readily apparent relationship between the *magnitude* of time distortion experienced by the practitioners and that experienced by their respective recipients. However, there is a very obvious correspondence between practitioners and their respective recipients in the *direction* of that time distortion. While there are several exceptions, the great majority (81%) of pairs of time distortions (ie, the practitioner and the recipient in any given session) are in the same

Table 1. Time distortion in practitioners (P) with their respective recipients (R) in sessions (S) 1 through 6

P & R Initials		S 1	S 2	S 3	S 4	S 5	S 6
SB	(P)	−4:58	−8:36	−2:48			
CB	(R)	−11:30	−11:14	−15:00			
SB	(P)	5:23	3:28	2:19	−4:43	−2:04	4:04
VD	(R)	2:38	3:28	3:19	−1:43	−4:04	:04
GA	(P)	− :57	−1:19	− :45	−4:01	−2:13	:00
MG	(R)	−3:57	−2:19	−3:45	−6:01	−4:13	−2:23
GA	(P)	−2:20	−1:05	:53	:14	−1:57	−2:04
GS	(R)	2:40	−2:05	− :07	−1:46	− :57	−2:04

direction. SB and her two recipients are striking in this regard, with a 100% congruence in both recipients. Of particular interest is the variation in the direction in the data for VD. This practitioner and recipient pair varied together in the direction of time distortion on alternate days. This varying together suggests that the observed pattern is not a stable or rigid response pattern but rather with a unique relationship that changes from treatment to treatment. Examining Figure 2 gives one a visual image of the "in sync-ness" or resonance that appears to have existed in these treatment sessions. It is as if the two participants are dancing or flowing together in consciousness.

In GA's two recipients, there are two patterns. In MG, there is a 100% congruence, and in GS, there is 50%. GS had the least magnitude of time distortion, in addition to presenting with a different pattern in terms of direction. It is possible that the ability of her system to shift into an expanded state of consciousness, and thus to experience the time distortion, was influenced by her antidepressant medication.

RECIPIENTS' EXPERIENCES

The data on time seem to suggest a "sharing" of expanded consciousness experienced by practitioners and recipients. In exploring the healing potential of this phenomenon, as healing has been defined herein, it is useful to consider the recipients' own stories. Each of the recipients was interviewed on the last day of the study. Of particular note are two responses that occurred across all recipients. They all felt relaxed, and they were all surprised by that. The surprise is particularly important in the context of healing as a creative emergence of something new. Some of the comments are included below to provide a sense of the recipient's experience of repatterning during the Therapeutic Touch process.

CB: . . . I think it has helped me—I really do . . . I think it's fascinating that you can turn me on and off . . . the first day I went home and felt just so relaxed and all I wanted to do was go to sleep, and then the next day I went home and I had a lot more energy . . . I just wish I was going to be here for the rest of the time; I really do feel like I've been cheated out of half of it . . . I wish I knew how to do it to someone else . . . I'm sure it helped me, I really am . . . I find it absolutely fascinating that my mood can change from a little bit of touch or treatment or whatever you want to call it.

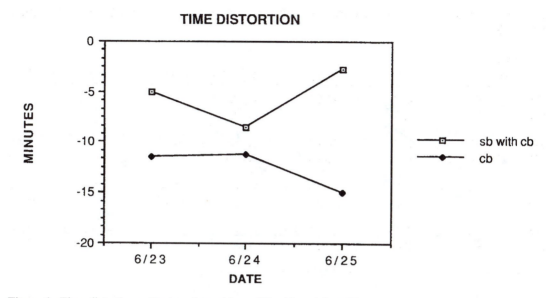

Figure 1. Time distortion estimates of practitioner SB with recipient CB.

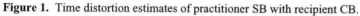

VD: . . . [my head clears] as time goes by [during treatment] it's nice . . . this is real quiet and it's sort of like getting up from a sleep . . . it's very calming and very restful; nonthreatening . . . I think that's nice if someone can make you feel like that in the middle of the day . . . I felt cared for, deeply cared for by . . . Hmmm, I don't even know her name.

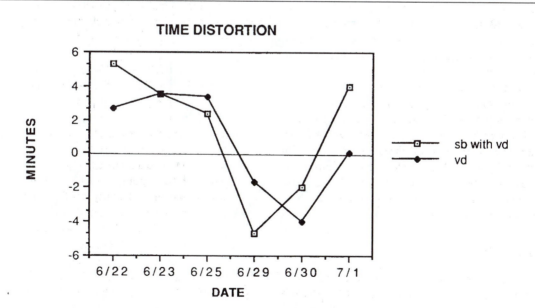

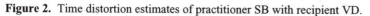

Figure 2. Time distortion estimates of practitioner SB with recipient VD.

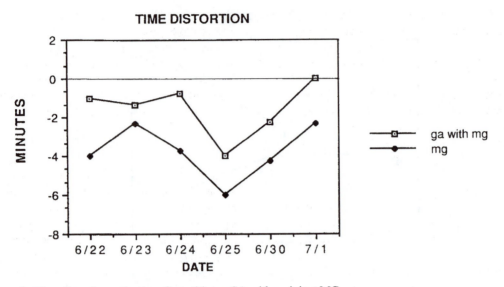

Figure 3. Time distortion estimates of practitioner GA with recipient MG.

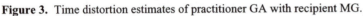

MG: . . . today I was very nervous all morning when I came in . . . Now I'm very calm, relaxed, and I don't know why but I am . . . I can tell, I don't believe it, but I can tell where her hands are; it seems like I can feel something like a weak radiant heat . . . I don't make sense, do I? . . . I get these feel-ings I think they're wrong, but I think coming here takes them out of me . . . it doesn't make sense, does it?

GS: . . . I do find it relaxing . . . whether it has any residual value, I don't know . . . it's very hard to evaluate . . . it's pleasant, it's very pleasant . . . it's pleasant and relaxing.

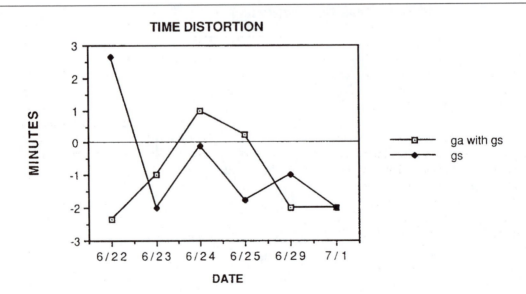

Figure 4. Time distortion estimates of practitioner GA with recipient GS.

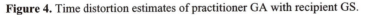

These comments support the other psychological findings of the study and suggest additional insights into the Therapeutic Touch process. The comment of VD that "I don't even know her name" is particularly telling. He was in the midst of describing a feeling of being deeply cared for/about and suddenly realized that he didn't know the name of the person doing the caring. This illustrates in quite a dramatic way the transpersonal nature of the healing interaction, which is an example of a "caring occasion," in Watson's language.[23(p59)] It is not an interaction based on a conditional connection of individual personalities, but rather involves the practitioner in engaging with the recipient on some deeper yet impersonal and unconditional level. In other words, the caring in the healing relationship takes place on a level that transcends individual personalities and identities. It is suggested here that the relationship occurs in the implicate order;[19] the underlying unified field in which the practitioner and the recipient are, in reality, already one. Therapeutic Touch allows both to experience this.

DISCUSSION

This pilot study included an exploration into the potential for resonance of two individual human fields of consciousness during a healing interaction. The findings suggest such a resonance. Therapeutic Touch has been used as an exemplar of the premise that the nurse can be the healing environment for the client during treatment. Yet the use of Therapeutic Touch is by no means the only way in which nurses can become healing environments. The singular premise of this article is that it is the intentional use of expanded consciousness that can allow a unique, healing human-environment process, regardless of the specific means or modality the nurse uses to knowingly participate in this process. The pivotal role of intentionality was supported in earlier work,[16] which demonstrated that patients receiving a mimic Therapeutic Touch treatment had no change in anxiety, whereas patients who received Therapeutic Touch, with its centering and intention to heal, had a dramatic decrease in anxiety following treatment.

The use of healing modalities that require the nurse to expand her or his consciousness also have the potential to create broader healing environments than the localized one surrounding a particular treatment. Our goal in the pilot study was to observe the outcomes of Therapeutic Touch in as natural and noninvasive a way as possible. The setting for this study was ideal. The suite of offices provided an environment that was separate from the noise and potentially negative associations of the hospital. More to the point, however, was the human caring environment that was created among the research team and that "overflowed" into the physical environment creating a safe place, a literal energetic cocoon, of caring and support into which the recipients entered each day. Because this was a descriptive study, no constraints were placed on the interactions of the investigator, the practitioners, and the recipients before, during, or after treatment. This means that the relationship between the practitioner and the recipient was not limited or prescribed as it has been in other Therapeutic Touch studies, but allowed to develop as it does in actual clinical use of the treatment. As the investigator of this study, I often found myself torn between worrying about "confounding" the study and yet knowing that this was the "real thing" as I watched (and took part in) deepening relationships with the recipients as they arrived and participated each day. Evidence of these deepening relationships was abundant. There was a dramatic increase in the amount of touching, hugging, back-patting, and so forth, that went on in the waiting room between the recipients, practitioners, and investigator. There was more smiling, more laughing, more conversation. There was more lingering and more interaction among the recipients. There was more inquiring into and sharing of personal lives coming from the recipients. The change in the affect, the facial and body language, and tone of voice of these people over the course of the study was quite profound. Subjects were never late and arrived (after the first day) always appearing delighted to be there and eager for their treatments to begin. Every recipient expressed sadness and disappointment when the study concluded. The healing that was experienced by all was obvious.

• • •

Inherent in the basic premise of this article is a challenge and a call to the nurse who aspires to practice out of a holistic, unitary framework. If we accept the basic premises of holism, of an interconnected universe, and of the fundamental inseparability of individuals one from the other, then we are called to look anew at how we knowingly participate in that universe. We can no longer view the environment solely as being "out there," amenable to our knowing participation in repatterning it yet somehow fundamentally other than self. We are the environment, for our patients, our colleagues, our communities, and our world. Dillbeck[51] reports on a series of studies on the effects of the number of people practicing transcendental meditation (TM) in various cities and the corresponding crime rates. The data demonstrate decreases in crime rate when more than 1% of the community meditate regularly. This effect has been termed the "Maharishi effect,"[26(p256)] since it was predicted by the Maharishi Mahesh Yogi, the founder of TM. What would be the effect in a single hospital if 1% of the nurses began to practice healing modalities using expanded consciousness?

The view put forth in this article would seem to demand much of us as nurses. Yet it is clear that in the process of expanding our own consciousness, of becoming healing environments, sacred spaces, we ourselves are healed. What could be more deserving of our intent and effort?

REFERENCES

1. Barrett EAM. Health patterning with clients in a private practice environment. In: Barrett EAM, ed. *Visions of Rogers' Science-based Nursing.* New York, NY: National League for Nursing; 1990.

2. Nightingale F. *Notes on Nursing.* New York, NY: Dover; 1969.

3. Barrett EAM. Rogers' science-based nursing practice. In: Barrett EAM, ed. *Visions of Rogers' Science-based Nursing.* New York, NY: National League for Nursing; 1990.

4. Quinn J. *An Investigation of the Effects of Therapeutic Touch, Done Without Physical Contact, on State Anxiety of Hospitalized Cardiovascular Patients.* Ann Arbor, Mich: University Microfilms; 1982.

5. Vaughn F. Transpersonal vision. *ReVision.* 1985;8(1):11–15.

6. Grof S. *Beyond the Brain.* Albany, NY: State University of New York; 1985.

7. Grof S. Modern consciousness research and human survival. *ReVision.* 1985;8(1):27–39.

8. Grof S. *The Adventure of Self Discovery.* Albany, NY: State University of New York; 1988.

9. Rogers ME. *An Introduction to the Theoretical Basis for Nursing.* Philadelphia, Pa: FA Davis; 1970.

10. Rogers ME. Science of unitary human beings. In: Malinski VM, ed. *Explorations on Martha Rogers' Science of Unitary Human Beings.* Norwalk, Conn: Appleton-Century-Crofts; 1986.

11. Rogers ME. Nursing: Science of unitary, irreducible, human beings: Update 1990. In: Barrett EAM, ed. *Visions of Rogers' Science-based Nursing.* New York, NY: National League for Nursing; 1990.

12. Newman M. *Theory Development in Nursing.* Philadelphia, Pa: FA Davis; 1979.

13. Newman M. Time as an index of expanding consciousness with age. *Nursing Research.* 1982;31(5):290–293.

14. Newman M. *Health as Expanding Consciousness.* St. Louis, Mo: Mosby; 1986.

15. Newman M. Newman's theory of health as praxis. *Nursing Science Quarterly.* 1990;3(1):37–41.

16. Quinn J. Therapeutic touch as energy exchange: Testing the theory. *Advances in Nursing Science.* 1984;6(2):42–49.

17. Quinn J. Therapeutic touch as energy exchange: Replication and extension. *Nursing Science Quarterly.* 1989;2(2):79–87.

18. Bentov I. *Stalking the Wild Pendulum.* New York, NY: Dutton; 1977.

19. Bohm D. *Wholeness and the Implicate Order.* London, England: Routledge & Kegan Paul; 1980.

20. Weber R. The enfolding-unfolding universe: A conversation with David Bohm. *ReVision.* 1978;1(3/4):24–51.

21. Pribram KH. Problems concerning the structure of consciousness. In: Globus G, ed. *Consciousness and the Brain.* New York, NY: Plenum Press; 1976.

22. Pribram KH. What the fuss is all about. *ReVision.* 1978;1(3/4):14–18.

23. Watson J. *Nursing: Human Science and Human Care.* New York, NY: National League for Nursing; 1988.

24. Sheldrake R. *A New Science of Life.* Los Angeles, Calif: JP Tarcher; 1981.

25. Dossey L. *Space, Time, and Medicine.* Boston, Mass: Shambhala; 1982.

26. Dossey L. *Recovering the Soul.* New York, NY: Bantam; 1989.

27. Gerber R. *Vibrational Medicine.* Santa Fe, NM: Bear & Co; 1988.

28. Gerber R. New frontiers in vibrational medicine: Technologies for diagnosing and treating illness using energy. In: *Energy Fields in Medicine.* Kalamazoo, Mich: Fetzer Foundation; 1989.

29. Karagulla S, Kunz D. *The Chakras and the Human Energy Fields.* Wheaton, Ill: Theosophical Publishing House; 1989.

30. Chopra D. *Quantum Healing.* New York, NY: Bantam; 1989.

31. Chopra D. *Perfect Health.* New York, NY: Harmony; 1991.

32. Jung CG. *Psychology and the East.* Hull RFC, trans. Princeton, NJ: Princeton University Press; 1978.

33. Metzner R. Resonance as metaphor and metaphor as resonance. *ReVision.* 1987;10(1):37–44.

34. Pert C. The wisdom of the receptors: Neuropeptides, the emotions and bodymind. *Advances.* 1986;3(3):8–16.

35. Weber R. Field consciousness and field ethics. *ReVision.* 1978;1(3/4):19–23.

36. Weber R. *Dialogues with Saints and Sages: The Search for Unity in Science and Mysticism.* London, England: Routledge & Kegan Paul; 1986.

37. Fox M. *Meditations with Meister Eckhart.* Santa Fe, NM: Bear & Co; 1983.

38. Fox M. *Illuminations of Hildegard of Bingen.* Santa Fe, NM: Bear & Co; 1985.

39. Wilber K. *The Atman Project.* Wheaton, Ill: Theosophical Publishing House; 1980.

40. Wilber K. *Eye to Eye.* Garden City, NY: Anchor Press, Doubleday; 1983.

41. Barrett EAM. *Visions of Rogers' Science-based Nursing.* New York, NY: National League for Nursing; 1990.

42. Malinski V, ed. *Explorations on Martha Rogers' Science of Unitary Human Beings.* Norwalk, Conn: Appleton-Century-Crofts; 1986.

43. Sarter B. *The Stream of Becoming: A Study of Martha Rogers' Theory.* New York, NY: National League for Nursing; 1988.

44. Grey A. *Sacred Mirrors.* Rochester, Vt: Inner Traditions International; 1990.

45. Quinn J. On healing, wholeness and the Haelen effect. *Nursing and Health Care.* 1989;10(10):553–556.

46. Krieger D, Peper E, Ancoli S. Therapeutic touch: Searching for evidence of physiological change. *American Journal of Nursing.* 1979;79:660–662.

47. Heidt P. Effect of therapeutic touch on anxiety of hospitalized patients. *Nursing Research.* 1981;30:32–37.

48. Cowling RW. A template for unitary pattern-based nursing practice. In: Barrett EAM, ed. *Visions of Rogers' Science-based Nursing.* New York, NY: National League for Nursing; 1990.

49. Quinn J, Strelkauskas A. *Psychophysiologic Correlates of Hands-on Healing in Healers and Healees.* Unpublished research report. 1988.

50. Krieger D. *The Therapeutic Touch.* Englewood Cliffs, NJ: Prentice Hall; 1979.

51. Dillbeck MC. Test of a field theory of consciousness and social change: Time series analysis of participation in the TM-Siddhi program and reduction of violent death in the United States. *Social Indicators Research.* 1990;22(4):399–406.

Caring for the Caregiver

Caring for self is a fundamental ingredient in caring for others. The authors of this section ask us to scrutinize seriously the personal self-neglect that nurses as a collective group have suffered throughout history. Somehow we have sustained the illusion that healing and caring involve continued self-sacrifice because of the misconception that others always come first. Yet, self-neglect ultimately leads to disillusionment, unmet personal needs, illness, and burnout.

To address this problem, a model of self-reflection is proposed (Lauterbach and Becker) to facilitate self-understanding and enhance the human experience of caring for others. The process of self-reflection is operationalized by several "how-to" recommendations: daily journaling, performing holistic self-health and -stress assessments, and implementing coping strategies such as healthy nutrition, exercise, and relaxation strategies. Likewise, self-care methods to sustain compassionate caregiving are emphasized in the article on awakening the inner healer (Wells-Federman). The process of healing, discussed as an integration and balance of one's physical, psychologic, social, and spiritual dimensions, leads one toward personal growth and development. Yet, before we are able to facilitate the process of healing in others, we must first acknowledge and nurture our own healer within.

Steps outlined to awaken the inner healer by caring for self include clarifying values and beliefs, setting realistic goals, challenging the belief that others always come first, and implementing specific guidelines and activities for managing stress. Systems energetics (Jenkins), represents yet another healthy framework for assimilating change in one's professional and personal life based on communication and developmental theories combined with traditional Chinese tenets of energy flow.

Another self-care strategy, humor, enables us to shift our perception to experience joy even in the face of adversity. Humor has therapeutic impact for the body-mind-spirit that positively affects psychoneuroimmunology, enhances perceptual agility, and nurtures spiritual energy. The first article (Wooten) presents an extensive literature review on the effects of humor with a comprehensive Humor Resources list. The uses, benefits, power, and criteria for appropriate use of humor are also described (Balzer) together with "how to do it" suggestions for developing a comic vision and building a humor kit.

The lesson here is fundamental and clear, yet often forgotten by nurses, educators, and administrators. Holistic nurses must first care for themselves before they can deliver transformational care to their clients.

Caring for Self: Becoming a Self-Reflective Nurse

Sarah Steen Lauterbach, EdD, RN
Associate Professor

Patricia Hentz Becker, EdD, RN
Associate Professor
School of Nursing
La Salle University
Philadelphia, Pennsylvania

The ultimate aim of nursing as a human caring art and science is to assist persons and society in becoming more fully human. This article uses work on caring for self based on a model of self-reflection[1] to articulate an educational/learning process. The model depicts the process of self-reflection to increase awareness and understanding. The primary thesis of this work is that caring for self is an essential component of caring for others. Through the experience of reflecting on oneself, one becomes more self-aware and understanding. Ultimately, through self-understanding one is guided to becoming more aware and understanding of experiences of others, of what it means to be human, thereby facilitating one's understanding of broader contexts of human experience in caring for others.

The goal of this article is to share an educational strategy for transforming nursing practice. Through promoting nurses' individual and collective self-understanding, the art and science of caring for humanity can be realized. The ultimate goal is an improved quality of meaningful life for all people.

BRIEF HISTORY OF THE WORK

The model of self-reflection described here was developed from the authors' teaching experiences with approximately 672 registered nurse/bachelor's-level nursing students in a clinical and theory course founded on nursing human systems experiencing stress. The model

Source: Reprinted from S.S. Lauterbach and P.H. Becker, *Holistic Nursing Practice,* Vol. 10, No. 2, pp. 57–68, © 1996, Aspen Publishers, Inc.

depicts a self-reflective learning process that focuses on developing caring attention and self-awareness of the nurse as a person. The theoretical course content includes a synthesis of stress and coping theory[2-10]; family, transition, and developmental theory; and holistic nursing intervention strategies and modalities.[11-19] The clinical experience includes an in-house laboratory and clinical experience focused on stress assessment, exploring and learning relaxation strategies, and other self-care modalities. The student completes a "self as client" clinical experience and also works with another individual, family, or human system experiencing stress.

Through our teaching experiences, we noted that important themes were articulated with greater and greater emphasis by students. As one student stated, "I have spent most of my life taking care of everyone else. Now, I really feel the need to spend as much time learning how to recognize and take care of my own needs, desires, and dreams." The costs and benefits of self-reflection were articulated by another student: "Even though self-reflection may seem like a painful and difficult process, it is one that offers solitude, inspiration, and growth." Finally, a student stated "Self-criticism hurts; self-understanding heals."

The process of reflecting on the course, its goals, teaching strategies, and outcomes unexpectedly evolved into an articulation of theory around the teaching/learning process of caring for self. In addition, the process of reflecting on teaching experiences has provided a voice for our students to share experiences and impressions about a process of transformation of caring experiences in their professional and personal lives.

Work on making explicit the learning process and the model of self-reflection began in the spring of 1991, and has resulted in uncovering theory grounded in teaching/learning experiences. Presented first as a poster at the 1991 National League for Nursing Biennial Convention in Nashville, Tennessee, this collaborative work has received great interest from nurses. It was selected for presentation in 1992, at the University of Wisconsin conference on transforming nurse education. It has been selected for presentation to a variety of educational conferences for undergraduate nursing programs, including registered nurse and bachelor's programs, generic programs, and 2-year associate degree curricula. It has also been presented to nurses in clinical practice.

In presentations and discussions with nurses, it has become apparent that the work validates the need for nurses in practice and education to care for themselves. In addition, the need for self-reflection and self-care is validated not only for adult student nurses but also for other mainstream population aggregates, such as women and other nurturing disciplines. Thus theory and clinical approaches to caring for self have been incorporated into discussions and workshops with the following groups: social work and nurse case managers in a long-term elder urban community care program, teachers and child care workers in Head Start programs in rural and urban settings, public health nurses in an urban setting, and staff of a primary care and public health nursing center in an urban setting.

AN IDEA THAT TRANSFORMS

The idea that caring for self is an integral part of caring for others is simple yet profound. It broadens and facilitates shifts of focus to include personal experience, and it humanizes caring work. It provides a strategy for widening and changing one's vantage point and perspective in caring. It offers the promise of a new, more personally chosen perspective and facilitates explorations, enabling nurses to see different choices for being and behaving in practice. It ultimately has the potential to enhance one's control over personal and professional actions. It is an idea that has the potential to transform and humanize caring.

For nursing, caring for self is becoming both a personal and a professional mandate. For nurses as persons, it has the potential to become a route for self-empowerment, self-fulfillment, and advocacy. It can also be a path for nurses connecting with nurses.

As a concept in nursing education, reflection has the potential to transform learning and personalize education. Using its generalizability, nurses' reflecting on their personal and professional experience, and nurses' focusing on understanding human experience, the process of self-reflection provides for understanding nursing practice experience. It promises greater depth and breadth of understanding the meanings and essences of caring for humanity.

PHILOSOPHICAL AND EDUCATIONAL UNDERPINNINGS

The work on the learning process is grounded in Dewey's[20] educational philosophy, particularly his thesis that there is a need for a theory of experience in education and his discussion concerning the continuum of experience. It is also grounded in principles of adult learning.

Dewey[20] stated that a person's growth and development are an exemplification of the concept of continuity of experience. He also stated:

> . . . every experience enacted and undergone modifies the one who acts and undergoes, while modification affects, whether we wish it or not, the quality of subsequent experiences. For it is a somewhat different person who enters into them.[20(p38)]

According to Dewey, discriminating between experiences that are educative and those that are miseducative becomes the task of the educator. The educator is assumed to have a maturity of experience that grounds him or her in facilitating the process of self-reflection. Nursing students, who are usually mature adults, often possess a maturity of experience. Discriminating between educative and miseducative experiences becomes a shared task between teacher and learner. Dewey further states:

> The student cannot be taught what he needs to know, but he can be coached: He has to see on his own behalf and in his own way the relations between

means and methods employed and results achieved. Nobody else can see for him and he can't see just by being "told," although the right kind of telling may guide his seeing and thus help him see what he needs to see.[21(p17)]

The model is also grounded in feminist pedagogy, including cooperative and connected ways of knowing such as intuition, subjective as well as objective learning, using personal and professional experience, and incorporating and integrating knowledge and experience.[22] The model attempts to bridge the gap between prevailing conceptions of nursing knowledge and the world of nursing practice.

THE PEDAGOGY OF CARING FOR SELF: THE TEACHER AS COACH, GUIDE, PARTNER, REFLECTIVE PRACTITIONER, AND FACILITATOR

Implied in Dewey's statements and assumptions concerning experience-driven education are pedagogic roles of the teacher as coach, partner, and guide. The role of teacher as a reflective practitioner proposed in this model makes the teacher a facilitator of reflection, a role that encompasses those of coach, partner, and guide. The reflective teacher needs to be practiced and involved in self-reflection and connected with a community of students and colleagues involved in conversations about learning. The teacher models the reflective process and mentors students in learning and developing—as Dewey called it, the habit of reflection.

THE NURSE AS A SELF-REFLECTIVE BEING

The model is also grounded in existential philosophy, especially phenomenology, which places value on lived experience, focusing on the meaning of one's living as a person within multiple life worlds. The nurse is viewed as a self-reflective being within this model. The view is a little different from that of Benner and Wrubel,[4] who use the work of Heidegger[23] for their view of the person as a self-interpreting being. Heidegger's concept of being includes viewing the person within his or her experience, actively involved in the world. Our definition of the nurse as a self-reflective being includes the view of the person as a self-interpreting being intimately involved with the world of life and nursing experience.

UNDERSTANDING EXPERIENCE: A PRELUDE TO ACTION

Using a phenomenologic perspective to view the world, this model uncovers and discovers meanings or essences in experience in an attempt to understand experience. According to Van Manen, "The essence or nature of an experience has been adequately described in language when the description reawakens or shows us the lived meaning or significance of the experience in a fuller or deeper manner."[24(p1)] In his work on "doing" phenomenology, Van Manen also writes that the phenomenologic perspective "is the attentive practice of thoughtfulness."[24(p1)] The ultimate aim of phenomenology is "to fulfill our human nature; to become more fully who we are."[24(p2)] Inquiry into experience as lived is necessary to understand humanity. Understanding meaning in experience becomes a prelude to action.

The vantage point of the phenomenologic view was well stated by one student:

> Assessing how I perceive my life and its stressors in a phenomenological view brings to light why and how I've come to be the person I am as well as why I perceive and feel things the way I do. Contemplating and studying my life phenomenologically is much like slowly weaving a meaningless tangle of thread into an intricate tapestry. The more I look at it and study it, the more I recognize important aspects that previously went unnoticed. Viewing my life phenomenologically has enriched and enhanced my own life as well as those with whom I am involved.

THE MODEL OF SELF-REFLECTION

The process of learning to care for self involves reflecting on oneself and becoming aware of the meanings of one's experience, and it results in increased awareness and increased depth and breadth of self-understanding. Figure 1 is a graphic depiction of the model of self-reflection.[1] This model depicts reflection as a process, a dynamic, multidimensional human process represented by a ribbon turning and looping, bending back to the world of self and experience. As awareness is increased, the reflective ribbon continues its movement, changing and initiating reflective action. As reflection leads to greater awareness of meaning in experience, it leads to self-understanding. The model depicts reflection as having the potential to change one's actions and behavior. In continuing the life processes of becoming and being a person within the world, one is informed about oneself.

The learning process is a transforming process for self, enabling the incorporation of new and past experiences and knowledge. After bending back to view self and experience, the ribbon never returns to its former position but rather continues onward. Reflection enables the person to see similar experiences differently, to incorporate old and new experiences and new reflections, and to project into future experience, providing a continuity of experience.

The depth and breadth of knowledge gained from reflection on experience are determined by one's life history, meanings, and values. The particular quality of experience helps one know and learn as well as balance competing ambiguities and understandings. One needs access to sufficient support and resources throughout the self-reflective process. Here, the role of the teacher as coach, guide, and participant in reflection is a supportive, facilitative one.

As a learning model, self-reflection becomes a critical process. It can begin at any time by persons at various levels of experience and expertise. As with other nursing skills and processes, guidance, coaching, and mentoring from a reflective practitioner assist and facilitate development.

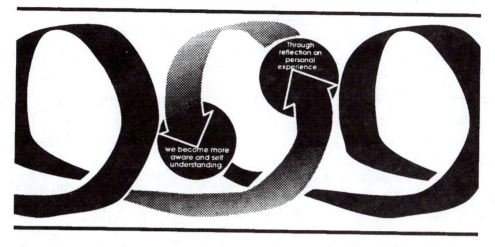

Through reflection on personal experience...

we become more aware and self understanding.

Figure 1. Model of self-reflection: Learning to care for self.

The process of self-reflection can be applied generally or specifically, depending on situational requirements, intent, and perceived or felt need. As a personal process, it is especially liberating and empowering for nurses because of value clarification and validation, affirmation, and personal commitment to self.

Reflection allows a person to arrive at a starting place and see it with new eyes, as if seeing it for the first time; this opens endless possibilities for interpreting meaning and responding. With reflection, it is possible to put bias in abeyance, to see things with different eyes and from different perspectives, and to develop new ways of responding. Self-reflection as a process promises an educative experience and demonstrates the underlying continuity of experience described earlier.

THE CONCEPT OF REFLECTION

One of the dictionary definitions of the word *reflection* is "bending or folding back," as of a ray of light. As a human process, and as used in this model, the metaphors of reflecting light and focus involve a bending back of attention to focus on self. This is experienced as validation for pulling back and taking time out for self. As one student stated:

I have learned to think of myself primarily on the basis of how others have treated me. Self-esteem has been developed and nurtured over time by those I have been closest to . . . my husband, my family, and friends. I have found that I need to meet my own needs in order to meet the demands that are placed on me by those around me.

Another student stated:

Unfortunately, nurses rarely take time to examine their own stress and coping patterns. Most could describe the interventions necessary for stress management for their clients, but few incorporate these techniques into their own lives. [Reflecting on myself] has allowed me to examine stress responses and develop coping strategies in handling a recent personal loss. It has permitted a self-examination and provided an opportunity for professional and personal growth.

SEEING SELF THROUGH ANOTHER LENS

The learning process is exemplified in the model using metaphors provided by photography, specifically that of focusing a portrait lens, to demonstrate reflection. Focusing the metaphoric portrait lens on self involves a magnification of aspects of self that heretofore were not visible to the naked eye; also, because of the relationship to the total picture, details of the portrait were previously difficult to see. The relationship of figure to ground—of self to world—is viewed differently through the portrait lens. A new perspective of self is facilitated by using the portrait lens. Figure 2 uses a magnifying glass to demonstrate visually the changes in the relationship of figure to ground when one is focusing on self.[1]

UNCOVERING THE SILENCE SURROUNDING SELF

The French phenomenologist Merleau-Ponty stated of phenomenology, "It is the things themselves, from the depths of their silence, that it wishes to bring to expression."[25(p4)] Merleau-Ponty posits that there is an atmosphere of silence surrounding the self and that it is from this world of silence that discovery of self will emerge. Becker[26] describes women's experiences of discovering and creating self resulting from uncovering the silence. Through reflection on self, self-inquiry and self-discovery begin. Grounded in teaching, professional experience, and reflective practice, the teacher guides the

learner toward greater awareness of self. Greater awareness of the possible meanings of experience is facilitated, and the opportunity to process clinical and personal meanings differently results in an expanded consciousness of the nurse as self within the world.

It is the world of silence surrounding nurses as persons that self-reflection in nursing education and practice addresses. Nurses often have practice and educational experiences that have encouraged silence. Many nurses have worked in hospital and health environments that are not conducive to developing a shared professional voice. In some settings, professional nursing autonomy and mature, adult, collaborative relationships and roles with nurses and other professionals are difficult.

Nurses are often just beginning to find their voices when they enter baccalaureate programs. Education provides an opportunity for nurses to learn new, more independent ways of seeing and responding. Many students become more self-reflective naturally when they return to school. An educational program that validates and focuses on caring for self and the tendency for students to be reflective make for a good fit between experience and education.

Developing the habit of self-reflection enables one to uncover other dimensions of experience, such as the hidden (as well as the explicit)

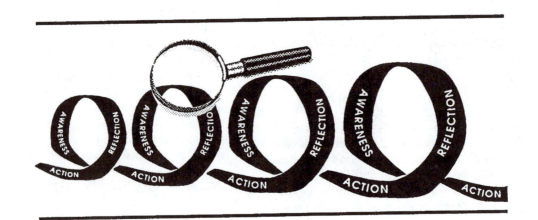

Figure 2. The reflective process.

meanings of behavior, experiences, values, thoughts, and feelings. Subtle changes in images achieved by varying the refractive angle provided by the metaphoric portrait lens often amount to important perceptual differences. Seemingly small qualitative changes in images can make all the difference in the world to the reflective, knowing person. Understanding meaning and experience as well as building better connections and interactions are possible among reflective practitioners. Herein lies the potential for transformation that becoming a self-reflective practitioner creates.

UNDERSTANDING, EXPANDED AWARENESS, AND EXPANDED CONSCIOUSNESS

Understanding, expanded awareness, and expanded consciousness are possible critical outcomes from self-reflection. Embedded within the process of self-reflection is connection with the larger social world. Nurses are temporally connected with people within the human world in a vital, caring way. Reflecting on the personal meanings of experience has the potential to connect nurses to patients, communities, aggregates, and groups. It connects nurses to each other, to institutions, and to other disciplines.

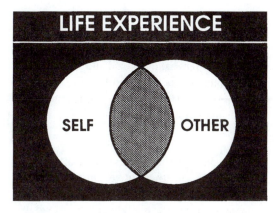

Figure 4. Human connection.

Figures 3 and 4 demonstrate the process of reflection on experience and the essential human connection with others' experience. In teaching nurses to become reflective about common, shared life experiences, nurses examine and interpret their experience, explicating similarities and differences in meanings.

Figure 4 demonstrates reflection on self as a prelude to learning to care for others. Reflection on experience is a connected experience for students, who have many current and past examples of common, collective, shared experience from practice. Understanding gained from reflection enables a person to assume responsibility for his or her experience within the world. The person experiences opportunities for choices that were previously unavailable and not conceptualized. Possibilities for action are increased from changing perceptions, perspectives, and priorities. Personal and professional risk taking behaviors are viewed differently. Choosing commitment provides greater control and enhanced success. The nurse, as person and self, experiences a clearer, more coherent sense of self within the world as well as an enhanced control over behavior, including behaviors of giving and receiving help and of advocacy.

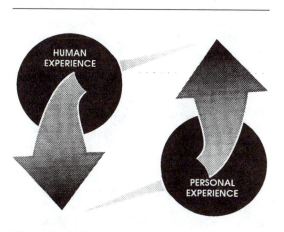

Figure 3. Reflection on experience. Through the context of our own life experience, we begin to understand the experience of others.

TO BECOME MORE FULLY HUMAN

The ultimate outcome of caring for self is to become more fully human, to understand what it means to be a person within the world, and to act on the increased understanding. The existential philosopher Sartre asserted that the goal of literature is "to reveal the world and particularly to reveal man to other men so that the latter may assume full responsibility before the object which has been thus laid bare."[27(p18)] He also stated:

> If you name the behavior of an individual, you reveal it to him; he sees himself. And since you are at the same time naming it to all others, he knows that he is seen at the moment he sees himself.[27(p16)]

A student shared her new sense of balance, shifts in perspective, and changing values when considering her life stress:

> My life, like most people, consists of a numerous array of small stressors. This includes the tendency to procrastinate, insufficient funds for furniture or a real bed, little time to take vacations or to socialize with friends. I feel these problems can be remedied with a relatively small amount of time and careful problem solving. To focus on such stressors would make them more than they are, causing me to lose my perspective on what is really important. Health, happiness, love, and the ability to enhance the quality of my life and others' lives are the only things I need to maintain a healthy, consistent sense of coherence.

Inherent in the process is a sense of shift in responsibility, a shift that enabled this student as a person to perceive and attend to the important and that enabled her to live more coherently, perhaps more gently, and one hopes, more humanly.

THE PRACTICE OF SELF-REFLECTION

Using a personal journal

The process of reflection is operationalized by journaling, which can be done by reflective thinking, evaluation, and processing of experience. There is a growing literature around the use of personal narratives in the nursing curriculum revolution.[28–31] Writing as a strategy to learn critical thinking and as a creative educational process is getting attention in the humanities as well as in nursing education literature. The use of a personal journal is proposed as a strategy for developing reflective thinking and for personalizing learning and knowing.[32–35]

Keeping a daily personal journal helps one establish the habit of self-reflection. Daily journal writing becomes daily reflective practice. It operationalizes the experience of bending back attention and focusing on self as client, nurse, and person. It may be helpful for nurses in uncovering silence, becoming more aware, and understanding themselves.

Many nurses talk about the benefit of writing as an integral process in learning and knowing. As one student stated:

> During the initial reading of my journal entries, I discovered how frequently I blamed my husband for our problems. I frequently wrote about what he was doing or not doing. After about two weeks of journaling, I realized this and started to change my thinking. I focused on what I was doing or not doing. This created a whole new perspective with many different situations. With a number of problems I could see ways to make positive changes.

Another student stated: "The journal opened my eyes to how I coped and opened the door to viewing different ways of coping."

Finally, a new convert to journaling stated:

Finding the time initially was a problem. How to squeeze something else into a busy schedule is a chore. But I had to because it was required for the course. As I journaled daily, I began to see patterns and things I ordinarily just acted on. Writing helped me to slow the reaction time down. Gradually, I began to see things differently. Now, I write for me. I write to clarify, to think through, to think about issues and about what I want out of life. If I don't write, I still go through the process. I am changing my life.

Increasingly, nurses are learning that they "write to learn."

Clinical experience of self as client

Nurses can begin the experience of caring for self with a "caring for self" clinical activity. In our classes, we encourage a holistic health assessment and an assessment of stress and coping strategies. We also assist in developing a plan for focus and intervention.

Taking care of self is often a transformational idea, especially for traditional and nontraditional nursing students because of the history of self-neglect that nurses as a group often describe. Personal neglect, overeating, lack of physical and leisure activities, distancing techniques (eg, compulsive shopping, inappropriate humor, and avoidance), the inability to say no, and screaming are some of the coping methods our students mentioned in early clinical discussions.

The best place to begin assisting nurses in learning to care for self is where they are. Nurses are encouraged to look at enhancing their resistance to stress by attending to their health habits, improved nutrition, and fitness activities. We suggest that part of each day (about 20 minutes) should be devoted to learning and practicing relaxation strategies, paying attention to one's physiologic responses to stress and relaxation, and learning to change one's responses to stress. Through getting in touch with their personal responses, nurses are sensitized to paying attention to themselves. In addition, there is a focus on cognitive and behavioral responses to stress and learning to gain control over these responses.

Attention to the person–environment relationship and to one's coping pattern provides an awareness of self that facilitates learning to balance and control one's personal responses. Nurses are assisted in reframing their personal goals from stress reduction to effective tension management and effective stress management. Nurses begin to see ways to balance life's demands through having greater control over their biologic responses to stress. By striving for a sense of well-being and maintaining a balance between demands and coping, students often feel empowered and energized.

Nurses also assess their distancing and palliative responses to stress and are assisted to look clearly at each situation using reflection. Support from reflective practitioners, guidance, and coaching assist nurses in knowing when and what kind of change in coping strategy is needed. Efforts are not made to minimize stress, but reappraisal assists in nurses' understanding stress within the context of other life experiences and may have that effect. Nurses learn, through reflective practice, to increase their sense of coherence, to become more farsighted, to enhance their rationality, and to develop flexibility in responding to demand.[3]

Comments from one student validate the potential of and the need for transformation that the clinical experience with self as client provides:

> Some of the changes I made were changes in my time schedule, seeing a family therapist, reading literature, increasing my physical activities, improving my dietary habits, and progressive muscle relaxation exercises. Overall, I have gained much insight

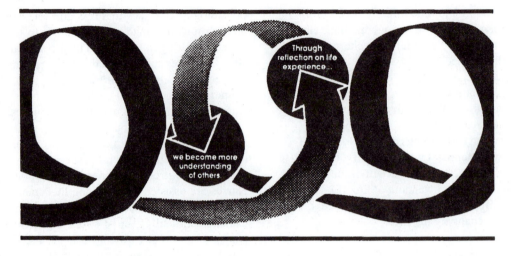

Figure 5. Model of caring for others.

into my stress and stressors. I have taken what I learned and applied it to my life and will continue to do so. My marriage has tremendously improved and become more satisfying. I give myself and my husband credit for this.

Another student stated:

When I first started this course, I thought that my major stress was time management. As I began journaling, I found that the areas that caused me the most stress and unhappiness were related to my living situation. These areas are also those that give me the greatest happiness.

FROM CARING FOR SELF TO CARING FOR OTHERS

As students uncovered experiences within their own lives and began to share their own personal stories, common shared themes among human conditions emerged. They were able to identify themes in their own experience that emerged as they chose a clinical focus. An understanding of self and others emerged from the clinical experience of caring for self. Under-

standing human conditions and personal meanings and caring for people experiencing stress became the organizing framework for further specific clinical applications. This process is depicted in Figure 5 as transforming the model of self-reflection to a model of caring for others.[1]

A TRANSFORMATION BETWEEN NURSES IN PRACTICE

Interestingly, we have found that the experience of self-reflection often helps nurses respond differently to colleagues and helps them develop caring, supportive relationships with each other. The experience of nurses becoming self-reflective appears to turn nurses to each other, building connections through personal and professional caring experiences. Engaging in conversations with nurses individually and collectively for the purpose of "calling out connecting conversations"[28] seems to happen with nurses around experiences of caring for self. The transformation involved in a single nurse caring for self seems to transcend self and becomes a transformation of a community of nurses, united through common interest and need in caring for each other as well as for humanity.

REFERENCES

1. Becker P, Lauterbach S. Learning to care for self. Poster presentation at the National League for Nursing Biennial Convention; June 9–13, 1991; Nashville, Tenn.

2. Antonovsky A. *Health, Stress, and Coping*. San Francisco, Calif: Jossey-Bass; 1979.

3. Antonovsky A. *Unraveling the Mystery of Health*. San Francisco, Calif: Jossey-Bass; 1988.

4. Benner P, Wrubel J. *The Primacy of Caring*. Reading, Mass: Addison-Wesley; 1989.

5. Cox T. *Stress*. Baltimore, Md: University Park Press; 1978.

6. Folkman S, Lazarus R. *Stress, Appraisal and Coping*. New York, NY: Springer-Verlag; 1984.

7. Jacobson S. *Nurses under Stress*. New York, NY: Wiley; 1983.

8. Monat A, Lazarus R. *Stress and Coping: An Anthology*. New York, NY: Columbia University Press; 1985.

9. Selye H. *The Stress of Life*. New York, NY: McGraw-Hill; 1956.

10. Selye H. *Stress without Distress*. New York, NY: Harper & Row; 1974.

11. Benson H. *Beyond the Relaxation Response*. New York, NY: Time Books; 1984.

12. Benson H. *The Relaxation Response*. New York, NY: Avon; 1975.

13. Davis M, Eshelmann E, McKay M. *The Relaxation and Stress Reduction Workbook*. Oakland, Calif: New Harbinger; 1988.

14. McKay K, Davis M, Fanning P. *Thoughts and Feelings: The Art of Cognitive Stress Intervention*. Oakland, Calif: New Harbinger; 1981.

15. Dossey B, Keegan L, Guzzetta C, Kolkmeier L. *Holistic Nursing: A Handbook for Practice*. Gaithersburg, Md: Aspen; 1995.

16. Grantz S, issue ed. *Holist Nurs Pract*. 1990;4(2).

17. Lachman V, issue ed. *Holist Nurs Pract*. 1990;4(4).

18. Lachman V. *Stress Management: A Manual for Nurses*. Orlando, Fla: Grune & Stratton; 1983.

19. Larkin D, Zahourek M, issue eds. *Holist Nurs Pract*. 1988;2(3).

20. Dewey J. *Experience and Education*. New York, NY: Macmillan; 1938.

21. Schon D. *Educating the Reflective Practitioner*. San Francisco, Calif: Josey-Bass; 1990.

22. Belenky M, Clinchy B, Goldberger N, Tarule J. *Women's Ways of Knowing: The Development of Self, Voice, and Mind*. New York, NY: Basic Books; 1986.

23. Heidegger M, Macquarrie J, Robinson E, trans. *Being and Time*. New York, NY: Harper & Row; 1962.

24. Van Manen M. *"Doing" Phenomenological Research and Writing*. Alberta, Ontario: University of Alberta; 1984.

25. Merleau-Ponty M, Lefort C, ed, Lingus A, trans. *The Visible and the Invisible*. Evanston, Ill: Northwestern University Press; 1968.

26. Becker P. Out of silence: Discovering and creating self. In: Munhall P, ed. *In Women's Experience*. New York, NY: National League for Nursing; 1995;2.

27. Sartre J, Frechtman B, trans. *What is Literature?* New York, NY: Harper & Row; 1965.

28. Baker C, Diekelmann N. Connecting conversations of caring: Recalling the narrative to clinical practice. *Nurs Outlook*. 1994;42:65–70.

29. Diekelmann N. The emancipatory power of the narrative. In: Schaperow R, ed. *Curriculum Revolution: Community Building and Activism*. New York, NY: National League for Nursing; 1991.

30. Gunby S, Chally P, Dorman R, Grams K, Kosowskim M, Pless B. Alice in Wonderland: A metaphor for professional nursing education. In: Schaperow R, ed. *Curriculum Revolution: Community Building and Activism*. New York, NY: National League for Nursing; 1991.

31. Krysl M. Sometimes a person needs a story more than food to stay alive. In: Schaperow R, ed. *Curriculum Revolution: Community Building and Activism*. New York, NY: National League for Nursing; 1991.

32. Bradley-Springer L. Discovery of meaning through imagined experience, writing, and evaluation. *Nurs Educ*. 1993;18:5–10.

33. Brown H, Sorrell J. Use of clinical journals to enhance critical thinking. *Nurs Educ*. 1993;18:16–19.

34. Lauterbach S. Journaling to learn: An educational strategy for developing self-reflection. In: Lauterbach S, Becker P, eds. *Understanding Human Experience*. New York, NY: National League for Nursing. In press.

35. Sedlak C. Use of clinical logs by beginning nursing students and faculty to identify learning needs. *J Nurs Educ*. 1992;31:24–29.

Awakening the Nurse Healer Within

Carol L. Wells-Federman, MEd, RN
Nurse Specialist
Division of Behavioral Medicine
Director of Clinical Training
Mind/Body Medical Institute
Deaconess Hospital
Adjunct Clinical Instructor in Nursing
Graduate School for Health Studies
Simmons College
Adjunct Instructor in Public Health
School of Medicine
Boston University School of Public Health
Boston, Massachusetts

The needs of the population we serve and the current health care agenda dictate that we make major shifts in the way we deliver care. The focus will be facilitating an individual's self-care management skills. Because nurses have always delivered care that facilitates self-care management and has an impact on the individual's mind, body, and spirit, this focus places nurses at the forefront in making a significant contribution to changing the health care system. Nurses have the responsibility, then, to understand a biopsychosocial-spiritual approach to care and to choose the most appropriate interventions to facilitate a person's growth and development toward wholeness of mind, body, and spirit.

Caring for and supporting individuals, families, and communities as they respond to and manage health and illness require skilled and compassionate application of scientific knowledge and technology. This knowledgeable and compassionate caring has biopsychosocial-spiritual correlates. As will be discussed, there is scientific evidence to support that caregiving interventions have quantifiable, reproducible physiologic effects.

If this caring is to be sustained, however, those who care must understand the role of healer and

The author wishes to thank Carol Lynn Mandle, PhD, RN, Susan Neary, MS, RN, CS, Eileen Stuart, MS, RN, CS, Carol Trockman, RN, Tricia Zuttermeister, MA, and Herbert Benson, MD, for their assistance in the preparation of this article.

Source: Reprinted from C.L. Wells-Federman, *Holistic Nursing Practice,* Vol. 10, No. 2, pp. 13–29, © 1996, Aspen Publishers, Inc.

recognize that they themselves do not create the change in others but rather participate in the process. Those who care must also recognize that, for knowledgeable and compassionate caring to be sustained, they must be willing to care for themselves and capable of doing so. In other words, they must be willing to awaken their healer within.

This article provides a framework for awakening the healer within by outlining the role of healer and introducing self-care methods necessary to sustain compassionate caregiving. The scientific evidence that supports the importance of caring in the healing process is presented next. Finally, the impact of awakening the healer within on creating the future of health care and nursing is discussed.

UNDERSTANDING THE ROLE OF HEALER

The word *healer* is often misconstrued as implying that a person and/or technique cures or heals. As far back as Hippocrates, however, it has been understood that the natural healing force within each of us is the greatest force in regaining health. Healing is an integration and balance of parts of oneself—physical and mental, emotional and spiritual, relationships and choices—leading toward personal growth and development.[1] Healing, therefore, is personal and not something that can be given to another. According to Quinn, "All healing, without exception, is self-healing."[2(p140)]

It has been our assumption that surgery, medication, acupuncture, or homeopathy cures or heals. These therapies may be necessary to remove barriers or stimulate healing, but they are not necessarily the cause of healing. Many of us know of patients who have died despite "successful" surgery. It is the person receiving the treatment, be it surgery, medication, or so-called "alternative" treatments, who does the healing. Healing is an intrinsic capacity of the patient, and as health care professionals we facilitate and support the healing process.

Healing, therefore, is not something the nurse gives to the patient; rather, the nurse facilitates the healing process through physical, psychosocial, technologic, and pharmacologic therapies and skills. As Nightingale is so often quoted as saying, "Nature alone cures . . . and what nursing has to do . . . is to put the patient in the best condition for nature to act upon him."[3(p33)] With this in mind, the nurse has no need to create dependence or monopolize wisdom. Instead, the nurse shows the patient, through compassionate caregiving, how to access his or her own inner wisdom and make health-promoting choices. In this way, the nurse becomes the educator in the true sense of the word (Latin *educare*, "to bring forth knowledge").[4]

Facilitating this process of healing in others dictates that we awaken the healer within ourselves. Awakening the healer within, however, requires us to face both the limitations and the miracles of our humanness and our work with balanced perspective. This balanced perspective requires a commitment to and practice of self-awareness and self-care. As Vaughan wrote:

> It is up to us, each one of us, to take responsibility for making the changes in our lives that will enable us to contribute to the well-being of the whole. If we aspire to optimum health either individually or collectively we must learn to pay attention to all aspects of physical, emotional, mental, existential, and spiritual well-being. Effective self-healing depends on taking all these into account.[5(p22)]

CARING FOR ONESELF AS A HUMAN BEING AND A NURSE

> *Live your life while you have it—life is a splendid gift. But to live your life you must discipline it. You must not fritter it away in fair purpose, erring act and inconsistent will.[3(p33)]*

It was my own struggle with burnout and the disillusionment with my profession that gave me the opportunity to focus my attention on self-care and change. Many nurses have experienced these same feelings of helplessness and loss of enthusiasm with their career. Much of mine stemmed from idealist beliefs and not knowing how to take care of myself while I cared for others. Having been through that disappointment, I am mindful now of the transformation this journey as a nurse, with all its challenges, frustrations, achievements, and passions, has made in my life. It has been a journey of growth and of owning the responsibility of taking care of myself and developing a balanced lifestyle.

Steps can be taken to increase career satisfaction and knowledgeable, compassionate caring that at the same time contribute to personal health and well-being. These steps, elaborated below, are clarifying values and beliefs, setting realistic goals, challenging the belief that others always come first, and learning to manage stress.

Clarify values and beliefs

Developing a balanced lifestyle means recognizing those things that are important to you and where you are in your life, evaluating what needs to be changed, and generating an action plan for that change. The first step is to identify what is important, meaningful, and valuable to you to assess whether your actions are consistent with your beliefs. What you believe in and value guide your actions by sanctioning certain behaviors and negating others. When you assess your values and beliefs, you begin to exercise your ability to make choices for yourself rather than relying on the beliefs and values imposed on you by others.

One method to help you identify what you value and ultimately clarify the relationship between your beliefs and actions is the "Ten Loves" exercise. Simon,[6] a pioneer in the field of values clarification, developed this exercise to help people evaluate the choices they were currently making. After reviewing the results, you, may find that there are certain things you enjoy doing, such as traveling, taking long walks, ballroom dancing, or playing with your children, that you have not been doing either because your time is being spent doing less important things or because you are constantly putting others

first. When you detect inconsistencies between your ideal life and your actual living habits, you can begin to develop a working plan for changing things rather than waiting for some miracle that will change them for you. This gives you back the control and choice in your life.

Set realistic goals

The first step in developing a working plan toward change is to identify your long-term goals and then determine the short-term goals or strategies that will assist you in meeting them. Be certain to make them realistic, positive, and behavior (activity) oriented. In other words, someone would be able to videotape you doing the activity (behavior). You might choose to read to your children every night before they go to bed, have dinner with the family at least five times a week, or spend an hour after dinner with homework or discussing what has happened during your children's day. The more specific you can be in setting goals, the easier it is to evaluate progress and success or to decide on what changes need to be made.

Challenge the belief that others always come first

Figure 1 is a list of questions to help you evaluate attitudes and behaviors that perpetuate the myth that there is healing in continued self-sacrifice. Healing, as discussed earlier, is personal and can only be facilitated by empowering the other person. The dictionary defines *facilitate* as "to make easier, to assist the progress of a person." This means a partnership; in other words, you are only *a part* of the process.

If your tendency is to become overinvolved with patients, boundaries between yourself and the patient can become unclear. Often, this leads to overwork and oversolicitous helping that ignores the responsibilities, autonomy, and resources of the patient. These are signs of helping to feel that you are in control and the world is safe. This overinvolvement and excessive activity are frequently a way to deal with anxiety.[7]

Answer the seven questions below with a *yes* or *no*. Try not to hedge. Choose the answer that's more accurate for you right now.

1) I will almost always listen to others who need emotional support, but I seldom ask anyone to pay attention to my emotional needs.   Y   N

2) When someone helps me I usually make sure I do as much or more to help them in return.   Y   N

3) When I don't respond to someone else's needs, I often feel selfish.   Y   N

4) I try hard not to hurt other people's feelings.   Y   N

5) Once I say "yes" people can count on me to get the job done, even if it costs me personally.   Y   N

6) I avoid conflict whenever possible.   Y   N

7) I tend to get myself in over my head by saying "yes" too much, too often.   Y   N

TOTALS

	YES	NO

Figure 1. Hooked on helping addiction test. *Source:* Reprinted from N.A. Tubesing and D.A. Tubesing, *Structured Exercises in Stress Management* (vol. 2, p. 44). Copyright © 1984, 1994 Donald A. Tubesing.

According to Benner and Wrubel, "The remedy for overinvolvement is not a lack of involvement but rather the right kind of involvement."[7(p375)] The art of nursing is to assume appropriate responsibility, not more responsibility than the situation requires. The results are not in your hands: Your responsibility is to offer what you can without imposing the outcome and at the same time to allow others their contributions. It takes courage and conscious awareness to know that what you offer may not be enough, however.

To facilitate a more balanced involvement, nurses need to develop a "clinical eye" to assess whether there needs to be some personal readjustment in perspective and behavior. Challenge the "caregiver fantasy," the belief that it is more important to take care of everyone else first. Burnout and disillusionment stem partly from the underlying beliefs and assumptions that fuel some of the "caregiver fantasy" thoughts that may run through your head. If never challenged, the beliefs that you must be all things to all people, that you must be perfect to be loved, or that your needs are not as important as others'

will keep you from hearing your innate wisdom and will erode the quality of your caregiving. Overinvolvement leaves little time for fulfillment of personal needs and often leads to resentment and blame. Because there is no humanness or room for error in this way of thinking, it distorts reality and wears away self-esteem.

These beliefs and thoughts can affect your health and well-being because they affect your mood, behavior, and physiology. This relationship among thoughts, feelings, behavior, and physiology is bidirectional. For example, a headache can affect your mood and in turn influence your thoughts. Conversely, focusing on a negative thought can affect your mood and in turn lead to increased muscle tension and eventually a tension headache. The headache may interfere with a planned social event that evening. Recognizing this cycle is important to challenging these beliefs and thoughts and subsequently changing the unrealistic and negative thinking that can lead to health consequences.

One way to challenge the "caregiver fantasy" is with affirmations. An affirmation is simply a positive thought, a short phrase, or a saying that has meaning for you. It can help change assumptions and beliefs that have negative consequences. Affirmations are important in reinforcing new ways of thinking and behaving from moment to moment. They are statements that you can select to reaffirm your new intentions, and they can help you increase the clarity of your goals and assume responsibility for your actions.

When you are starting to feel upset, anxious, frustrated, sad, or overwhelmed, stop and examine what you are saying to yourself and simply challenge that monologue with language that is more affirming, such as

- I can ask for what I need.
- I can take care of myself.
- I'm doing the best I can.
- I can find alternatives to problems.
- I can meet my needs.
- I care for myself and I care for others.

Initially, this may seem superficial and uncomfortable, but as you continue to change this inner dialogue, you will begin to notice changes in your behavior and in your environment. Practice self-talk that celebrates your unique contribution as an individual who has both strengths and weaknesses.

Learn to manage stress

Nurses are not immune to stress-related illnesses or health-risking behaviors. Some alarming statistics support this fact[8]

- Nurses are 30 to 100 times more likely than the general population to become chemically dependent.
- Nurses have an inordinately high burnout rate compared with most other professions.
- Physicians and nurses are the two types of professionals who are most likely to develop addiction to hard narcotics, such as demerol and morphine.

Learning to manage stress is a prerequisite to promoting health and well-being. Managing stress requires acknowledging the mind–body connection, eliciting the relaxation response,

practicing personal presence, taking care of your body, and building a support network.

Acknowledge the mind–body connection

When you acknowledge the mind–body connection and learn that there is a relationship among thoughts, feelings, behaviors, and physiology, healing can occur. Healing can become blocked in times of stress because of the bidirectional feedback loop between mind and body. The stress response is triggered when you perceive that a situation is a threat to your physical and psychologic well-being and that you are unable to cope effectively with the demand.[9] This generates a cascade of biochemical events initiated by the central nervous system that affect the body. Most specifically, the autonomic nervous system via the sympathetic branch produces a generalized arousal of the body, including increased heart rate and blood pressure, heightened awareness of the environment, shifting of blood from the visceral organs to the large muscle groups, increase in muscle tension, altered lipid metabolism, increased platelet aggregability, and increased respirations. This basic adaptive response to physical stress was named the fight or flight response by Cannon in the early 1900s.[10]

The musculoskeletal system is also affected by the stress response. Neural messages are transduced through the nervous system via motor pathways to increase muscular tension and rigidity. This increase in muscle tension is again a primitive adaptive response to meet the challenge of physical stress. The musculoskeletal system is also activated by the sympathetic nervous system during the stress response.

In response to stress, the psychoneuroendocrine system (hypothalamic–pituitary–adrenal axis) is also affected. Threat or stress causes the hypothalamus to secrete corticotropin-releasing hormone, thus stimulating the anterior portion of the pituitary gland to secrete corticotrophin, which in turn causes the adrenal cortex to secrete corticosteroids. Corticosteroids are responsible for increased blood sugars, sodium retention, alterations in lipid metabolism, increased antiinflammatory response (acutely), and, over time, a decrease in immune function. Similarly, other hormones regulated by the psychoneuroendocrine system, such as reproductive and growth hormones as well as endorphins and enkephalins, can be affected by the stress response.

These innate automatic physiologic responses to stressful stimuli are necessary to meet the demands of physical stress. The stress response is repeatedly triggered, however, as we face the challenges of daily hassles. Acutely, the stress response may cause or exacerbate symptoms such as anxiety, angina, cardiac dysrhythmias, pain, tension headaches, insomnia, and gastrointestinal complaints. With repeated or prolonged exposure to physical or psychologic stress, the stress response can cause diseases or exacerbate symptoms of diseases that are influenced by central nervous system stimulation, precipitating arousal of the musculoskeletal system, autonomic nervous system, or psychoneuroendocrine system. Research confirms the link between the stress response and such diseases as the common cold,[11] chronic pain,[12] cancer and other diseases influenced by the immune system,[13,14] hypertension, infertility, and diabetes,[15] to name a few.

Over time, chronic excessive exposure to stress can lead to physical, psychologic, social-behavioral, and spiritual consequences (see the box titled "Biopsychosocial-Spiritual Effects of Stressful Events"). Just as stress affects your physiology, so too does it affect how you think, feel, and act. Stress often increases negative mood states, such as anxiety or depression, and can affect your thinking and ability to concentrate or problem-solve effectively.

Your behavior can change when you are under stress. Acts that you would ordinarily be able to control, such as overeating or excessive drinking of alcohol, are much more difficult to control under stress. This inability to control health-risking behavior as a result of increased stress is called stress disinhibition. In other words, you are no longer inhibited from participating in that behavior because your defenses are down.

Biopsychosocial-Spiritual Effects of Stressful Events

Biologic
  Musculoskeletal system
  Sympathetic nervous system
  Peripheral nervous system
Psychologic
  Increase in negative mood states
Social-behavioral
  Stress disinhibition
  Increased health-risking behaviors
Spiritual
  Disruption in personal belief system

Stressful events or illnesses can challenge personal beliefs. When an event appears to be inconsistent with your spiritual belief or your sense of meaning and purpose, it can leave you feeling vulnerable and unsafe. These are often times when it may be necessary to evaluate a need for a shift in values, beliefs, and actions important for personal growth and development. This may require an openness to new possibilities and changing health-risking behaviors. Stressful events may be perceived as either challenges that lead to positive growth or threats that can lead to negative consequences.

To manage stress effectively and counteract these health consequences, it is important to identify early warning signals. Stress warning signals differ from individual to individual, but Benson and Stuart[15] list some common ones. Early recognition of stress warning signals gives you an opportunity to elicit the relaxation response, therefore decreasing the sympathetic arousal that in turn exacerbates these symptoms.

The relaxation response

The relaxation response is the antithesis of the stress response. It is an integrated physiologic response originating in the hypothalamus that leads to a generalized decrease in central nervous system arousal. In 1971, Wallace and colleagues[16] first described the relaxation response after observing a hypometabolic state in people practicing transcendental meditation. They described the relaxation response as a state of deep rest brought about by focused attention on a simple mental stimulus, such as a word, phrase, or image. This focused attention is associated with decreased sympathetic nervous system activity, resulting in lower heart rate, blood pressure, respiratory rate, metabolic rate, and muscle tension. In other words, as shown in Table 1, the relaxation response is the physiologic opposite of the stress response.

The changes in sympathetic nervous system activity are considered acute physiologic changes and occur when the relaxation response is elicited. Studies also suggest that there are benefits of eliciting the relaxation response that extend beyond the acute response, providing a carryover effect.[17,18] These studies show a reduced end-organ responsivity to norepinephrine under stress after regular elicitation of the relaxation response, suggesting a more long-term physiologic effect.

To the extent that stress causes or exacerbates a symptom or illness, eliciting the relaxation response can break the stress–symptom cycle. The immediate physiologic effects are a decrease in heart rate, blood pressure, respiratory rate, and muscle tension. The long-term physiologic effect is a decrease in central nervous system arousal with its concomitant decrease in musculoskeletal system, sympathetic nervous system, and psychoneuroendocrine system arousal.

In addition to these physiologic changes, psychologic and behavioral changes may also occur, as shown in Table 1. Subjective states associated with eliciting the relaxation response have been described as a sense of well-being and peace of mind during and after the response.[19] After eliciting the relaxation response, you can more easily focus attention and appraise attitudes and assumptions in a more conscious, objective way. You can then begin to replace ways of thinking and behaving that have not served you well with new, more positive, health-promoting thoughts and behaviors.[6,19,20] This allows for an openness to new possibilities and for

Table 1. Physical, psychologic, and social changes of the stress response compared with the relaxation response

Stress response	Change	Relaxation response
↑	Metabolism	↓
↑	Heart Rate	↓
↑	Blood pressure	↓
↑	Respirations	↓
↑	Muscle tension	↓
↑	Negative mood states	↓
↑	Health-risking behavior	↓

changing behaviors in more healthful ways, creating a greater alignment between your values and lifestyle choices.

This state of mind may also help you develop a spiritual perspective that can engender a shift in values and beliefs important to personal growth and development. A study conducted by Kass and colleagues[21] found that a significant number of subjects who regularly elicited the relaxation response, regardless of method, reported an increase in positive attitudes associated with spirituality. This increase in positive attitudes contributed to a decrease in frequency of medical symptoms and an increase in health and well-being.

Because the relaxation response is an innate physiologic response, it can be elicited using a number of techniques that involve mental focusing. Techniques commonly used are diaphragmatic breathing, autogenic training, progressive muscle relaxation, repetitive prayer, mindfulness, meditation, and yoga stretching. All these techniques have two basic components: the repetition of a word, sound, phrase, prayer, image, or physical activity, and the passive disregard of everyday thoughts when they occur during the practice. Audiotapes are recommended to help guide you through this process. Further guidelines can be found in the box titled "Guidelines for Eliciting the Relaxation Response."

Guidelines for Eliciting the Relaxation Response

Maintain a passive mental attitude to intruding thoughts.

Repeat a simple mental stimulus (a word, phrase, image, or prayer).

Practice once a day for 20 minutes (alternative: twice a day for 10 minutes each).

Practice it in the same place every day.

Do it first thing in the morning.

Try not to lie down; chances are you will fall asleep.

Take the phone off the hook.

Tell your family, secretary, etc not to bother you.

Don't use an alarm clock; set a watch in front of you or put a pillow over an alarm clock so that it rings softly.

It is normal for thoughts to come and go; simply note that your mind has wandered, passively ignore the thoughts, and go back to what you were focusing on.

Try to elicit the relaxation response immediately after you exercise; the sense of deep relaxation should come more easily.

Don't do it after a large meal.

Regular elicitation of the relaxation response will help you feel less anxious and stressed for some time after those 10- to 20-minute sessions. It is important, however, to intervene in your health and well-being throughout the day. What can you do to counteract those daily minor irritations and hassles? How can you keep the minor stress warning signals of jaw and shoulder tension from developing into a painful tension headache? One way is to monitor stress warning signals and practice "mini-relaxations" to break the stress cycle. A mini-relaxation response can be anything from a few conscious, deep, diaphragmatic breaths to several minutes of sitting quietly. This simple practice is one of the most effective ways to utilize the relaxation response more fully; it is a practical way to reduce tension and anxiety, improve concentration, and increase your ability to relate more easily with others. The following are two suggestions for mini-relaxations:

1. As you inhale, count slowly up to four. As you exhale, count slowly back down to one. Thus as you inhale, say to yourself "one, two, three, four"; as you exhale, say to yourself "four, three, two, one." Do this several times.

2. Take a few deep, diaphragmatic breaths, and as you do so begin to recall something that would bring a smile to your face. This could be the image of your child's face, your favorite pet, or another loved one, or it could be the memory of a favorite place, food, or event in your life.

Practice mini-relaxations throughout the day to counter the harmful effects of arousal from the stress response.

Develop the skill of personal presence

Another important stress management intervention is to develop the skill of personal presence. Presence is a nursing intervention described by Gardner as a "physical 'being there' and a psychological 'being with' a patient for the purpose of meeting the patient's health care needs."[22(p.191)] It is the gift of self through availability and attention to needs. To be available to others in this way, you must practice the skill of being present to yourself. Being physically and psychologically present means that you completely experience the moment and do not allow yourself to be distracted, hurried, or fragmented. Mini-relaxations are an excellent way of practicing the skill of being present.

Another effective way of developing this skill is through mindfulness. This is the ability to focus attention on what you are experiencing from moment to moment.[23] The practice of mindfulness can be particularly useful in allowing you to extend the benefits of eliciting the relaxation response to more areas of your daily life. It comprises the combination of slowing down and bringing your full attention (thoughts, feelings, and bodily sensations) to the activity you are doing at the moment.

Some ideas for practicing personal presence (mindfulness) are as follows[23]:

- Every morning as you awaken, bring your full attention to your breathing. Gradually allow your awareness to expand out into the room, and then slowly begin to listen to the sounds of the outdoors.
- Peel an orange, take one section, and carefully examine it through all your senses: sight, smell, touch, taste, and the sound of each bite. Enjoy mindfully each new experience.
- On your way to work, focus on how you walk, drive, or ride the transit. Take some deep, diaphragmatic breaths, and relax your body as you travel.
- Before entering a patient's room, take a second or two to attend to your breathing, relax your body, and focus your mind.
- Allow the repetitive events of the day to become cues for a mini-relaxation: answering the ringing telephone, auscultating a heartbeat, answering a call light, and before, during, and after rounds or reports.
- Make a conscious transition as you return home from work. Be certain to leave work thoughts and worries at work, and be mindful of your home environment each day.
- As you go to sleep, once again focus on your breathing, and become completely aware of your surroundings. Practice consciously letting go of today and tomorrow as you allow your mind and body to get some much needed rest.

Take care of your body

You must take care of your body to manage stress. Because the mind and body are connected, you cannot ignore one while paying attention to the other. The body requires rest, healthy nutrition, and exercise. People who exercise on a regular basis rate their bodies more positively than those who are inactive.[24] Physical activity has been shown to have a positive effect on morbidity and mortality[25,26] and to lead to improved appearance and psychologic changes. Exercise has been shown to reduce anxiety, tension, and fatigue; to relieve depression; and to increase vigor and self-esteem.[27]

Exercising regularly can help you adopt a more active lifestyle as you begin to feel better physically and emotionally. These positive effects can be obtained with exercise of only moderate intensity. For example, a brisk walk of 30 to 60 minutes three to five times a week is sufficient to produce the fitness standard that promotes health and decreases risk of disease.[28] Being physically active on a daily basis is what is important. One way to begin is to increase the number of healthy activities in your routine. Some ideas to help with this are as follows:

- Play active games with your children.
- Garden on the weekends.
- Walk or bicycle to work.
- Take the stairs instead of the elevator.
- Park your car at the farthest point in the parking lot at work.

You can gain tremendous physical and psychologic rewards by simply changing some of your daily routine. It is also important, however, to develop a regular FITT exercise program that involves the following parameters[28]:

- F (frequency): Aerobic exercise three to five times a week, muscle toning two times a week.
- I (intensity): Moderate (by heart rate and perceived exertion); able to complete 8 to 12 repetitions of each toning exercise.
- T (time): 20 to 60 minutes, plus warm-up and cool-down, 15 to 20 minutes to complete a series of 8 to 10 muscle toning exercises.
- T (type): Aerobic (eg, walking, bicycling, or swimming), muscle toning (eg, weight machines, free weights, or calisthenics).

With these FITT guidelines in mind, you can establish an exercise prescription specific to your needs. Remember to begin slowly and build up gradually. If you are older than 45 years or have cardiovascular risk factors (eg, hypertension or diabetes) or pulmonary disease, it is recommended that you have a complete work-up, including an exercise test, before beginning an exercise program.

Taking care of your body also requires that you eat healthy, balanced meals. The American lifestyle has made it increasingly difficult to practice healthy eating habits. One of the frustrations of nursing practice is trying to help others develop these habits. Therefore, you must learn how to manage this in your own life. This, of course, takes planning, choosing a variety of foods, and maintaining a diet low in fat, saturated fat, and cholesterol with plenty of vegetables, fruits, and grain products. The current US dietary guidelines call for 6 to 11 servings a day from the bread, cereal, rice, and pasta group; 2 to 4 servings from the fruit group; 3 to 5 servings from the vegetable group; 2 to 3 servings of meat, poultry, fish, beans, eggs, or nuts; 2 to 3 servings of milk, yogurt, or cheese; and a minimal amount of fats, oils, and sweets. Following these simple guidelines can pay large health dividends.

A healthy diet combined with a regular exercise routine has many health benefits. One of the most effective ways to lose weight is to combine exercise with nutritious eating. Exercise and proper nutrition can improve your cholesterol profile, reduce blood pressure, and improve your overall cardiovascular profile.

Develop a support network

One of the most effective ways to reduce distress and burnout is to develop a social support network with fellow nurses.[29] Fellow colleagues can provide the insights and perspectives necessary to cope with commonly shared experiences. Nurses are repeatedly exposed to tragedy, death, and even, in the case of violence, the presence of cruelty. Coping may range from laughter to overinvolvement, from detachment to elaborate self-protective maneuvers. These can only grant temporary reprieve. Acknowledging the pain

and seeking support from others are the most enduring long-term coping strategies.[7]

Practicing collegiality is a way of fostering this social support network. It is a way of building an atmosphere at work where you can support your colleagues and they you. It is Thoreau who reminds us in his writings that it is far more important to carve and paint the atmosphere in which we work than to be able to carve a statue or paint a picture.[30]

Building a supportive work environment requires conscious awareness of and action toward valuing yourself and your colleagues. According to Uustal, "collegiality is the ethic of caring shared among nurses and is a natural extension of the ethic of caring that also focuses on patient care and self-care for the caregiver."[31(p46)] The following are some suggestions for shaping the quality of the atmosphere in which you work and developing a strong support network[31]:

- Find someone doing something right, and acknowledge him or her.
- Expect the best from yourself and those with whom you work.
- Model the values you believe. Take responsibility for your health and well-being, and encourage others to do the same.
- Establish a mentoring or buddy system.
- Make decisions based on nursing's ethical values.
- Establish a support group to help deal with the feelings that can arise from professional practice.
- Be supportive, but refer colleagues to professional support when needed.

Summary

Learning to manage the stress in your life is integral to your capacity for sustained, compassionate caregiving. Understanding and practicing healthy behaviors impacts on your ability to encourage those practices in others. Prioritizing your needs and managing stress will give you personal insights into the importance of compassionate caring and will be the foundation of your practice.

ACKNOWLEDGING THE IMPORTANCE OF COMPASSIONATE, KNOWLEDGEABLE CARING

It is a peculiarly modern mistake to think that caring is the cause of burnout and that the cure is to protect oneself from caring to prevent the "disease" called burnout. Rather, the loss of caring is the sickness and the return of caring is the recovery.[7(p373)]

When the importance of caring in nursing is not understood, it is a serious problem. It costs nursing and patients a great deal when we fail to value our traditionally feminine history. The feminine principle concerns itself with nurturing. Nurses must continue to integrate traditional feminine nursing foundations within a scientific, task-oriented, cost-contained environment.

If we look at the current needs in health care, we can readily see how nursing can contribute in its unique way to meeting these demands. In 1979, the Surgeon General's Report[32] stated that as many as half the premature deaths in the United States may be due to unhealthy behaviors or lifestyles. Seven of the 10 leading causes of premature death in our country, according to this report, could be reduced if Americans altered health-risking behaviors, such as smoking, eating foods high in saturated fat, consuming a poor diet, misusing alcohol, maintaining a sedentary lifestyle, and responding unhealthily to tension and stress.

The emphasis in health care has shifted to those with chronic illness. Although the average life expectancy of the American population as a whole has increased, recent morbidity and mortality data point to the continuing need for a better understanding of how to implement healthy behavior change strategies as well as prevention and health-promotion interventions for individuals with chronic illness.[33]

At the same time, it has been reported that 70% to 80% of visits by the average patient to the average primary health care provider are self-limiting, meaning that the treatment is nonspecific or the symptom would go away on its own.[34] In a health care system that is not equipped to meet the demands of the population it serves, patients often get labeled as inappropriate utilizers. They are not inappropriate utilizers, however; rather, it is their care that is inappropriate.

Nursing can make a valuable contribution to these health care demands. It is through our caregiving interventions, our unique understanding of the human as a biopsychosocial-spiritual being, and our ability to look beyond the symptom to the causes of that symptom that place us in such an important position. Interventions that nurses have traditionally used for centuries, such as relaxation, touch, imagery, social support, listening, prayer, empathy, compassion, and education, are important parts of that process.

When nurses show compassion and understanding, give a back rub, or coach patients using breath focus; when we teach patients to use relaxation, imagery, or music therapy; when we listen empathically, foster social support, or teach self-care skills—we change the patient's perceptions and increase his or her ability to cope. This in turn affects perceptions and decreases the attendant physiologic arousal, creating the best possible environment for healing.

Although we have always believed that these nursing interventions have therapeutic properties, these properties have been difficult to quantify. Pioneering research on the mind–body connection by nursing, behavioral medicine, and psychoneuroimmunology has implications for nursing practice, providing empirical evidence that our nursing interventions have quantifiable, reproducible physiologic effects.

Interventions that access the mind–body connection can be used across the health care continuum, including acute, ambulatory, chronic, rehabilitative, home care, and hospice settings. The needs of the patient, his or her diagnosis, and the setting and feasibility of implementation will determine the specifics of the intervention. Effective treatment is dependent upon a comprehensive assessment of the patient's biopsychosocial, behavioral, and spiritual factors that affect health and illness and the ability of the nurse to determine differentially which intervention would best access the mind–body connection and address the underlying problem. It is, of course, important to involve the patient in any treatment decisions and plans.

As discussed earlier, relaxation techniques can reduce sympathetic arousal and help counter the stress response. These techniques, therefore, can be used to coach patients during treatment, or patients can be taught a technique for use at home.

Interventions such as therapeutic touch and therapeutic massage can be used with patients who are unable to participate actively in learning and practicing relaxation exercises. Therapeutic touch has been found to reduce anxiety in hospitalized patients,[35–38] to reduce tension headaches,[37] and to decrease the need for postoperative pain medication.[38] Physiologic effects of therapeutic massage have been studied on patients with acute myocardial infarction,[39] normotensive women,[40] and middle-age and elderly adults.[41] Groer and colleagues[42] found a statistically significant increase in salivary immunoglobulin A concentration in subjects who received a 10-minute back massage compared with control subjects. These preliminary findings suggest that therapeutic massage may enhance immune function.

Other nursing interventions used in the treatment of health problems have been found to influence the stress–symptom cycle and directly affect muscular tension, anxiety, cardiovascular arousal, and the psychoneuroendocrine indices. Social support has been found to be related to a decrease in minor illnesses and absenteeism,[43] a decrease in heart disease in middle-age men,[44] an increase in longevity among women with metastatic breast cancer,[45] and an increase in longevity in individuals with malignant melanoma.[46] Frasure-Smith[47] demonstrated that providing emotional and social support to patients recovering from myocardial infarction, through only 6 hours of nursing contact (on average), correlated with a 50% reduction in subsequent death rates. It was postulated that positive changes in the patient's emotional state modulated the stress response.

Journal writing is another nursing intervention that has been found measurably to improve physical and mental health.[48] When care is empathic, it has been found to increase care satisfaction and empowerment and to decrease anxiety and depression.[49] Thus interventions that address self-esteem, autonomy, self-care, peace of mind, and well-being begin to assume empirical, physiologically based importance in addition to their inherent value.

There are a myriad of interventions that nurses can use to promote adaptation, self-care, empowerment, and a sense of control that draw their empirical value from accessing the mind–body connection and interrupting the stress–symptom cycle. The difference that this caregiving can make in the life of another can often be profound.

CREATING A VISION FOR THE FUTURE OF HEALTH CARE AND NURSING

If millions of nurses in a thousand different places articulate the same ideas and convictions about primary health care, and come together as one force, then they could act as a powerhouse for change. I believe that such a change is coming, and that nurses around the globe, whose work touches each of us intimately, will greatly help to bring it about.[50(p130)]

Other disciplines, including medicine, are beginning to realize that the current health care agenda requires a paradigm shift. They also must view patients in a more comprehensive, holistic manner. Changes in medical school curricula and practice and new approaches have been suggested. What is not recognized, however, is that the new health care model is here now and has been for centuries: It is called nursing. Nursing must develop a stronger voice and take its rightful place in shining the light toward the future for other disciplines to follow. We can create a new environment because we have the unique ability to bring a biopsychosocial-spiritual perspective to treating human responses to actual or potential health problems in the traditional biomedical setting in which we practice.

Within nursing, comprehensive care that includes care of the caregiver has many implications for nursing education, practice, research, administration, and policy. Nursing education can begin to add self-development courses at both the baccalaureate and master's level. Caring can be introduced into the nursing curriculum at all levels of education, including faculty–student–administration relationships.

In the practice environment, self-development can be fostered and maintained with systematic, continued support and mentoring through staff development and postgraduate fellowships. Programs can be made available to promote and provide exercise, nutrition counseling, stress management, and support. Research that continues to study the phenomology of caring as it relates to healing would further both knowledge and skill. Administration can further the development of ideas within practice that increase health outcomes for both nurses and patients. Nursing must also work to promote health care coverage that provides direct payment for caregiving. In schools, with nurses as primary providers and health promotion leaders, health programs can introduce care-based curricula that promote health and self-care.

•   •   •

As we move into the 21st century, the health care delivery system will be more technologi-cally sophisticated, more organizationally complex, and more cost controlled than ever before. Our most important responsibility will be to continue to create a healing space for patients and for ourselves within this complex environment. There are many challenges in clinical practice, but nurses should continue to create a new vision based on traditional feminine nursing interventions integrated with technology and pharmacology because this will increase our satisfaction with our work, improve our health and well-being, and promote satisfaction, health, and well-being among our patients.

Nursing always has been, and always will be, full of surprises and challenges. The need for change and continued growth is nothing new to nursing. Nightingale[3] recognized this a century ago when she cautioned us as nurses not to be satisfied that we have learned all that we can learn because nursing is a progressive art. Her words continue to be meaningful today as we move further toward developing nursing as a science in its own right. The uniqueness of nursing is that we focus on promoting health for people and their world. We must remember, however, that if health is to be sustained, those who provide the help must be capable of caring for both themselves and others.

There are so many possibilities and experiences available to all of us. Pause now, look inside, and acknowledge the importance of *you* as a human being and of your work as a nurse. Plan and design your future, and help plan the future of nursing. Make certain your voice is heard. Awaken the nurse healer within you.

REFERENCES

1. Dossey BM, Keegan L, Guzzetta CE, Kolkmeier LG. *Holistic Nursing: A Handbook for Practice.* 2nd ed. Gaithersburg, Md: Aspen; 1995.

2. Quinn JF. Healing: The emergence of right relationship. In: Carlson R, Shield B, eds. *Healers on Healing.* Los Angeles, Calif: Tarcher; 1989.

3. Nightingale F. *Notes on Nursing: What It Is, and What It Is Not.* Philadelphia, Pa: Lippincott; 1992.

4. Schwarz J. Healing, love, and empowerment. In: Carlson R, Sheild B, eds. *Healers on Healing.* Los Angeles, Calif: Tarcher; 1989.

5. Vaughan F. *The Inward Arc.* Boston, Mass: Shambhala; 1986.

6. Simon SB. *Meeting Yourself Halfway: 31 Value Clarification Strategies for Daily Living.* Niles, Ill: Argus Communications; 1974.

7. Benner P, Wrubel J. *The Primacy of Caring: Stress and Coping in Health and Illness.* Reading, Mass: Addison-Wesley; 1989.

8. Summers C. *Caregiver, Caretaker: From Dysfunctional to Authentic Service in Nursing.* Mount Shasta, Calif: Commune-a-Key; 1992.

9. Wells-Federman C, Stuart E, Deckro J, Mandle CL, Baim M, Medich C. The mind/body connection: The psychophysiology of many traditional nursing interventions. *Clin Nurs Spec.* 1995;9:30–37.

10. Cannon W. The emergency function of the adrenal medulla in pain and the major emotions. *Am J Physiol.* 1914;33:356–372.

11. Cohen S, Tyrrell DA, Smith AP. Psychological stress and susceptibility to the common cold. *N Engl J Med.* 1991;325:606–612.

12. Turner JA, Clancy S, Vitaliano PP. Relationships of stress, appraisal and coping, to chronic low back pain. *Behav Res Ther.* 1987;25:281–288.

13. Hillhouse J, Adler C. Stress, health, and immunity: A review of the literature and implications for the nursing profession. *Holist Nurs Pract.* 1991;5:22–31.

14. Houldin AD, Lev E, Prystowsky MB, Redei E, Lowery BJ. Psychoneuroimmunology: A review of literature. *Holist Nurs Pract.* 1991;5:10–21.

15. Benson H, Stuart E, eds. *The Wellness Book: A Comprehensive Guide to Maintaining Health and Treating Stress-Related Illness.* New York, NY: Simon & Schuster; 1993.

16. Wallace RK, Benson H, Wilson AF. A wakeful hypometabolic physiologic state. *Am J Physiol.* 1971; 221:795–799.

17. Hoffman JW, Benson H, Arns PA, et al. Reduced sympathetic nervous system responsivity associated with the relaxation response. *Science.* 1982;215:190–192.

18. Morrell EM, Hollandsworth JG Jr. Norepinephrine alterations under stress conditions following the regular practice of meditation. *Psychosom Med.* 1986;48:270–277.

19. Stuart E, Deckro J, Mandle CL. Spirituality in health and healing: A clinical program. *Holist Nurs Pract.* 1989;3:35–46.

20. Benson H. *Your Maximum Mind.* New York, NY: Time Books; 1987.

21. Kass JD, Friedman R, Leserman J, Zuttermeister PC, Benson H. Health outcomes and a new index of spiritual experience. *J Sci Stud Relig.* 1991;30:203–211.

22. Gardner DL. Presence. In: Bulecheck GM, McCloskey JC, eds. *Nursing Interventions: Essential Nursing Treatments.* Philadelphia, Pa: Saunders; 1992.

23. Hoblitzelle OA, Benson H. Eliciting the relaxation response. In: Benson H, Stuart E, eds. The *Wellness Book: The Comprehensive Guide to Maintaining Health and Treating Stress-Related Illness.* New York, NY: Simon & Schuster; 1993.

24. Freedman R. *Bodylove.* New York, NY: Harper & Row; 1989.

25. Blair SN. Physical fitness and all cause mortality: A prospective study of healthy men and women. *JAMA.* 1989;262:2395–2401.

26. Blair SN, Kohl HW, Gordon NF, Paffenbarger RS Jr. How much physical activity is good for health? *Annu Rev Public Health.* 1992;13:99–126.

27. Blumenthal J, Williams R, Needels T, Wallace A. Psychological changes accompanying aerobic exercise in healthy middle aged adults. *Psychosom Med.* 1982;44: 529–536.

28. Huddleston JS. Move into health. In: Benson H, Stuart E, eds. *The Wellness Book: The Comprehensive Guide to Maintaining Health and Treating Stress-Related Illness.* New York, NY: Simon & Schuster; 1993.

29. Norbeck J. Coping with stress in critical care nursing: Research findings. *Focus Crit Care.* 1985;12:36–39.

30. Thoreau HD. *Walden.* In: Howarth W, ed. *Walden and Other Writings.* New York, NY: Random House; 1981.

31. Uustal DB. Rx: Holistic caring for the caregiver. In: Dossey BM, Guzetta EE, Kenner CV, eds. *Critical Care Nursing: Body–Mind–Spirit.* Philadelphia, Pa: Lippincott; 1992.

32. US Department of Health, Education and Welfare. *Healthy People: The Surgeon General's Report on Health Promotion and Disease Prevention.* Washington, DC: Government Printing Office; 1979. DHEW publication 7 79-55071.

33. Sullivan LW. Partners in prevention: A mobilization plan for implementing Healthy People 2000. *Am J Health Promot.* 1991;5:291–297.

34. Ingelfinger FJ. Medicine: Meritorious or meretricious. *Science.* 1978;200:942–946.

35. Heidt PR. Effect of therapeutic touch on anxiety level of hospitalized patients. *Nurs Res.* 1981;30:32–37.

36. Quinn JF. Therapeutic touch as energy exchange: Testing the theory. *Adv Nurs Sci.* 1984;6:42–49.

37. Keller E, Bzdek VM. Effects of therapeutic touch on tension headache pain. *Nurs Res.* 1986;35:101–106.

38. Meehan TC. Therapeutic touch and postoperative pain: A Rogerian research study. *Nurs Sci Q.* 1993;6:69–78.

39. Bauer WC, Dracup KA. Physiologic effects of back massage in patients with acute myocardial infarction. *Focus Crit Care.* 1987;14:42–46.

40. Longworth JC. Psychophysiological effects of slow stroke back massage in normotensive females. *Adv Nurs Sci.* 1982;4:44–61.

41. Reed BV, Held JM. Effects of sequential connective tissue massage on autonomic nervous system of middle-aged and elderly adults. *Phys Ther.* 1988;68:1231–1234.

42. Groer M, Mozingo J, Droppleman P, et al. Measures of salivary secretory immunoglobulin A and state anxiety after a nursing back rub. *Appl Nurs Res.* 1994;7:2–6.

43. Lynch JJ. *The Broken Heart: The Medical Consequences of Loneliness.* New York, NY: Basic Books; 1977.

44. Orth-Gomer K, Unden AL, Edwards ME. Social isolation and mortality in ischemic heart disease. A 10-year follow-up study of 150 middle-aged men. *Acta Med Scand.* 1988;224:205–215.

45. Spiegel D, Bloom JR, Kraemer HC, Gottheil E. Effect of psychosocial treatment on survival of patients with metastatic breast cancer. *Lancet.* 1989;2:888–891.

46. Fawzy FI, Fawzi NW, Hyan CS, et al. Malignant melanoma. Effects of an early structured psychiatric intervention, coping, and affective state on recurrence and survival 6 years later. *Arch Gen Psychiatr.* 1993;50:681–689.

47. Frasure-Smith N. Long-term follow-up of ischemic heart disease: Life-style monitoring program. *Psychosom Med.* 1991;51:485–512.

48. Pennebaker JW, Kiecolt-Glaser JK, Glaser R. Disclosure of traumas and immune function: Health implications for psychotherapy. *J Consult Clin Psychol.* 1988;56:239–245.

49. Squier RW. A model of empathic understanding and adherence to treatment regimes in practitioner–patient relationships. *Soc Sci Med.* 1990;30:325–339.

50. Roode J, Rogers ME, eds. *Changing Patterns of Nursing Education.* New York, NY: National League for Nursing; 1987.

Systems Energetics: Holistic Model for Advanced Practice Nursing

Jennifer Jenkins, MBA, RN, CNAA
Principal
Jenkins and Associates
Senior Consultant
Healthcare Concepts, Inc.
Memphis, Tennessee

We know that absence of change is death. Even at rest, living organisms are undergoing small homeostatic changes to preserve balance, equilibrium, and renewal. Change, for many people, is energizing. For others, it is energy depleting. What makes some people welcome and seek change and others avoid it? When does change becomes so overwhelming that it threatens the health and well-being of an individual?

For advanced practice nurses (APNs), many things can threaten personal and professional balance. Health care payers (employers, insurance companies, health maintenance organizations [HMOs]) too often reward providers based on the number of clients seen or procedures done, rather than desired outcomes. This creates a dilemma for a values-driven clinician. Multiple tasks and roles tug at the clinician's ability to organize time and sequence activities effectively. APNs may find themselves working with a physician who is a workaholic and who expects the same from the nurse. Families may not appreciate the work demands of the nurse and may make unrealistic demands on the roles expected of the nurse at home. For the nurse in solo practice, cash flow management may compromise the effectiveness of both personal and professional decisions, minimizing growth opportunities.

Source: Reprinted from J. Jenkins, *Advanced Practice Nursing Quarterly,* Vol. 2, No. 1, pp. 67–74, © 1996, Aspen Publishers, Inc.

The author thanks Nancy Post, PhD, who created Systems Energetics; for her support and mentoring in the use of the model. Dr. Post is president of Post Enterprises, Inc. of Philadelphia, PA.

To maintain balance, the following objectives were mentioned as critical by nearly every APN interviewed by the author:

- a clear purpose and goals
- the ability to utilize effective planning and decision making
- negotiation of roles, responsibilities, expectations, and schedules with coworkers, family, and significant others
- setting priorities, sorting activities, managing time, and focusing effort
- keeping a healthy sense of humor
- using comfortable routines and systems;
- periodically evaluating personal and professional life and "cleaning house"; and
- working and living with others who have similar values, purpose, approaches, and methods

How can one learn to incorporate all these suggestions in a healthy and energizing way? One very effective way is through a health-based model that can be applied to individuals, groups, and systems, called Systems Energetics. The Systems Energetics model stems from Dr. Nancy Post's experience with work groups in multicultural settings and her desire to develop a practical model of healthy functions in organizations (Post, 1993). The model integrates communication and developmental methodologies derived from modern American HR/OD theory while effectively incorporating the tenets and practices from systems in the Far East. The model equates change with healing while acknowledging that change is frequently painful. Applied to groups and communities it follows the normal cycle of organizational life: generation, growth, synergy, stabilization, and completion.

ASSUMPTIONS

This model incorporates several important assumptions

1. Everything is energy.
2. Potential and kinetic energy act in cyclical and complementary relationships.
3. Life is a result of the movement of energy.

Everything is energy

Each person is imbued with a life energy at conception. The Chinese would call this "chi" or "qi." Animate and inanimate objects are made of energy. Energetically then, if energy is life, all matter is alive.

Western culture has a great deal of trouble understanding this approach. It is the dilemma of trying to understand how a machine works by taking it apart and studying the parts. Rather, one can only understand by knowing how the machine interacts with the energy source that drives it. In health care, it is like trying to learn how the brain works by studying its parts. Instead, we need to ask how it interacts with everything else. Energy moves in predictable ways. It can be used and it can be replenished. This is the relationship and balance between potential and kinetic energy.

Potential and kinetic energy act in cyclical and complementary relationships

As individuals progress through life, they consume much of their energy with little regard for the need to replenish. For some, it is a process as brief and explosive as a roman candle. These individuals focus on the outcome, quickly achieve often spectacular results, and then, burn out early. Complete attention to process without outcomes results in stagnation—individuals so caught up in doing that they forget (or never know) their purpose. They just spin their wheels.

Others have learned to conserve and recycle their energy so that they are more in balance. They mellow and age like fine wine. It is obvious to them that to achieve enduring value, they must go through the necessary steps and time to achieve balance.

It is a choice every person must make—outcome, process, or both. It may mean the difference between fleeting success, prolonged and agonizing existence, or thriving and making lasting contributions.

Life requires movement of energy

The principles of energetics require that energy move in order to sustain life. This is not as simple as it may sound. At times energy needs to collect and develop potential. Other times it needs to move and disperse stored energy. Both activities occur simultaneously. This balance is reflected in Western science by the principles of potential and kinetic energy; in China, by the concepts of yin and yang.

Kinetic energy is very easy to see. Just watch a young child, puppy, or kitten play and you will see the vitality and exuberance of this energy. In springtime, new growth shoots out of the earth and flowers burst into bloom. In summer, when life seems to be at its peak, the sun burns its brightest and life seems full and boundless.

Then the children suddenly stop and are content to sleep. Kittens take one of their 90 naps each day. The days grow shorter, the nights longer. Resting is the new paradigm.

Resting gives us the opportunity to replenish depleted energy stores. It allows us time to create patterns and rhythms, which, like habits, take less energy once learned and practiced. It gives us time to reflect on what we like and don't like; what is helpful and what is not; what we want to continue doing and what we want to leave behind. If you

have experienced late summer and fall, you will recognize the slower pace, a gathering in, and the clarity of the air. As leaves begin to color and then fall, we can almost see nature contracting and mobilizing for the long winter ahead.

ENERGY FLOWS

We know that energy flows in our bodies through defined pathways or meridians. Acupuncturists have used this knowledge for years to stimulate and adjust the flow so that no blockages occur or persist that will lead to physical, emotional, and mental signs of imbalance.

Energy flows in predictable patterns, which are cyclical, like the seasons of the year. This cyclical pattern is organized into what is commonly known as the five element model, with energy flowing in a clockwise direction unless impeded (see Figure 1). Kinetic energy dominates the left-hand side and potential energy, the right.

In Chinese cultures metaphors are used to help describe and explain their beliefs. This is like the Westerner's use of right- and left-brain activities to stimulate learning on both sides of

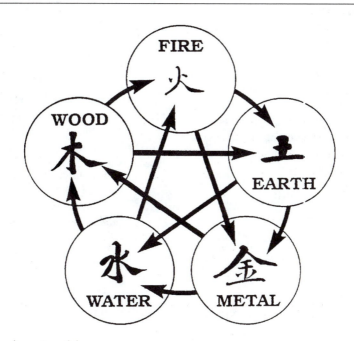

Figure 1. The five element model.

the brain, enhancing and facilitating short- and long-term memory. With this in mind, there are five elements (right brain) and five basic functions (left brain) related to them.

Metaphors for the elements are water, wood, fire, earth, and metal. Functions are generation, growth, synergy, stabilization, and completion.

Water is the metaphor for the uncertainty of beginnings and start-up. Anxiety and fear mix with the excitement of new directions and purpose. Resources are very important to sustain not only this stage but also the journey ahead.

Wood represents growth. New directions, mission, and purpose are developed into plans and visions. Decisions are made so forward movement can occur. As the change becomes more concrete, emotions run high and disagreements are common as each person tries to get his or her agenda included.

With implementation, a lightness comes to the project. Fire represents synergy—a state in which the sum of all the inputs is greater than the sum of each one taken singularly. Synergy results from effective communication, problem-solving, coordination, and control. People often laugh during this phase as they experience the excitement of finally getting the project going and begin to see early results.

Earth takes over as the change becomes more ingrained, more stabilized. Growth is slower and more predictable. Systems (e.g., information systems) and routines simplify the work and make it more predictable, requiring less energy to complete. Productivity, nurturing, and ease of movement are evident. Individuals begin to empathize with each other and appreciate the contribution from each person.

Finally, as the project nears completion, the element of metal exerts itself. We evaluate what we set out to do, whether we did it, and how well it was done. We decide if we were true to our values. We "clean house" by asking what we want to take with us as we move on and what we want to stop doing because it is not helpful. We distill down to the essence of what is important and we grieve the ending of one cycle even as we anticipate a new one.

USING SYSTEMS ENERGETICS IN SETTING UP AND MANAGING YOUR PRACTICE

Systems Energetics is a model that can be used to guide and track your practice. It follows nature's change cycles and reflects healthy business practices. Energy moves in a clockwise direction. Elements feed the next one and drain the one behind. Each element crosses the cycle to control excesses in another (e.g., wood controls earth, water controls fire). Seasons are associated with each element and activities related to that element often take less energy when done in the corresponding season (see the box entitled "Seasons and the Five Elements").

Water element

Water is the element of generation, beginning life, drive.

Many of us sit in January with the seed catalogues and think about the garden we are sure we will plant. This is analogous to the energetic element of water, which begins with reflection and moves to action. It is about assessing resources, allocating them, and deciding on a direction or mission.

When you first start into practice, you may feel you have too many choices and not enough resources to do them all. You have to decide upon a specific goal and then search the job market for the right position. You may make many lists—revising, adding, and deleting before you feel comfortable with your decision. For some of you, the ambiguity is too much and the first defined, structured position available is accepted.

Seasons and the Five Elements

Water	Winter
Wood	Spring
Fire	Summer
Earth	Late summer
Metal	Autumn

Others get excited negotiating an individualized job description with a variety of opportunities and much more ambiguity.

Once you have accepted a position, a period of waiting occurs until you actually start work. What happens in the waiting? Do you worry is this the right job? Will I have the time to do this? What if I don't like it? What if I can't do this? What if they don't think I am right for the job? Will I have wasted money or time?

Ambiguity may cause you to grow disenchanted, and by the time you start, your anxiety may prevent you from mobilizing the energy to do a good job. For those better able to "go with the flow" the time of waiting is one of growing anticipation and planning that explodes in activity once you start work.

The water stage feels like being dropped in the middle of the ocean. You can't touch bottom and you can't see land. The questions will be: Can I find shore? Will I be able to swim to safety? What can I hold on to? Will I survive? All these questions have an element of fear associated with them, which is the emotion of the water element.

People in this energy over long periods experience anxiety, depression, and withdrawal. Getting out of bed is nearly impossible. Normal activities sap strength. Opportunities are rejected because there is insufficient energy to take advantage of them.

Those of you who started a new practice probably experienced a degree of anxiety, if only for a short time. Changes in reimbursement, family commitments, work arrangements all may trigger a degree of fear. When you mobilize your resources and get clarity on what is most important, you move out of fear and into action. You make the necessary transition to the next element, wood.

Wood element

Returning to the garden analogy, you have received your seeds and it is now warm enough to plant. For weeks you have read the weather forecasts and readied your garden tools. You plotted out the garden on graph paper and have measured and tilled the garden. Your mind can picture the garden as it will become in summer. You just can't wait to get your hands dirty, and your first day out, you work until exhausted.

This is wood energy. Focused, planned, with a vision for the future and the necessary decisions made. It is a kinetic time. It is like school-age children who play for hours in the surf and build castles in the sand.

Action—this is truly the byword of the wood element—visioning, planning, delineating roles, and making decisions. It is a time when differences of opinion are evident and anger (or frustration) is the characteristic emotion.

As you develop your practice, you begin to see new opportunities and have a clearer sense of how you want your practice to develop. You are excited and eagerly anticipate making the changes necessary to "grow" your practice. As your plan develops, you begin to make decisions about how you will proceed, and then you meet the roadblocks.

Your partner disagrees; your family resents the amount of time it will take from them; the reimbursement institutions deny payment; HMOs expect you to see a higher volume of patients. You experience the anger and frustration of the wood element.

However, just as mighty trees weather storms if they are healthy and flexible, so can you. View obstacles as opportunities. Examine your options, get other opinions, rearrange your plan in creative ways to find newer and better ways of reaching your goal. If you insist on rigidity, you may break. Pick and choose your battles. Fight on principle, but give and take on process. The old adage is true—there is more than one way to reach any goal.

Fire element

By remaining flexible, you can mobilize your energy and move into the element of fire for many of your solutions. The fire element function is to develop synergy through negotiating, networking, marketing, coordinating, sorting, and problem solving. Humor and laughter are essential components of fire energy and go a long way in draining off the anger and frustration you may feel in the growth (wood) phase.

As you negotiate with family and coworkers you can find win-win solutions that respect the needs of all. Communicating openly with everyone will keep intentions clear and misunderstandings at a minimum. Working together as a team will enhance the synergy needed for this phase of your development. By pooling ideas and talent, you will be able to achieve much more than if each of you worked separately.

When you have worked comfortably in this phase long enough to be effective, it will be easy to move into earth energy.

Earth element

Picture yourself during the "dog days" of summer. It is hot and the air is thick with humidity. Grass and gardens are growing slower and you move more slowly. Sipping lemonade under a fan while swinging back and forth on the swing is heaven. Life goes on as you sit and reflect. Things seem to all be fitting together and you are vaguely aware of the rhythms of nature. You barely exert the energy to notice a fat bee buzzing at the flowers at your feet.

Your practice has flowered and has become almost routine. You balance home and work with an ease that often surprises. You manage time, resources, and activities with a minimum of effort. You have office systems in place that automate much of your work. Your routine is comfortable, not monotonous. Clients and coworkers relax in your presence and sense both your confidence and competence. You are able to empathize with them but draw a line that permits you to remain your own person. You have begun the process of "cleaning house," both personally and professionally so that you have room for new directions that you feel are coming soon. Life is good. This is earth energy at its strongest, and it is preparing you for the final stage of this cycle, metal.

Metal element

Your practice has been fulfilling, and yet. . . .

You are in the autumn phase of your practice. Just as cold winter nights drain the leaves and leave the colorful metallic elements that are so beautiful in the crystal clear sun of the shortening days, so it is time for reflection and clarification in your life.

You clearly sense the need to strip it down to essential components and to free yourself for new opportunities that will require much reflection and thought. Is this the practice you wish to continue? What aspects would you like to keep? To leave behind? Where will you go next? What new experiences, education, and resources will you need?

You feel a mixture of sadness about this phase ending and a certain happiness at what you have achieved, and, yet, there is a degree of anxiety and excitement about beginning a new phase. You take a deep breath and begin anew.

ENERGETICS, HEALTH, AND YOU

Systems Energetics is a natural way of working with your career and your personal life.

In the beginning of this article, several things were identified by APNs as being essential to staying balanced in both their personal and professional lives. Systems Energetics provides a simple way of knowing what needs to be done at each stage of change so that your energy moves forward at a sustainable pace.

During generation, water energy slowly builds and bursts into kinetic energy as it makes the transitions to growth or wood energy and then to fire or synergetic energy. It is during the fire stage that energy flows begin to slow, not unlike a fire with glowing embers. Reflection and renewal become more important as the transition to earth and finally metal occur. By gathering in and becoming more efficient, one gains the reserve energy to evaluate and set out in new directions. Let us see how each of the suggestions fit into the model.

Clear purpose and goals (water element)

Having a clear purpose and goals is like having your ship's compass focused on your destination. No matter what winds blow or problems arise, you can always get back on course if you know the proper coordinates of your destination.

Know what you want to achieve and keep that goal in front of you. Post it in your office; put it in your calendar. Review your resources to ensure that you have what you need to be successful. This may be time, cash flow, reserves, skills, support systems, people, or space. Be sure that your resources are present and properly allocated. Know how to access additional resources if needed.

If you experience difficulty in managing the energy in this phase of developing your business, you may feel thirsty, fearful, passive, aimless, lack clarity, or experience back pain. It may seem that you have trouble hearing people's responses or their messages are confusing (almost like how sounds are distorted under water). Any of these, or several together, should trigger the question from earth energy, "What do I need to feel more confident?" (see Figure 1). Determining how to take care of yourself contains your fear and allows you the footing (ground, earth) to collect the power to move forward. Another approach is to use the wood element to drain excess water. Asking, "What needs to be done next so I can get started?" begins the growth phase of wood.

Ability to utilize effective planning and decision making (wood element)

Have a workable plan that takes your purpose and goals and gives them detail or vision. Your goal may be to set up a clinic for unwed mothers. Resources may include grants, fund raisers, interested and talented staff, a vacant building, and a network of supporters.

Your plan or vision will develop all the details necessary to make your venture work—action plans, timetables, assignments, start date, procedures and policies, and job descriptions. Decisions will have to be made to put it all into action. They should be timely and made with confidence so that you do not agonize over them.

Negotiation of roles, responsibilities, expectations, schedules, etc., with co-workers, family, and significant others (wood to fire element)

For any successful venture involving more than one person, synergy is desirable. That is, achieving a greater outcome by working effectively together than could be achieved by each working solo. To do this one must communicate, negotiate, coordinate, sort, control, and solve problems.

As your practice grows, you will experience differences of opinion and problems will arise, both anticipated and unanticipated. Left unresolved, you can become stuck in wood energy. This can manifest in one-sided headaches, tautness and rigidity, eye strain, or excessive or suppressed anger. If you feel any of these sensations, ask, "What values are driving my decisions?" This question, coming from metal energy, permits you to stay true to those things most central to you (see Figure 1). By ensuring that your decisions are principle based, you will be more consistent and able to determine where you can negotiate and where you need to stand firm. Others will respond with respect and you will have a sense of who you are.

To continue the growth of your practice, communication within the business must be matched with effective marketing outside. Ask your patients/clients what they need and develop products and services to meet their needs. If your professional coworkers have different expectations than you, you must air both views and find win-win solutions. Find out what your partner needs, identify what you need, and find common ground. Respect the needs of your family and negotiate roles and responsibilities that are acceptable to all.

Setting priorities, sorting activities, managing time, focusing effort (fire element)

As your practice grows, begin to set priorities and sort activities. For example, which of your activities are essential, nice to do, and nonessential? Which can be done by someone else? How can you organize your time to focus on what is most important? Which activities can be grouped together so that they can be accomplished in less time?

Without the discipline these questions trigger, your practice may resemble a wildfire out of control and burning up your energy. If you feel dry, frantic, unable to sit still, tired, suffer from insomnia, your heart races or skips beats, or your blood pressure is high, you may be suffering from imbalance in your fire energy.

Perhaps the most important question to ask when you are feeling burned out is, "What is my goal (purpose, mission)?" By using this question from water energy, you can more effectively control the activity of your fire energy (see Figure 1). Another solution is to draw excess fire energy to earth. A question to do this might be, "How can I make this system more predictable (stable) and productive?" By doing this, you begin the reflective (potential) side of the cycle. You are controlling the activity of your practice by beginning to fine tune through evaluation and adjustment.

Keeping a healthy sense of humor (fire element)

Perhaps one of the best ways to stay healthy is to have a great sense of humor. Laughter is characteristic of fire energy. It can be used to drain excess wood energy, allowing you to move to fire. Alternatively it can be used to soften the sharpness of metal energy, which can be hypercritical, overly hierarchical, or morose. It helps you balance the serious nature of your business with a healthy respect for the relative insignificance of this moment in the continuum of eternity.

Healthy humor is not used in abusive or hurtful ways, but seeks to find the absurdity and make it lighter so that it can be corrected or eliminated. Humor prevents deterioration. It is said that for every 15 minutes a day of laughter, you add an hour to your life. The field of psychoneuroimmunology is demonstrating the positive impact humor has on the immune system. So go ahead . . . laugh! You may find you will have more time to do all the wonderful things you want to do.

Using comfortable routines and systems (earth element)

Earth energy is evident when your practice has reached a degree of maturity and you are enjoying the opportunity to have more time to explore new possibilities. This is done in a languid way. That is, as opportunities present themselves, you leisurely explore them. You probably will not take full advantage of all of them, but will choose only those that are fun and fulfill your greater mission.

You will have systems in place that automate some aspects of your practice—information systems, scheduling systems, reminder postcards for patients' appointments, or an excellent office manager. Your freed time will be involved with many charity activities that bring value to you and to those you consider important.

The danger in this phase is to become enamored of systems to the exclusion of outcomes or to find yourself tending too much to the needs of others and not enough to yourself. This will be likely if you experience sudden changes in weight, excessive feelings of sympathy and worry, muscle weakness, poor concentration, a strong sweet tooth, or apathy.

Often in this case, it is helpful to use the controlling element, wood, to trigger movement. Key questions would be, "What is the plan and what decisions do I need to make?" If this does not seem to help, perhaps draining excess earth energy to metal can be accomplished by asking,

"What of this is helpful or not helpful? What do I need to keep (stop) doing?" This house-cleaning set of questions makes room for you to do what is most important and keeps energy moving forward, although at a slower pace than on the left side of the cycle.

Periodically evaluating personal and professional life and "cleaning house" (metal element)

At some point in any change, whether it be personal or professional, there comes a time for closure. At its healthiest, the metal energy phase is characterized by the ability to evaluate results critically and objectively. There is an ability and readiness to eliminate work, ideas, or job categories that are no longer helpful to the mission and purpose. This is done cleanly, with compassion and foresight.

You feel restless and are ready to move on.

It may be to a new practice or position, or it may simply be time to evaluate where you are, refine it, and continue on. In either case, you may experience a mixture of sadness that this phase is ending and an excitement or anxiety about moving on.

If you linger too long in this phase, the metallic energy can manifest in exacerbation of allergies or asthma, excessive or deficient grief over attention to details and evaluation procedures, a need for hierarchy, and a sense of isolationism. Bringing the heat of fire energy (see Figure 1) to the picture by asking, "What is important and what is not?" or "How can we lighten this up?" may take the edge off. A good joke, going to a funny movie may be helpful. Or drain off excess energy by asking, "How can we use what we have learned to start a new project?" or "What resources do we have that we can use to help this other group?"

Endings are beginnings, beginnings are endings. Keeping that thought is very important as you balance the need to achieve closure with the need to be sensitive to the feelings of those involved. If you close your practice, it may be a wonderful new beginning for you—retirement or a new practice, but for your employees it may mean job insecurity or lack of financial resources. Your patients will need reassurance that they will have the same care from the new practitioner and that they can trust the two of you to communicate the necessary information so care is seamless.

Working and living with others who have similar values, purpose, approach, methods

Finally, Systems Energetics is a health-based holistic model. By living and working with others who share values, purpose, approach, and methods, you can begin to build a wonderful practice and life. This is only part of the answer.

The secret is to recognize that holistic health is dynamic. Too much familiarity will cause stagnation. Differences of opinion, style, process all are vital to the continued evolution of our systems. Therefore, always include people who may not share the same values, purpose, approach, and methods. The diversity of the two will enrich you and keep you vital.

CHANGE IS LIFE

In health there is a dynamic balance that self-corrects and energizes. There is time for both the energy expenditure required of the water-wood-fire half of the cycle, as well as the renewal of the fire-earth-metal side. Both are necessary. When one or the other is out of balance, adjusting the energy flow can ensure health.

Change is life.

Knowing how to recognize and work with the phases of change may be the difference between life and death; certainly between health and disease. Systems Energetics is a natural, healthy way of incorporating change into your career and your personal life. By paying attention to your body, the cycles of nature, and common sense, you will welcome change and stay balanced, healthy, and vital.

REFERENCE

Post, N. (1993). *Elements of organization.* Philadelphia, PA:
Post Enterprises.

SUGGESTED READING

Beinfield, H., & Korngold, E. (1991). *Between heaven and earth.* New York, NY: Ballentine Books.

Chia, M., & Chia, M. (1989). *Fusion of the five elements I.* Huntington, NY: Healing Tao Books.

Kaptchuk, T.J. (1983). *The web that has no weaver.* New York, NY: Congdon & Weed.

Humor: An Antidote for Stress

Patty Wooten, BSN, RN, CCRN
Founder and President
Jest for the Health of It Services
Davis, California

Source: Reprinted from P. Wooten, *Holistic Nursing Practice,* Vol. 10, No. 2, pp. 49–56, © 1996, Aspen Publishers, Inc.

Humor is a quality of perception that enables us to experience joy even when faced with adversity. Stress is an adverse condition during which we may experience tension or fatigue, feel unpleasant emotions, and sometimes develop a sense of hopelessness or futility.[1–3] Nurses work in stress-filled environments that place demands upon their physical, emotional, and spiritual well-being.[1,3–5] Responding to these demands while protecting ourselves from their potentially harmful impact will help us remain healthy. This article describes the therapeutic consequences of using humor as a self-care tool to cope with stress. It describes research showing that humor can stimulate the immune system, enhance perceptual flexibility, and renew spiritual energy.

Selye,[6] a pioneer researcher in psychosomatic medicine, defined stress as the rate of wear and tear within the body as it adapts to change or threat. Chronic exposure to job stress can lead to burnout, which Maslach defines as "a syndrome of emotional exhaustion and cynicism that occurs frequently among individuals who do 'people work' of some kind."[1(p3)]

Nurses are compassionate and caring individuals working with people who are suffering; and thus they are at risk for job stress and burnout. We may have feelings of failure when our efforts are ineffective, anger and frustration arise when patients reject our care or are noncompliant with treatment, and we feel grief when patients die.[7] The constant experience of these emotions leads to stressful changes within our body. Finding humor in a situation and laughing freely with others can be a powerful antidote to stress. Our sense of humor gives us the ability to find delight, experience joy, and release tension.[8] This can be an effective self-care tool.

HISTORICAL PERSPECTIVE ON HUMOR AND HEALTH

Humor is a word of many meanings. It derives from the Latin word *umor*, meaning liquid or fluid. In the Middle Ages, humor referred to an energy that was thought to relate to a body fluid and an emotional state. This energy was believed to determine health and disposition (eg, "He's in a bad humor").[9] A sanguine humor was cheerful and associated with blood. A choleric humor was angry and associated with bile. A phlegmatic humor was apathetic and associated with mucous. A melancholic humor was depressed and associated with black bile.[10] In modern dictionaries, *humor* is defined as "the quality of being laughable or comical" or as "a state of mind, mood, spirit." Humor, then, is flowing, involving basic characteristics of the individual and expressed in the body, emotions, and spirit.

The word *heal* comes from the Anglo-Saxon word *hælen*," which means "to make whole." Bringing together the body, mind, and spirit can be healing. As Socrates once commented on the medical theory of his day, "As it is not proper to cure the eyes without the head, nor the head without the body; so neither is it proper to cure the body without the soul."[10]

HUMOR AND EFFECT ON THE SPIRIT

In the Christian tradition, the soul is the cradle of the spirit. Spirit can be defined as the vital essence or animating force of a living organism; often it is considered divine in origin. This energy is referred to as *ch'i* in the Chinese tradition and as *ki* in the Japanese tradition. It can be visualized with Kirlian photography or felt during the application of healing touch. Spirit can be influenced by the feelings of joy, hope, and love.[2] The experience of laughter momentarily banishes feelings of anger and fear and provides moments of feeling carefree, lighthearted, and hopeful.[11]

When the spirit is depleted, nurses can experience what is known as compassion fatigue, a feeling that they have little left to give.[1,12] Usually this occurs when the nurse's self-care program has been inadequate. Finding humor in our work and our life can be one way to lift the spirit's energy level and replenish ourselves from compassion fatigue.[13–15]

NORMAN COUSINS' EXPERIENCE LEADS TO MODERN RESEARCH

Norman Cousins first called the attention of the medical community to the potential therapeutic effects of humor and laughter in 1979, when he described his utilization of laughter during his treatment for ankylosing spondylitis.[11] Believing that negative emotions had a negative impact on his health, he theorized that the opposite was also true: that positive emotions would have a positive effect. He believed that the experience of laughter could open him to feelings of joy, hope, confidence, and love. Cousins spent the last 12 years of his life at the University of California at Los Angeles Medical School in the Department of Behavioral Medicine exploring the scientific proof of his belief. He established the Humor Research Task Force, which coordinated and supported worldwide clinical research on humor.[2]

Cousins, although one of the best known proponents of using positive emotions to improve health, was certainly not the first to assert such a relationship. As early as the 1300s, Henri de Mondeville, professor of surgery, wrote "Let the surgeon take care to regulate the whole regimen of the patient's life for joy and happiness, allowing his relatives and special friends to cheer him, and by having someone tell him jokes."[16(pp147–148)] The difference is that we now have scientific studies of that relationship.

HUMOR AND LAUGHTER AFFECT THE BODY

Stress has been shown to create unhealthy physiologic changes. The connection between stress and high blood pressure, muscle tension, immunosuppression, and many other changes has been known for years.[17] We now have proof that laughter creates the opposite effects. It appears to be the perfect antidote for stress.

Berk,[17,18] at Loma Linda University School of Medicine's Department of Clinical Immunology, has conducted carefully controlled studies showing that the experience of laughter lowers serum cortisol levels, increases the amount of activated T lymphocytes, increases the number and activity of natural killer cells, and increases the number of T cells that have helper/suppressor receptors. In short, laughter stimulates the immune system, offsetting the immunosuppressive effects of stress.

This research is part of the rapidly expanding field of psychoneuroimmunology, which defines the communication links and relationships between our emotional experience and our immune response as mediated by the neurologic system.[19–21] For example, we know that during stress the adrenal gland releases corticosteroids (which are quickly converted to cortisol in the bloodstream) and that elevated levels of these have an immunosuppressive effect. Berk's research demonstrates that laughter can lower cortisol levels and thereby protect our immune system.[17,18] Activation of T cells provides lymphocytes that are awakened and ready to combat a potential foreign substance. Natural killer cells are a type of immune cell that attacks viral or cancerous cells and does not need sensitization to be lethal. These cells are always ready to recognize and attack an aberrant or infected cell. This becomes important in the prevention of cancer. Cells within our bodies are constantly changing and mutating to produce potentially carcinogenic cells. An intact immune system can function appropriately by mobilizing these natural killer cells to destroy abnormal cells.[22]

Receptor sites are important as a communication link between the brain and the immune system. Emotions can trigger the release of neurotransmitters from neurons in the brain. These chemicals then enter the bloodstream and "plug into" receptor sites on the surface of an immune cell. When this occurs, the cell's metabolic activity can be altered in either a positive or a negative direction.[23] Many cells within the body have different receptor sites on their surface; of particular interest in this research are those sites on the immune cells.[24]

Other investigators have supported these findings. Locke,[22] at Harvard, showed that the activity of natural killer cells was decreased during periods of increased life change that were accompanied by severe emotional disturbance, whereas subjects with similar patterns of life change and less emotional disturbances had more normal levels of natural killer cell activity. At the VA Medical Center in San Diego in 1987, Irwin and colleagues[25] noted that natural killer cell activity decreased during depressive reactions to life changes. At the Ohio State University School of Medicine, Glaser[26] and Glaser[27] studied the cellular immunity response patterns of medical students before examinations. Their work showed a reduction in the number of helper T cells and a lowered activity of the natural killer cell during the highly anxious moments just before the examination.

Salivary immunoglobulin A (IgA) is our first-line defense against the entry of infectious organisms through the respiratory tract.[28] At the State University of New York at Stony Brook, Stone et al[29] revealed that the salivary IgA response level was lower on days of negative mood and higher on days with positive mood. This finding was quickly confirmed by two other groups of investigators. Dillon and Baker,[30] working at Western New England College, found that subjects showed an increased concentration of salivary IgA after viewing a humorous video; while Lefcourt and coworkers,[31] from the University of Waterloo in Ontario, showed that subjects who tested strong for appreciation and utilization of humor had an even stronger elevation of salivary IgA after viewing a humorous video.

All this research, done in the last 10 years, helps us understand the mind–body connections. The emotions and moods we experience directly affect our immune system. A sense of humor allows us to perceive and appreciate the incongruities of life and provides moments of joy and delight. These positive emotions can create neurochemical changes that will buffer the immunosuppressive effects of stress. Laughter can provide a cathartic release, a purifying of emotions, and a release of emotional tension. Laughter, crying, raging, and trembling are all cathartic activities that can unblock energy flow.[32]

HUMOR AND THE EFFECT ON THE MIND

Selye[33] clarified that a person's interpretation of stress is not solely dependent on an external event; it also depends upon his or her perception of the event and the meaning that he or she gives it. In other words, how you look at a situation determines whether you will respond to it as threatening or challenging.[3,34–36]

Because different people respond differently to the same environmental stimuli, some people seem to cope with stress better than others.[1,4,12] Kobassa[35,36] has defined three hardiness factors that can increase a person's resilience to stress and prevent burnout: commitment, control, and challenge. If you have a strong commitment to yourself and your work, if you believe that you are in control of the choices in your life (internal locus of control), and if you see change as challenging rather than threatening, then you are more likely to cope successfully with stress.[34] One theme that is becoming more prominent in the literature is the idea that a causative factor in burnout is a sense of powerlessness.[1]

In this context, humor can be an empowerment tool. Humor gives us a different perspective on our problems, and, with an attitude of detachment, we feel a sense of self-protection and control in our environment.[37,38] As comedian Bill Cosby is fond of saying, "If you can laugh at it, you can survive it."

HUMOR AND LOCUS OF CONTROL

It is reasonable to assume that if locus of control measures strongly as internal, that a person will feel a greater sense of power and thus be more likely to avoid burnout.[5,35] Research presented in 1990 at the 8th International Conference on Humor in England documented changes in locus of control and appreciation of humor related to a humor training course.[5] Using the Adult Nowicki-Strickland Scale,[39] with proven reliability and validity studies, Wooten assessed the locus of control in 231 nurses in Pennsylvania, Kentucky, and California. She then administered Svebak's Sense of Humor Questionnaire,[40] using only the subscales that have been proved to be reliable and valid. The experimental group then completed a 6-hour humor training course; subjects were given permission and techniques for appropriate use of humor with patients and coworkers. The control group had no such humor training. The same survey tools were then readministered to each group 6 weeks later to determine changes in locus of control and appreciation of humor.

Using the Wilcoxon matched pairs signed-ranks test, Wooten found that there was a significant decrease in the measure for external locus of control in the experimental group ($P = 0.0063$, two-tailed t test). Using the same analysis for the control group, she found no significant change. Wooten also examined the potential difference in initial locus of control scores between the experimental and control groups using the Mann-Whitney U test and the Kolmogorov-Smirnov test and found no significant differences between the two groups.

This study indicates that, if one is encouraged and guided to use humor, one can gain a sense of control in one's life. Use of humor represents what Kobassa[35] calls cognitive control. We may not be able to control events in our external world, but we

Humor Resources

American Association for Therapeutic Humor
222 Meramec, Suite 303
St Louis, MO 63105
(314) 863-6232
  Networking source for application of humor in caregiving professions; excellent bimonthly newsletter and annual conference.

A Chance To Cut Is a Chance To Cure
Rip Pfeiffer, MD
171 Louiselle Street
Mobile, AL 36607
  A funny book about medicine, surgery, hospitals, and patients written by a cardiovascular surgeon (price: $5.00).

Chordiac Arrest
527 East Third Street
Lockport, IL 60441
  Barbershop quartet of physicians singing funny songs about medicine (audiotape: $10.00).

Clown Camp
c/o University of Wisconsin at La Crosse
1725 State Street
La Crosse, WI 54601
(608) 785-6505
  Clown training, week-long intensives, traveling camp.

Clown Supplies
c/o M.E. Persson
17 Chesley Drive
Barrington, NH 03825
(603) 664-5111
  Catalog sales of a wide variety of clown supplies, props, and gags.

Humor and Health Letter
PO Box 16814
Jackson, MS 39236-6814
(601) 957-0075
  Excellent newsletter about laughter research and applications; published bimonthly for $25/year.

Humor Project
110 Spring Street
Saratoga Springs, NY 12866
(518) 587-8770
  Publishes *Laughing Matters*, a quarterly journal; excellent catalog of humor books.

In Your Face Cards
4091 Splendor Way
Salt Lake City, UT 84124
(800) 377-8878
  Hilarious cards, calendars, and T-shirts with hospital humor.

Incomplete ICU Nurse's Disorientation Guide
JANE Press
12088 Anderson Road, Suite 114
Tampa, FL 33625
  Hilarious guidebook for all nurses, written by Jane McKay (price: $5.00).

Jest for the Health of It Services
c/o Patty Wooten
PO Box 4040
Davis, CA 95617
(916) 758-3826 (voice)
(916) 753-7638 (fax)
jestpatty@mother.com
  Presentations about humor and laughter for health professionals; consultation for creating humor programs and laughter libraries.

Journal of Nursing Jocularity
Doug Fletcher, RN, Publisher
PO Box 40416
Mesa, AZ 85274
(602) 835-6165
73314.3032@compuserve.com
  Hilarious quarterly publication about the funny side of nursing; subscriptions: 5615 Cermak Road, Cicero, IL 60650-2290 ($14.95/year).

Nursing Notes
c/o Larry Brennan, RN
253 Winthrop Road
Syracuse, NY 13206
(315) 463-8971
  Barbershop quartet of nurses singing funny songs about hospitals and nursing (audiotape: $10.00).

Too Live Nurse
PO Box 201
Canaan, NY 12029
  Audiotape of funny songs about dysrhythmias and advanced cardiac life support protocols (price: $17.00).

Whole Mirth Catalog
1034 Page Street
San Francisco, CA 94117
  Catalog with many humorous items, toys, gags, and books.

have the ability to control how we view these events and the emotional response we choose to have to them.[3] Further research is needed to determine how long these effects persist.

Humor perception involves the whole brain and serves to integrate and balance activity in both hemispheres. Derks, at the College of William and Mary in Williamsburg, Virginia, has shown that there is a unique pattern of brain wave activity during the perception of humor.[41] Electroencephalograms were recorded on subjects while they were presented with humorous material. During the setup to the joke, the cortex's left hemisphere began its analytic function of processing words. Shortly afterward, most of the brain activity moved to the frontal lobe, which is the center of emotionality. Moments later the right hemisphere's synthesis capabilities joined with the left's processing to find the pattern, to "get the joke." A few milliseconds later, before the subject had enough time to laugh, the increased brain wave activity spread to the occipital lobe, the sensory processing area of the brain. The increased fluctuations in delta waves reached a crescendo of activity and crested as the brain "got" the joke and the external expression of laughter began. Derks' findings shows that humor pulls the various parts of the brain together rather than activating a component in only one area.

LEARNING TO LAUGH

How does one go about laughing? How can one get that humor perspective that can so affect the spirit, body, and mind? How does a nurse learn to access the lighter side of the self in the often tragic world of nursing?

Laughing at yourself is not always easy. Frequently one is too immersed in a problem to find any humor in it. It can help to seek out people with that special flair for seeing the funny side of a situation, to use the available talent to aid one in the quest for laughter and comic release.

There are many great resources for nursing humor (see the box). One of the best is the quarterly *Journal of Nursing Jocularity*. Subscribing to the journal will give you the opportunity to read true stories of hilarious nursing encounters as well as cartoons, parodies, jokes, reviews of humorous books, and interviews with professional humorists. The journal also holds an annual conference on humor skills for health professionals.

Another way to keep ourselves laughing is to stay in touch with our "inner clown," that playful, childlike nature that we all have but perhaps fail to acknowledge because of the seriousness of our work. Many resources and training programs exist. One can even go so far as actually to become a professional clown.

Humor and laughter can be effective self-care tools to cope with stress. They can improve the function of the body, the mind, and the spirit. An ability to laugh at our situation or problem gives us a feeling of superiority and power. Humor and laughter can foster a positive and hopeful attitude. We are less likely to succumb to feelings of depression and helplessness if we are able to laugh at what is troubling us. Humor gives us a sense of perspective on our problems. Laughter provides an opportunity for the release of uncomfortable emotions that, if held inside, may create biochemical changes that are harmful to the body.

People can increase their beneficial laughter by adding exposure to humorous material. Caregivers can consciously change their behaviors to provide more laughter and cheer in their work settings. Humor resources are plentiful. Laughter training exists. We *can* become our own best medicine.

REFERENCES

1. Maslach C. *Burnout—The Cost of Caring*. Englewood Cliffs, NJ: Prentice-Hall; 1982.

2. Cousins N. *Head First—The Biology of Hope*. New York, NY: Dutton; 1989.

3. Seligman M. *Helplessness*. New York, NY: Freeman; 1975.

4. Keane A. "Stress in ICU and non ICU nurses." *Nurs Res*. 1985;34:231–236.

5. Wooten P. Does a humor workshop affect nurse burnout? *J Nurs Jocularity*. 1992;2:42–43.

6. Selye H. *The Stress of Life*. New York, NY: McGraw-Hill; 1956.

7. Montgomery C. *Healing through Communication*. Newbury Park, Calif: Sage; 1993.

8. Lefcourt H, Martin R. *Humor and Life Stress*. New York, NY: Springer-Verlag; 1986.

9. Wooten P. Laughter as therapy for patient and caregiver. In: Hodgkin J, Connors G, Bell C, eds. *Pulmonary Rehabilitation*. Philadelphia, Pa: Lippincott; 1993.

10. Moody R. *Laugh after Laugh*. Jacksonville, Fla: Headwaters; 1978.

11. Cousins N. *Anatomy of an Illness*. New York, NY: Norton; 1979.

12. McCranie E. Work stress, hardiness, and burnout among hospital staff nurses. *Nurs Res*. 1987;36:374–378.

13. Robinson V. *Humor and the Health Professions*. 2nd ed. Thorofare, NJ: Slack; 1991.

14. Wooten P. Interview with Sandy Ritz. *J Nurs Jocularity*. 1995;5:46–47.

15. Ritz S. Survivor humor and disaster nursing. In: Buxman K, ed. *Humor and Nursing*. Staten Island, NY: Power Publications; 1995.

16. Walsh J. *Laughter and Health*. New York, NY: Appleton; 1928.

17. Berk L. Neuroendocrine and stress hormone changes during mirthful laughter. *Am J Med Sci*. 1989;298: 390–396.

18. Berk L. Eustress of mirthful laughter modifies natural killer cell activity. *Clin Res*. 1989;37:115.

19. Ader R. *Psychoneuroimmunology*. New York, NY: Academic Press; 1991.

20. Soloman G. Psychoneuroimmunology: Interactions between the central nervous system and the immune system. *J Neurosci Res*. 1987;18:1–9.

21. Guillemin R, Cohn M, Melnechuk T. *Neural Modulation of Immunity*. New York, NY: Raven; 1985.

22. Locke SE. Life change stress, psychiatric symptoms, and natural killer cell activity. *Psychosom Med*. 1984;6:441–453.

23. Pert CB, Ruff MR, Weber RJ, Herkenham M. Neuropeptides and their receptors: A psycho-somatic network. *J Immunol*. 1985;35:820s–826s.

24. Berk L. Interview with JR Dunn. *Humor Health Lett*. 1994;3:1–8.

25. Irwin M, Daniels M, Bloom E, Smith T, Weiner H. Life events, depressive symptoms, and immune function. *Am J Psychiatr*. 1987;144:437–441.

26. Glaser JK. Psychosocial moderators of immune function. *J Behav Med*. 1987;9:16–20.

27. Glaser R. Stress-related impairments in cellular immunity. *Psychiatr Resident*. 1985;16:233–239.

28. Martin RA, Dobbin JP. Sense of humor, hassles, and immunoglobulin A: Evidence for a stress-moderating effect of humor. *Int J Psychiatr Med*. 1985;18:93–105.

29. Stone A, Cox DS, Neale JM, Valdimarsdottir H, Jandorf L. Evidence that secretory IgA antibody is associated with daily mood. *J Pers Soc Psychol*. 1987;52:988–993.

30. Dillon K, Baker K. Positive emotional states and enhancement of the immune system. *Int J Psychiatr Med*. 1985;5:13–18.

31. Lefcourt H, Davidson-Katz K, Kueneman K. Humor and immune system functioning. *Int J Humor Res*. 1990;3:305–321.

32. Goodheart A. *Laughter Therapy*. Santa Barbara, Calif: Stress Less Press; 1994.

33. Selye H. *Stress without Distress*. New York, NY: Lippincott & Crowell; 1974 .

34. Lefcourt HM. *Locus of Control: Current Trends in Theory and Research*. Hillsdale, NJ: Erlbaum; 1982.

35. Kobassa SC. Personality and social resources in stress resistance. *J Pers Soc Psychol*. 1983;45:839–850.

36. Kobassa SC, Maddi SR. *The Hardy Executive: Health and Stress*. Homewood, Ill: Dow-Jones Irwin; 1984.

37. Klein A. *Healing Power of Humor*. Los Angeles, Calif: Tarcher; 1989.

38. McGhee P. How To Develop Your Sense of Humor. Dubuque, Iowa: Kendall-Hunt; 1994.

39. Nowicki S. A locus of control scale for college as well as non-college adults. *J Pers Assess*. 1974;38:136–137.

40. Svebak S. Revised questionnaire on the sense of humor. *Scand J Psychol*. 1974;15:328–331.

41. Dunn JR. Interview with P. Derks. *Humor Health Lett*. 1992;4:1–7.

Humor: A Missing Ingredient in Collaborative Practice

Julia W. Balzer, MN, RN
Independent Consultant
Staff Educator
Training and Development
Baptist Medical Center
Jacksonville, Florida

Roses are red
Violets are blue
I have this problem . . .
and so do you!

Humor with positive intent can be a nondefensive, creative way to set the stage for effective communication and problem solving between disciplines. Collaborative practice is a serious endeavor that can promote trust and respect between disciplines, but transition to a collaborative practice model may not be smooth. All too frequently, turf issues surface when members of various disciplines struggle to define complementary roles in the delivery of care.

COMMUNICATION

Prescott and Bowen[1] describe the process of effective nurse–physician communication. This process applies to any struggle between disciplines.

> When physicians and nurses work together optimally, relationships are positive, disagreements are collaboratively resolved to the benefit of the patient, and patient care flows smoothly and efficiently. In contrast, poor relationships and inadequate resolution of disagreement have potentially serious consequences for patient care.[1(p127)]

When one member of a team has a problem communicating with another, patient care may

Source: Reprinted from J.W. Balzer, *Holistic Nursing Practice,* Vol. 7, No. 4, pp. 28–35, © 1993, Aspen Publishers, Inc.

suffer. Then everyone has a problem. Consider the following example. A surgeon in an intensive care setting was chiding a nurse, saying "Nurses at hospital X bring me coffee when I come to the unit." The nurse retorted lightly, but with clear, serious intent, "Now, Doctor, which would you rather have, the excellent patient assessment and care we provide on this unit or a cup of coffee." Working together does not always have to be serious. Humor may be an essential ingredient in tough times.

Devereux[2] identified five considerations for nursing practice in collaboration: clinical competence, legal definition of increased independence, assertive not aggressive communication, interpretation of an appropriate nursing role, and willingness to assume responsibility. Clear communication and the ability to manage stress are essential ingredients in all of these considerations. Humor is a useful intervention as well. A part of the humor movement is to introduce play and creativity into the work setting.

The introduction for nurses and physicians to the concept of collaborative practice and primary nursing in one pediatric hospital was conducted in a retreat setting. A local resort was used to add an informal note to stimulate shared ideas. Later, the 6-month evaluation was conducted in conjunction with a dinner meeting to celebrate in a festive atmosphere. To introduce the concept to other pediatric staff in the community and to continue dialogue, a skit was presented at grand rounds, attended by pediatric nurses and physicians throughout the city. The skit was written by the nurses and physicians working on the collaborative practice unit. A spoof on the nurse–physician relationship, the skit became an ice-breaker for initiating serious discussion about the progress on the unit and the joint practice issues that the operation of the unit raised.

When interviewed about their experience on this unit, nurses identified playful banter as a form of humor that relieved tension while acknowledging the problems nurses and physicians experience in the struggle to deliver patient care in a more collegial manner. Some physicians struggled with the change (eg, nurses writing on traditional physician's progress notes). One physician became so accustomed to a particular nurse's attention to detail that he countered, "Let's go over these notes together or you'll beat me to death!" Another physician nicknamed a nurse "Trouble" when she confronted him regarding several issues. They resolved the issues and, although he teased her with a nickname, she did not find it offensive. Instead, she chose to view it as his way of smoothing over the conflict. She had met her goal and received effective resolution of the issue.

When interviewed after 6 months, nursing staff members concluded that they had determined which physicians were open to humor on an individual basis. As they gave examples of humorous interchanges, it became clear that taken out of context it would be hard to sort positive from negative humor. Written anecdotes could be read as questionable even when nursing staff involved found them appropriate—truly a case of "you had to be there." An important criterion of any humorous interchange, however, continues to be positive intent.

Malcolm Kushner, an attorney and corporate humor consultant, points out that a prime rule of communication is "over time, content fades, but the relationship remains."[3(p108)] If the intent is positive and that is what is communicated, then the actual words are less important. That is, the risk of humor is worth taking. He cites a study by Baron,[4] a psychology professor at Rensselaer Polytechnic Institute, that confirms the value of humor for creating positive relationships. Conclusions of the study included the idea that confrontation at work often depends on how one may say things rather than on what one may say. Baron hypothesized that people cannot experience anger and amusement at the same time. In the study students performed role play of business communication encounters. In some cases conflict was introduced; in others, humor was introduced. The students completed questionnaires about feelings toward role play participants. Results showed that "using humor often reduced anger and produced a more positive encounter. . . . Humor put subjects in a better mood . . . and increased the likelihood that they would choose a constructive approach to resolving conflicts."

CAVEATS IN THE USE OF HUMOR

An important caveat in the use of humor is to distinguish between positive and negative humor. Positive humor intends to bring people closer together. It adds needed perspective and, in effect, says "we are all in this together." Positive humor diminishes the impact of a stressor. For example, Erma Bombeck uses the positive humor intervention of exaggeration to describe the plight of the homemaker. Negative humor is demeaning and serves to distance people. It may be thinly veiled anger, racism, or sexism. Its recipient, actually its target, feels diminished in stature by the humor.

Assertive use of humor involves being able to distinguish between its use and abuse. Women have too often been passive victims of humor at their expense. Vestiges of antifemale humor still invade the nurse–physician relationship. Humor that ridicules any specific group need not be passively accepted. It is appropriate to say, "I don't think that is funny," when legitimate concerns are minimized. For example, one female nurse trying to communicate concerns about a patient's condition to a male physician was teased about "worrying her pretty head" and "getting all emotional like a woman."

Using humor as a substitute for effective confrontation may seem easier, but it may not achieve the desired result. If a concern or complaint is raised in a humorous way, the other person is not obligated to take it seriously.

Similarly, sarcasm may mask anger that could be used to energize problem solving. Anger is best expressed directly and with appropriate, serious body language, words, and intent. Humor that focuses on a personal characteristic creates a victim and may disguise anger about another issue that needs resolution.

Humor that gently pokes fun at oneself may allow staff members to admit their own imperfections and free them to take needed risks to offer creative solutions to problems. Humor that perpetuates stereotypes invites further victim-

ization such as, "I can't figure out this budget—isn't that just like a woman?"

FUNCTIONS OF HUMOR

Robinson[5] identified social and psychologic functions of humor in the health care setting. These functions included establishing relationships, coping with social conflict, promoting group solidarity, and relieving tension.

During the 7 years this author has presented humor workshops and consultations, three recurring functions of humor in staff relationships have been identified:

1. *Prevention*—a playful attitude at work where people can enjoy their work, where humor is an accepted ingredient of the work day, sets a tone for team work that is a preventive measure for tough times. A court jester can be appointed on a rotating basis to plan an activity that helps staff members see each other as people. Baby picture contests have been well received by many teams, others have posted one staff baby picture and have staff members guess the identity.

2. *Interruption of negative expectations*—when staff is stressed, communication may not be smooth. One nurse supervisor kept a huge pair of sunglasses in her office. When tension mounted on the unit, she would put them on and walk down the hall. Likewise, a magic wand can be used to cheer staff. "Abracadabra! Now you will have a better day!" One critical care unit labeled its candy jar "grump beans" and offered them as necessary. Emergency department staff members report calling out a punch line to a well-known joke when the staff was struggling to meet multiple priorities. Not only did the punch line lighten the mood, it served to strengthen relationships by illustrating that even in tough times, a common ground existed.

3. *Perspective*—humor can help "keep the big picture." Computer-generated certificates can be used as awards, even for noting small amounts of progress. A group of health care managers took clown noses to a budget meeting and put them on during tough negotiations. The ensuing laughter assisted the participants to problem solve during the budget process. In an-

other institution, a nurse who directed a variety of hospital departments took many different hats to a meeting, exchanging hats according to departmental topics. She used humor to represent her awareness of differences and her ability to respond to the needs of nonnursing, as well as nursing, departments. Putting needs in perspective helped her to initiate discussion about equal treatment for all departments effectively.

Dr Watzlawich of the Mental Research Institute of Palo Alto, California, says humor can defuse conflict by a change in expectation. He feels that "When a conflict is escalating, things seem to be going inexorably in an anticipated direction. But if something completely unexpected happens, then things can't continue this way and a change must occur."[3(p110)]

This notion of change in expectation is the way a joke works. That is to say, a punch line destroys the expectation built by the narrative of the joke. Shattering the expectation forces the listener to perceive the issue in a different context, to envision a different meaning.[3] For example, a nurse facing a barrage of hostility from a physician was puzzled because she usually has a smooth working relationship with him. Once the nurse recognized that the anger was not directed at her personally, she responded, "Doctor, did you have nails for breakfast?" The physician's expectation of an angry retort to hostility was unmet. The physician apologized, recognizing that his anger was displaced toward the nurse, and actually was in response to a difficult day. Confronted with humor, he was enabled to laugh at himself. Once staff members can laugh at a problem they are one step closer to creative solutions. Consider the most effective brainstorming session: uncensored, from its extremes arise some of the most unique approaches. Burns identified three functions of humor in the workplace. These functions are to

1. Reinforce the rules and boundaries of an established group.
2. Help break down the boundaries of a group into which you would like to be accepted
3. Ease tensions between groups.[7(p134)]

Benefits of humor identified by participants in the author's work are listed in the box entitled "Benefits of Humor in Collaborative Practice."

Barreca[7] identified strategies for successful use of humor including humor that expresses self-confidence, such as the comment about nursing assessment versus coffee; humor that is a signature, a unique representation of self; and humor that creates consensus.

Other examples of the constructive use of humor illustrate the concept. The director of a school for radiation technology is known for her outlandish sense of humor, her own signature behavior. When asked to participate in a teaching conference at 9 o'clock, she assumed the conference was in the morning. When she learned it was at night she retorted, "If I have to teach that late, I'll come in my jammies." She did just that, arriving in huge pink fuzzy slippers and a bathrobe over her uniform. The attendees were laughing and energized; participation was high. In another illustration, one hospital invited me to do a workshop on humor for a biannual nurse–physician educational offering. At the event, after the presentation I distributed clown noses. When the 100 participants donned their clown noses, there was that "moment of agreement when everyone is in sync."[7(p142)]

Benefits of Humor in Collaborative Practice

Adds perspective
Builds trust
Creates a positive work environment
Decreases defensiveness
Deflects anger
Enhances team work
Energizes staff
Invites openness
Permits imperfections and humanness
Promotes job satisfaction
Reframes difficult situations
Relieves tension
Underscores common goals

THE POWER OF HUMOR

Dr True, who has worked with humor and communication for 25 years, found that humor had the power to "fix communications breakdowns, influence and inspire others, and win liking and trust."[8(p99)] He suggests that you

- Share laughter with others, to help them understand that you and they have objectives in common.
- Open up, and admit that you, too, make mistakes.
- Think funny about yourself, and take your honors and rewards lightly.

Collaborative practice is based on the common objective of quality patient care. The ability to make mistakes and the lack of omnipotence are shared by all disciplines. Each discipline has its fair share of practitioners who take themselves, or their own point of view, too seriously. When team members consciously make an effort to "lighten up" in the spirit of improving the outcome of patient care, the joint venture becomes more palatable and more of a growth experience.

CRITERIA FOR APPROPRIATE USE OF HUMOR

Leiber[9] identified three criteria for the appropriate use of humor in the clinical setting. These criteria are: timing, receptivity, and content. They apply in staff-to-staff relationships in the manner described in the text that follows.

Timing

Working as a member of an emergency department staff team demands efficient, serious intervention. When the staff reviews a particular crisis and the interventions selected, humor may serve to relieve tension and initiate discussion of needed improvement in response. To illustrate this point, consider the following example. An agitated man came into the emergency department brandishing a gun. A resident physician, focusing on the danger to other patients and to staff, took the gun away from the man. After the crisis passed, he realized this intervention was quite dangerous. He used humor to critique his actions by writing on the unit chalkboard in Olympic scoring style "Patient Take Down, Form 9.5, Style 8.0."

In another example, if a staff member is rushed or a meeting agenda is tight, humor may be ill-timed. If a staff member is moody or irri-

---

Developing the Comic Vision

1. Start with yourself. Laugh at yourself. Give yourself permission to be human. If you trip, laugh out loud.
2. Read the comics and political cartoons in newspapers as examples of comic vision. Look at local newspapers when traveling to find local perspectives on current issues and regional humor.
3. Read cartoons and humorous letters to the editor or editorials in other professional journals.
4. Start an album of cartoons that track current work issues and encourage all team members to contribute.
5. Attend funny movies and comedy clubs.
6. Listen to humorous audiocassettes on the way to work to begin your day looking for humor.
7. Collect humorous one-liners that are "inside" jokes with your team.
8. Experiment with building a humor kit at work. Start with only a few items and encourage participation and a feeling of ownership.
9. Laugh at others for what they do, at their incongruities as they mirror your own.
10. Share your comic vision to make other people laugh. Laughter is contagious and adds much-needed joy in ourselves and our colleagues.

Source: Copyright © Julia W. Balzer Riley, RN, MM, Constant Source Seminars, Cumming, Georgia.

table and these reactions are shared by other staff, a humorous intervention might be timely to "save the day." An emergency "run" to the coffee shop for chocolate chip cookies has been the ice-breaker needed in one training and development department. In the same department, each team member was provided with small bottles of bubbles to blow for stress relief. These activities serve to relieve staff tension without being offensive if other staff enters the office.

Receptivity

As the staff on the pediatric collaborative practice unit noted earlier, not all people have a sense of humor. Some professionals choose to draw a clear distinction between the serious business of health care and the informality of their personal life, and these boundaries need to be honored. Whenever appropriate, however, shared humor strengthens ties.

Content

Humor that is offensive or deals with people in stereotypic ways does not build relationships and may invite aggression. This type of humor includes sexist, racist, or ethnic humor. Whenever a personal response to humor is negative, the staff member needs to consider if the humor is of an offensive nature and, if so, call this observation to the attention of the colleague. Laughing at humor reinforces it and may promote negative humor.

People vary greatly in what is considered funny. The gallows humor that serves to decrease tension in the operating room may not be amusing to the patient or the family. A staff member who has a family member whose alcoholic behavior has been disruptive may be sensitive to disparaging comments made about alcoholism. If this sensitivity interferes with a working relationship with a colleague, sharing this sensitivity may be helpful.

DEVELOPING THE COMIC VISION

A comic vision seems to come naturally to some people, those who always see the light side even in the most difficult of times. Personal ex-

perience with crises and tragedy fosters the development of this perspective for some. Participants of workshops on humor report that often the keeper of the morale at work has had the toughest life when their personal story is told. Most people have the capacity to build on their sense of humor, to allow themselves to see the humorous side of problems, and to share this gift (see the box entitled "Developing the Comic Vi-

---

Building a Humor Kit

The first step is to raise your humor consciousness. Be on the lookout for funny things.

- Sources include: toy stores, clown supply stores, party stores, magic shops, Halloween and other seasonal displays, souvenir or joke counters, teacher or school supply stores, children's discards, and garage sales.
- Bubbles. When you have nothing measurable or observable for a day's work, bubbles lighten the mood.
- Whistles and small noisemakers. Useful to begin meetings in a novel way to set the tone for team work.
- Funny hats or noses. These items relieve tension.
- Clown supplies. Includes items such as huge sunglasses.
- Cartoons. Cartoons can communicate current issues; use on bulletin boards, in memos, or in minutes of meetings.
- Laughter box. Use when a good laugh is needed.
- Funny buttons. Buttons express a concern or the mood of the unit.
- Stickers. They bring out the inner child.
- Posters. Either motivational or humorous are helpful.
- A magic wand. It provides endless possibilities.

Source: Copyright © Julia W. Balzer Riley, RN, MM, Constant Source Seminars, Cumming, Georgia.

sion"). A humor kit in the health care setting can give staff the permission and the tools with which to begin to develop a comic vision (see the box entitled "Building a Humor Kit").

●   ●   ●

The positive use of humor helps us keep perspective, laugh at life's incongruities, or poke gentle fun at ourselves, acknowledging our lack of perfection and setting a tone of trust and acceptance among colleagues. Always remember, take your work seriously, but yourself lightly.

REFERENCES

1. Prescott PA, Bowen SA. Physician–nurse relationships. *Annals of Internal Medicine.* 1985;103:127–133.

2. Devereux PM. Nurse–physician collaboration: nursing practice considerations. *The Journal of Nursing Administration.* 1981;11(9):37–39.

3. Kushner M. *The Light Touch: How to Use Humor for Success in Business.* New York, NY: Simon & Schuster; 1990.

4. Baron R. Reducing organizational conflict: an incompatible response approach. *Journal of Applied Psychology.* 1984;69(2):272–279.

5. Robinson VM. *Humor and the Health Care Professions.* Thorofare, NJ: Charles B. Slack Co; 1977.

6. Burns T. Friends, enemies, and the polite fiction. *American Sociological Review.* 1953;18(6):654–662.

7. Barreca R. *They Used to Call Me Snow White . . . But I Drifted: Women's Strategic Use of Humor.* New York, NY: Penguin; 1991.

8. True H. *Humor Power: How to Get It, Give It, and Gain.* Garden City, NY: Doubleday; 1980.

9. Leiber DB. Laughter and humor in critical care. *Dimensions of Critical Care.* 1986;5(3):162–170.

Integrating Holism within the Client's Cultural and Environmental World

I have long believed that many problems in delivering holistic nursing care have been created because of the way we assess clients. Most of us have learned to assess clients using a traditional, standardized medical database with some sporadic psychosocial questions tacked on at the beginning or end to lend a holistic perspective. Because the client is assessed primarily from a medical point of view, a holistic assessment of the client's body-mind-spirit needs does not take place. In reality, we are collecting only part of the data we need. If all appropriate data are not obtained, we miss things.

Addressing cultural issues is a good example of this assessment dilemma. Because most nursing assessment tools do not include culturally sensitive questions, except perhaps ethnic and religious affiliation, it is no surprise that we are collecting inadequate cultural data. If culturally appropriate health care issues (problems) are not identified, a plan of care with culturally sensitive interventions will never materialize. As a result, even the most meticulously planned nursing interventions will fall short of their outcomes if they collide with how the client thinks, acts, and feels.

The poignant case studies by Cooper illustrate how nursing interventions fall apart when we assess only part of the whole patient. To confront this problem, a cultural health care assessment blueprint is outlined (based on Leininger's Sunrise Model) that can be used in clinical practice to assess the cultural dimension of our clients. Likewise, Morris presents a case study using Rosenbaum's cultural assessment guide as another tool and another method by which to assess culture. Although it is unlikely that most of us will become experts in every culture we encounter, we need to include culturally appropriate questions as a part of our nursing assessment and acquire a knowledge base of various cultures (e.g., African-Americans [Morris] and Jews [Beck and Goldberg]) as well as an understanding of cultural beliefs about health topics (e.g., death and grief [Esposito, Buckalew, and Chukunta]).

In addition, even the most meticulously planned nursing interventions will fall short if they collide with an unhealthy client environment. It is no surprise to learn, for example, that the level of hospital noise still exceeds the Environmental Protection Agency's recommendations (Griffin) that were established in 1974. The outcome of disturbing hospital noise has profound psychophysiologic effects on patients, including anger, sleep deprivation, sensory overload, increased pain, and ICU psychosis. Strategies to eliminate, reduce, or control structural, mechanical, and personnel noise need to be identified and implemented. Likewise, environmental light also is a variable that affects health and illness. In an outcome study of neonates, altering light was useful in patterning day-wake and night-sleeping of infants in a nursery (Girardin).

Holistic nurses do not underestimate the impact of culture or environment on the client's body-mind-spirit. Culture and environment are powerful variables that must be factored into the equation of providing holistic patient care.

Culturally Appropriate Care: Optional or Imperative

Teresa P. Cooper, MSN, RN, CPNP, CTN
Coordinator
Community Health Outreach with the
Department of Pediatrics
Division of Community Pediatrics
University of California San Diego
San Diego, California

Source: Reprinted from T. Cooper, *Advanced Practice Nursing Quarterly,* Vol. 2, No. 2, pp. 1–6, © 1996, Aspen Publishers, Inc.

CASE STUDY: MARIA

Maria is a 17-year-old pregnant, English-speaking, Mexican American who presented for her prenatal appointment with her "mother." Maria has lived with a monolingual, Spanish-speaking, 65-year-old woman from rural Mexico she calls "Grandmother" since she was abandoned by her biological mother at 3 months of age. Maria, now 8 months pregnant, had missed at least half of her prenatal appointments. On this, her 8th-month visit at a Teen Obstetric Clinic, the staff expressed concerns about her missed appointments. Her blood pressure was very elevated and she was found to have a marked increase in weight. The examining physician advised that she be admitted to the hospital for some tests due to concerns about the infant. The physician, confident that she had given clear and understandable instructions to the patient, left to schedule the necessary tests.

Maria and her grandmother began to cry silently, but inconsolably at this news.

Maria had numerous consults during her 3-day hospitalization. No one could understand why her hematocrit level was 15–17 and her platelet and blood count were pathologically low. A hematology consult could provide no further insight regarding the abnormal blood levels. Maria was transfused with a pint of blood.

An interning physician from the South, familiar with traditional and alternative health beliefs and practices, asked Maria one question: Was she eating anything other than normal food? Maria responded that she was eating eight bars of Magnesia de Carbonada (chalk) each day because it tasted like dirt and she had been craving dirt and ice (pica) as well as suffering from heartburn and vomiting. She related that her grandmother had given her the Magnesia de Carbonada to cleanse her stomach and prevent her from eating ice because her grandmother believed that eating ice would give her and the infant pneumonia and bronchitis.

This case study demonstrates many of the problems that arise when health care professionals fail to understand the implications that "routine" care can have for individuals from other cultures. Moreover, it underscores the need for these professionals to be aware of the role alternative health practices and beliefs can play in the clinical picture.

Perhaps the first question that this case study raises concerns the missed prenatal appointments and the inconsolable crying elicited by the physician's decision to admit Maria. While the clinic staff were performing their duties employing the best traditions of American medicine, their ignorance of the Mexican culture, particularly as it relates to pregnancy and hospital care, triggered a whole range of emotions for Maria and her "mother."

In Mexico's rural areas, pregnancy is considered a natural phenomenon, and prenatal care is rarely given. Infants are usually born at home, and any abnormality is not seen as preventable but rather as controlled by God. Hospitals are used only by the dying. For Maria, keeping her appointments for prenatal care at the hospital involved overcoming enormous culturally related fear. Moreover, the suggestion of a hospital admission, from Maria's and her grandmother's perspective, meant only one thing: the mother or the child (or both) was going to die. In addition, the concerns expressed by the staff about the missed prenatal visits tended to promote incredible feelings of guilt in these people whose cultural values include pleasing authority figures and equate pleasing authority with respect. Caught between two cultures, Maria and her grandmother needed in-depth, detailed explanations and they needed someone who could not only understand and respect their differing health beliefs but also bridge both cultures to allay their fears.

Likewise, the importance of nonethnocentric, culturally aware health care professionals is dramatically brought home by the incidents surrounding the hematological findings. One culturally astute question ascertained in minutes what 3 days of costly tests, consults, and hospitalization could not.

Ethnocentrism (the belief that one's own ways are the best, the most superior, the more preferred, or the only way) and cultural imposition (the tendency to impose one's beliefs, values, and patterns of behavior on another culture for varied reasons, often because of ethnocentrism, cultural blindness, or ignorance) in an advanced nursing practice are not only ineffective practice but also can cause irreparable cultural clashes. Moreover, they result in care that is neither high-quality nor cost-effective. In contrast, nurses prepared in transcultural nursing, who recognize the importance of cultural variations in health beliefs and incorporate this knowledge in their area of advanced practice, are, beyond a doubt, both quality-effective and cost-effective health care providers.

TRANSCULTURAL NURSING

During the past decade, the need for transcultural nursing knowledge has become imperative. With increased migration and movement of people worldwide, the profession of nursing is providing care to immigrants, refugees, and people from almost every point of the globe. The nurse interacts with clients who hold world views and health values very different from his or her own. The most carefully planned nursing intervention can be unacceptable to the client if the client's cultural attitudes, beliefs, and values are not assessed and incorporated into the nursing plan. Understanding culture is unquestionably essential to understanding people and meeting their health needs.

Madeleine Leininger (1995), founder of transcultural nursing, defines culture as "the learned and shared beliefs, values, and lifeways of a designated or particular group which are generally transmitted intergenerationally and influence one's thinking and action modes" (p. 9). Culture can be conceptualized as the blueprint that guides a person's lifeways and predicts patterns of behavior. Culture pervades a person's being so completely that seldom is the time taken to identify the cultural components of attitudes, habits of living, or world views.

Perhaps in no other area of life is culture so significant as in health care beliefs and health-seeking behavior. Cultural values influence the entire continuum of decisions made from child-birth, to medication taking, to self-care, to care of the dying. A culturally competent nurse be-comes aware of and respects the reasons for cul-tural practices and decisions for self and others and develops an understanding of why some choices are made by patients and other choices rejected. Individuals who do not conform to the health practices of Western medicine are often viewed by health providers as peculiar, strange, uncooperative, or noncompliant.

Consider, for example, the visit of a Chinese couple, the Chans, who brought their 2-year-old son to the children's clinic. The nurse was frus-trated because the parents had not taken the child's temperature at home. All remarks were addressed to Mrs. Chan, who would not respond to the nurse's inquiries. The Chans were not happy because, pending the result of a throat cul-ture, they did not receive medication for the child. And, because the nurse addressed Mrs. Chan, Mr. Chan felt deprived of the respect he anticipated as a member of a culture that desig-nates the male as the decision maker.

This interaction represents a health care expe-rience between members of two cultural groups in which little communication or understanding occurred (Boyle & Andrews, 1989). Is it not eas-ily understood, then, why the Chan family would neither trust this health care provider nor return to this clinic?

In transcultural nursing, differences and pref-erences in health care are expected and viewed as part of the normal variation observed in cul-turally diverse populations. A transculturally competent nurse would have been sensitive to the nuances of the Chans' behavior, more pre-pared to anticipate differences in health views and beliefs, and aware of spoken or unspoken cultural conflict arising out of the Chans' visit to the clinic. Nursing interventions that are cultur-ally relevant not only decrease the possibility of stress and noncompliance arising from cultural misunderstandings, but also increase compli-ance and mutual respect. There are often prob-lems (many times unspoken) when nurses and clients from different cultural backgrounds in-teract, unless the nurse is willing to learn and adapt to the values of the client.

An important component of increased trans-cultural understanding is the sensitivity of the nurse to his or her own cultural beliefs and val-ues. Advanced practice nurses must identify their own personal values, biases, and ideas to illuminate conscious and unconscious attitudes. While this need is cogently applicable in all nursing settings, advanced practice nurses as a group seem to possess middle-class American values, beliefs, and attitudes yet typically pro-vide health care to the multiethnic, low-socio-economic, "hyphenated" American people. Thus it is imperative that these nurses "set aside per-sonal values, biases, ideas, and attitudes that are judgmental and may negatively affect care" (Giger & Davidhizar, 1991, p. 22). It is only through self-awareness and understanding of one's own cultural values and beliefs that accu-rate client assessments, interpretations, and de-cisions can be made (Leininger, 1995).

Leininger (1995) defines transcultural nursing care as:

> A formal area of study and practice in nursing focused upon comparative ho-listic cultural care, health, and illness patterns of individuals and groups with respect to differences and simi-larities in cultural values, beliefs, and practices with the goal to provide cul-turally congruent, sensitive, and com-petent nursing care to people of di-verse cultures (p. 4).

An assumption basic to the practice of transcultural nursing is the belief that caring is a universal phenomenon that varies only in form and manifestation. Caring for others is found in all cultures, but the methods by which it is done and the meaning that caring conveys are as diverse as the groups that define it. What is valued and judged as "good" care is culturally based; members of a particular cultural group describe what constitutes good care for them to a more meaningful degree than can those outside that cultural group. The more closely nursing care integrates the client's perception of care, the more accepted it will be.

CULTURALOGICAL HEALTH CARE ASSESSMENTS

In order to discover how culture care factors contribute to attitudes toward health, nurses need to develop skill in conducting culturalogical health care assessments. Leininger (1995) defines culturalogical assessment as "the systematic identification of the culture care beliefs, meanings, values, symbols, and practices of individuals or groups within a holistic perspective including the worldview, life experiences, environmental context, ethnohistory, and social structure factors" (p. 118). The nurse needs to identify which care values are similar or different to those of the client and those of other cultures.

Leininger's Sunrise Model provides a comprehensive guide for the nurse to use in conducting culture care assessment (Figure 1). The major areas of the Sunrise Model are the world view and social structure dimensions that include the following:

1. culture values and lifeways
2. religious, philosophical, and spiritual beliefs
3. economic factors
4. educational factors
5. technological factors
6. kinship and social ties
7. political and legal factors

The world view of the client and the social structure in which he or she lives are fruitful areas to explore when assessing the client. Material and nonmaterial resources of the client are also important in getting a holistic view of the client, as are uses of space, need for privacy, and group cohesiveness.

The nurse can initiate the assessment anywhere in the model and proceed to the different areas as indicated by the client's responses. The reality of the clinical day often requires the nurse to conduct the assessment at intervals over a period of time. This approach permits the nurse to reflect on the information the client has shared and to determine areas requiring further exploration. Essential ingredients of an effective cultural assessment are the ability of the nurse to engage in active listening, use open-ended questions, reflect nonjudgmentally on what the client has shared, and determine areas that the client deems important.

The nursing assessments routinely conducted as part of the nursing process are an outgrowth of the Western medical model. They fail to address the needs of many ethnic-specific people in the client population. Moreover, most nursing assessments are biomedically focused and do not consider cultural terms and conditions that need to be explored in order to deliver effective and culturally appropriate nursing care.

According to Leininger (1995), "The major focus of culturalogical assessment is on ascertaining culture care patterns, expressions, and meanings that reflect the client's care needs and well-being, or that influence the client's patterns of illness, disabilities or death" (p. 118). The process of culturalogical assessment requires time, patience, knowledge, and skills to explore and validate what the client says and does. Although the assessment model varies to accommodate the client's world view and manner of expressing ideas to the nurse, it generally includes cultural factors, beliefs and relationship to care, language statements and the meanings the client attaches to an idea, nonverbal communication, the use of space, and religious beliefs regarding healing.

There are three major modalities that can guide nursing plans and interventions so as to provide culturally appropriate care that is ben-

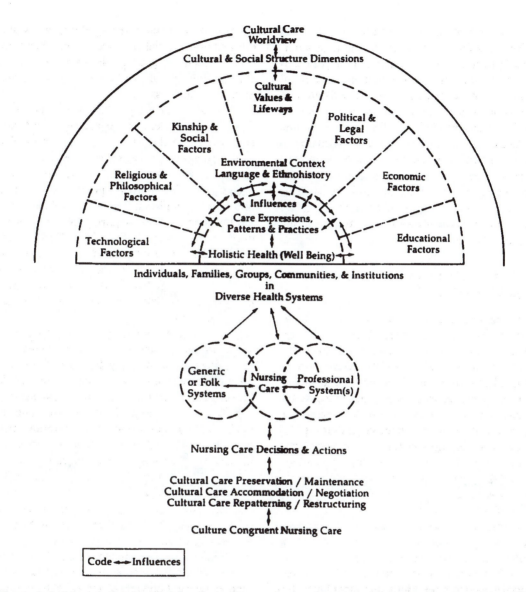

Figure 1. Leininger's Sunrise Model to depict theory of cultural care diversity and universality. *Source:* Reprinted with permission from Leininger, M. *Culture Care Diversity and Universality: A Theory for Nursing,* © 1991, National League for Nursing Press.

eficial. According to Leininger (1991), these three modes are (1) cultural care preservation and/or maintenance, (2) cultural care accommodation and/or negotiation, and (3) cultural care repatterning or restructuring. The culturally competent nurse plans care with the client using those modes of action indicated by the data obtained from the cultural assessment. Only one dominant mode of action may be necessary. The drinking of herbal tea by an Asian client to relieve tension or including all members of the Mexican-American family in health care decisions illustrate cultural preservation. Cultural care accommodation is indicated when, for example, a Muslim woman, following the tenets of her culture, requests that her care be provided exclusively by female health care providers. As much as it is possible to do so in the clinical setting, this request can be accommodated or negotiated by the culturally competent nurse. Cultural care repatterning may be indicated in situations where the client engages in practices that are deleterious to health and well-being. Repatterning of care requires a sensitivity to people's lifeways and an extensive cultural knowledgebase. Cultural repatterning is inherent in empowering clients to perform self-care, prevent illness, or negotiate American society effectively. Transcultural nursing skills are imperative to accomplish these objectives successfully and effectively.

CASE STUDY: ESTELLA

The following case study poignantly describes effective cultural repatterning. In California, a new state-funded program called Cal-Learn is being implemented in several cities. Cal-Learn is designed to help pregnant and parenting adolescents who receive Aid to Families with Dependent Children (AFDC) return to school and graduate in order to reduce their chances of long-term welfare dependency.

The case manager assigned to Estella, an 18-year-old, first-generation Mexican-American mother of a 7-month-old child, met with seemingly unexplainable obstacles when attempting to accomplish the task of enrolling Estella in school. After detailed explanations by the case manager to a very interested Estella, who appeared to have an enthusiastic response to school reenrollment, the case manager became completely frustrated when, despite repeated positive contacts, Estella failed to enroll in school.

The case was presented at a Community Health Case Conference, led by the program's health consultant, a certified transcultural nurse. This nurse was able to clarify the events that had transpired in this case as well as suggest an approach to help the family repattern their beliefs and values.

In Estella's Mexican-American belief system, once a young woman has a child, motherhood is her primary responsibility. While Estella truly did want to return to high school and complete her studies, her cultural values of motherhood would not allow her to take on another primary responsibility. Such a role would jeopardize her motherhood role. To complicate matters further, the case manager infused her own cultural values, which promote independence and self-sufficiency, and employed Western methods that called for her to address the adolescent alone and in private so that the adolescent could be empowered to make her own decisions. The case manager did not realize that the Mexican-American value system dictated that a decision such as this had to involve the entire family.

As much as Estella desired to return to school, she could not make this decision alone. Her family would need to be part of the decision-making process and would have to be included when the detailed explanations of this program were given to Estella. Not wanting to be disrespectful to the case manager (who is both an authority figure and an elder), she always said "Yes" when questioned about enrolling in school.

Rather than causing Estella to be caught between two cultures, it was suggested that the case manager act as an advocate for Estella's well-being in this country by explaining to her family that unlike the practice in some other countries, a high school diploma is required for Estella to have a better life and to be able to provide for herself and her child. Thus it was up to the case manager to facilitate repatterning for Estella's family.

The case manager began by going to Estella's home and asking her parents to be present at her next appointment (cultural care accommodation). Here the case manager would re-present the goals of the program to the family, ask for their support with Estella's school enrollment, explain the importance of their involvement, and ask if a family member could provide child care (cultural care preservation).

Estella is now enrolled in school (cultural care repatterning), and her mother is providing child care. All cultural obstacles have been overcome, and everyone is feeling good about the decisions made.

●   ●   ●

All care modalities require collaboration of the nurse, client, and family to plan, implement, and evaluate care for cultural congruence. In order to learn about the cultural values and beliefs of people and to understand their specific needs and expectations, the nurse needs to integrate culture care assessment into advanced practice.

There is much to learn. It is no easy task to repattern our thinking and abandon stereotypical attitudes and beliefs. An openness to diversity is the first essential step for all professional nurses committed to effective delivery of care to ethnically specific people in sensitive and caring ways. An awareness of one's own values also brings respect, acceptance, and openness to learn about the values of others. The process of awareness and acceptance enables advanced practice nurses to not only enrich their own worlds but also enrich the lives of the clients they serve by meeting their health care needs in a culturally appropriate way.

REFERENCES

Boyle, J., & Andrews, M. (1989). *Transcultural concepts in nursing care.* Glenview, IL: Scott, Foresman & Co.

Giger, J., & Davidhizar, R. (1991). *Transcultural nursing: Assessment and intervention.* St. Louis, MO: Mosby–Year Book.

Leininger, M. (1991). *Cultural care diversity and universality: A theory of nursing.* New York, NY: National League for Nursing Press.

Leininger, M. (1995). *Transcultural nursing: Concepts, theories, research and practices.* New York, NY: McGraw-Hill.

Bridging Cultural Boundaries: The African American and Transcultural Caring

Rita I. Morris, PhD, RN
Associate Professor
School of Nursing of San Diego State
*   University*
Adjunct Faculty Member
University of Phoenix
San Diego, California

The transcultural nursing movement has been developing culture care theories, cultural assessment and analysis tools, and guidelines for culturally sensitive care over the past four decades. Yet, culture care lags behind the medical model of care in the nation's institutions. It is generally acknowledged that "health care providers cannot be experts on every culture with which they are likely to come into contact" (Jackson, 1993, p. 30). How then do we bridge boundaries and identify differences that matter? This article discusses how advanced practice nurses (APNs) can better understand and serve African-American clients by doing the following:

1. examining the influences of culture in health care
2. tracing cultural trends among African Americans
3. evaluating the importance of cultural assessment in clinical practice, and
4. teaching cultural assessment and cultural caring

The nation's cultural composition is rapidly becoming more diverse and more complex as global immigration grows. An enduring element in this diversity is the African-American culture. African Americans comprise about 12% of the population of the United States. It is estimated that their number will double to approximately

Source: Reprinted from R.I. Morris, *Advanced Practice Nursing Quarterly,* Vol. 2, No. 2, pp. 31–38, © 1996, Aspen Publishers, Inc.

Acknowledgments are due to Nancy Gardetto, MSN, FNP, who conducted the LH interview.

65 million by the year 2050 (U.S. Bureau of the Census, 1983). Are we in the nursing profession developing transcultural skills to serve this growing population effectively?

In practice, the nurse must remember that all cultures exhibit considerable variation and that individuals whose appearance may at first suggest one culture may in fact identify with a different culture or with an unexpected variant.

INFLUENCES OF CULTURE ON HEALTH CARE

Many African Americans perceive illness as a natural occurrence resulting from disharmony and conflict in some aspect of their life. This belief involves three general areas: (1) environmental hazards, (2) divine punishment, and (3) impaired social relationships. Another belief is that everything has an opposite. For every birth there is a death, for every illness someone must be cured (Cherry & Giger, 1991).

There are still some Black Americans in the rural South who practice folk medicine based on spirituality, including witchcraft, voodoo, and magic. Black folk medicine survived not only as a manifestation of African cultural heritage but also as a necessity when African Americans could not gain access to the modern health care delivery system. Furthermore, they could not afford the high cost of modern medicine (Giger & Davidhizar, 1991). Today, even though they have access, many refuse to use the system, citing reasons of past experience, insensitive treatment on the part of caregivers, and escalating costs.

Low-income and less educated families often view high-technology medicine as appropriate only in trauma situations. The leading causes of morbidity and mortality in the African-American population include violent assault and accidental death and injury (U.S. Department of Health and Human Services, 1985). Willis (1992) points out that, "High technology care is also encountered all too frequently in neonatal intensive care units, because of the disproportionately high numbers of African-American babies born with conditions such as low birth weight, prematurity, and the effects of high risk behaviors and lifestyles" (p. 140).

It is well known that people of various cultures have different health care beliefs, values, and expectations for their health care. Every year, millions of the nation's health care dollars are wasted due to a lack of cultural sensitivity. There have been many incidents where cultural practices were mistaken for abusive practices. For example, a Caucasian public health nurse (PHN), on the day she visited an African-American family, observed that the extended family members were bawling at each other. Fearful that the infant of the 14-year-old, single mother was in danger, the nurse reported the incident to Child Protective Services. This family felt betrayed and refused further services from the PHN. Margaret Andrews (1992) points out that "a serious conceptual problem exists within nursing in that nurses are expected to know, understand, and meet the health needs of culturally diverse people, without any formal preparation for doing so" (p. 7).

There is increased interest in introducing cultural concepts both in education and in practice but the process is slow and outcomes are poor. These results may be due to the fact that theoretical knowledge alone is not enough. Application of theory in field practice requires not only knowledge but also a change in attitude, an open mind, and a willingness to listen and examine other ways of doing things. Communicating across cultures is a complex skill. Neiderhauser (1989) explains the variations of styles of communication in different cultures as follows:

> Cultural groups differ in the way that information is perceived and understood. . . . Perceptions are important to consider in communication, because actions are generally based on the interpretation of information. If information is perceived differently or inaccurately then the desired response will not occur (p. 569).

Many minorities are extremely sensitive and unless health providers separate their own health care values and beliefs, without unconsciously imposing them on the patient, their interventions will not be successful. In supervising community health nursing students, this author has repeatedly heard students say "My client will not open up to me." My immediate response is always, "What is your client's cultural background? Let's do a visit together."

On one occasion, a student and the author visited a young African-American mother who was pregnant and unmarried. She had a history of hypertension, chain smoking, and past episodes of drug abuse. She was expecting her fourth child. It was apparent that this client was very worried. The author commented that she looked worried and asked whether she would like to relate her concerns. Nonverbally, the author conveyed to her genuine interest in her welfare. After the preamble of questions on the progress of her pregnancy, she had the opportunity to validate whether there was genuine concern, and she decided to open up. She spoke about her diabetic mother, who was living with her. She was her mother's sole caretaker, as her siblings living in the area were too irresponsible.

In the postconference meeting, the student remarked that the client was a different person, willing to open up. The student felt more comfortable and hopeful that she could continue caring for this client in a more meaningful way. What was the difference? Concern, understanding, and a willingness to listen to her were key factors in gaining her cooperation. We were viewed as an available resource, persons she could trust and turn to if she needed guidance.

AFRICAN AMERICANS: PAST, PRESENT, AND FUTURE CULTURAL TRENDS

Most African Americans are descendants of slaves brought to the United States in past centuries. Life experiences under slavery have shaped the internal attitudes and belief systems handed down in African-American families. The subsequent obstacles to equality have also influenced the lives of African Americans in the United States. Many of the problems that African Americans now face are more closely associated with economic status than with race. Discrimination and poverty reinforce social and psychological barriers arising from the difference of culture, which is itself shaped by discrimination and poverty.

In the past, African Americans were viewed as a group apart, physically present in America, but culturally distinct because of appearance, origin, and experience with slavery. Little was done to assist African Americans to obtain education, housing, and employment. The impact of prejudice, poverty, and segregation continues to affect many African Americans disproportionately to the present day (Spector, 1991; Willis, 1992).

In particular, the number of African-American males incarcerated is rapidly increasing. In 1993, out of over 932,000 inmates, 418,900 (45%) were Black males and 27,900 (3%) were Black females (U.S. Department of Justice, 1995). Two questions arise from these numbers: Why do African Americans constitute half of the inmates when they comprise only one eighth of all Americans? Will culture care strategies reduce incarceration?

Communication

The English dialect spoken by most African Americans, often called Black English, has served as a unifying factor in maintaining ethnic identity. Many African Americans use standard English in a professional capacity and Black English when socializing and interacting in all-Black settings. Black English and standard English often use different slang words to convey the same meaning. For example, the word chilly or chillin' in Black English means sophisticated, whereas a White individual may use the word groovy or cool to convey the same meaning.

Colloquial speech changes within different cultures at different times and in different ways. Therefore, APNs must be alert to both the existing differences and the changes as they emerge, in Black English as in any other language.

Speech among African Americans usually is very colorful and dynamic. Communication involves body movements, such as facial gestures, hand and arm movements, expressive stances, handshakes, and hand signals, along with verbal interaction. Sounds, such as an emphatic "oo-wee" or "uh-huh," are also used in conversations. Most African Americans use Black English in a systematic way that can be predictably understood by others. Thus Black English should not be regarded as substandard or ungrammatical, but as an expression of a separate identity and as a unifying factor (Cherry & Giger, 1991).

Music is an integral aspect of African-American culture. It is experienced interactively by following the words, dancing, tapping, or bobbing to the rhythm; or, it may be experienced passively as a part of the environment (Willis, 1992). Because of the relatively continuous presence of words or music among African Americans, they are sometimes characterized as loud or shallow. This pejorative characterization reflects perceptions stemming from a different set of values, as well as a lack of understanding of the African-American culture.

Religion

Early African religion was animist, centered on the concept of a supreme God who created the world and who was present as a life force in all things. The worship of ancestors and the spirits of nature coexisted. It was believed that the ancestral spirit remained with the family. Elaborate funerals may be, in part, a legacy of traditional concern to maintain affiliation with the dead.

No doubt, the practice of ancestral worship was imported from Africa, where it is a very strong custom to this day. Strategies to promote healthy behaviors must take into account the importance of ancestor worship. An example of a barrier to health promotion in West Africa will illustrate this concept.

Diarrheal diseases are the leading cause of infant mortality, which ranges from 110 to 150 deaths per 1,000 live births. In one West African village, bore hole wells with hand water pumps were built to provide pure water. The foreign developers predicted that the use of clean water would cut down on diarrheal diseases. But, the villagers continued to use the water from the open streams. Dialogue with the people showed that they believed that the spirit of their ancestors lived in the water that flowed in the streams. Abandoning the stream water would bring down the wrath of the ancestors.

A creative response was then developed. The villagers were shown how the same water from the streams blessed by their ancestors filtered deep down and was brought up by the pumps. Rational explanations consistent with their beliefs brought about the change. Cultural beliefs are often the reason for noncompliance. It takes time and patience to observe, listen, and find out why clients do what they do. The outcomes will be rewarding.

Family values

Values related to family remain rooted in African traditions. The extended family is viable. The family is the reflection of the African-American culture. It has been the source of strength, resilience, and survival. The value of group effort for the common interest is taught as a more enduring strategy for the survival of the African-American community, as opposed to individual effort for private gain. Private gain is well respected, but there is an expectation that it will be shared in reasonable measure with the larger community. The value of independence is instilled (i.e., the ability to stand on one's own feet). This concept may be in conflict with the group ethic, but it actually extends that ethic when responsibility to the group is accepted.

African-American families place a high value on respecting and obeying older persons. There is a high value placed on obedience to parents as well as other older persons, including an older sibling.

It may appear that there is a breakdown in the modern African-American family. No doubt, African-American lifestyles are undergoing tremendous evolution, but the extended family plays a very important role in supporting the teenage adolescent mother. In the United States, "Black teens are only 14% of the teenage population, yet they account for 28% of all adolescent births and 47% of all births to unmarried teens" (Williams, 1991, p. 9).

Teenage mothers usually live with their mothers, and these grandmothers hold a central and integral place in the family structure. The African-American grandmother is a source of wisdom, strength, and leadership. Jones (1991) described the role of the Black grandmother as "an authority on the mysteries of life—having babies and caring for them, curing common illnesses, preparing tasty meals from meager food . . . she was respected and esteemed for her knowledge . . . and willingly helped neighbors, as well as her own kin" (p. 50). In the 1990s, this role continues, with grandmothers often the sole caretakers, as their children are lost to drug addiction and incarceration.

Many African Americans are more focused on the present situation and are not future-oriented. Some believe that time is flexible and that events will begin when they arrive. Some African Americans believe that planning for the future is hopeless, because of their previous encounters with racism and discrimination (Poussaint & Atkinson, 1970). Their concept of the future is colored by their strong religious belief that there will be happiness and freedom from pain after death. Therefore, the sufferings and tribulations on earth become more bearable (Giger & Davidhizar, 1991).

THE IMPORTANCE OF CULTURAL ASSESSMENT IN CLINICAL PRACTICE

Nursing care to clients of multiethnic backgrounds is often problematic. The United States has been referred to as the "melting pot" of myriad races and creeds. The concept of melting pot emerged largely from a combination of cultural ideas of equality and the European ethnocentric perspective. Yet each ethnic group strives to remain pure, largely due to the desire to retain traditional rituals and mores. Over the past two centuries, there has emerged a generic American culture, with its ethnocentric views prominent in the delivery of health care. Stan-

dardization, mass production, and reliance on technology permeate mainstream American culture, but they are not characteristic of traditional cultures. Therefore, gauges, such as the Denver II (a simple test to assess the development of children under the age of 6 in the areas of personal/social, fine motor/adaptive, language, and gross motor development), are often misused when they are applied without allowing for differences in culture. For example, in many African-American households, it is customary for infants to sleep with their mothers or grandmothers; this practice is often disturbing to mainstream health care providers.

The American health care system has focused on generalization of client needs, and it has become sorely lacking in assessment of ethnic differences among patients. Cultural differences are often at the root of poor communication, interpersonal tensions, ineffective working relationships, and poor assessment of health problems. Nurses need to understand the client's values, beliefs, family life patterns, and forms of communication in order to provide relevant care. Recently, ethnicity has been recognized as an important consideration for effective health care delivery (Tripp-Reimer & Afifi, 1989). In fact, over the past four decades, transcultural concepts have emerged and been recognized as essential to effective nursing in an intensely multicultural world (Leininger, 1995).

Today, cultural assessments are viewed as essential in caring for clients with diverse backgrounds. They go beyond "the traditional psychomotor, physiological, or mental health assessments to the broad holistic aspects of culture with multiple factors influencing people's behavior" (Leininger, 1995, p. 118).

PREPARATION FOR CULTURAL ASSESSMENT

How then, can nurses be prepared to perform cultural assessments? Both educators and service providers should rise to the challenge and provide knowledge and skills, enabling nurses to perform cultural assessments. Leininger (1995) points out, "to label a client's behavior and needs in ways that are inaccurate creates ethical problems" (p. 120). According to Boyle and Andrews (1989), collecting information about an individual's cultural background allows the nurse to modify interventions to mesh with the individual's cultural constraints and resources.

Health care practitioners who want to use cultural data in planning programs and interventions must decide how and what data to collect. Several models of cultural assessment tools are discussed in the literature, but no one tool is fully applicable.

Several cultural assessment tools are now available to help nurses in their everyday practice. Some more commonly used tools are

- Bloch's (1983) cultural assessment guide. It contains four major areas of data collection: cultural, sociological, psychological, and biological/physiological.
- Leininger's (1991) acculturation health care assessment. It is based on her culture care theory and Sunrise Model.
- Rosenbaum's (1991) cultural assessment guide. It addresses the areas of cultural affiliation, health care beliefs and practices, illness beliefs and customs, interpersonal relations, spiritual practices, and a world view and other social structures category.
- Tripp-Reimer and Afifi (1989) and Tripp-Reimer, Brink, and Saunders' (1984) cultural assessment guide. It assesses the cultural content of a client's system in a series of three stages that revolve around values, beliefs, and customs.

The content and comprehensiveness of each tool vary. The usefulness of these tools depends on the nurse's ability to select one that is appropriate for the client's health needs and concerns. For many clients, a thorough cultural assessment may not be necessary. Basic cultural data include ethnic affiliation, religious preference, family roles and functions, child-rearing practices, food patterns, and ethnic health care practices. An initial assessment will indicate whether further assessment of cultural factors is needed.

CASE STUDY OF AN AFRICAN-AMERICAN HOMELESS CLIENT

Rosenbaum's (1991) cultural assessment guide was modified and used in the cultural assessment of LH, a 50-year-old African-American homeless man with a presenting history of hypertension and angina.

The student gave affiliation information and asked the client's permission to learn more about his culture. It was explained that his participation in the interview was voluntary and that he was free to refuse to answer any questions or stop the interview at any time if he felt uncomfortable.

Health care beliefs and practices

Question: Can you tell me what care means to you, and how care is shown by people in your culture?

Response: Care means helping one another and sharing. The way things are now, there's not too much care. Not only Black people don't care, but nobody cares. In Colorado, we had rent parties if people could not pay the rent. We got together in our community and threw a party, charged some money, and the money raised was given to the family that needed help with the rent. We had painting parties. If someone's house burned, like what happened in the Los Angeles riots, everybody pitched in and helped that person.

Question: I'd like to understand what health means to you. Imagine yourself totally healthy. Explain what that would be like for you. Tell me how you would know when you are healthy. How do people in your culture stay healthy?

Response: Health means good physical condition with no aches and no pains. You wake up feeling good. My brother was sick before he died. He was always angry and upset. I'm not tense. People in my culture need to learn how to eat. They eat big meals with a lot of meat and highly seasoned foods. These are not very healthy. Few Black people eat vegetables, except some green leafy vegetables, string beans, and cabbage.

Question: What does food mean to you? Can you tell me the types of food you eat, how food is prepared, when your mealtimes are, and who you share your meals with?

Response: I share my meals with nobody. The types of foods I try to eat are chicken, fish, and turkey. Vegetables—I like all except cabbage; it does not like me. I love okra. I like cheese, but stay away from it because it's not good for my heart. I try to broil my food and stay away from fried foods. Because I am homeless, my mealtimes and the foods I eat are not on regular schedules. I have been eating much more prepared restaurant food because it's easy and hot.

Question: Can you tell me about activities or sports that were performed by you or your family to keep people healthy?

Response: In my culture, people do not usually do activities or sports to stay healthy. When I was young we would bike, play softball, and lift weights to get bigger and stronger. Those were the only activities we did to be healthy. Many Black men believe if you're strong, you're healthy.

Question: I would like to hear about your beliefs and practices regarding special life events such as birth and marriage. Can you tell me what getting older means to you and how older people are cared for in your culture?

Response: [Declined to answer the question regarding life events, saying it was too painful.] I don't know how older people are cared for. I don't mind getting old, as long as I am capable of taking care of myself. I want to age gracefully and die naturally. I don't want to be killed early and have another man decide my fate.

Illness: Beliefs and customs

In LH's family, drinks with lemon, honey, and castor oil were given to sick family members to help clean the phlegm and sickness from the body. The sick family member was rubbed down with Vicks or often hot mustard plasters. These treatments drew the illness out of the body. LH's mother made lye soap and family members used it to clean the skin, so infections did not occur. Today, LH drinks the lemon and honey with whiskey. He did not like the castor oil. It made him nauseated, and he hated the Vicks treatment.

Question: Can you tell me your culture's practices regarding illness?

Response: In the Black culture people don't talk about illness, they keep it to themselves. Just like loss, if they are about to lose something, their job or their house, they don't tell anyone until it's gone. Illness is the same way. When you hear that someone died, you say I did not even know he was sick. When something is wrong with a Black man, it's his own business.

Question: I would like to know more about your experiences with health professionals and your beliefs about when to go to them for help.

Response: I have good doctors. I have had good luck with my health care. If something is wrong and lasts over a week, then I know it's time to go to the doctor. Except this tooth. It's been hurting for a long time and you and the doctor have told me to go to the dentist, but I don't go. I don't know why I don't go to the dentist. Probably because I have had a bad experience.

[There are no folk healers and no evil eye according to LH.]

Interpersonal relations

Question: What is your philosophy of raising children, and what is their place in the family?

Response: I was raised with a strong belief in God, the Bible, and the church. God was instilled in our souls. The kids today are different. They are irreverent and rude. Their parents don't make them go to church and learn about God or the Bible. They have no rules, and they don't know how to behave. These days there's no place in the home for children; they are bad. But it is the parents' fault for not bringing the kids up with the belief of God and the Bible.

Spiritual practices

Question: Tell me more about your religious beliefs and your spiritual self.

Response: As I have told you before, I believe strongly in God and the Bible. I believe in God of the Living Church. When no living person can help me, I go to God and tell him my problems.

Question: Tell me about your feelings about life and death.

Response: Life's been good to me. I have made mistakes in life. But I can't blame anyone but myself for where my life is. I live life day-by-day. It's something we all have to do. No one in my family has ever gotten killed. My daughter died a tragic death, but she's the only one.

Question: Can you tell me about your beliefs and practices related to the death of a loved one? How do people in your culture mourn? Do you believe in spirits and the afterlife? I also want to know when it is appropriate for men and women to express their feelings when a loved one dies.

Response: When people die, the family grieves together. They take care of the funeral. They sing and pray all day because it is a way to let go of the pain they feel. I don't believe in afterlife or spirits. In my culture, the man never shows his feelings in public. They don't even show their women or kids their feelings. You just leave a man alone when he grieves, because he's angry and hurt inside. The women carry on and cry all day long, sometimes for weeks. My sister she never got over my mother's death. Never! That's the way it is in the Black culture.

Question: Please tell me about the duties of men and women in your religion and church.

Response: The men are deacons, pastors, preachers, and ushers. They take the offerings. There is a man's choir, a woman's choir, and a combined choir. The women don't do much in church. They are in the choir, and they take care of the children.

World view and other social structures

Question: Can you tell me how you see life in relation to the world around you?

Response: Poor! But as long as I am able and the world around me does not affect me, I enjoy life. I don't care what the world around me does.

Question: What in life is important to you?

Response: A good relationship with a woman. I haven't had that in a long time and I miss that.

Question: Tell me the kinds of jobs members of your family have had and how finances have influenced your life.

Response: Most of my people have been domestic types. My brother and myself were cooks. My older brother worked for the water department. My sister and my mother were domestic helpers. I don't know about the finances, we've always been poor. The finances haven't influenced my life any.

Question: Can you tell me what education means to you? Describe the education you received and what education you hope your children will receive.

Response: I did not finish high school. I always regret not having an education. I want my children to get an education. I worry that their grandmother is too old to push them hard and with boys you have to push them hard. I want my two sons to get a college education. Every one in my family got their high school education, except me and I don't want my children to be like me.

Outcome of interview

The insights gained from this interview yielded improved understanding of the client as a person and helped in the planning of interventions. LH was assisted in finding a place to live. He was able to cook and eat healthy meals, and his cardiac condition has improved. His progress is a tribute to nursing education and transcultural caring.

REFERENCES

Andrews, M.M. (1992). Cultural perspectives on nursing in the 21st century. *Journal of Professional Nursing, 8*(1), 7–15.

Bloch, B. (1983). Bloch's assessment guide for ethnic/cultural variations. In M. Orque, B. Bloch, & L. Monnroy (Eds.), *Ethnic nursing care: A multicultural approach.* St. Louis, MO: Mosby.

Boyle, S., & Andrews, M. (1989). *Transcultural concepts in nursing care.* Boston, MA: Scott/Foresman & Company.

Cherry, B., & Giger, J.N. (1991). Black Americans. In J.N. Giger & R.E. Davidhizar (Eds.), *Transcultural nursing.* St. Louis, MO: Mosby–Year Book.

Giger, J.N., & Davidhizar, R.E. (1991). *Transcultural nursing* (1st ed.). St. Louis, MO: Mosby.

Jackson, L.E. (1993). Understanding, eliciting and negotiating clients' multicultural health beliefs. *Nurse Practitioner, 18*(2), 30–32, 37–43.

Jones, F.C. (1991). The lofty role of the Black grandmother. *Crisis, 80*(1), 41–56.

Leininger, M.M. (Ed.). (1991). *Culture care diversity and universality: A theory of nursing.* New York, NY: NLN Press.

Leininger, M.M. (1995). *Transcultural nursing: Concepts, theories, research & practices.* New York, NY: McGraw-Hill.

Neiderhauser, V.P. (1989). Health care of immigrant children: Incorporating culture into practice. *Pediatric Nursing, 15*(6), 569–574.

Poussaint, A., & Atkinson, C. (1970). Black youth and motivation. *Black Scholar, 1,* 43–51.

Rosenbaum, J.N. (1991). A cultural assessment guide: Learning cultural sensitivity. *Canadian Nurse, 87*(4), 32–33.

Spector, R.E. (1991). *Cultural diversity in health and illness.* (3rd ed.). Englewood Cliffs, NJ: Prentice Hall.

Tripp-Reimer, T., & Afifi, L. (1989). Cross-cultural perspectives on patient teaching. *Nursing Clinics of North America, 24*(3), 613–619.

Tripp-Reimer, T., Brink, P., & Saunders, J. (1984). Cultural assessment: Content and process. *Nursing Outlook, 32*(2), 78–82.

U.S. Bureau of the Census. (1983). General population characteristics—Part I. In *United States summary 1980 census of population* (Vol. 1). Washington, DC: Government Printing Office.

U.S. Department of Health and Human Services. (1985). *Health status of minorities and low income groups* (DHHS Publication No. [HRSA] HRS-P-DV 85-1). Washington, DC: Government Printing Office.

U.S. Department of Justice. (1995). *Prisoners in 1994 (Bureau of Justice Statistics Bulletin* NCJ-151654). Washington, DC: Author.

Williams, C.W. (1991). *Black teenage mothers: Pregnancy and childrearing from their perspective.* Lexington, MA: Lexington Books.

Willis, W. (1992). Families with African-American roots. In E.W. Lynch & M.J. Hanson (Eds.), *Developing cross-cultural competence.* Baltimore: Brookes.

The World Bank. (1990, June). *World development report 1990: Poverty.* New York: Oxford University Press.

Jewish Beliefs, Values, and Practices: Implications for Culturally Sensitive Nursing Care

Sharon E. Beck, DNSc, RN
Assistant Hospital Director
Nursing Education and Quality Improvement
Temple University Hospital
Philadelphia, Pennsylvania

Evelyn K. Goldberg, MS, RN
Community Health Educator
Tru Care Home Health Agency, Inc.
Philadelphia, Pennsylvania

Source: Reprinted from S. Beck and E.K. Goldberg, *Advanced Practice Nursing Quarterly,* Vol. 2, No. 2, pp. 15–22, © 1996, Aspen Publishers, Inc.

Tevya, in a song from *Fiddler on the Roof,* proclaims "Tradition! Tradition! We have a tradition for everything—how to sleep, how to eat, how to work, and even how to wear clothes." Much of what Jews do can be considered tradition. The tradition, though, is based on three millennia of religious and cultural experiences. Knowing what some of these traditions and practices are can help nurses provide culturally sensitive care to their Jewish patients.

Of the 258 million people in the United States, only 2.3% identify themselves as Jewish (U.S. Bureau of the Census, 1994). Worldwide, only about 0.25% identify themselves as Jewish (Johnson, 1994). The majority of American Jews live in and around large metropolitan areas.

Judaism is passed from mother to child. Thus, if a woman is Jewish, her child is Jewish. A Jewish man must marry a Jewish woman or a religiously converted woman in order to have Jewish children. This requirement has been observed for about 3,500 years, causing some to characterize the Jewish people as a race.

Many of the laws Jews follow, practices they do religiously and culturally, affect every aspect of daily life, from waking in the morning with special prayers, to retiring at night with more special prayers. These laws encompass such things as Jewish men wearing fringed shawls under their shirts, ritually washing the hands before eating, covering one's head, keeping a kosher diet, and making ethical decisions in business and personal relationships.

The Jewish religion is monotheistic, that is, teaching that there is only one God. This God revealed himself to Moses and all those present at Mt. Sinai and gave the Jewish people the Ten Commandments and the entire Torah, or Five Books of Moses (Old Testament). The word *Torah* means teaching or instruction (Wigoder, 1989, p. 709). The Torah, which is central to the Jewish religion, is said to contain all that one needs to live a happy, healthy, and ethical life. Thus is derived the idea that Judaism is a way of life as well as a religion. Throughout Jewish history there have been many rabbinical commentators who have written explicit and detailed interpretations of the Torah. One's interpretation will affect the level of observance of the 613 commandments, or instructions (laws), found in the Torah. Religious observance of Jewish laws might be placed on a continuum, with extremely strict observance on the right end and little-to-no observance on the left end. Figure 1 depicts how the continuum might look.

The purpose of the laws of the Torah is to make each person act in an ethical manner toward fellow humans, and toward all of God's creatures. It is said that Rabbi Hillel of the first century B.C.E. (Before the Common Era) was asked to tell, while standing on one foot, what Judaism is all about. He is said to have replied, "Do not to others that which you would not have others do to you" (Heifetz, 1991, p. 73). Thus, Judaism is a religion and a complete system of ethical living. Following the laws and doing ethical acts is called doing a *mitzvah* or a good deed. Examples of *mitzvot* (plural form) are saying a prayer before eating, honoring one's parents and teachers, saying a kind word to the patient in the next bed or to the nurse, taking care of one's body, and teaching one to earn a living.

As the Orthodox define strict religious observance based on the Torah, the information presented here will be from that perspective. Please keep in mind, though, that one may see many different levels of observance; they are all Jewish.

BELIEFS AND ETHICAL PRINCIPLES

Preservation of life and health

Jews believe that God created the world and that we were created in His image. The body is only a loan from God, and one is required to care for it (Lebeau, 1983). Hence we find that Jews make in-depth use of the medical system, wanting to exhaust all possibilities. Hand washing is part of a religious ritual, with a special prayer being said along with the act. This ritual was observed long before microorganisms were discovered. Caring for one's body is considered a mitzvah. Jews also believe that illness is not a coincidence. It is a time to reflect and do soul searching to improve oneself and to express regret (S. Caplan, personal communication, January 2, 1996).

In Judaism, the preservation of life takes precedence over all other values. With only three exceptions, every Jewish law may be disobeyed if it can be demonstrated that keeping it would be life-threatening. The exceptions are idolatry, murder, and sexual immorality such as incest and rape (Kertzer, 1993). Therefore, all ritual laws and religious observances are suspended if they have the potential to be harmful to life. If, for example, fasting on a fast day would induce medical harm or decrease life in any way, then one is obligated not to fast (Bleich, 1981). Patients often need help from the professional in understanding this principle so that they can do what is necessary to sustain life without feeling guilty. In addition, it is the Jewish health professional's responsibility to preserve life at all costs. A goal of medicine for the Jewish physician is to improve the quality of life. However, the quality of life is never a factor in determining

Reformed	Reconstructionist	Conservative	Orthodox

Figure 1. Continuum of observance of Jewish laws.

whether a patient should live or die. Pain and suffering require compassion, support, and pain medication, but not the termination of life. Thus, making the decision to remove life supports that have already been instituted is not an option (Rosner, 1991).

Aging is not considered a disease. Thus a 90-year-old has the same right to life as someone who is 10 or 30. Respect for the aged is important, and the value of life is not predicated on utility (Meier, 1991). It is incumbent on the individual to seek medical treatment when ill because taking care of oneself is mandated. Physician and patient are considered "partners with God." Jews are expected to be responsible for both themselves and their neighbors (Rosner, 1991).

Orthodox patients will often need to consult with their rabbi before making medical decisions. If the rabbi finds the problem difficult to answer, consult with a rabbinical medical specialist, such as a bioethicist who is also an Orthodox rabbi. Such a specialist is learned in medicine, Torah, law, and ethics. Contemporary rabbinical commentators strive to answer biomedical ethical dilemmas relating to modern medical advances, such as: As Jews are prohibited from eating blood, can blood transfusions be used to save a life (*The Holy Scriptures,* 1956)? What does Torah say about the use of gene therapy, fetal tissue, and organ transplantation?

Truth-telling

Part of the ethical system in Judaism is the obligation to tell the truth and not engage in falsehoods. As in every ethical system, however, there are exceptions. Because preservation of life takes precedence over truth-telling in the treatment of terminal illness, the decision of how and what to tell the patient must be weighed against the need to preserve the patient's physical and mental well-being. Patients should be made aware that an illness is serious so that they can get their affairs in order (Rosner, 1986). On the other hand, an important obligation is to do no harm. Continuing to care for the patient and administering medication that might not be use-ful could be done for the psychological effect of fostering hope. Jewish law deems it important not to hasten death by disclosure (Bleich, 1981).

Confidentiality

Judaism has very strict rules about disclosure of confidential information. It is recognized, however, that there are situations in which confidential information may need to be disclosed. The overriding principle is the need to know coupled with the need to do no harm. "Respect for privacy and the inviolability of the professional relationship certainly do not take precedence over protection of lives and the safety of others" (Bleich, 1981, p. 35). The recipient of such information is obligated to reveal it in order to save lives or property.

JEWISH PRACTICES AND RITUALS

A distinctive feature of Judaism is its great variety of rituals that cover every aspect of the life cycle. Practices become symbolic and move beyond the ordinary to the holy. Legal requirements are called halachah, which means "the Jewish way of walking in the world." Many customs are associated with these legal requirements and rituals (Kertzer, 1993). One example is the legal requirement of circumcision and the rituals surrounding the ceremony. Another example is the legal requirement to procreate.

Birth

A number of beliefs, practices, and rituals surround birth. Some of these are

- Sexual intercourse arises from the commandment to multiply; therefore, it is a holy act. Humans are born pure (without sin) from this holy act, and each child is considered a blessing.
- During childbirth a woman is considered in the category of someone ill; therefore, any Jewish law that would put her in danger is set aside (Abraham, 1990).

- A male Jewish child is circumcised and named on the 8th day after birth, never before. If the infant is sick or weak, he may not be circumcised until it is safe to do so. If one twin has died within 8 days of birth, the other infant may not be circumcised until 31 days (Abraham, 1990).
- Circumcision on the 8th day may take place on the Sabbath, but if it is delayed for health reasons, it may not take place on the Sabbath (Bleich, 1981).
- Circumcision is performed by a mohel, a religious man specially trained to perform this ritual. Ideally it takes place in the home and is witnessed by 10 Jewish men. Godmothers and godfathers are chosen and take part in the ceremony.
- When a female child is born the father is called to read the Torah in the synagogue. Modern Jewish families have made this event a celebration as well (Trepp, 1980).
- Abortion is an option if there is danger to the mother's life from the continuance of the pregnancy. An unborn fetus is not considered a person until born; the fetus is considered part of the mother's body and not separate until the head has emerged. At that time the child cannot be harmed for any reason. A stillborn fetus is buried, not discarded. It is preferable, if an abortion is necessary, that it be performed within the first 40 days after conception (Abraham, 1990).
- A woman is considered impure whenever blood is coming from her uterus, on the occasion of birth or menstruation. Her husband is not permitted to have physical contact with her until she has gone to the ritual bath (mikvah).
- Orthodox men may not touch any woman other than their wife, daughter, or mother (Carson, 1989). It would be inappropriate for a female nurse to extend her arm for a handshake.

Visiting the sick

It is the duty of every Jew to visit the sick. This duty includes taking care of the physical and emotional needs of the patient and praying on the patient's behalf. Close relatives visit first, and more distant friends and relatives visit after 3 days. If, however, the illness has occurred suddenly, all may visit at once. Jewish families are usually close; therefore, it is not unusual for many visitors to come and stay with the family. This extra attention helps both the patient and the family cope with the illness. When a person recovers from a serious illness, there is a special prayer that is recited (Rosner, 1986).

Dying and death

Death is considered part of life. There is constant awareness that life is finite. The only acceptable determination of death is irreversible cessation of breathing and heartbeat. Absence of brain waves does not indicate death. It is very important to know the precise time of death because it is used to determine both the mourning period (Shiva) and the annual honoring of the dead (yahrzeit).

Jewish law requires that the body be treated with utmost respect. Limbs must be straightened, not crossed; the eyes must be closed; the lower jaw must be bound; and the body must be covered (Abraham, 1990).

Autopsies required by civil law or those that may lead to information that will contribute to the preservation of life are permissible, but must be limited; the remains must be treated with respect at all times. For example, an autopsy would be warranted if a patient were receiving an experimental drug and the autopsy would provide information about that drug in order to aid others. Limbs and organs that are removed should preferably be buried with the body. Bed linens and clothing stained with blood lost in death may also be required for burial. The body is "guarded" from the time of death to that of the burial. The guard stays with the body at all times, even at the funeral home. The body is ritually washed, usually by an independent group associated with the community. The body is clothed in simple white linen (Bleich, 1981).

Cremation and embalming are prohibited by Jewish law. If a person mandates cremation then he or she may not be buried in a Jewish cemetery. Cosmetic treatment of the body is also forbidden as is the public viewing of the body. Burial takes place as soon as possible after death unless a delay is necessary in order to allow close relatives to be present (Bleich, 1981). A plain wooden coffin is used for burial, and no flowers are permitted. Funeral services are not elaborate, thereby preventing ostentation and embarrassment and creating equality (Wigoder, 1989). Legal euthanasia at the request of someone incurably ill and in pain is against tradition. While it is prohibited to remove life sustaining devices, there is no mandate to apply the equipment (Kertzer, 1993).

Deathbed confession begins with a prayer for healing and ends with an affirmation of God. Rabbis cannot pardon sins; only God and the person who was sinned against can grant a pardon. It is therefore encouraged at the end of life for the individual to make amends to the aggrieved party. A sin against God can only be reprieved through repentance and a resolve not to repeat the transgression (Kertzer, 1993). A witness must be present when a person prays for health so that if death occurs, God will protect the family and the spirit will be committed to God. Extraneous talking about death is not encouraged unless it is initiated by the patient (Carson, 1989).

The first period of mourning (Shiva), which is commemorated by the wearing of a torn black ribbon, begins immediately after the funeral. Shiva is not observed from sundown Friday evening to sundown Saturday, or on holidays. The length of the mourning period is usually 7 days. The immediate family are obliged to sit Shiva and to do no work. During this week, friends and family visit to offer help and condolences. Food is brought so that the mourners do not have to cook. One of the greatest good deeds is to contribute to the mourners' first meal. It is customary today for friends and relatives to make or send food during the entire period of Shiva.

Ill persons are not informed of the death of close relatives if it is likely to lead to deterioration of their own health (Abraham, 1990). It is customary to cover all mirrors during the Shiva period and to wash one's hands before entering the house for the first time. Mourning rituals are meant to strengthen and support the family and honor the dead (Kertzer, 1993).

After the first week of mourning, a general period of mourning ensues for 11 months. At a convenient time before the first anniversary of death, a memorial stone is unveiled at the graveside. After the first year, anyone who has ever been a mourner recites a memorial prayer on the anniversary of the death and at certain holidays.

Special clothes

The kippah, or skullcap, is worn to pray. Most Orthodox men wear this head covering at all times. It is seen as a sign of respect for God. Orthodox married women wear hats or wigs over their hair as well as long dresses and long sleeves as signs of feminine modesty. Orthodox men wear small tailit, or prayer shawls, under their shirts and larger versions when praying. Many Orthodox men also wear long black coats and black hats (Kertzer, 1993).

Education

Education and scholarship are highly valued by the Jewish populace. The Jews have long been known as "the people of the book." Study of Torah is done in a very systematic way. Three times each week, a specific portion is ritually read from the Torah scroll and then studied. It takes exactly 1 year to complete the reading and study of the entire Torah scroll; the process is begun again on the day of completion. Each year that the reading and study are completed, the person gains new wisdom since the Torah is being perceived through the eyes of one who is a year older than the last. Jewish parents generally want their children to be better off than they are in terms of education, health, and wealth. Education is seen as the chief means to that goal, and many Jewish children attend highly rated public or private schools.

Questioning everything is in keeping with the nature of Judaism, even to questioning God. It is through questioning and looking beyond what is visible that creative problem solving and discovery occur. Jewish patients may ask many questions, sometimes asking the same question over and over again, trying to gain new insight.

Sabbath

The Jewish Sabbath starts at sundown on Friday and ends at sundown on Saturday. All days begin with the evening sunset and continue to the following sunset. Friday evening Sabbath dinner is a time for family togetherness. Whole families may pray, learn, eat, and communicate on this holy evening. Orthodox Jews observe this day strictly; other Jews observe it less so, to varying degrees. Some do not use the telephone on the Sabbath, do not work, drive, do housework, or sew. They do nothing that tears something apart (like toilet paper on a roll) or puts something together (like fixing or mending). Also included are such things as writing and handling money. Sabbath candles are to be lit by the Jewish woman even in the hospital.

An article (Sommer, 1995) written about the practices in Maimonides Medical Center in Brooklyn, New York, which has a large Orthodox Jewish population, describes a number of accommodations that have been instituted for this group for the Sabbath. For example, a Jewish patient who comes into the emergency department does not have to sign a written consent until after the Sabbath is over. Because Orthodox Jewish patients do not ride on the Sabbath, they are permitted to stay in the hospital or emergency department until after sundown on Saturday. The hospital has a Sabbath elevator that automatically stops on all floors so that buttons do not have to be pushed. Orthodox nurses and physicians are given the appropriate time off for both Sabbath and holidays. Privacy for prayers is also provided.

Operations not considered urgent are not performed on the Sabbath nor are preparations for these operations, such as blood tests, shaving, and so forth (Abraham, 1990). Jews are required to set aside the laws of the Sabbath in case of possible danger to life.

Keeping kosher

The word kosher means "fit or proper"; that is, the food must be made ritually fit for human consumption (Kolatch, 1990, p. 106). Jews consider "keeping kosher" a way of transforming the mundane, physical act of eating into a holy act that requires one to think about and to praise God (Dresner & Siegel, 1959; Jacobs, 1987; Klein, 1979; Prager & Telushkin, 1975). Keeping kosher also "encompasses aspects of discipline, and of behaving humanely and ethically toward people and animals" (Goldberg, 1994).

Observance of kosher laws could be placed on the previously mentioned continuum from reform to orthodoxy (see Figure 1). Basically, all fresh fruits, vegetables, and legumes are kosher. Fish with both scales and fins, such as tuna, salmon, flounder, and cod, are kosher. Animals that both chew their cud and have split hooves, such as cows and sheep, as well as domesticated fowl, such as chicken, turkey, duck, and goose, are all considered kosher (Jacobs, 1987).

Kosher foods are divided into three main categories: meat, dairy, and parve. Foods made from milk components are called dairy. These foods include milk, cream, ice cream, cheeses, butter, and all products that contain dairy components, such as whey, lactose, and casein. These substances are often found in some breads and salad dressings as well as other commonly consumed foods (Freedman, 1970).

Foods made from animal components are called meat. Meat products are those items made using acceptable animals and fowl (as described previously). The animal must be killed by a specially trained person, called a shoket, in the most humane way possible (usually by cutting both the jugular and the carotid with a smooth-edged, ultra-sharp blade). The meat is then salted in order to remove the blood. Jews are absolutely forbidden to eat blood because it is the symbol of life (Klein, 1979). The meat may then be prepared as steaks, chops, roasts, patties, soups, hot dogs, and so forth.

Milk (dairy) products and meat products are not eaten together at the same meal. Parve foods are those that are neither meat nor dairy. This group includes fruits, vegetables, grains, legumes, eggs (without any blood spots), and acceptable fish. Fish does not include any shellfish because of the requirement to have both scales and fins.

Ingredients in a food product may render it unkosher. Hard cheeses, such as Swiss and muenster, contain "rennet," which is made from the intestines of an animal. If it was a kosher animal that was slaughtered in a kosher manner, then the cheese is kosher (Eidlitz, 1992). Soups are another example. Many soups, such as minestrone and vegetable, contain a meat or chicken base. If the meat or chicken is a kosher animal that was slaughtered in a kosher fashion, then the soup is considered a meat. Cream of broccoli soup and other cream soups are usually made with a chicken base. Because chicken is considered a meat, and it may not be eaten with dairy, the soup is not kosher. Non-dairy creamer is another example. It often contains sodium caseinate, a milk protein, and therefore it is a dairy product that may only be served with a dairy meal.

The Jewish community has an elaborate system of overseeing organizations that supervise and certify that a product is kosher. Each organization has its own symbol, which is placed on the product. Some symbols seen commonly are Ⓤ, Ⓚ, Ⓚo, ⟨Ⓚ⟩, Ⓚ, CRⒸ, Ⓚ, K, ☩. Products certified by strict religious Orthodox rabbinical organizations are accepted by most Jews as being "strictly" kosher. A kosher product that contains a dairy component, such as a bread containing whey, may have a tiny "D" next to the Kosher symbol, thus, Ⓤᴅ. The symbol on a parve product, such as egg noodles, might look like this, Ⓤᴘ (Kolatch, 1990).

Orthodox Jewish patients have a very strict interpretation of biblical law and will not eat foods that are prepared in a hospital kitchen. Family members can bring in the foods required by the patient in order to supplement any kosher foods available from the dietary department. The nurse can use this opportunity to teach the patient and family about his or her nutritional requirements. A hypertensive patient, for example, might be placed on a sodium-free, low-fat diet. The family could make salt-free chicken soup with rice, boiled chicken without the skin, boiled potatoes, and broccoli spears, all without salt. This meal would be a meat meal, and any accompanying coffee or tea would not have milk or cream. The box provides an example of a 2-day meal plan using dairy and parve foods. Orthodox patients

---

Two-Day Meal Plan

Day 1

Breakfast
  Orange juice
  Cold cereal, 1 serving
  Milk
  Coffee, tea, herb tea

Lunch
  Garden salad
  Bagel with cream cheese
  Fresh fruit salad
  Soda or iced tea

Dinner
  Cottage cheese on lettuce
  Broiled flounder
  Baked potato with margarine
  Mixed vegetables
  Whole wheat bread
  Prepackaged kosher cake
  Soda or hot tea

Day 2

Breakfast
  Fresh grapefruit half
  2 hard-boiled eggs
  Toast and jelly
  Coffee, tea, milk, herb tea

Lunch
  Cream of potato soup
  Cooked noodles with cottage cheese
  Steamed vegetables
  Soda or hot chocolate

Dinner
  Vegetarian lasagna
  Green beans with almonds
  Roll
  Frozen yogurt
  Hot tea or coffee

and their families would be unlikely to eat meat meals outside their home, unless they were specially packaged kosher frozen meals that could be heated and served to the patient in their own disposable tray.

IMPLICATIONS FOR CULTURALLY SENSITIVE PATIENT CARE

Sarah Greenfeld, a 59-year-old patient newly diagnosed with insulin dependent diabetes, anxiously informs you that she must speak to her rabbi before taking her prescribed pork insulin. The family of 22-year-old David Grossman, a trauma victim, is being asked to donate his heart and corneas. They, too, say they must speak to their rabbi before making a decision. The nurse finds Mr. Cohen standing, facing the window with a prayerbook in his hand. She comes up to him and asks him to take his medications. He motions for her to leave and continues to pray. Each of these patients has identified themselves as Jewish.

What does each situation mean to you, the nursing professional? Each represents a common circumstance that the nurse could encounter. The information presented in this article will give the nurse some understanding of these situations, but due to the wide variation in Jewish practices, even within the various groups, it is important for the nurse to ascertain from the patient and family exactly what their particular beliefs and practices are. A good rapport with the patient and good communication skills are very useful in eliciting this information.

Sarah Greenfeld might cringe at the thought of taking pork insulin. After all, she would never eat pork. The culturally sensitive nurse might help her call her rabbi. The rabbi most likely would explain to her that she is permitted and even required to take this insulin for three reasons: (1) her life is dependent on taking the medication; (2) it is in a form that is unrecognizable from its origins; and (3) she will be injecting the insulin, not ingesting it. After Mrs. Greenfeld's conversation with the rabbi, she probably would feel freer to verbalize other concerns about her disease process to her nurse.

The distraught family of David Grossman, at the suggestion of their nurse, might speak to their rabbi about organ donation. Their rabbi would explain that organ donation has been approved by the Orthodox movement's Rabbinical Council of America, if the organs are harvested in accord with the highest standards of dignity (Rosenberg, 1991). They most likely would be grateful for the deference shown to their beliefs at such a difficult time.

Furthermore, if a nurse is aware that morning and afternoon prayers are an important part of a Jewish person's day, seeing Mr. Cohen with prayerbook in hand would be a clear signal not to interrupt. The nurse could leave quietly and return in 15 minutes with the medication. Being culturally sensitive to Mr. Cohen's needs would not only individualize his plan of care but also facilitate cooperation.

● ● ●

As advanced practice nurses, it is important to recognize that Jewish patients have many different beliefs and customs that have the potential to influence their care. As Judaism is a way of life, all aspects of care may be influenced by rituals, beliefs, and practices. It is therefore essential that nurses understand that these practices exist and find out from the patient and family the customs and beliefs to which they adhere.

REFERENCES

Abraham, S.A. (1990). *Comprehensive guide to medical halachah.* Jerusalem, Israel: Feldheim.

Bleich, J.D. (1981). *Judaism and healing.* Hoboken, NJ: Ktav.

Carson, V. (1989). *Spiritual dimension of nursing practice.* Philadelphia, PA: W.B. Saunders.

Dresner, S., & Siegel, S. (1959). *The Jewish dietary laws.* New York, NY: Burning Bush Press.

Eidlitz, E. (1992). *Is it kosher?* New York, NY: Feldheim Publishers.

Freedman, S. (1970). *The book of Kashruth: A treasury of kosher facts.* New York, NY: Bloch.

Goldberg, E.K. (1994, September 19). When your patient requires a kosher diet. *Nursing Spectrum, 3*(19), 18.

Heifetz, M. (1991). A concept of ethics. In L. Meier (Ed.), *Jewish values in health and medicine.* New York, NY: University Press.

Jacobs, L. (1987). The dietary laws. In L. Jacobs (Ed.), *The book of Jewish practice.* NJ: Behrman House.

Johnson, O. (Ed.). (1994). *Information please almanac 1995.* New York, NY: Houghton Mifflin.

Kertzer, M.N. (1993). *What is a Jew?* New York, NY: Collier Books.

Klein, I. (1979). *A guide to Jewish religious practice.* New York, NY: Jewish Theological Seminary.

Kolatch, A. (1990). The foods we eat. In A. Kolatch (Ed.), *The Jewish home advisor.* New York, NY: Jonathan David Pub.

Lebeau, J. (1983). *The Jewish dietary laws: Sanctify life.* New York, NY: United Synagogue of America.

Meier, L. (1991). Three cardinal principles of Jewish medical ethics. In L. Meier (Ed.), *Jewish values in health and medicine.* New York, NY: University Press.

Prager, D., & Telushkin, J. (1975). *Eight questions people ask about Judaism.* New York, NY: Tze Ulmad Press.

Rosenberg, S. (1991). Organ donation: The ultimate tzedakah. *Jewish Exponent, 190*(21), 2x–3x.

Rosner, F. (1986). *Modern medicine and Jewish ethics.* Hoboken, NJ: Ktav.

Rosner, F. (1991). The patient–physician relationship: Responsibilities and limitations. In L. Meier (Ed.), *Jewish values in health and medicine.* New York, NY: University Press.

Sommer, B. (1995). How we do it: Special considerations for Orthodox Jewish patients in the emergency department. *Journal of Emergency Nursing, 21*(6), 569–570.

The Holy Scriptures. (1956). Philadelphia, PA: The Jewish Publication Society.

Trepp, L. (1980). *The complete book of Jewish observance.* New York, NY: Behrman House.

U.S. Bureau of the Census. (1994). *Statistical Abstract of the United States, 1994.* Washington, DC: Government Printing Office.

Wigoder, G. (Ed.). (1989). *The encyclopedia of Judaism.* New York, NY: Macmillan.

Cultural Diversity in Grief

Linda M. Esposito, RN, MPH
Assistant Coordinator

Pamela Buckalew, RN, CNS, C
Coordinator

Tabiri Chukunta, BA, MA
Manager of Safety and Coordinator of
  Diversity
New Jersey Sudden Infant Death Syndrome
  Resource Center
Department of Neonatology
St. Peter's Medical Center
New Brunswick, New Jersey

Source: Reprinted from L. Esposito, P. Buckalew, and T. Chukunta, *Home Health Care Management and Practice,* Vol. 8, No. 4, pp. 23–29, © 1996, Aspen Publishers, Inc.

Diversity is a part of the natural order of things, as natural as the trillion shapes and shades of the flowers of spring or the leaves of autumn.

—Gene Griessman

Culture, as defined by Brock, "is what makes you a stranger when you are away from home."[1(p.ix)] It includes, as Brock further explains, "all those beliefs and expectations about how people should speak and act which have become a kind of second nature to you as a result of social learning."[1(p.ix)] Consequently, when a person is exposed to an alien society, the result is "a disturbing feeling of disorientation and helplessness that is called 'culture shock.'"[1(p.ix)] This concept is significant in the United States, since America is one of the most ethnically diverse nations in the world. As America's culturally diverse population continues to increase rapidly, the need for a more culturally competent caregiver workforce also rises. According to the US Census Bureau, the population of Asian and Pacific Islanders in the United States increased by 87% from 1981 to 1991. Similarly, Hispanics increased by 50%; American Indians, Eskimos, and Aleuts by 42%; blacks by 15%; and whites by 7%. The bureau went on to project that in the next century, the greater number of people living in the United States will belong to groups now referred to as "minorities."

This article is written with the conviction that cultural sensitivity is not just another fad of the

1990s; it is the untapped resource for new skills needed to care for the increasingly diverse patient population. By reexamining attitudes toward patients of different cultures and gaining understanding of their cultures and psychosocial environment, the caregiver begins to develop cultural competence in dealing with cross-cultural issues.

ARGUMENT AGAINST CULTURALLY SENSITIVE CARE

The question some caregivers ask is "Won't pointing out cultural differences make things worse?" "If you point out differences won't the caregiver develop stereotypes?" "Isn't it safer to emphasize that everyone is the same?"

Concerns about addressing differences arise from the mistaken notion that differences in themselves are negative or, at best, without value. Color and culture blindness assume that "we are all the same." Sameness attitude arose as a progressive argument against racial bigotry, which ranked races, putting "white" on top and everyone else following. However well intentioned, it is not the adequate and effective response to the patient's realities, since it establishes the culture of some as the norm, while ignoring the cultures of others.

Another offshoot of "sameness" attitude is the misguided notion that sameness is synonymous with equality. This equality-as-sameness assumption has created major dilemmas for groups from different cultures, who are expected to completely deny and forget their culture (and identity) in order to "fit in."

A caregiver who assumes that all patients are of the same culture assumes that all needs could be met outside the realm of the patient's cultural identity. In some respect this assumption is like expecting left-handed patients to write with their right hands because they receive care in cultures dominated by right-handed people.

LITERATURE REVIEW

Grief assessment and assisting families through the process of their grief is a challenge to the home health care nurse. Current theories and practice stress the importance of being aware of the family's specific culture, which can help the nurse effectively meet this challenge. It is important to realize that sudden infant death syndrome (SIDS) and other diagnoses that are acceptable in the biomedical perspective may not necessarily be congruent with other health belief models.[2]

The nurse will need to assess varied aspects of the family's belief system, such as the degree to which the specific culture affects the family's ability to cope in its grief process. Is the culture one of a spiritual or biomedical orientation? What resources does the family have? Does the family mesh and intertwine with American cultural beliefs in the grief process or are they distinctly different? How long have they been residing in the United States? Rural and urban locations may also affect the family's belief system. Similarly, it is of equal importance for the nurse to become in touch with his or her own belief system and attitudes toward death and grief.

The following represents a literature search of current beliefs and coping behavior of people from varied cultures. Although preliminary, they may provide the information needed for the nurse to become culturally sensitive to the family's grief needs and orientation.

Native Americans

Lawson[2] defines the term Native American as encompassing diverse tribal groups with distinct characteristics and styles. The Native American culture has varied degrees of influence from contemporary American culture. Strobe[3] addresses the mourning practices of the Navajo people as being limited to 4 days, and the bereaved are expected to return to normal life.[3] Excessive emotion is not encouraged within these 4 days. The Navajo people believe speaking of the deceased or of their emotions concerning the loss can do harm to the living due to the power of the deceased individual. In family life children have great value and may be the only achievement they possess in life. Religious ceremonies are based on living with nature; wakes are long, with food and memorial gifts distributed. Many Native Americans believe that the spirit of the dying person cannot be freed unless the family is with them.[4] Miller and Schoenfeld[5] explored the occurrence of the pathologic grief-work hypothesis. In the Navajo people the cultural norms do not endorse the grief-work hypothesis. It is doubtful that this suppression of grief does not have an effect on the individual in terms of depression. Often suspicious of individuals of European descent, Native Americans may respond to an approach of sensitivity and respect for their spiritual beliefs. The Navajo are private grievers, and expressing grief is believed harmful to the spirit of the deceased. The nurse's grief assessment should include the entire family. Listening and providing support to the family or community may be more effective than use of an interview style.

Mexican-Americans

Mexican-Americans are defined in the literature as people who have migrated from Mexico to the United States and those people who are their descendants.[2] Usually Spanish is their first language and the one commonly used in the home. Ross[4] identified Spanish-speaking peoples' thoughts on death as punishment from God for evil deeds. Spanish people accept a strong need to engage in penance in a way of suffering during their grief process. It is unthinkable to send a dying relative to the hospital or an aged family member to a nursing home.[5] Language consideration is an important area to address in providing grief counseling. It should not be assumed that the language the patient speaks is also what he or she can read. Interpreters may be necessary. Some Spanish families may be reluctant to accept home visits because they may possess inadequate proof of legal status. Religion and ceremonies play an important part in working through Spanish peoples' grief. The family is the major support system.

Southeast Asians

The term Southeast Asians encompasses a diverse group of people. Included are a number of different ethnic groups, languages, and religions, as well as nations of origin. According to Yamamoto,[6] the Japanese people's grief belief system is not based on working through their grief, but on a need to feel a continued sense of the deceased individual's presence and effects on the survivors' lives. They speak to their ancestors and work toward maintaining the relationship. McGoldrick et al[7] describe the Chinese family as having a similar belief system concerning death: one is classified as a "good death" if certain rituals are followed and as a "bad death" if rituals are not followed. A good death is expected either by a medical disease process or advanced age; the family has a chance to say goodbye to the loved one. The last experience the deceased has is viewing his or her loved ones. The family is allowed to exhibit great emotion at the time of death. Mourning is 49 days, strips of black cloth are worn by men on the arm, and women are expected to place simple floral arrangements made of wool in their hair. According to McGoldrick et al,[7] "Following the mourning period, two special memorial days, one in March and the other in September, are set aside for surviving family members to pay their respects at the gravesites."[7(p35)]

A bad death is sudden, unexpected, untimely, or violent and is believed to place shame on the Chinese family. These deaths are thought to be caused by ancestors' transgressions. Mourning is inhibited and a working through of the grief does not take place. This is a valuable concept to acknowledge, particularly when working with families who have adopted Western philosophies concerning death but whose support systems follow the strict Chinese beliefs from their country. For example, sudden infant death syndrome (SIDS) is considered a bad death based on Chinese definition. In a bad death, speaking of the deceased is avoided. Parents of a SIDS baby require great support from their families to reconcile and cope with the loss of their infant. A conflict may arise when they attempt to verbalize their grief and seek support from their parents or grandparents. Language assessment is again an important aspect of effective counseling. Familiarities with Western concepts vary with all individuals. The Asian population may have a combination of spiritualism and biomedical beliefs. Some Chinese-Americans may fear hospitals, feeling that if the loved one dies in a hospital, his or her spirit may become lost.[4] A proper way for some Asian families to show respect is through smiling and head nodding, which can be erroneously interpreted as understanding. Therefore other methods of evaluation should be used to determine comprehension of the information and counseling given.

Hispanic

Hispanic cultures include Puerto Ricans and Spanish descendants. Grabowski and Frantz[8] conducted a 2x2 multivariate analysis of variance and determined that Latinos grieving sudden death have a significantly greater grief intensity than Latinos grieving expected death and than Anglos grieving either kind of death. In the Latino population the intensity of grief was not affected by funeral rituals, closeness of relationship, time since death, or participation in novenas. Puerto Ricans place great importance on resolving conflicts, seeing the dying relative, and completing relationships that will free him or her to enter the afterlife. Curses and visions of the deceased are common within this culture. Feelings of guilt or unresolved issues in the relationship of the deceased and survivor will manifest themselves in this manner.[9] For example, in some Hispanic families the father is expected to pick up or display attention to the child upon returning home from work; if this is not done, it is believed that something will happen to the child. In the case of SIDS, it is important to assess if guilt feelings arise from a deviation from the above expected belief.

African American

The African American population, by history, has experienced tragic and unexpected deaths. They achieve support through their religious beliefs. A strong community and church support system exists. Initial reactions to grief are accepted; however, prolonged grief is not tolerated.[7] McGoldrick et al state, "there are no prohibitions about the public expression of grief, particularly by women and children in the African American culture. At the funeral moving spirituals are sung about the pain and suffering of this life, the joy of reuniting with deceased relatives and achieving final peace."[7(p32)] The concept of being "strong" is held in high regard in the cultural guidelines of grief. Usually, however, the African American will rely upon his or her family and church for support and avoid organized, professionally run groups.

Muslim

Wilkan[10] contrasted two Muslim societies, the Balinese and the Egyptians. Grief work is encouraged in the latter society but not in the former. In Egypt, grieving is encouraged and prolonged, and Bali "manage the heart" in grief, going on with their normal life functions.[10] Laughter and cheerfulness conceal their sorrow and help them to avoid reminders of the deceased. The Egyptians grieve in an opposite manner, immersing themselves in the sorrow of the loss. Interesting to note, whether individuals work through their grief or manage their hearts, both are equally effective in the respective culture.[3] Bereavement practices of other cultures may be unthinkable to Anglo-Western culture; however, they prove to be as effective in enabling the bereaved to survive the death of a significant other.

ETHNICITY

A family's ethnic and religious identity completes its family profile. To understand families during bereavement, their history, beliefs, and rituals must be recognized and understood. Ethnic background is an important part of family history taking. However, erroneous conclusions can occur if visible signs of ethnicity based on skin color, surname, nationality, or religion are assumed to yield identical information for each member of an ethnic group. Group values do not stereotypically apply to all families within that ethnic group.

A specific tradition may be followed by families in a similar ethnic group; however, the variations in diversity may be numerous. Multigenerational families may have a special ethnic ritual, but may exhibit individual family differences that deviate from the custom. Conversely, families from different ethnic groups may have similar characteristics or behavior, particularly in foods, attitudes, beliefs, and customs, if many ethnic groups live in the same neighborhood. Many cultures take pride in acculturation and in being unrecognizable from their culture of origin.

Nurses must be able to identify a family's ethnic background and assess how this resembles the family's ethnic heritage. By recognizing and understanding a family's cultural ancestry, nursing care can be planned according to a family's ethnic framework.

Families that do not identify with or participate in the customs of their ancestors are still affected by them. The historic makeup of an individual is affected by ethnic characteristics that are passed on from generation to generation. Even families that attempt to sever themselves from their families of origin are subtly influenced by their ethnic background.

Ethnic identity includes attitudes, beliefs, and a world view that is passed on from one generation to the next in an almost unconscious fashion without necessitating verbal explanations.[11] Behaviors often continue after the belief system has been gone. The Chinese disperse hard candy with a coin inside, called "lucky money," to mourners at a funeral. Some Jewish families cover the mirrors in the house of mourning, and Greek Orthodox families may provide koliya (boiled wheat) to mourners.[11] These rituals are rooted in the core of their ethnic heritage.

Unresolved family issues may have originated from ethnic beliefs, and reframing them in ethnic terms may assist in integration. When working with families, five aspects of ethnicity should be examined: (1) attitudes toward life and death; (2) expression of pain, suffering, and grief; (3) acceptance of outside authority; (4) expectations of family responsibility; and (5) gender roles.[11]

The way in which a family views life and death is a family belief system that has its core in the ethnic heritage of that family. A family's basic disposition toward the meaning of life and death is expressed behaviorally. Some families may consider life of any kind better than death, and this may make families cling to life in the worst pain and suffering. For example, some people may accept the death of an infant to SIDS by saying, "This happens to infants and there is nothing that we could have done differently to have prevented this from happening." People of Irish descent may take a philosophic approach to life and death, such as "The baby died because it was meant to die."[11] In addition, the Irish believe in hard work, and women usually tend to take on total responsibility for their self-care. In working with families of Irish descent, a nurse can reframe the therapeutic approach by involving significant family members and explaining that it is fate that will get them through their grief with emphasis on hard work as a part of working through their grief. The Irish believe that life is full of suffering, but if fate brings suffering, it must be accepted with stoicism.[11]

Puerto Ricans believe that the journey into the next life requires as much spiritual assistance as a family can obtain. Faith healers, spiritualists, and extended family members may be called upon to provide emotional support to a family.[11] Some families may wish to have their infant or loved one buried in their native country to call upon family support. Visiting nurses may not be able to make an initial home visit to a family until after the deceased is buried and the family returns to the United States from their native country. This may take 2 weeks to a few months.

According to Lawson, "Migrants, who may have suffered social, economic, and cultural dislocation as well as discrimination and poverty in their area of resettlement, are already experiencing profound grief. Death of an infant or loved one can overwhelm their already limited resources."[2(p77)]

Nurses need to be aware of conflicts that may arise in families. When choices are made that are counter to the ancestral ethnic and religious beliefs of the family, conflict may occur, resulting in the need for conflict resolution. Each culture has its own unique mourning rituals. The women of the Gusii cultures of Kenya are seen wailing loudly for an extended period of time at gravesites in a distinctive cultural style. Wailing begins when someone is dying and occurs for several days until the women of the deceased are exhausted. There is no difference between wailing and spontaneous crying. A woman performs a slow dance in rhythm to the lament, arms stretched and palms turned upward. She sings an extemporaneous lament that is sometimes designated toward the deceased and sometimes to the people at the funeral. Women distantly related to the deceased may join in the rhythmic dance, wailing, and singing laments with tears. When the grave diggers are finished, the women explode in grief and hurl themselves onto the grave, crying and singing together for hours. The women who are closest to the deceased become publicly exhausted.[12]

Gusii men behave differently than Gusii women. Men are not allowed to express their grief. They are expected to prepare and direct the funeral ceremonies and observe the women in their grief. The womens' wailing makes the men feel mournful, and it is important for them to visualize the women's expressions of grief.[12]

The manner in which families perceive illness and pain needs to be assessed by nurses. In the case of a SIDS death, often parents will ask "Did my baby suffer?" It is important for nurses to respond and reassure families that the baby did not suffer and was not in pain at death. SIDS parents who witnessed the death of their infants reported that their infants did not suffer at the time of death. An understanding of a family's beliefs and expressions of pain and suffering according to their ethnic background is important to assist them with their grief. Many Mediterranean cultures, Puerto Ricans, and blacks express their grief openly.[11] The exhaustion from wailing and screaming can lead to fainting by mourners at Puerto Rican or Iranian funerals. It may be considered poor etiquette to show no emotion at a funeral. Other ethnic groups may not display their grief in public or private. An Irish funeral may seem like a party more than a funeral, with drinking and joking. Crying is permitted but is quickly suppressed with humor.[11]

White Anglo-Saxon Protestants do not express their grief publicly nor have rituals for the expression of grief. Nurses need to encourage these families to talk about their feelings of grief as well as give them permission to do so. Repressed feelings may lead to complicated grief reactions. Asian cultures may contain their expressions of grief but have structured rituals for mourning.[11] The public expression of personal feelings is improper in the Japanese culture, but Japanese are expected to participate in the public mourning ritual. A culturally appropriate framework is provided for families with an acceptable outlet for the expression of grief.

Medical personnel usually represent authority to families. Various ethnic groups respond to health care professionals in a variety of ways. Some groups may obey and acquiesce with directives; others may question and be oppositional to authority; many may be suspicious of authority figures, depending on their past experiences with health care and social service agencies. The nurse may come in contact with a family's acceptance of outside authority. Some families may welcome a home visit, others may question and challenge the reason for the visit, while others may refuse a visit altogether or not be available when the nurse arrives at the home for the scheduled appointment.

Similar to Puerto Ricans, Mexicans, and Hispanics, West Indians will be more verbal and comfortable if extended family members are included in the home visit. Jewish families respect authority when they are assured of the highest standards. They may question the nurse about her credentials and expertise in providing bereavement counseling. Irish families will not question the authority of the nurse and may feel that it is not appropriate to question the nurse's credentials.

Some ethnic groups relate to authority figures when they feel some thread of connection with the health care professional. The use of an interpreter who can speak a family's native language in a face-to-face interview or telephone call helps the nurse connect with a family.

Family boundaries that have been established between a family and other social groups determine how the family views authority figures. Ethnic groups that have rigid boundaries between the family and the environment and who rely only on other family members for support most likely will not accept a home visit. Some families feel that they have enough support from their family and do not request a home visit. Other groups may feel that it is not acceptable within their family mores to receive outside support. All ethnic groups are similar in terms of gender roles, with minor variations.

Women are usually expected to be the matriarchal caretakers of a family, while men are usually the providers of financial support. It may be necessary for the nurse to assess a family's beliefs in male and female roles within a particular family in terms of ethnicity and grief.

Some women during their grief may not have energy to complete household tasks such as laundry, cooking, or cleaning. Alternative plans to provide assistance to a mother during the initial crisis stage may need to be explored. Men tend to grieve differently from women and are usually not as verbal about expressing their grief. They may want to return to work soon after the death of their baby, which may present difficulty for the wife, who may feel that her husband is not emotionally available to her.

•   •   •

The expanding, culturally diverse population in the United States is offering new challenges in the provision of health care, especially in bereavement counseling to families. Cultural differences and similarities and their impact on individual therapeutic approaches need to be recognized and understood when working with families. Suggestions have been made to enhance the caregivers' cultural sensitivity but do not represent a "cookbook" approach on how to render care to specific populations. Using caution not to stereotype ethnic groups despite their antecedent culture will help to individualize emotional support to families.

Assessment of a family's beliefs, attitudes, and world view will help the nurse to be culturally sensitive to a family's grief needs and orientation. A family's beliefs and attitudes toward using support systems outside the family network will determine how a nurse or health care provider is accepted. Connecting with a family is determined through understanding and communicating within their ethnic framework.

> Diversity brings new solutions to an everchanging environment, and that sameness is not only uninteresting but limiting.
>
> —Gene Griessman

REFERENCES

1. Brock, P. (1970). *Culture Shock*. New York: Alfred A. Knopf.

2. Lawson, L. (1990). Culturally sensitive support for grieving parents. *Maternal Child Nursing*, 15, 76–79.

3. Strobe, M. (1992–1993). Coping with bereavement: a review of the grief work hypothesis. *Omega*, 26(1), 19–42.

4. Ross, M. (1981). Societal/cultural views regarding death and dying. *Topics in Clinical Nursing*, October: 1–15.

5. Miller, S.I., Schoenfeld, L. (1973). Grief in the Navajo: psychodynamics and culture. *International Journal of Social Psychiatry*, 19, 187–191.

6. Yamamoto, J., et al. (1969). Mourning in Japan. *American Journal of Psychiatry*, 125, 74–79.

7. McGoldrick, M., Hines, P., Lee, E., Preto, N. (1986). Mourning rituals. *Networker*, November: 29–36.

8. Grabowski, J., Frantz, T. (1992–1993). Latinos and Anglos: cultural experiences of grief intensity. *Omega*, 26(4), 273–285.

9. Cancelmo, J., Millan, F., Vazquez, C. (1990). Culture and symptomatology—the role of personal meaning in diagnosis and treatment: a case study. *The American Journal of Psychoanalysis*, 50(2), 137–149.

10. Wilkan, U. (1988). Bereavement and loss in two Muslim communities in Egypt and Bali compared. *Social Science and Medicine*, 5, 451–460.

11. Platt, L., Perisco, V. (1993). *Grief in Cross Cultural Perspective*. New York: Garland Publishers.

12. Rosen, E. (1990). *Families Facing Death*. New York: Lexington Books.

The Impact of Noise on Critically Ill People

Joyce P. Griffin, PhD, RN, OCN
Director
Clinical Nursing Research
Naval Hospital
Portsmouth, Virginia

The hospital environment has been a subject of study for many years. Florence Nightingale, in 1860, identified hospital noise as disturbing to the patient. She also described how individuals can vary in their response to noise:

> Unnecessary noise, or noise that creates an expectation in the mind, is that which hurts a patient. It is rarely the loudness of the noise, the effect upon the organ of the ear itself, which appears to affect the sick . . . There are certain patients, no doubt . . . who are affected by mere noise. But intermittent noise, or sudden and sharp noise, in these as in all other cases, affects far more than continuous noise.[1(p44)]

An individual, while confined in the unfamiliar, hostile environment of the intensive care unit (ICU), is exposed to sounds of varying intensity, duration, and frequency—most with little meaning. Patients may perceive these noises as disruptive and frustrating, particularly because they cannot eliminate the source of the sound. Although hospital personnel become accustomed to alarms and equipment noises, patients may be repeatedly startled. Response to noise is a complex area for study, as the same noise level elicits varying responses among persons.[2–3]

NOISE

Noise is defined as any unwanted sound.[2] Objective noise is measured in hertz (Hz) and deci-

Source: Reprinted from J.P. Griffin, *Holistic Nursing Practice,* Vol. 6, No. 4, pp. 53–56, © 1992, Aspen Publishers, Inc.

bels (dB). Frequency of sound waves refers to the number of vibrations per second, measured in units of Hz.[2] Sound levels, or intensity, are measured in units of dB. In measuring intensity, an A-weighted sound level meter is generally used, as it resembles the human ear in sensitivity to noise composed of varying frequencies. It measures in units called dBA.[2]

Loudness of sound is defined as the subjective intensity of sound, and is highly correlated with the unwantedness of a sound.[3] Annoyance is a psychological response to noise, and signifies one's reaction to the sound based both on its physical nature and its emotional content.[2,3] In general, noises described as annoying are high pitch, intermittent, of long duration, impulse in character, greater than 60 dBA, and increasing in level.[3–5] Sounds reaching a high peak very abruptly, such as a cardiac monitor alarm, are judged to be very noisy. An individual's hearing will adapt to a continuous noise, such as the hum of machines, but will be disturbed by intermittent noises, such as laughter.[3]

Objection to noise also increases with the unwantedness of sound, its potential for speech interference, and the degree to which it disturbs sleep.[6] Noise begins to interfere with the understanding of everyday speech at 37 to 45 dBA.[2]

INFLUENCING VARIABLES

A personality attribute, noise sensitivity, may influence the reaction to hospital noise. Noise sensitivity is defined as an individual difference variable characteristic of the person, consisting of the subjective awareness of noise and reaction to it.[7,8] Weinstein[7] and Topf[8] found noise sensitivity to be of sufficient power and generality to predict the degree of disturbance to noise. Griffin,[9] however, found no relationship between noise sensitivity and disturbance due to hospital noise in acutely ill people.

Age influences individual response to noise. Older adults are more disturbed by noise than are younger adults,[10] and are more likely to be awakened from sleep.[10–12] Hearing acuity and severity of illness may also influence response to noise.

HOSPITAL NOISE

The US Environmental Protection Agency[13] (EPA) recommends that hospital noise should be maintained at 40 to 45 dBA or lower to prevent annoyance adequately during the day, and levels less than 35 dBA are recommended for sleep. Intermittent sounds rising to 50 dBA on 100 or more occasions during an 8-hour period are compatible with undisturbed sleep in hospitals.[13,14]

A number of studies,[5,15–19] have documented hospital noise as greater than 45 dBA. Using precision sound-level meters, researchers discovered the average 24-hour sound level in a 17-bed recovery room was 57.2 dBA;[15] in multi-bedded rooms, 53 to 80 dBA;[5,20–21] and in ICU, 58 to 72 dBA.[5,15–16]

In all studies, hospital noise levels were of sufficient intensity to interfere with rest and sleep. Loud noises over 70 dBA were common in all areas, but especially in the ICU, where they occurred on average every 9 minutes.[15] Another study[18] measured intermittent sounds over 50 dBA over 300 times between the hours of 5:30 AM to 6:30 AM. A recent study examining noise levels in patient-care areas of a regional naval medical center found similar results (Griffin J. 1991. Unpublished data). Noise levels in the ICU and on multibedded wards were consistently well in excess of levels recommended by the EPA. Measurements in the ICU, taken with a precision sound-level meter, ranged from 50 to 80 dBA over the course of 24 hours. Stairwell noise ranged from 70 to 110 dBA. On multibedded wards, the patient beds closest to the nurses' station registered sound levels from 60 to 70 dBA.

Conversation among staff and, to a smaller extent, equipment are responsible for the majority of hospital noise. Staff communication was found to be often needlessly loud and unrelated to patient care.[15,19,22]

IMPACT OF HOSPITAL NOISE ON CRITICALLY ILL PEOPLE

Numerous studies have documented the disturbing effect hospital noise has on patients—reactions ranging from anger to frustration.[3,16,18–19,21,23] Research reveals that this noisy environment can potentiate behavioral changes in the critically ill.[24] Hospital noise has been associated with sleep deprivation,[25–28] sensory overload,[3–6] increased perception of postoperative pain,[28] and ICU psychosis.[24] Physiological effects, such as an increased heart rate, have also been noted.[8] The stress from noise is particularly important in hospitals because it could impede healing.[18]

Populations considered to be particularly vulnerable to adverse effects of continual loud sound are infants, especially premature infants in incubators; persons with heightened cardiovascular or psychological reactivity to unwanted sound; and persons taking ototoxic drugs.[29]

In a series of works, Topf has studied the effects of aversive physical characteristics of the environment on health.[8,17,30] Her model, modified from Moos,[31] is limited to the major variables influencing the impact of the environment on health. These variables are personality attributes, age, seriousness of illness, perceived control over hospital noise, and socioeconomic status. The model includes the possibility of interventions, such as instruction for control over hospital noise.[8] Her studies have looked at patient outcomes in the form of postoperative recovery and disturbance due to hospital noise.[17,30] The experimental condition, instruction for control over noise, did not account for significant amounts of variance in disturbance due to hospital noise or recovery.

Griffin and colleagues[32] studied the effects of progressive muscular relaxation on disturbance due to hospital noise. A sample of 100 acutely ill patients hospitalized in a critical care area were randomly assigned to an experimental or control group. The experimental group was instructed in relaxation; the control group received a short visit to control for placebo effects. Results revealed the experimental group had significantly lower levels of disturbance from hospital noise after being instructed in the use of the relaxation technique than prior to the intervention. Control group subjects demonstrated no such change.

•   •   •

Modifying the environment can greatly decrease sound levels. Closing the patient's door reduces the noise levels generated outside the room. Using chairs with wheels reduces noise from chairs scraping against floors. Setting telephones and alarms to low volumes, and answering them promptly will greatly reduce noise levels. Choose quieter equipment, and inform the manufacturers that sound levels were an important criterion in selection. Computer printers can be placed away from patient rooms, or soundproof covers can be installed. Patients can be given earphones so they can listen to radio or television without disturbing others.[22] Most importantly, we can lower our voices when speaking to colleagues or patients. Inservice training can raise consciousness about this important issue.

REFERENCES

1. Nightingale F. *Notes on Nursing: What It Is and What It Is Not.* New York, NY: Dover; 1969.

2. Kryter K. *The Effects of Noise on Man.* New York, NY: Academic Press; 1985.

3. Baker C. Sensory overload and noise in the ICU: Sources of environmental stress. *Critical Care Quarterly.* 1984;6(4):66–80.

4. Surry J. *Industrial Accident Research: A Human Engineering Appraisal.* Toronto, Ontario: Ontario Ministry of Labor; 1974.

5. Bentley S, Murphy F, Dudley H. Perceived noise in surgical wards and an intensive care area: an objective analysis. *British Medical Journal.* 1977;2:1503–1506.

6. Hansell H. The behavioral effects of noise on man: the patient with ICU psychosis. *Heart and Lung.* 1984; 13(1):59–66.

7. Weinstein N. Individual differences in reaction to noise: a longitudinal study in a college dorm. *Journal of Applied Psychology.* 1978;63(4):458–466.

8. Topf M. A framework for research on the aversive physical aspects of the environment. *Research in Nursing and Health.* 1984;7:35–42.

9. Griffin J. *The Effects of Progressive Muscular Relaxation on Subjectively Reported Disturbance due to Hospital Noise.* New York, NY: New York University; 1987. Doctoral dissertation.

10. Lukas J. Noise and sleep: a literature review and a proposed criterion for assessing effect. *Journal of the Acoustical Society of America.* 1976;58:1232–1240.

11. Thiessen G. Disturbance of sleep by noise. *Journal of the Acoustical Society of America.* 1978;64:216–220.

12. Williams H, Williams C. Nocturnal EEG profiles and performance. *Psychophysiology.* 1966;3:164–166.

13. US Environmental Protection Agency. *Information on Levels of Environmental Noise Requisite To Protect Public Health and Welfare with an Adequate Margin of Safety.* Washington, DC: US Government Printing Office; 1974. #550/9-74-004.

14. Walker J. Noise in hospitals. In: May D, ed. *Handbook of Noise Assessment.* New York, NY: Van Nostrand Reinhold; 1978.

15. Falk S, Woods N. Hospital noise levels and potential health hazards. *New England Journal of Medicine.* 1973;289:774–781.

16. Turner A, King C, Craddock J. Measuring and reducing noise. *Hospitals.* 1975;49:85–90.

17. Topf M. Noise induced stress in hospital patients: coping and nonauditory health outcomes. *Journal of Human Stress.* 1985;11(3):125–134.

18. Hilton A. Noise in acute patient areas. *Research in Nursing and Health.* 1985;8:283–291.

19. Hilton A. Noise: who says hospitals are quiet places? *Canadian Nurse.* 1986;82(5):24–28.

20. Topf M. Noise pollution in hospitals. *New England Journal of Medicine.* 1983;309:53–54.

21. Haslam P. Noise in hospitals: its effect on the patient. *Nursing Clinics of North America.* 1970;5:715–724.

22. Hilton A. The hospital racket: how noisy is your unit? *American Journal of Nursing.* 1987;87(1):59–61.

23. Noble M. *The ICU Environment: Directions for Nursing.* Reston, VA: Reston Publishers; 1982.

24. Hansell H. The behavioral effects of noise on man: the patient with ICU psychosis. *Heart and Lung.* 1984;13:59–65.

25. Snyder-Halpern R. The effect of critical care unit noise on patient sleep cycles. *Critical Care Quarterly.* 1985;7(2):41–51.

26. Helton M, Gordon S, Nunnery S. Correlation between sleep deprivation and the ICU syndrome. *Heart and Lung.* 1980;9:464–468.

27. Hilton A. Quantity and quality of patient's sleep and sleep disturbing factors in an ICU. *Journal of Advanced Nursing.* 1976;1:453–457.

28. Minckley B. A study of noise and its relationship to patient discomfort in the recovery room. *Nursing Research.* 1968;17(3):247–250.

29. Williams M. The physical environment and patient care. In: Fitzpatrick J, Taunton R, Benoliel J, eds. *Annual Review of Nursing Research.* New York, NY: Springer; 1988.

30. Topf M. Personal and environmental predictors of patient disturbance due to hospital noise. *Journal of Applied Psychology.* 1985;70(1):22–28.

31. Moos R. *Coping with Physical Illness.* 2nd ed. New York: Academic Press; 1984.

32. Griffin J, Myers S, Kopelke C, Walker D. The effects of progressive muscular relaxation on subjectively reported disturbance due to hospital noise. *Behavioral Medicine.* 1988;2:37–42.

Lightwave Frequency and Sleep-Wake Frequency in Well, Full-Term Neonates

Barbara W. Girardin, PhD, RN
Graduate Lecturer
Division of Nursing
California State University
Carson, California

Alterations in lighting intensity is a typical nursing intervention to facilitate comfort and sleep. However, the frequency of lightwave emissions may also relate to sleep in neonates. It was the purpose of this study to test a hypothesized relationship between lightwave frequency and sleep-wake frequency in well, full-term, Hispanic neonates in a well-baby, hospital nursery.

THEORETICAL FRAMEWORK

The relationship between the frequency of human and environmental field patterns is proposed in Rogers'[1] "Science of Unitary Human Beings." The conceptual-theoretical-empirical structure[2] for this study is as follows: Given that "manifestations of field pattern emerge out of the human and environmental field mutual process,"[1(p5)] and "manifestations of speeding up of human field rhythms are coordinate with increasing frequency of environmental field patterns,"[1(p7)] and sleep-wake frequency is a manifestation of human field pattern, and lightwave frequency is a manifestation of environmental field pattern, then higher frequency (HF) sleep-wake is associated with HF lightwaves (blue), and lower frequency (LF) sleep-wake is associated with LF lightwaves (red).

The hypothesis tested was that neonates experiencing HF (blue) lightwaves have greater sleep-wake frequency than do neonates experiencing LF (red) lightwaves.

Source: Reprinted from B.W. Girardin, *Holistic Nursing Practice,* Vol. 6, No. 4, pp. 57–66, © 1992, Aspen Publishers, Inc.

Rogers also proposes the correlates of human patterning[3(p9)] that describe change as moving toward higher frequency, more diversity, and more waking. A further purpose of this study was to answer the research question, what is the relationship between sleep-wake frequency, the variability in sleep-wake frequency, and the amount of waking?

RELATED LITERATURE

There is extensive lighting literature, mostly with adults and with light that is visually perceived. The visual perception of light in adults involves a learned response to light, dark, and colors, a response based on color preference and a physiological response. In the neonate, color preference does not operate,[4] nor is there a learned response to light and color. In this study, light was perceived dermo-optically, because neonates' eyes were primarily closed during sleep. Nevertheless, the lighting literature concerning adults and visually perceived light is useful in identifying relationships of lightwave frequencies and measures of activation.

In the adult, visually perceived lightwave frequencies have been related to respiratory rate, frequency of eyeblink, and systolic blood pressure;[5] galvanic skin response;[6,7] anxiety and tension;[5,8] arousal;[7] physical performance;[9–12] perceived duration of time passage;[13,14] and general satisfaction.[15] The results of these studies demonstrate a relationship of LF (red) lightwaves to measures of greater activation. However, in the early studies, there was questionable control over the precision of the lightwave variable, the learned response to light and color preference.

A second set of literature addresses dermo-optic perception of light in subjects unaware of the lightwave frequency. Without an awareness of lightwave frequency, the potential confound due to the learned response and color preference is eliminated. Smith[16] and Lysenko and Barilo[17]

supported a relationship between LF (red) lightwaves and measures of greater activation.

Smith[16] found more crying and greater amounts of activity in neonates with their eyes primarily closed while in LF (red) lightwaves, compared with HF (blue) lightwaves. However, there was a possibility of a crossover effect. When exposing just the hands of 70 adult subjects to LF (red) strobe lighting, Lysenko and Barilo[17] demonstrated significant alpha waveform changes in the electroencephalogram (EEG). The 70 subjects had their eyes closed and were unaware of the lightwave frequency. However, the effect of the strobe on measures of activation is unclear, separate from the lightwave frequency of that strobe.

A third set of literature supports the predicted relationship and concludes that LF (red) lightwaves relate to measures of lower activation, and HF (blue) lightwaves relate to measures of higher activation.[18–20] These adult subjects had dermo-optic perception of light and were unaware of the lightwave frequency administered.

Nelson[18] and Thomas and colleagues[19] concurred that HF (blue) lightwaves related to the time experience of "time flies" and a longer production estimate. Ludomirski[20] found a positive relationship between lightwave frequency and the subjective measure of human field motion in blind and sighted adults who were unaware of the lightwave experience. Ludomirski[20] concluded that vision is not required for a response to lightwaves, as evidenced by the same results in blind and sighted subjects. She also concluded that HF (blue) lightwaves, in contrast to LF (red) lightwaves, relate to measures of greater activation.

In summary, lightwave frequency does relate to various measures of activation, even with dermo-optic perception of light in subjects unaware of the lightwave frequency administered. However, there is conflicting evidence about the direction of the relationship of lightwave frequency and sleep in adults; in neonates, the relationship has been relatively unexplored.

METHOD

Definitions

Lightwave frequency. Lightwave frequency is the identifying number of cycles per second emitted by a light source. LF and HF were 20 footcandles (ftc) intensity at the neonate. LF lighting had a peak wavelength of approximately 650 nm.[21] It was produced by six Philips preheat fluorescent red tubes, F20 T12/R. HF lighting had a peak wavelength of approximately 450 nm.[21] It was produced by two Philips preheat fluorescent special blue tubes, F20 T12/BB. Six LF (red) fluorescent tubes were used in the one group to equal the intensity of the two HF (blue) tubes used in the other group.

Ambient light. Ambient light was produced by cool white fluorescence at 20 ftc at the neonate, the standard for the well-baby nursery.[22]

Sleep-wake frequency. The value was obtained by counting the number of alternations from a sleep state (quiet sleep or active sleep) to a wakeful state (nonalert waking, alert, or fuss-cry) in a sleep period. Sleep and waking observations were based on Thoman's[23] behavioral criteria.

Sample

Potential neonatal subjects were recruited from all well neonates having at least one Hispanic parent and admitted to the well-baby nursery of an urban, county hospital in Southern California. Those qualifying neonates and mothers formed the sampling frame from which two neonates per night of data collection were randomly drawn. Selecting the Hispanic neonate population with their darker skin tones was intended to improve skin absorption of light[24] and to standardize absorption of light among subjects because of their similar skin tones.

The subjects met the selection criteria if they were normal by routine laboratory test and physical exam, 37 to 42 weeks gestation, appropriate for gestational age, at least 6 hours of age,

female or uncircumcised male, and had an Apgar of 7 or greater.

Assignment to groups was conducted just prior to the experimental lighting. The first of two neonatal subjects per night were randomly assigned to one of the two randomly selected groups (LF-red or HF-blue). The second subject was assigned to the remaining group (LF-red or HF-blue).

The age of the neonates ranged from 6.1 hours to 5.4 days with a mean age, in hours, of 23.9 (SD = 21.5). The older neonates were available for the study because they remained hospitalized with their mothers who had planned cesarean section deliveries. The variance in the age of the neonates did not relate to sleep-wake frequency as evidenced by an insignificant *t*-test between neonates less than 12 hours of age and those greater than 12 hours of age. The mean birthweight was 7.6 pounds (SD = 1.2). There was no significant difference between the two groups in age, birthweight, gender, head and skin features, volume of formula consumed, comforts provided, mode of birth (vaginal or cesarean), the number of neonates being fed by breast and bottle, and the number being fed with bottle only. Accidental stimuli received and the noise levels were similar between the groups because subjects from each group were observed concurrently.

Ninety-two neonates had parents who were both Hispanic. Eight neonates had a Hispanic parent and a Caucasian or Asian parent. The head of the household typically had 1 year of high school education and was a field or common laborer. The mean household income was $11,037. Mothers were from 15 to 36 years of age, with a mean age of 25.3 (SD = 5.2).

Design

The study was a two-factor, repeated-measures, experimental design. LF (red) and HF (blue) lightwaves were the two levels of the grouping factor with 50 neonates per group. The three sleep periods were the three levels of the repeated-measures factor. The timing and the duration of the sleep periods in the nursery were determined by the hospital routine. Sleep periods in the nursery alternated with feed periods in the mothers' rooms. The light in Sleep Period 1 consisted of cool white fluorescent nursery light. Sleep Period 1 was the control period for comparing the two groups prior to the experimental lightwaves. Sleep Period 2 consisted of LF (red) or HF (blue) experimental lighting. Sleep Period 3 consisted of cool white nursery lighting.

The extended observations of approximately $2\frac{1}{2}$ hours in each of the three sleep periods were indicated to

- allow for relatively naturalistic, undisturbed sleep for observations, consistent with the nursery routine;
- maximize the lighting effect because the neonates' eyes were primarily closed, and their bodies were covered, limiting the direct interface between the lightwaves and the neonates;
- improve the possibility of a light effect, given the low 20 ftc intensity; and
- heed previous studies[25-27] that recommended increasing the duration of the lightwave experience to at least 30 minutes.

Procedure

Approval to conduct the study was obtained from the appropriate institutional review board for the protection of human subjects.

The steps in the procedure were organized around the every-4-hour feeding routine, when the neonates were taken from the nursery to their mothers' rooms. The three consecutive $2\frac{1}{2}$-hour sleep periods for observations began after the 4 PM, 8 PM, and 12 midnight feedings. Limiting the observations to the evening and early morning helped to avoid the array of sleep interruptions in the nursery during the day and minimized the threat from sunlight variations. It was appropri-

ate to limit observations to a 12-hour period because sleep-wake frequency is symmetrical around the clock until the age of 6 weeks.[28-30] All the sleep-wake observations for each neonate were recorded only during the three consecutive sleep periods in the nursery by a single data collector. Every night of data collection, two neonates were observed. The neonates were located side by side in the nursery to help equalize the environmental stimuli, like noise. There was a white reflective room divider between the two subjects when they were receiving the LF (red) or HF (blue) lightwaves.

Instruments

The measurement of sleep-wake frequency was based on observations of the six sleep-wake states as identified by Thoman[23] in the Sleep-wakefulness Infant State Instrument for clinical research.

The six states ranged from quiet sleep to fuss-cry, as determined by observations of movement, eyelid position, respiration, and sound production. The every-10-second recording of the sleep-wake state was recommended[23] to capture the rapid changes in sleep-wake in neonates. The recording began with the first sleep state following the neonates being repositioned in the crib at the beginning of the sleep period. The count ended approximately 5 minutes before each feed period.

Intrarater reliability by percentage of agreement was estimated at 91% to 94%. The every-10-second recordings from an actual observation period of three consecutive sleep periods were compared with the every-10-second recordings from an audiovideo recording of the same three consecutive sleep periods on the same neonate by the same rater. This procedure was conducted on a randomly chosen subject within the first 50 and second 50 subjects.

LF (red) or HF (blue) lighting were the two experimental lighting types, as described in the definitions. The experimental lightwave tubes were secured in a standard fixture located 22 inches above the neonate. A Plexiglas diffuser limited ultraviolet transmission and dispersed the bright light. The intensity of the LF (red) and HF (blue) lightwaves was maintained at 20 ftc, at the level of the neonate. The difference between the groups in lighting intensity and duration of observations was statistically insignificant.

RESULTS

Hypothesis

The hypothesis that neonates experiencing HF (blue) lightwaves have greater sleep-wake frequency than do neonates experiencing LF (red) lightwaves was supported, as tested with the group by sleep period linear interaction of the $2 \times (3)$ mixed analysis of variance, $t (1) = -2.169, p < .05$. This critical test of the hypothesis contrasts the linear trends over the three sleep periods between the two groups.[31] The simple main effects in the HF group, across the three sleep periods, $F (2, 196) = 9.06, p < .001$, re-

vealed a significant acceleration in sleep-wake frequency values. Table 1 indicates the actual change in mean values of sleep-wake frequency. The LF (red) group demonstrated an increase in the mean values of sleep-wake frequency of 1.02 cycles across the three sleep periods. The HF (blue) group demonstrated an increase of 4.32 cycles across the three sleep periods.

The mean difference between the two groups in sleep-wake frequency values during Sleep Period 1 was insignificant. The random assignment of subjects to groups after Sleep Period 1 supports that the difference in means is due to chance and not to observer bias.

Research Question

The research question was, what is the relationship between sleep-wake frequency, variability in sleep-wake frequency, and the amount of waking? Descriptive findings indicate that

Table 1. Means and standard deviations of sleep-wake frequency and the number of observations of sleep and waking levels

Lighting group	Sleep period		
	1	2	3
Lower frequency			
Sleepwakefulness frequency			
Mean	7.38	7.28	8.40
SD	6.30	5.15	6.52
Range	0–30	0–22	1–28
Number of sleep levels			
Mean (%)	721 (80)	728 (84)	686 (76)
Number of waking levels			
Mean (%)	162 (18)	130 (15)	207 (23)
Higher frequency			
Sleepwakefulness frequency			
Mean	5.46	6.86	9.78
SD	4.78	5.27	7.13
Range	0–22	0–23	0–29
Number of sleep levels			
Mean (%)	782 (88)	721 (83)	672 (73)
Number of waking levels			
Mean (%)	104 (12)	137 (16)	235 (26)

less sleep-wake frequency is associated with less variability in sleep-wake frequency and more sleep. Greater sleep-wake frequency is associated with more variability in sleep-wake frequency and more waking.

In the LF (red) group, relative to the HF (blue) group, there was less of a change across the sleep period or a lower sleep-wake frequency, less change in the standard deviation or less variability, and more sleep. Lower sleep-wake frequency was evidenced by a flattened slope in the mean values across the three sleep periods, an acceleration of 1.02 cycles. (See Table 1.) There was a maximum change of 1.37 in the standard deviation across sleep periods. The amount of sleep increased during the experimental lighting of Sleep Period 2 from 80% to 84% (see Table 2). This trend of increasing sleep in the LF (red) lightwaves did not extend to Sleep Period 3.

Relative to the LF (red) group, the HF (blue) group demonstrated greater sleep-wake frequency, greater variability, and more waking. Mean sleep-wake frequency in the HF (blue) group increased 4.32 cycles across the three sleep periods (see Table 1). The standard deviation in the HF group increased 2.35 across the three sleep periods. The amount of waking increased by 14% from Sleep Period 1 to Sleep Period 3, as the amount of sleep decreased by 15% (see Table 2). This means there is a rela-

tionship between sleep-wake frequency, the variability in sleep-wake frequency, and sleep or waking.

Related Findings

The number of wakings in both groups did not increase at the end of the sleep period, as the scheduled feeding approached. This means that waking and feeding were not synchronized with the every-4-hour hospital feeding routine.

DISCUSSION

Practice

The practice implications are notable because the study was conducted in a relatively naturalistic nursing setting, and nurses make similar observations of sleep and waking.

It is possible that the LF (red) and HF (blue) lightwaves may be useful in patterning day-waking and night-sleeping in neonates. LF (red) lightwaves were associated with less sleep-wake frequency and more sleep. Therefore, LF (red) lightwaves may contribute to night-sleeping. HF (blue) lightwaves were associated with greater sleep-wake frequency and more waking and may contribute to day-waking or be useful for undesirably sleepy neonates.

Results of this study contribute specific sleep-wake frequency criteria for assessing neonates' sleep and rest patterns. The total sample mean for sleep-wake frequency was 6.42 (SD = 5.54). This mean value corroborates the previous findings of 0 to 8 in a 4-hour sleep period.[32–35] When nurses find that sleep-wake frequency in a sleep period reaches 17 to 18, representing two standard deviations from the mean, they have support to describe a neonate as wakeful.

The amounts of sleep, transition, and waking (Table 2) in the cool white nursery lighting in Sleep Period 1 are similar to previous findings,[35–37] but are specific to cool white fluorescent nursery lighting. The values may be useful

Table 2. Percentage of time in sleep, transition, and waking states in the three sleep periods

Lighting group	Sleep period		
	1	2	3
Lower frequency			
Sleep	80	84	76
Transition	2	1	1
Waking	18	15	23
Higher frequency			
Sleep	88	83	73
Transition	0	1	1
Waking	12	16	26

in beginning to establish norms of sleep-wake behavior in specific lighting environments.

The duration of sleep-wake change in the LF (red) and HF (blue) lightwaves was demonstrated. The LF (red) lightwave experience was associated with more sleep during the experience, whereas the HF (blue) lightwave experience was associated with more waking, lasting hours after the lightwave experience. Demonstrating this different duration of action between the LF (red) and HF (blue) lightwaves helps clarify the therapeutic effects of lightwaves.

The number of wakings did not increase as the scheduled feeding time approached. This gives reason to reconsider the every-4-hour feeding routine if waking and hunger are the rationale for the feeding routine.

Theoretical implications

The study results contribute to Rogers'[1] Science of Unitary Human Beings by supporting the following:

- the theoretical statement relating the frequency of human and environmental patterns
- the description of the human field in terms of pattern
- the description of the human energy field as unitary, and
- the association of three postulated correlates of human patterning

Theory support

The accelerating pattern of sleep-wake frequency demonstrated in the HF (blue) lightwave group, relative to the LF (red) lightwave group supports Rogers'[1] propositional statement that, "manifestations of speeding up of human field rhythms are coordinate with increasing frequency of environmental field patterns."[1(p7)] This result contributes empirical support to the relationship among these frequencies in Rogers' Abstract System.[1]

Pattern

Rogers[1] emphasizes pattern identification in describing the human field. The results of this study demonstrate that pattern identification requires extended and frequent recordings and statistical testing appropriate to comparing the long-term pattern in two groups. Here, sleep-wake states were recorded for three sleep periods of $2\frac{1}{2}$ hours each, and the recordings taken every 10 seconds during those sleep periods provided a distinct, rhythmical, and nonrepeating pattern.

The statistical test of the hypothesis—the group by sleep period linear interaction—was sensitive enough to demonstrate a significant difference in the long-term sleep-wake frequency pattern in the groups. The analyses of variance, group effect, and simple effect at each sleep period were not sensitive enough to demonstrate significance. The group effect collapses across the sleep periods, and the simple effect uses only part of the long-term pattern, so neither are sensitive to whole pattern identification.

The unitary nature of the human field

The significant results in neonate subjects who perceived the lightwaves primarily dermo-optically support the irreducible and unitary nature of the human field. The lightwave experience involves more than the visual system, color preference, and learned response to color.[17,19,21] Limiting the explanation of the lightwave experience to the visual mechanism may result in conclusions that are misleading.

Three postulated correlates of human patterning

The descriptive study results support the relationship among Rogers'[2] three postulated correlates of human patterning, such that LF sleep-wake relates to less diversity of sleep-wake frequency and more sleep (see the box entitled "Rogers' Postulated Correlates of Human Patterning"). Also, HF sleep-wake relates to greater diversity of sleep-wake and more waking.

Research

The major research-related recommendations are as follows:

- Continue observations following the experimental lightwave experience for 12 hours in order to describe the extended pattern of sleep-wake changes.
- Provide a lighting experience of 2 to 3 hours when the intensity is low, in order to improve pattern identification in the sleep-wake variable.
- Use separate groups for each of the lightwave alternatives, thus avoiding a po-

tential crossover effect from the long-term changes that occur in sleep-wake following a lightwave experience.

● ● ●

Lightwave frequency does relate to sleep-wake in well neonates, such that HF (blue) lightwaves are associated with more waking episodes in contrast to LF (red) lightwaves. Therefore, alternatives in lightwave frequency may be useful in patterning day-waking and night-sleeping. Results support Rogers'[1] propositional statement from which the hypothesis was derived and Rogers' postulated correlates of human patterning. Further research should continue to use only the one lightwave experience per group and monitor sleep-wake for an extended period of 12 hours.

REFERENCES

1. Rogers ME. Science of unitary human beings. In: Malinski VM, ed. *Explorations on Martha Rogers' Science of Unitary Human Beings*. Norwalk, Conn: Appleton-Century-Crofts; 1986.
2. Fawcett J, Downs F. *The Relationship of Theory and Research*. Norwalk, Conn: Appleton-Century-Crofts; 1986.
3. Malinski VM, ed. *Explorations on Martha Rogers' Science of Unitary Human Beings*. Norwalk, Conn: Appleton-Century-Crofts; 1986.
4. Adams RJ, Maurer D, Davis M. Newborns' discrimination of chromatic from achromatic stimuli. *Journal of Experimental Child Psychology*. 1986;41:267–281.
5. Gerard R. *Differential Effect of Colored Light on Psychophysiological Function*. Los Angeles, Calif: University of California, Los Angeles; 1958. Doctoral dissertation.
6. Jacobs KW, Hustmyer F. Effects of four psychological primary colors on galvanic skin resistance, heart rate and respiratory rate. *Perceptual and Motor Skills*. 1974;38:763–766.
7. Wilson GD. Arousal properties of red versus green. *Perceptual and Motor Skills*. 1966;23:942–949.
8. Jacobs KW, Suess JF. Effect of four psychological primary colors on anxiety state. *Perceptual and Motor Skills*. 1975;41:207–210.
9. Chance RE. *The Effects of Two Ranges of Fluorescent Light Spectra on Human Physiological Performance.*

Gainesville, Fla: University of Florida; 1982. Doctoral dissertation.
10. Cortes TA. *An Investigation of the Relationship Between Light Waves and Cardiac Rate*. New York, NY: New York University; 1975. Doctoral dissertation.
11. Lovett-Doust JW, Schneider R. Studies on the physiology of awareness: The different influence of color on capillary oxygen saturation. *Journal of Clinical Psychology*. 1955;11:366–370.
12. Mass J, Jayson J, Kleiber D. Effects of spectral differences in illumination on fatigue. *Journal of Applied Psychology*. 1974;39:524–526.
13. Smets G. Time expression of red and blue. *Perceptual and Motor Skills*. 1969;29:511–514.
14. Ali MR. Pattern of EEG recovery under photic stimulation by light of different colours. *Electroencephalography and Clinical Neurophysiology*. 1973;35:550–552.
15. Flynn J, Spencer T. The effects of light source color on user impression and satisfaction. *Journal of IES*. 1977;6(3):167–179.
16. Smith C. The relative brightness values of three hues for newborn infants. *Studies in Infant Behavior III*. 1936;12:91–94.
17. Lysenko N, Barilo G. Dermo-optic sensitivity of human beings in the long range of the visible spectrum. *PSI Research*. 1983;2:39–43.
18. Nelson M. *An Investigation of the Relationship of Visual Lightwave Frequency and Man's Time Estimation*. New

York, NY: New York University; 1976. Doctoral dissertation.

19. Thomas SD, Graney M, Burgess E, Allen EK. *Experimental Test of Human Response to Lighting.* Unpublished manuscript; 1991.

20. Ludomirski G. *The Relationship Between the Environmental Energy Wave Frequency Pattern Manifested in Red and Blue Light and Human Field Motion in Adult Individuals with Sensory Perception and Those with Total Blindness.* New York, NY: New York University; 1984. Doctoral dissertation.

21. North American Philips. *Color Selection Guide for Fluorescent Lamps.* PW-1215. Bloomfield, NJ: North American Philips; 1985.

22. James L, Muirhead D, eds. *Standards and Recommendations for Hospital Care of Newborn Infants.* 6th ed. Evanston, Ill: American Academy of Pediatrics; 1986.

23. Thoman EB. *Sleep and Waking States of the Neonate.* Rev ed. Storrs, Conn: Department of Psychology/Behavioral Neuroscience, University of Connecticut; 1985.

24. Duplessis Y. Dermo-optical sensitivity and perception: Its influence on human behavior. *International Journal of Biosocial Research.* 1985;7:76–93.

25. Kolanowski AM. *The Relationship Between Two Types of Artificial Lighting and Restlessness as Manifested by Level of Activation and Motor Activity in the Elderly.* New York, NY: New York University; 1990. Doctoral dissertation.

26. Malinski VM. *The Relationship Between Hyperactivity in Children and Perception of Short Wavelength Light.* New York, NY: New York University; 1980. Doctoral dissertation.

27. McDonald SF. *A Study of the Relationship Between Visible Lightwaves and the Experience of Pain.* Detroit, Mich: Wayne State University; 1981. Doctoral dissertation.

28. Faienza C, Capone C, Galgano M, Sani E. The emergence of the sleep-wake cycle in infancy. *Italian Journal of Neurological Sciences.* 1986; suppl 5:37–42.

29. Hellbrugge T. The development of circadian and ultradian rhythms of premature and full term infants. In: Scheving LE, Halberg F, Pauly J, eds. *Chronobiology.* Tokyo, Japan: Igaku Shoin Ltd; 1974.

30. Minors DS, Waterhouse JM. *Circadian Rhythms and the Human.* Boston, Mass: Wright Publishers; 1981.

31. Winer BJ. *Statistical Principles in Experimental Design.* 2nd ed. New York, NY: McGraw-Hill; 1971.

32. Anders T. Neurophysiological studies of sleep in infants and children. *Journal of Child Psychology and Psychiatry and Allied Disciplines.* 1982;23:75–83.

33. Stern E, Parmelee AH, Akiyama Y, Schultz M, Werner W. Sleep cycle characteristics in infants. *Pediatrics.* 1969;43:65–70.

34. Watt J, Strongman K. The organization and stability of sleep states in fullterm, preterm and small for gestational age infants: A comparative study. *Developmental Psychobiology.* 1985;18:151–162.

35. Webb W. The rhythms of sleep and waking. In: Scheving L, Halberg F, eds. *Chronobiology.* Tokyo, Japan: Igaku Shoin Ltd; 1974.

36. Dreyfus-Brisac C. Ontogenesis of brain bioelectric activity and sleep organization in neonates and infants. In: Faulkner F, Tanner J, eds. *Human Growth (Vol 3): Neurobiology and Nutrition.* New York, NY: Plenum; 1979.

37. Hoppenbrouwers T, Hodgman J, Arakawa K, Geidel S, Sterman M. Sleep and waking studies in infants: Normative studies. *Sleep.* 1988;11:387–401.

UNIT IV

Health Promotion for Clients with Selected Lifestyle Alterations/Abuse

More likely than not, clients with selected lifestyle alterations such as tobacco, alcohol, drug, and sexual abuse will not necessarily seek out the professional guidance of a healthcare provider for their problem. We will often encounter such clients because of other primary health reasons (e.g., the elderly patient admitted to the coronary care unit for congestive heart failure). But we will discover lifestyle alterations and abuse only if we have the foundational knowledge to assess such problems. The articles chosen for this unit present both research and practical "how-to" suggestions for understanding some of the hidden alterations and abuse issues our clients experience.

The hidden problems associated with smoking in the elderly are described (Baer) and supported via the results of a survey that profiles 108 elder smokers. Details of two smoking cessation programs developed by the Visiting Nurses' Association (based on the National Cancer Institute's Smoking Cessation Model for Primary Care Sites) are presented. The author delineates the educational, assessment, treatment, and research components of these programs. A useful mini-assessment tool to identify smokers and refer them to cessation counselors is included.

The hidden or unrecognized problem of alcohol abuse in the elderly also is outlined (Ruppert) related to its causes, adverse effects,

assessment, and treatment. Often alcoholism goes undetected in the elderly because such clients deny the problem, do not fit our alcoholic stereotype, or we incorrectly attribute the physiologic or mental deterioration of alcoholism to a part of the aging process. A alcoholism screening test has been provided for geriatric patients to detect alcoholism in older adults. Physical and mental signs of alcoholic deterioration also are described. Such knowledge and practical tools will equip us routinely to assess older adults for alcohol abuse and recognize subtle physical and mental signals of alcoholism for early intervention.

The qualitative study reporting the experiences of 23 incarcerated women (Muller and Boyle) who reported engaging in sex with multiple partners to purchase drugs lends a rich perspective on how this little-known population views HIV and condom use. Because many of the HIV studies have been conducted on gay men, the findings describing the relationship of high-risk behaviors in women to poverty, lack of economic opportunities, discrimination, and sexual inequality lends insight into interventional programs that might be developed to empower women to alter high-risk behaviors.

Hall and Kondora provide us with the understanding and empirical knowledge base by which to understand another hidden problem—childhood sexual abuse (CSA). This article comprehensively focuses on the role of memory and remembrance in the healing process of women CSA survivors. Practical suggestions for remembering including reminding, reminiscing, recognition, body memory, place memory, and commemoration are described as interventional strategies to facilitate the recovery and rehabilitation of such clients. It is likely that these strategies could be used with other clients who have experienced traumatic events.

Smoking Assessment and Intervention: An Essential Part of Disease Treatment

Carol Ann Baer, PhD, RN
Nurse Researcher
Wellness Division
VNA Care Plus
Danvers, Massachusetts

Smoking is responsible for an estimated 434,000 deaths per year in the United States.[1] Its relationship to cardiovascular disease, cancer, and respiratory dysfunction is well established. Despite these facts, tobacco assessments and interventions are not a standard of care. Although 70% of smokers see their doctor each year,[2] only 40% say they receive counseling.[3]

Elder smokers are counseled even less often.[4] They are part of the "more than 65 population" projected to reach 67 million by the year 2050.[5] Though living longer, they are often afflicted with chronic disease and disability.[6] The elderly consume the largest share of public health dollars and comprise most of the home care caseloads.

Nursing, in its Social Policy Statement,[7] defines its responsibility to patients as extending beyond the traditional disease model. Nursing is "the diagnosis and treatment of responses to actual or potential health problems."[7(p9)] Issues of practice regulation and service reimbursement can impede nurses' mission. Although the profession has defined advance practice and secured limited reimbursement, health promotion and teaching services related to patient responses such as smoking are not part of "standard" treatment.

Consistent with nursing's social commitment to extend care beyond the disease model, VNA Care Plus has expanded traditional services. (VNA Care Plus is the diversified services entity of VNA Care Network, a family of Medicare/Medicaid certified, Joint Commission on the

Source: Reprinted from C.A. Baer, *Home Health Care Management and Practice,* Vol. 9, No. 2, pp. 64–70, © 1997, Aspen Publishers, Inc.

Accreditation of Healthcare Organizations-accredited agencies serving more than 100 communities on a broad corridor from southern New Hampshire to Stoughton, Massachusetts.) The Wellness Division Manager has successfully written and secured grants for health promotion programs. Three of these are tobacco control projects funded by the Massachusetts Department of Public Health, Health Protection Fund. Together these grants form a continuum of care ranging from tobacco use prevention to smoking cessation services.

Smoke Free Circles develops community leadership to encourage the prevention of tobacco use and to limit exposure to secondhand smoke. Women of childbearing age from the community receive training and are paid stipends to provide educational groups in their homes or other community locations. *Smoking Cessation at Primary Care Sites* promotes assessment of smoking status upon admission and offers education and resources directed toward cessation for homebound and clinic clients, as well as for smokers in the general community. *It's Never Too Late* assesses the habits, knowledge, and views of elder smokers to develop tailored programmatic interventions and contribute to cessation research.

The latter two grant projects are based on the National Cancer Institute's (NCI) Smoking Cessation Model[8] and the stages of change for cessation.[9] The NCI model identifies four major interventions for providers

1. *Ask* about smoking at every opportunity.
2. *Advise* all smokers to stop.
3. *Assist* smokers in stopping.
4. *Arrange* follow-up.

The change model identifies five points along a continuum from which smokers may move over time and suggests different interventions for each stage.

Outcomes for the two programs geared toward cessation (*Smoking Cessation for Primary Care Sites* and *It's Never Too Late*) will be described in relation to practice, education, and research. Recommendations based on programmatic experience will be made.

EDUCATION

Health information

The Wellness Division recognized the importance of educating providers and clients about tobacco use and its impact on health. Scientific literature, pamphlets, and audiovisuals were reviewed; distributed as appropriate; stored in the wellness library; and used in instructional programs for consumers, clients, and providers.

Assessment and treatment skills

Staff hired through the grants were selected for their interest and background in public health education. Staff included two Smoking Cessation coordinators and a clinical research director. As part of their orientation they attended lectures, workshops, and facilitator training sessions to develop skills in smoking assessment, cessation facilitation, and other related treatment modalities. Training on the NCI model for Smoking Cessation in Primary Care Sites was provided by the Massachusetts Department of Public Health (DPH). Other workshops were sponsored by organizations such as the American Lung Association and American Cancer Society.

The Smoking Cessation coordinators then worked with the Massachusetts DPH to provide educational programs on the NCI model for smoking cessation to agency staff and to other health professionals from the community, all of whom can significantly influence smokers as they progress along the cessation continuum.

Developmental opportunities

Agency, community, and statewide educational forums provided clients and staff a wide window of opportunity, from developing skills in community leadership to scientific sessions and leadership development. The assistance was invaluable for educational support as well as encouraging change related to tobacco cessation.

PRACTICE

Assessments

Systematic evaluation of clients' smoking was begun shortly after the tobacco control projects became part of the Wellness Division. A mini assessment tool was constructed (Figure 1) to identify smokers on admission and refer to agency cessation counselors. As with any organizational change, there were issues around use of the smoking assessment form that had to be addressed. Smoking Cessation coordinators worked with administrative and clinical staff to identify any impediments and ease the transition.

A detailed assessment tool was developed for the purpose of learning more about elder smokers and their views through the research and demonstration project. The tool included items on demographics, perceived benefits and barriers to cessation, and the General Health Status Survey (SF 36).[10] Benefits and barriers are the individual's perception of factors that affect their cessation efforts. General Health Status

---

1. Do you now smoke cigarettes?
   _ yes _ no
   Other tobacco products?
   _ pipe _ snuff _ cigar _ chewing tobacco
2. Does anyone in your household smoke?
   _ yes _ no
3. How many cigarettes do you smoke a day?
   _____ # of cigarettes
4. How soon after you wake up do you smoke your first cigarette?
   _ within 30 minutes
   _ more than 30 minutes
5. How interested are you in stopping smoking?
   _ not at all
   _ somewhat
   _ very

Our smoking cessation coordinator is available for support for you and your family. She will be in touch with you to introduce herself.

Figure 1. Tobacco use assessment.

Survey is a standardized measure containing 36 items representing eight health concepts.

Identification and recruitment of smokers

Smokers from VNA caseload and from the communities were recruited and offered assistance. Outreach efforts occurred through public media, mailings, advertising, community activities, physicians' offices, telephone calls, and personal contact. Between July 1995 and March 1996, smoking cessation for primary care staff contacted or treated 382 smokers. This number includes those homebound clients referred by nursing staff and other community residents.

An additional 108 smokers were recruited for *It's Never Too Late*'s detailed research and demonstration project. Admission criteria required that participants understand English, be more than 65 years of age, smoke cigarettes, and be mentally competent. Survey administration took place at each site during a time that was convenient for study participants. Confidentiality, informed consent, the estimated time for completion of the survey, and the potential benefits of participation were discussed.

Elder smokers were difficult to recruit. Contacts with approximately 2,000 individuals yielded 108 participants. Contacts were made through Councils on Aging, social/community organizations, retirement organizations, physicians' offices, elderly housing, nursing homes, bingo halls, housing authorities, restaurants, and elderly health clinics.

Recruitment difficulties may be related to several factors: fewer smokers among the elderly; hesitancy of older individuals to share information with "strangers"; embarrassment about admitting their smoking habit; concern that they would be coerced into cessation despite assurances to the contrary; and the attitude that "if I have lived this many years smoking, why should I quit?"

Formalized referral/treatment system

Smoking assessments are now done on every client admitted to the VNA caseload, whether homebound or seen in the clinics. Contacts with clients vary in frequency and format. They are dependent on clients' mobility status, motivation, and treatment plans. Staff recommendations are tailored to the individual place on the change continuum, nicotine dependency, lifestyle, and health status. Treatment is provided in a variety of ways: mailing, telephone, personal encounter, individual counseling, and group work. The actual number, type, and length of interventions per client were tracked on the individual client records. An aggregate compilation of this data would provide valuable program information.

Cessation groups

The purpose of the groups was to help, support, and inform participants in their cessation efforts. The Wellness Division supplied educational and motivational materials plus nicotine supplemental therapy to those who met the criteria. Cessation groups were free of charge to participants, lasted from 5 to 8 weeks, and continued throughout the year.

The first cessation group was formed in response to volunteers for the *It's Never Too Late* study. Initial recruits were "highly motivated to quit" and asked for immediate assistance with cessation. Although the project plan was to design interventions after data collection and analysis, a sense of clinical responsiveness to clients superseded the research design. The curriculum for the groups was based on the *Benefits Beyond Retirement* (BRET) instructional manual[11] that focuses on older adults. Three groups for the study participants were conducted during the year. Seventeen (19.5%) of the study participants successfully completed cessation groups. Twelve were smoke free at the end of the sessions.

Another 10 groups were facilitated by the primary care grant staff between July 1995 and March 1996: one for women, several for employees, and others "open" to any age or status. Most groups used content based upon the American Lung Association's Freedom From Smoking curriculum.[12]

Experience is limited with homogenous subgroups. The staff facilitator of the women's group identified more openness and sharing in that particular group than in several others she has run. The number of seniors successfully completing *It's Never Too Late* groups is impressive, since they initially agreed to the survey, not cessation. Success is attributed to the BRET curriculum and the holistic focus of the facilitators who tailored cessation efforts to participants' life and health status. These combined factors empowered patients and promoted success. Postgroup evaluation forms verified staff perceptions.

Staff now believe groups are the most costefficient and effective way to intervene with smokers. The bonding, socialization, and group sharing that takes place motivate and support individuals in their quitting attempts. Specific cessation, relapse, and treatment evaluation data for each group are not available.

Newsletter

The *It's Never Too Late* research and development project constructed newsletters mailed quarterly to all participants. Content was based on learning needs identified through the survey. Newsletters included information on health risks associated with smoking, resources, and tips for "success with cessation." Successive issues built on participants' knowledgebase, encouraged ongoing participation, promoted "movement" along the cessation continuum, and described survey results.

RESEARCH/CONCLUSIONS

It's Never Too Late was designed to elicit clients' views on smoking and assess their personal smoking habit. Survey items include demographics; smoking history/pattern; nicotine dependency; factors affecting cessation efforts or "benefits and barriers" (Figure 2); and health status (see box entitled "Elder Smokers Profile").

In summary, the participant profile represents an aging population living alone and seriously

How True or False is each of the following statements for you?
DT = Definitely true
MT = Mostly true
DK = Don't know
MF = Mostly false
DT = Definitely false

It is never too late to quit smoking.
Even after 40 or 50 years of smoking, the body can repair much of the damage from smoking.
Stopping smoking is worthwhile at any age.
Smoking low tar and nicotine cigarettes, compared to regular cigarettes, lowers the risk of illness.
My future health would improve if I quit smoking.
The following will happen if I quit smoking:
I will sleep better.
My circulation will improve.
I will be able to breathe better.
I will be able to walk farther.
The bone loss that smoking causes will slow down.
I will feel more "in control" of my life.
I will be able to taste things better.
My sense of smell will improve.
My blood pressure will improve.
I will save money.
The likelihood of a fire in my home will decrease.
I will inspire others who want to quit.
I will be a positive role model for others.
My risk of having a stroke will decrease.
My risk of having lung disease will decrease.
My risk of having a heart attack will decrease.
My risk of having a hip fracture will decrease.
Others will no longer be offended by my smoke.

It would please my family if I quit.
It would please my friends if I quit.
It would please my doctor if I quit.
It would please my nurse if I quit.
I am too addicted to nicotine to quit.
Quitting smoking will cause me to be irritable.
I will experience nicotine withdrawal symptoms.
I will gain weight.
Smoking helps me to concentrate.
I am too nervous to quit.
Smoking gives me something to do.
My friends who smoke would not like it if I quit.
Family members who smoke would not like it if I quit.
Smoking is how I socialize.
Smoking makes my teeth yellow.
Smoking cessation programs are too expensive.
Nicotine patches are too expensive.
It is too much trouble to get a nicotine patch prescription from my physician or nurse.
It is too much trouble to leave home to go to a smoking cessation program.
I don't know of a cessation program in my area.
Transportation to a program is a problem.
My health care provider does not mind my smoking.
If I were to join a smoking cessation program, a morning session would be more convenient.
If I were to join a smoking cessation program, an afternoon session would be more convenient.
If I were to join a smoking cessation program, an evening session would be more convenient.
If I were to join a smoking cessation program, I would like it to be a group program.
I prefer to quit by doing a program on my own at home.
My vision is too poor for reading.

Figure 2. Benefits and barriers.

addicted to nicotine for most of their long lives. They smoke in their homes as they awaken, despite the concern of accidental fire. Although they believe cessation would improve their health and fill their pocketbook, many seeing themselves as "too addicted" have never tried to quit. Most have never had professional cessation assistance, with half of them believing it's too expensive.

Elder smokers health status perception

The SF-36 Health Survey[10] was developed to measure health status from the patient's point of view. The SF-36 measures eight health concepts that are relevant across age, disease, and treatment groups: (1) limitations in physical activities because of health problems; (2) limitations in usual role activities because of physical health problems; (3) bodily pain; (4) general health perceptions; (5) vitality (energy and fatigue); (6) limitations in social activities because of physical or emotional problems; (7) limitations in usual role activities because of emotional problems; and (8) mental health (psychologic distress and well-being). The survey's standardized scoring system yields a profile of eight health concept scores.

The SF-36 was part of the *It's Never Too Late* survey. Analyses show relationship between SF-36 subscores and other participant characteristics. Older smokers had higher scores on bodily pain than younger smokers. Respondents who had more "quit" attempts had lower bodily pain scores and were likely to smoke within the first 5 minutes of awakening. Those for whom the first

Elder Smokers Profile

Demographics
- 108 participants
- Average age 69.3 y with a range to 90 y
- 66% females and 34% males
- 70% widowed, separated, or divorced

Smoking pattern
- Average of 46 "pack" years
- 74% have first cigarettes within 30 minutes of waking
- 28% smoke "even if they are sick enough to be in bed most of the day"
- 3 was average number of quit attempts
- 22% had never quit, even for 1 day

Environment
- 95% smoke in home
- 79% agreed they would save money by not smoking
- 81% acknowledged quitting would reduce risk of fire
- 73% did not find it difficult to refrain from smoking in places where it is forbidden

Health implications
- 77% believe that "it is never too late to quit"
- 75% agree quitting is worth it at any age
- 60% believe weight gain would result from quitting
- 49% said it was "definitely true" that their health would improve with cessation
- 50% felt they would "definitely" be able to "breathe better" and "walk farther"

- 30% responded "do not know" to one or more of 14 health outcomes associated with cessation, such as improving circulation and bone density and decreasing the incidence of high blood pressure, heart attack, and stroke

Relationships
- 77% believed it would please their family if they quit
- 63% said it would please their friends if they quit
- 77% believed it would please their doctor
- 46% said it would please their nurse if they quit

Tobacco dependency
- 44% believe they are "too addicted to nicotine to quit"
- 55% believe they "will have nicotine withdrawal symptoms"
- 51% believe they "will be too irritable to quit"

Knowledge of resources
- 87% of the participants had not tried a support group or professional quitting program
- 45% said they would prefer quitting "on their own at home"
- 51% believe cessation programs are too expensive
- 44% said that nicotine patches were too expensive

cigarette was "the most difficult to give up" had lower physical function, role emotion, and social functioning scores. This could mean that cigarette smoking negatively and significantly affects their health or that smoking is used to "reduce" the existing physical and emotional stressors. Participants "most likely to smoke in bed" and "to smoke even when they are sick in bed" have lower physical function scores, implying a relationship between nicotine dependency and poorer health.

The "younger" smokers were more likely to "light up" within the first 5 minutes of awakening. This finding may be consistent with the escalating amount of nicotine put in cigarettes in more recent years. Besides looking at smokers' health status perception scores in relation to other variables, average health subscale scores were compared with national norms. (Table 1).

Follow-up information

Fifteen participants responded to an abbreviated second survey. Four of them were smoke-free. Comparison between first and second surveys showed a significant increase in knowledge regarding smoking risks.

When funding for the *It's Never Too Late* program was extended to a second year, it was decided to continue with the original participants rather than recruit additional numbers. This would provide opportunity to "move" participants along the change continuum and expand and refine survey data through qualitative inquiry. Eight agreed to be interviewed. Findings are as follows:

Table 1. Elders health status perception scores

SF 36 subscale	National norm*	Smokers average
PF	69.3	63.52
RP	64.54	74.5
BP	68.49	75.8
MH	76.87	70.22
RE	81.44	79.12
SF	80.61	86.27
VIT	59.9	57.16
GHPE	62.56	61.8

Abbreviations: Physical Function (PF) is the ability to perform physical activities. Role—physical (RP) is the extent of problems (eg, with work) due to physical health. Bodily pain (BP) is pain or limitations due to pain. Mental health (MH) is the degree of feeling nervous or happy and calm all of the time. Role emotional (RE) is the extent of problems with work or other daily activities due to emotional problems. Social function (SF) is the ability to perform social activities without interference due to physical or emotional problems. Vitality (VIT) is the feeling of tiredness or energy all of the time. General Health Perception (GHPE) is evaluation of personal health.

*This column represents the average scores of 442 men and women 64 to 75 years of age (smoking status unknown). Ware, Snow et al. 1993.

- Seven showed movement along the cessation continuum.
- Five of the seven had attended VNA support groups and remained nonsmokers.
- One significantly cut down.
- One is back to his level of smoking (history of severe depression with psychotropic medications).

In addition, the interview data provides rich, detailed information about the experience of smoking, treatment, cessation, and relapse. Categories are motivators to quit; to stay quit; smoking as a new nonsmoker or smoker post-treatment; evaluation of positive and negative aids during quit; and current view of overall health. As analysis proceeds, the qualitative data enhance the surveys, providing more colorful, vibrant pictures of the clients. Mrs C, for example, responded to the newspaper advertisement inviting participation in *It's Never Too Late*: "It was like God had sent me a message, it really was. Here was the thing in the paper. We want you. Oh, praise the Lord! . . . If I hadn't run into that, it [cessation] wasn't something I could do for myself." Mrs C successfully completed the group and remains a nonsmoker nearly 2 years. Her former smoking husband has joined her in quitting. She says in summary: "I truly believe that my life is saved. . . . I know I couldn't have stopped alone. I just feel so good health-wise. . . . I appreciate being there—taking the time to listen, 'stay with us,' and help."

RECOMMENDATIONS

Standardized protocol

Given the relationship between smoking and disease, it seems imperative that all health care providers extend their treatment of disease to include health promotion for tobacco use. They should systematically ask patients about smoking and their readiness to quit, advise all smoking patients to quit, and help them in the process. By standardizing assessment and other treatment forms, data could be more easily collected and compared.

Consistent interventions from providers

Far greater impact on smoking populations may be made if direct care providers consistently address the use of tobacco in their ongoing clinical encounters with patients. Such consistency conveys to patients that smoking is a serious matter that negatively affects health. It also verifies that quitting is possible and preferable. Combining these strategies with what the smoker sees within his own life and health as motivations to quit are the building blocks for tobacco education and cessation.

Tips in treating elder smokers

According to Marcel Proust, "the real voyage of discovery consists not in seeking new landscapes but in having new eyes." I have rediscovered through smoking elders that clinical outcomes need to be "stepped" along the continuum. Empowering clients to make informed choices requires their commitment as much as ours. We may want them to take giant steps when baby steps are the most they can manage. Here are a few "tips," or general principles, to apply.

- Elder smokers often have habits older than those of us caring for them. Be patient.
- Remember that when they began smoking it was viewed as social, sophisticated, romantic, and healthy.
- Understand, inform, and offer treatment (or refer) for their addiction. Addiction is a difficult fact for older people, in particular, to accept.
- Recognize their anger toward a society that "hooked" them into smoking. Help them convert that energy into goals toward health.
- Appreciate, acknowledge, and patiently support elders' efforts in the context of their rich life experience. At their age, they may have to "move" slowly.

Further investigation

Further investigation of smokers would be valuable. Possibilities for continued study include more detailed analysis of assessment data; a qualitative or ethnographic study to expand on smokers' beliefs and views about smoking; and rigorous program and outcome evaluation.

Analysis of assessment data may include relationships among motivation, health status, interventions, and outcomes. Such analysis could help us to answer the following questions:

- How do smokers who say they "want to quit" compare to those who say they "have no interest?"
- Are there differences in terms of health status, views on smoking, smoking history?
- Do they have higher cessation rates?

Intervention studies may limit participants to those "ready for cessation." Although this would exclude smokers less "ready for change," it would improve program cessation rates. Comparative intervention data within and between individuals at the same stage of readiness would then be available.

What is the percentage of "treated smokers" who progress toward cessation, quit, or relapse? Are there personal, health, or psychologic characteristics that respond more to tapering, nicotine replacement therapy, group support, or individual counseling? Are the programs cost-effective?

What should be done with smokers who do not want treatment? Can smokers who do not want treatment be moved toward cessation? How? What interventions are successful for what subgroups? The extent of the impact on smokers by our interventions is unclear. More detailed comparative information would show change within individuals over time and is critical to the analytic evaluation of program outcomes.

Survey responses suggest a lack of understanding of many health risks associated with continued smoking. Is this lack of understanding based on need for additional information or denial of personal risk? Health care providers, committed to education, practice, and research components of tobacco use, can empower their patients to answer those questions and "move" toward cessation. Thus treatment of diseases caused by tobacco use is not complete without treating the smoking.

REFERENCES

1. U.S. Environmental Protection Agency. Respiratory health effects of passive smoking: fact sheet. 1993.
2. Wilson E. Enhancing smoke free behavior: prevention of stroke. *Health Rep.* 1994;6(1):100–105.
3. Lewis C. Disease prevention and health promotion practices of primary physicians in the United States. *Am J Prev Med.* 1988;4:9–16.
4. Cox J. Smoking cessation in the elderly patient. *Clin Chest Med.* 1993;14(3):423–428.
5. U.S. Congress, Office of Technology Assessment. Life sustaining technologies and the elderly. OTA-BA-306. Washington, DC: US Govt Printing Office; 1987.
6. Pifer A, Bronte L, eds. *Our Aging Society Paradox and Promise.* New York, NY: WW Norton and Company; 1986.
7. American Nurses' Association. *Nursing: A Social Policy Statement.* Kansas City, Mo: American Nurses' Association; 1980.
8. National Cancer Institute smoking cessation model. In *Smoking Cessation Training and Technical Assistance Manual.* Massachusetts Tobacco Control Program; 1994.
9. DiClemente C, Prochaska J, Gibertini M. Self-efficacy and the stages of self-change of smoking. *Cog Ther Res.* 1985;9(2):181–200.
10. Ware J. *SF-36 Health Survey.* Boston, Mass: Medical Outcomes Trust; 1993.
11. Feldman. *BRET Benefits Beyond Retirement: It's Never too Late to Quit Smoking.* College Park, MD: University of Maryland; 1992.
12. American Lung Association. *Freedom from Smoking: Guide for Clinic Facilitators.* #0118. New York, NY: American Lung Association; 1993.

Alcohol Abuse in Older Persons: Implications for Critical Care

Susan D. Ruppert, PhD, RN, CCRN, FNP
Associate Professor
Division of Critical Care and Transplantation
The University of Texas-Houston Health
   Science Center
School of Nursing
Houston, Texas

Alcohol abuse and dependence in older adults have received relatively little attention in recent nursing literature and in health care education. However, an estimated 10% to 15% of older people are affected by alcoholism, with approximately 3 million alcoholic people over age 60.[1–3] An estimated 10% to15% of older patients who seek health care have alcohol-related problems.[4] Up to 20% of older patients in acute care hospitals have a problem with alcoholism.[2] These prevalence reports may actually represent an underestimation of the often hidden, unrecognized, or undiagnosed problem of alcohol abuse in this population. However, what is clear is that these older patients often require critical care. Recognition of the problem of alcoholism in this population is vital in preventing consequences related to alcoholism and acute withdrawal.

FACTORS CONTRIBUTING TO ALCOHOL USE IN OLDER ADULTS

Reasons for alcohol abuse in the older population are numerous and often complex. Multiple physiologic and psychosocial theories have been proposed for the use and abuse of alcohol. Although heredity may contribute to lifelong patterns of drinking in some individuals, other factors contribute to alcohol abuse in this population. Multiple stresses of aging encountered by older adults include planned or unplanned retirement, loss of a productive role, declining health, chronic pain or disability, financial diffi-

Source: Reprinted from S.D. Ruppert, *Critical Care Nursing Quarterly,* Vol. 19, No. 2, pp. 62–70, © 1996, Aspen Publishers, Inc.

culties, lack of social support, and death of a spouse or other loved ones.[2,5,6] Widowers have the highest rate of alcoholism in the older population.[2] Because women frequently outlive their spouses, this group is particularly vulnerable. Faced with multiple losses, the older individual may experience boredom, loneliness, and extreme depression.[6] Depression and alcohol dependence in older adults are significant risk factors associated with suicide.[4] Additionally, the normal physiologic changes that occur with aging lower the tolerance for alcohol. Even if the older individual has had a long history of alcohol use without loss of function, physiologic and metabolic changes may now lead to serious problems with alcoholism.

Onset of alcohol use in older adults may be early or late. Two-thirds of older alcoholic patients have had drinking problems since their early years.[6] These individuals tend to have more alcohol-related declines in physical and mental health. Because of organ system changes, this group faces a significant problem with life-threatening illnesses and severe withdrawal symptoms. Late-onset alcohol-abusing patients include persons who begin excessive drinking after age 40.[6] Some sources define this group as those who either began drinking after age 60 or within the past 10 years.[2,5] Frequently, life stressors associated with aging trigger the drinking. This group is more likely to keep the problem hidden.[2] Some individuals may have had intermittent episodes of drinking since early years. Recurrence of drinking in later years is also triggered by experienced losses.

ADVERSE EFFECTS OF ALCOHOL IN OLDER PERSONS

Age-related physiologic changes result in pronounced effects of alcohol in older adults. These changes produce an increased biologic sensitivity and susceptibility to the adverse effects of alcohol. An increased alcohol concentration in the blood for any given amount of alcohol occurs as a result of physiologic changes in absorption, distribution, and elimination.

Absorption is affected by a decrease in gastrointestinal (GI) blood flow and motility coupled with cellular changes in the GI tract. A loss of protective mucus in the stomach results in a heightened risk for gastric irritation and injury. With aging, a decrease in total body water occurs as a result of a decrease in lean body mass and an increase in body fat. Thus, the distribution of water-soluble alcohol is decreased in the older individual because of a reduction in fluid volume. Alcohol is metabolized by the liver and excreted by the kidneys. Age-related decreases in hepatic blood flow result in a reduction in the enzyme activity needed for metabolism. A decline in renal glomerular filtration and in tubular function affects the kidneys' ability to excrete metabolized substances, including alcohol.

With these changes in absorption, distribution, and excretion, even a relatively small amount of alcohol can result in a significant blood alcohol concentration. Body tissues and organs are at greater risk for exposure to higher levels of alcohol for longer periods of time. Over time this exposure can predispose the older individual to significant health risks and disease manifestations that may result in admission to the intensive care unit (ICU) and most certainly complicate the presenting illness picture. For example, alcohol abuse may seriously contribute to hypertension in this population. Decreased lymphocyte production and decreased overall white blood cell function can occur with chronic alcohol use, impairing the immune response. Coupled with age-related changes in the immune system, an increased susceptibility to infection (eg, pneumonia, tuberculosis, hepatitis) exists.

Mental status changes may occur as a result of the effects of alcohol consumption. Such cognitive impairments or dementias may be the consequence of blood alcohol concentration, alcohol–drug interactions, malnutrition, sleep deprivation, and organ system inflammation or damage resulting from alcohol abuse (eg, cirrhosis, hepatitis, pancreatitis, cardiomyopathy, cerebellar degeneration).

Insomnia is common in older persons. A reduction in rapid eye movement (REM) sleep and total nighttime sleep normally occurs with aging. Chronic use of alcohol disorganizes sleep patterns by further shortening REM periods, reducing non-REM sleep, and increasing awakening times.[7] Lack of sleep may result in further cognitive impairments, mood alterations, and decreased immune function.

Alcohol can also induce breathing disturbances such as obstructive sleep apnea, occasional apnea, and snoring, which result in hypoxemia and hypercapnia. Breathing changes during sleep occur as a result of alcohol-induced increases in upper airway muscle atonia, depression of hypoglossal nerve activity, altered carotid body chemoreceptor function, and depression of the arousal response.[7]

Nutritional status may be negatively affected by the use of alcohol. Inadequate nutritional intake in older adults caused by age-related appetite decreases, altered eating habits, and reduced income may be further affected by the consumption of "empty" calories from alcohol. Chronic alcohol consumption inhibits the absorption of folic acid, niacin, thiamine, and riboflavin. Fat absorption also may be impaired. In addition, magnesium, calcium, and zinc are lost.[7] Deficits of nutritional elements can result in the development of anemias, blood dyscrasias, and mental status changes. A decrease in clotting factors and platelets can contribute to coagulation impairments. Acute thiamine deficiency may result in the development of Wernicke-Korsakoff syndrome. This neurologic condition is associated with nystagmus, ataxia, confusion, decreased recent memory, and the tendency to fabricate stories to fill memory gaps.[8]

Older adults are frequently polydrug users. This population receives 25% to 30% of all written prescriptions and has the highest use of sedatives, tranquilizers, and hypnotics.[9] Concomitant use of alcohol with these medications has an additive depressant effect on the central nervous system (CNS), resulting in impaired psychomotor abilities and behavior. Adverse reactions between alcohol and analgesics, antihypertensives, anticonvulsants, antibiotics (most notably metronidazole), antidiabetic agents, and H_2 receptor antagonists (ie, cimetidine) can occur.[7] When combined with many common over-the-counter medications, alcohol may contribute to other health problems in older people. Syncope, sedation, and hypotension may occur when alcohol is used in combination with antihistamines. Many older individuals take aspirin for pain relief. Alcohol enhances the anticoagulant effects of aspirin. Additionally, alcohol in combination with a nonsteroidal anti-inflammatory drug (including aspirin) may increase the risk for gastric irritation, peptic ulcers, and GI bleeding.[7]

RECOGNIZING THE PROBLEM

Screening

A comprehensive history is essential in detecting alcohol abuse in older patients. Information should be elicited concerning past and present drinking patterns, reasons for drinking, and feelings about drinking. Inquiry concerning the type, frequency, and amount of alcohol consumed should be incorporated into the history. Specific details can be discovered by inquiring about where the patient drinks and the time of day that drinking occurs. Questions should be asked in a matter-of-fact, nonjudgmental manner.

Several screening instruments are available for assessing alcoholism.[10–12] One or more of these instruments should be incorporated into any comprehensive history. These screening instruments are brief, reliable, and valid measures that can be used easily by health care providers. Because some providers have little experience in alcohol abuse screening, these tools provide an understandable and comfortable means for gathering data.

The CAGE questionnaire is a short, four-question assessment tool designed to assess alcohol abuse.[10] One positive answer indicates that further evaluation is warranted; two positive responses indicate that alcohol abuse is likely. The 13-question Short Michigan Alcohol Screening Test (SMAST) is another screening tool.[11] This test examines both drinking patterns and the consequences of drinking. In an older population the tool has been found to have a sensitivity of 72% and a specificity of 98%.[12] Recently, this instrument has been adapted for use in geriatrics (MAST-G) (See Box titled "Michigan Alcoholism Screening Test—Geriatric Version"). Although longer in length, the MAST-G is specifically designed to detect alcoholism in older adults.

In addition to specific information about alcohol use, data concerning overall health status, medical and surgical conditions, present medications, and a history of past or present trauma or injuries should be obtained. History of injuries such as burns, cuts, falls, vehicular accidents, or home accidents warrants further investigation concerning alcohol use. Of particular

concern are the identification of memory losses or gaps concerning such injuries and the events leading to them. Because depression is often linked to alcohol abuse in older people, assessment of depression using an established scale may be helpful in uncovering a hidden or unrevealed problem.

Critical illness, mental status changes, or denial may render the patient an unreliable source of information; therefore, family members or significant others should be included in the history interview. Information concerning specific knowledge of alcohol use, behavioral changes, and past or present injuries should be obtained. Although this area may be a sensitive one that family members are reluctant to discuss, the

Michigan Alcoholism Screening Test — Geriatric Version (MAST-G)*

1. After drinking have you noticed an increase in your heart rate or a beating in your chest?
2. When talking with others, do you underestimate how much you actually drink?
3. Does alcohol make you so sleepy that you often fall asleep in your chair?
4. After a few drinks, have you sometimes not eaten or been able to skip a meal because you didn't feel hungry?
5. Does having a couple of drinks help decrease your shakiness or tremors?
6. Does alcohol sometimes make it hard for you to remember parts of the day or night?
7. Do you have rules for yourself that you won't drink before a certain time of the day or night?
8. Have you lost interest in hobbies or activities you used to enjoy?
9. When you wake up in the morning, do you ever have trouble remembering part of the night before?
10. Does having a drink make you sleepy?
11. Do you hide your alcohol bottles from family members?
12. After a social gathering, have you ever felt embarrassed because you drank too much?
13. Have you ever been concerned that drinking might be harmful to your health?
14. Do you like to end an evening with a night cap?
15. Do you find your drinking increased after someone close to you died?
16. In general, would you prefer to have a few drinks at home rather than go out to social events?
17. Are you drinking more than in the past?
18. Do you usually take a drink to relax or calm your nerves?
19. Do you drink to take your mind off your problems?
20. Have you ever increased your drinking after experiencing a loss in your life?
21. Do you sometimes drive when you have had too much to drink?
22. Has a doctor or nurse ever said they are worried or concerned about your drinking?
23. Have you ever made rules to manage your drinking?
24. When you feel lonely, does having a drink help?

*Scoring: 5 or more "yes" responses are indicative of an alcohol problem. *Source:* Reprinted with permission from University of Michigan Alcohol Research Center, © The Regents of the University of Michigan, 1991. For more information contact: Frederic C. Blow, Ph.D., University of Michigan Alcohol Research Center; 400 E. Eisenhower Pkwy, Suite A; Anne Arbor, Michigan 48108; 734-998-7952.

critical care nurse needs to assure the relatives and friends that the information is vital in planning and delivering holistic, safe care.

Several barriers may exist that prevent health care providers from recognizing and detecting alcoholism in older people. First, a lack of knowledge about alcoholism in older adults may preclude the critical care nurse from including this aspect in initial history taking. The older individual may not fit the stereotype of what the nurse views as "the alcoholic patient." Second, physical and mental changes noted by the critical care nurse or family members may be attributed to the "normal" deterioration that occurs with aging. Third, the older individual may deny that a problem exists.[13] The nurse will need to be persistent, yet nonjudgmental in eliciting information from the patient that confirms the existence of substance abuse. Finally, cognitive, physiologic, or illness-related changes may make obtaining the information from the patient difficult, if not impossible. In all cases, information should also be collected from family members and significant others about the use of alcohol by the patient.

PHYSICAL MANIFESTATIONS

Physical findings during assessment may depend on the duration of alcohol abuse and subsequent organ system involvement. However, alcohol addiction can affect literally every body system. A thorough physical assessment by the critical care nurse may raise suspicion of alcohol abuse even in light of a negative history.

Neurologic changes may be evident as altered mental status. Impaired judgment, coordination, headache, and confusion may be seen. Differential diagnosis based on dementia can often be difficult in older patients owing to numerous contributing factors. Nystagmus, ataxia, and impairment of recent memory can be related to Wernicke-Korsakoff syndrome.[8]

Gastrointestinal signs and symptoms can include nausea, vomiting, anorexia, epigastric or abdominal pain, and diarrhea. Fifty percent of cirrhotic alcoholic patients develop parotid gland enlargement.[14] Nutritional deficiency may result in stomatitis, glossitis, and cheilitis. Additionally, muscle inflammation and wasting may be present. Hepatic involvement can manifest with hepatomegaly, spider angiomas, palmar erythema, jaundice, ascites, and GI bleeding.

Cardiovascular symptoms can result from alcohol-related changes to the heart muscle. As a result, cardiomyopathy and dysrhythmias occur. Inefficient pump action leads to a decreased cardiac output. Alcohol precipitated coronary spasm can cause variant angina. In addition, significant alcohol consumption is associated with hypertension.

Laboratory findings

The best laboratory marker for alcohol abuse is the gamma-glutamyl transferase (GGT) level. An elevated GGT is seen in an estimated 75% of heavy drinkers.[15,16] Because elevations in the gamma-glutamyl transferase may also occur with certain medications (ie, anticoagulants, anticonvulsants), trauma, obesity, diabetes, gallbladder disease, nonalcoholic liver disease, and heart or kidney disease, results should be interpreted in combination with history and physical assessment data.[17] Chronic alcohol use may also be associated with elevations in the transaminase hepatic enzymes (eg, AST [SGOT] and ALT [SGPT]). An elevated serum ammonia level can be seen in patients with cirrhotic encephalopathy. Increased erythrocyte mean corpuscular volume (MCV) may occur because of folic acid or B_{12} deficiencies seen with chronic alcohol abuse. Moderate to heavy alcohol consumption can also lead to hypercholesteremia with elevated serum high-density lipids (HDL) and low serum low-density lipids (LDL). Prolonged prothrombin time and partial thromboplastin time may be seen. An elevated serum amylase and serum lipase and a decreased calcium occur if pancreatitis is present. Although laboratory findings may raise suspicion of alcohol use, none of these tests is highly sensitive or specific to alcoholism. Blood alcohol levels are only useful if recent drinking is suspected and in formulating a differential diagnosis for neurologic impairment.

TREATMENT OF ACUTE WITHDRAWAL

The alcoholic patient may be admitted to the critical care setting for treatment of a coexisting disease or condition or directly because of alcohol-related organ system damage. Factors such as malnutrition and compromised immune function related to alcoholism serve to complicate the critical illness. A physical dependence on alcohol occurs with chronic use; therefore, alcohol withdrawal symptoms may occur in as little as several hours after abstinence. Certainly, withdrawal during the course of hospitalization from either known or hidden alcoholism affects the course of recovery for the older individual. Prompt recognition and immediate treatment of withdrawal symptoms are needed.

Older patients with coexisting conditions and critical illnesses are more likely to exhibit more severe manifestations. Clinical manifestations of withdrawal can be divided into three categories.[18] In the first category, symptoms include elevation in blood pressure, tachycardia, diaphoresis, anxiety, insomnia, nausea, vomiting, and the "shakes." Hand tremors may persist for several days. Neuronal excitement in the second category produces seizures. The third category includes sensory–perceptual disturbances such as confusion, agitation, hallucinations, and delirium tremors.[18] Hallucinations can be tactile, olfactory, visual, or auditory.[19] The confusion and hallucinations seen in the older population are sometimes difficult to distinguish from other causes such as hypoxia, cognitive changes, drug interactions, reaction to anesthesia, sleep deprivation, and ICU psychosis. Astute recognition by the critical care nurse of the other physiologic changes associated with withdrawal is necessary to establish a differential diagnosis. Delirium tremors often occur suddenly within 3–4 days after abstinence and can persist for 4–7 days. A 5% to 25% mortality rate is associated with delirium tremors.[18,19] Hyperthermia or vascular collapse may lead to death.[18]

Care for the patient during alcohol withdrawal consists of pharmacologic treatment, correction of metabolic alterations, nutritional support, and environmental control. Pharmacologic treatment for withdrawal includes the use of benzodiazepines. Longer acting preparations such as chlordiazepoxide (Librium) or diazepam (Valium) are usually preferable during detoxification because of the drugs' ability to self-taper. However, shorter acting agents such as lorazepam (Ativan), oxazepam (Serax), or midazolam (Versed) are more often used in older patients and those individuals with impaired hepatic function.[20] Large loading doses are given initially with a 25% dose tapering over the next 3–4 days. Although standard dosing protocols are cited in the literature, dosing often needs to be individualized to prevent over- or underdosing in older patients.[20] Phenytoin (Dilantin) may be necessary if seizures occur. Haloperidol (Haldol) can be used in managing alcohol withdrawal psychosis.[18] However, because this agent potentiates orthostatic hypotension and tachycardia and can cause delirium in older persons, its use may not be desired.

Nutritional support is vital during both the illness and the recovery phases. Supplements with thiamine, folic acid, magnesium sulfate, and multivitamins are necessary in treating deficiencies. During critical illness, fluid volume and trace elements are usually replaced through total parenteral nutrition. Vitamin K may need to be supplemented if the prothrombin time is increased. Safety is a particular concern during withdrawal. Restraints and padded siderails may be indicated during periods of confusion and agitation. The patient should be placed in a quiet, private environment to reduce stimulation. Frequent reorientation is necessary.

PREVENTION AND LONG-TERM TREATMENT

Primary prevention should be directed at lowering the incidence of alcohol use in this population and in identifying individuals at risk for developing a problem with alcohol abuse.[6] Referral to groups that provide the older individual with retirement planning assistance, health promotion education, and coping strategies for life changes is essential.

Comprehensive discharge planning for the inpatient should include referral to a community-based substance abuse program. The critical care nurse should collaborate with other members of the health care team to find a program that will meet the unique needs of the patient and family. Involvement of the patient and his or her significant others is critical to the patient's success in such a program. Decisions concerning treatment options should be based on the severity of the problem, degree of social support, degree of psychologic impairment, presence or absence of other medical problems, and relapse history.[13]

Self-help groups such as Alcoholics Anonymous (AA) can provide the patient with support and assistance during recovery. Additionally, AlAnon or Adult Children of Alcoholics groups are available in many communities to provide support for family members and significant others. Specialized AA groups offered at senior citizens centers are particularly helpful to older adults. Treatment occurs within the mainstream of peer socialization and activities. Other beneficial and needed services such as access to meals and transportation may also be available at these senior centers.[13] Organically impaired older adults may benefit more from less structured programs and one-to-one counseling.[21]

Outpatient or inpatient treatment centers are other options. Although outpatient programs allow patients to remain in their usual environment, this option does not remove patients from the possible recurrent use of alcohol.[13] Patients may also have difficulty in securing transportation to such centers. Inpatient centers provide 24-hour care, but at higher cost. Planning for such referrals includes investigating which programs have payment plans, have discounts or sliding scale fees, or accept Medicare. Halfway houses may provide another option for some. However, these residential programs are usually not equipped to handle any concurrent medical or psychiatric conditions.[13] Some of these programs do not accept adults over age 65.

●   ●   ●

The health care risks and problems associated with chronic alcohol use predispose this vulnerable population to critical illnesses. Systemic damage from chronic use may seriously complicate even minor illnesses. Certainly, safety issues are posed in critical illnesses during detoxification. The critical care nurse must be prepared to assess older adults routinely for alcohol abuse problems. Recognition of subtle clues can result in early intervention that improves the short- and long-term outcomes for the patient. An interdisciplinary team approach is vital in formulating plans of care that address the immediate and posthospitalization needs of the older alcoholic patient. A thorough understanding of this often hidden problem in older adults will allow comprehensive and individualized care to be provided.

REFERENCES

1. Gupta K. Alcoholism in the elderly: uncovering a hidden problem. *Postgrad Med.* 1993;93(2):203–206.

2. Dube CE, Lewis DC. *Project ADEPT: Special Populations; Curriculum for Primary Care Physician Training.* Providence, RI: Brown University; 1994.

3. Bloom P. Alcoholism after sixty. *Am Fam Physician.* 1983;28(2):111–113.

4. Curtis L, Geller G, Stokes E, Levine D, Moore R. Characteristics, diagnosis, and treatment of alcoholism in elderly patients. *J Am Geriatr Soc.* 1989;37:310–316.

5. Schonfeld L, Dupree L. Antecedents of drinking for early and late-life onset elderly alcohol abusers. *J Stud Alcohol.* 1991;56(6):587–592.

6. Hoffman A. Alcohol problems in elder persons. In:

Stanley M, ed. *Gerontological Nursing*. Philadelphia, Pa: FA Davis; 1995.

7. Dufour M, Archer L, Gordis E. Alcohol and the elderly. *Clin Geriatr Med*. 1992;8(1):127–141.

8. Schuckit M. *Drug and Alcohol Abuse: A Clinical Guide to Diagnosis and Treatment*. New York, NY: Plenum Press; 1989.

9. Gomberg E. Drugs, alcohol, and aging. In: Kozlowski L, Annis H, Cappell H, et al, eds. *Research Advances in Alcohol and Drug Problems*. New York, NY: Plenum Press; 1990.

10. Ewing JA. Detecting alcoholism: the CAGE questionnaire. *JAMA*. 1984;254(14):1,905–1,907.

11. Selzer ML, Vinokur A, Evon Rooijen L. A self-administered Short Michigan Alcoholism Screening Test (SMAST). *J Stud Alcohol*. 1975;36(1):117–126.

12. Willenbring ML, Christensen KJ, Spring WD, Rasmussen R. Alcoholism screening in the elderly. *J Am Geriatr Soc*. 1987;35:864–869.

13. Marcus M. Alcohol and other drug abuse in elders. *J ET Nurs*. 1993;20(3):106–110.

14. Burns C. Early detection and intervention for the hidden alcoholic: assessment guidelines for the clinical nurse specialist. *Clin Nurse Spec*. 1994;8(6):296–303.

15. Lieber CS. Hepatic, metabolic, and toxic effects of ethanol: 1991 update. *Alcohol Clin Exp Res*. 1991;15(4): 573–592.

16. Pandey GN. Biochemical markers of predisposition to alcoholism. *Alcohol Health Research World*. 1990; 14(3):204–218.

17. United States Preventative Task Force. *Guide to Clinical Preventative Services*. Baltimore, Md: Williams & Wilkins; 1989.

18. Antai-Otong D. Helping the alcoholic patient recover. *Am J Nurs*. 1995;95(8):22–29.

19. Marcus M, Look D, Oswald L. Nursing care of clients with substance abuse in the hospital. In: Sullivan E, ed. *Nursing Care of Clients with Substance Abuse*. St Louis, Mo: CV Mosby; 1995.

20. Littrell R, Hyde G. Pharmacologic therapies in surgical patients with drug and alcohol addictions. In: Miller N, Gold M, eds. *Pharmacologic Therapies for Drug & Alcohol Addictions*. New York, NY: Marcel Dekker; 1995.

21. Canter W, Koretzky M. Treatment of geriatric alcoholics. *Clin Gerontol*. 1989;9(1):67–69.

"You Don't Ask for Trouble": Women Who Do Sex and Drugs

Rachel Beaty Muller, RN, MSN
Doctoral Student

Joyceen S. Boyle, RN, PhD, FAAN
Department of Community Nursing
School of Nursing
Medical College of Georgia
Augusta, Georgia

Although the literature on human immunodeficiency virus (HIV) and its transmission has burgeoned with information about the disease process, treatment, and epidemiology, there is still little understanding of the social behavior of high-risk groups, especially those who exchange sex for drugs or money.[1] Interventions with clients at risk for HIV have involved education about risk behaviors and condom use; such measures are currently the most effective means to limit the spread of HIV. But attempts to change or influence sexual behavior must take into account the context in which behavior occurs as well as multiple social, cultural, and environmental factors.

The study described in this article focused on a group of women who exhibited high-risk behavior—women who engaged in sex with multiple partners primarily for money to purchase drugs. The purpose of this research was to understand the context and experiences of a select group of high-risk women, all of whom were in jail on charges of prostitution or being a "public nuisance." In particular, data were elicited about the women's lifestyles, drug use, and sexual experiences, including the use of condoms.

Source: Reprinted from R.B. Muller and J.S. Boyle, *Family & Community Health,* Vol. 19, No. 3, pp. 35–48, © 1996, Aspen Publishers, Inc.

The authors acknowledge the contributions to this study by Gerald Bennett, RN, PhD, FAAN, who read and commented on earlier drafts of this article.

RELATED LITERATURE

Although there are reports of changes in sexual patterns and knowledge related to HIV transmission, little is known about the specific factors that reduce risk and maintain changes in behavior.[2] Studies have indicated that attitudes, values, and beliefs among various cultural and ethnic groups must be taken into account when planning intervention strategies.[3–7] However, many of these studies have major shortcomings when findings are applied to the women in this study. Gender issues are problematic because many of the studies on risk behavior and HIV have examined sexual practices of gay men, and such findings cannot be generalized to women.[8]

The effects of an individual's consumption of alcohol and drugs are also of concern in HIV transmission. Studies have found increased risk behaviors with the use of drugs and alcohol.[9–11] A recent study assessing sexual behavior, sexually transmitted diseases, and cocaine use in inner-city women reported that each of the HIV-positive women acknowledged crack cocaine use.[12] Another recent study of women enrolled in an inner-city drug treatment program concluded that drug use and HIV disease and acquired immune deficiency syndrome (AIDS) "permeate the subjects' sexual, familial, and household relationships."[13(p271)]

Heterosexual HIV transmission has accounted for the largest proportionate increase in reported AIDS cases, with women representing the larger proportionate increase.[14] Heterosexual contact has become the predominant mode of HIV exposure among women. Prostitutes and their sexual partners have been identified by the Centers for Disease Control[15] as being at increased risk for HIV infection. Many intravenous drug users report prostitution as a means of financial support for their drug use and thus are at risk for HIV infection from intravenous drug use as well as unprotected sex.[16,17] Exchanging sex for drugs or money with the concomitant higher risk for sexually transmitted diseases and HIV infection has also been observed in the crack cocaine culture.[18–22] In addition, prostitutes (as well as other women) are at risk if their steady, nonpaying sexual partners use drugs or engage in behaviors that are likely to expose them to sexually transmitted diseases.[17,23]

Several studies[16,23,24] suggest that many women at high risk do not take adequate protective measures when engaging in sexual activities with someone who is known to them. For example, condoms are not likely to be used by prostitutes with their nonpaying sexual partners. Similarly, heterosexual respondents who reported sexual behavior changes in response to the AIDS epidemic acknowledged continued unprotected intercourse.[25] In contrast, a number of studies[9,16,17] report that many prostitutes require the use of condoms by their customers, a practice that reportedly started in the 1970s in response to the risk of acquiring other sexually transmitted diseases, especially herpes.[9,16,17] Condom use appeared to act as a mechanism that separated a prostitute's professional practice from personal sexual relationships.[26,27]

Pressure from sexual customers as well as economic concerns of the more desperate and vulnerable women make it difficult for them to comply with safer sexual practices. Women in a drug treatment program developed strategies to reduce the risk of sexually transmitted infections; however, they were unable to sustain risk-reduction efforts.[28] After reviewing studies on women and HIV infection, Smeltzer and Whipple[29] concluded that models for interventions must consider empowerment of women because "women who are most at risk of HIV infection are often disadvantaged and disenfranchised."[29(p255)] Personal empowerment has been suggested as an integral concept in attempting to help drug-dependent African American women.[30–33]

Interventions that address risk behaviors only at the individual level and teach strategies that attempt to change personal behavior without confronting issues and structures that foster risky behavior may be incomplete.[1] Individual behavior change may well be enhanced and supported by incorporating important population-level determinants of risk that include physical, cultural, and environmental considerations.[5,8]

Poverty, lack of economic opportunity, discrimination, and sex inequality and their relationship to HIV risk behaviors have yet to be fully explored. Overall, the AIDS epidemic has been disastrous for poor minority women—in part because of the prevalence of intravenous drug use and crack cocaine in their communities.

METHODS

This study was conducted in a city jail located in a southeastern city in the United States. An ethnographic approach described by Spradley[34,35] was selected to meet the purpose of the study. Ethnography is ideal for the discovery of cultural meaning and facilitates description of the ways that social activities are conducted.[34] An ethnographic design facilitates an understanding of the participants' world and seeks to discover the implicit assumptions and cultural rules that guide behavior.

Data for the study were collected over a 3-month period using interviews and participant observation with 23 women during the time they spent in jail. The focus of the study, however, was on the experiences and context of the women's lives before their incarceration.

Sample

The convenience sample of 23 participants was selected from the jail population. All of the participants admitted to having several sexual partners and had received money or drugs from men for sexual activities. Some of the women reported serial monogamous sexual relationships in the past. Two male participants who were transvestite prostitutes were also interviewed. They reported that they considered themselves women, identified themselves socially by feminine names, dressed as women outside of the jail, were on hormone therapy before incarceration, and functioned as women with their "dates." The data provided by these two male participants about their sexual behavior were consistent with the data provided by the female participants. Although some of the women did not consider themselves prostitutes, all acknowledged being close to the prostitution subculture by virtue of their familiarity with "street life" (ie, knowing how to "sell" sex to obtain money). Drug use, predominantly alcohol and crack cocaine, was an integral part of their daily lives.

The sample consisted of 5 white and 18 African American participants from 18 to 49 years of age. Four of the women were married at the time of the study; 14 participants reported a mean income from prostitution as slightly over $1,500 per month. Of the 14 participants who reported prostitution as a steady means of income, 4 reported practicing prostitution less than 1 year; 5 had been prostitutes from 2 to 5 years, and 3 others had been "in the life" for 5 to 10 years. This study was conducted under conditions of informed consent. Participants were permitted to use initials rather than their full name on the consent form; all tapes were destroyed at the completion of the study.

Data collection and analysis

Data collection and analysis occurred simultaneously; Spradley's[34] approach to ethnographic interviews categorizes the data as it is collected. Interviews were conducted in a private area of the jail. All interviews were audiotaped. The interviews began with "grand tour" questions that elicited a broad view of the women's lives including drug use, sexual practices, and knowledge of HIV disease. The participants were asked such questions as, What can you tell me about AIDS? How do you protect yourself against AIDS? What does your man think about using a condom with him? How do you feel about using a condom? Later, as "insider" language was learned, the questions reflected this knowledge. Tell me how you use your "works." How do you choose your "running partners"? How do you get "paper" for your "stuff"? Tell me about your "old man" and your "friends on the side." What about "freaking and geaking"?

Questions were constructed to categorize data by developing taxonomies based on exclusiveness and inclusiveness. Contrast questions searched for attributes and relationships among the terms and elicited labels, definitions, or examples. Toward the end of each interview, further questions elicited details that had not been sufficiently described by the participants. Women who were knowledgeable about selected topics were interviewed several times to facilitate interpretation of data and expand the initial findings. The jail setting posed some limitations; a few women were released before they participated in additional interviews.

Tapes from 14 participants who reported income from prostitution were transcribed verbatim for analysis. The remaining tapes were scanned for corroborating and atypical data. All interviews were conducted by one of the investigators. The 14 transcripts were read by both investigators for initial insights about the women's lifestyles as well as how they viewed HIV disease and their descriptions of sexual practices and drug use. A total of 71 domains were identified in the initial analysis; these domains were then scrutinized to identify components to expand the description of the domain. For example, the domain "ways to get drugs" was explored to identify the different ways that participants used to obtain drugs. "Having it given to you," "freaking and geaking" (sex and drugs), "doing anything" (becoming a junkie), "stealing," "dating" (prostitution), and "roasting" (con games) were explored to expand the description of the domain. Then ethnographic themes were formulated to explain relationships among the domains.

Qualitative evaluation criteria as defined by Leininger[36] were used to enhance the rigor of this study. Credibility and confirmability were strengthened through repeated inquiry and exhaustive exploration of each domain until theoretical saturation was achieved. The experiences and relationships described by the participants were shared and corroborated by the participants after the initial analysis. This process was followed to ensure that the true significance of actions, symbols, and events were interpreted accurately and reflected the meaning and values of the participants. Meaning-in-context and saturation occurred through extended interviews over a significant period of time as well as frequent reinterviewing and member checks with participants. Findings from this study may have transferability to other women in contexts and situations comparable to those described here.

The method, design, and rationale for conducting an ethnographic analysis have been reported in detail by Spradley.[34,35] Spradley[34] urged the use of the participants' own words and terminology to describe and understand the meaning of experiences. Whenever possible, we have tried to use participants' terminology if we thought it enhanced understanding; on the other hand, we tried not to go overboard with the use of what could be considered "street language." The four themes presented here examine relationships between sex and drugs, sex and money, women with multiple sexual partners, and lastly the use of condoms.

Limitations of the study include the sample and site of the research; only women who were incarcerated in the city jail could be sampled for theoretical saturation. In addition, the study was conducted in a small facility, and the sample was restricted to informants who happened to be incarcerated at the time of the interviews. The participants were asked to describe events that had occurred before their incarceration; there was no opportunity for the investigators to observe their behavior outside of the restricted jail environment.

FINDINGS

Doing sex and drugs

All of the participants reported the use of crack cocaine and multiple sexual partners. Sex and drug use were closely related; sex was used by the women to obtain drugs and to generate money for other needs. The women described an environment where drugs were readily available and everyone used them. The close link between drugs and sexual behavior was explicitly and graphically described by the participants. One participant described a scenario that illustrated how sex and drugs—in this instance crack co-caine—were intimately linked:

> We all were in the room and this guy came in with some dope. So we went into the bathroom to cut it up. He asked me, "Who is the bitch with the green pants?" I said, "I don't even know her, she came here with X." So he said, "Go tell her I want to do something with her." I wouldn't tell her nothing, I just say he want to talk with her in the bathroom. She was one of the ones who said she wouldn't do that, but I knew the guy, right. She stayed in the bathroom and I could hear him say, "Look bitch, if you ain't going to do nothing, you can get out. Don't you want this rock?" She ended up doing it.

"Freaking and geeking" are activities that were described in a recreational context; for example, a party usually involved several persons participating in sexual activities while smoking large quantities of crack cocaine. "Freaking" refers to sexual activity; "geeking" is getting high and still wanting more drugs. Freaking and geeking fulfilled social and emotional needs as well as providing a way to obtain drugs. Ménage à trois was described as a common arrangement during these sessions. Freaking and geeking usually began in a social gathering among friends and over time, friends of friends or other acquaintances joined the group. The result was a mix of people participating in drug use and sexual activities in a casual way. One of the participants, a 23-year-old African American named "Star," described how freaking and geeking happens:

> Like me and some friends get to-gether. We might meet up with some men; might not even know them, you know how people is. They say, "We got something to get high with, y'all want to go freak and geek a little bit?" Or, me and my friend had a room, so

> we meet these guys; one had just picked up the other one who was a drug man. They go in the room and the first guy says, "Why don't you all get comfortable" and stuff like that. They start, for example, one of the guys like kinda talked to me and the other say nothing. My girlfriend she was preg-nant, she was smoking but they didn't want her, they wanted me. So, we started, both of them steady giving me pieces, both of them wanted me, I was steady smoking. . . .

Other women started on drugs in a slightly different manner. At first they were able to buy cocaine themselves for their personal use. However, when they had no money or they wanted larger quantities of cocaine, freaking and geek-ing were easy and viable ways to obtain drugs, especially crack cocaine. It was generally under-stood by everyone that women could engage in sex to obtain drugs or money. Getting together with others led to participation in sexual activi-ties and the use of drugs. These social aspects of freaking and geeking were important to women. Having sex for drugs (as opposed to money) was not viewed as prostitution or considered high-risk behavior by the participants because of the social aspects of the interaction. After all, they were just freaking and geeking with "friends."

Friends on the side

Some of the participants described a different kind of lifestyle, one that involved "friends on the side," or men with whom they had sex to supplement their income. Sometimes money ex-changed hands, but it was just as common for the women to receive household goods such as gro-ceries, diapers, clothes, or whatever else was needed. Often men would pay rent or utility bills or simply give the women money. Women with friends on the side were not involved in "street activities" or freaking and geeking. Usually, women who had friends on the side were older and more settled, although they occasionally used drugs. Having friends on the side to help pay the bills was not considered prostitution, and it certainly was not considered high-risk behavior by the participants. It was simply a way of making ends meet. One of the participants named Susie said, "I know girls that go out . . . it ain't no everyday thing like running the streets. A friend might come over and pick them up; they go do a little something and come back with some money. I don't call that prostituting." Because the women knew the men and considered them friends and important members of their support system, they did not believe that having sex with them involved risky behavior.

Many times the women knew that their "friends" were having sex with other women, but they still did not consider the men or themselves at risk for HIV infection. The men could usually be counted on for help when a woman needed it. Breaking off a sexual relationship with them would compromise a woman's financial stability and jeopardize her intimate relationships.

Multiple sexual partners

The participants classified the women they knew into seven categories:

1. just has relationships
2. whore
3. freak
4. junkie
5. has friends on side
6. con artist
7. prostitute (professional or part-time)

Each category identifies characteristics that illustrate the women's status and roles. The ways in which women classified their behaviors and the men with whom they associated were closely tied to decisions about condom use. The conventional definition of having sex for financial gain or even in exchange for drugs was not always considered prostitution. Although the participants had been arrested for prostitution or solicitation, many of them were offended when the term "prostitution" was applied to them.

Women who "just had relationships" were not paid for sex, because these kinds of relationships were based on emotional and social ties to their sexual partners. These relationships were seen as "normal," and women who "had relationships" were usually not involved in street life. "Whores" were differentiated from other women because they were not paid money or anything else in exchange for sexual favors. They were described as women who "gave it away." A whore was the kind of woman who engaged in sex because she thought it would make men like her. The participants considered whores to be at high risk for HIV infection, but they were not "real" prostitutes.

Women who participated in freaking and geaking, or "freaks," generally were not considered prostitutes. They were considered lucky to have friends who could help them obtain drugs. The recreational and social aspects of freaking and geaking were emphasized. One woman explained it this way: "It's all just fun and they want the drug. They going to do what they can to get that drug. Let's go have some fun. Freaking's all in the game with the geaking."

Junkies were freaks who would "do anything" even for a small amount of crack cocaine. A junkie was a step down from a freak in the social order. No participant in this study considered herself a junkie; junkies were described as "too far gone." All the participants maintained that they would never become a junkie because they could control their drug use. Women with "friends on the side" had regular steady relationships that provided support and security.

Another kind of woman with multiple sexual partners was called a "con artist." A con artist promised sexual services but did not follow through if at all possible. For example, con artists pursued targets that were unfamiliar with street life or men who were very drunk or high on drugs. A con artist would promise a man to "go out and get some drugs for a little fun," then take the man's money and not return.

Prostitutes were of two categories: professional and part-time. The women who said they were part-time prostitutes sold sex for money but said they were not financially dependent on prostitution. They only engaged in sex for money when they wanted drugs or to get something for their children. Prostitution was something they initiated, yet they had little control over the actual situation. For example, they did not feel comfortable in setting limits, such as asking the man to wear a condom, because they had not made careful plans for the sexual encounter. On the other hand, professional prostitutes considered that prostitution was "work," and they went about it in a methodical manner. They budgeted their time, not rushing customers but setting time limits. Prostitutes planned their workdays carefully, scheduling "regulars" during the day whenever possible and "turning tricks" at night. Drug use was considered a threat to protecting themselves from unscrupulous "johns," and its use exposed the women to the possibility of getting arrested. Rosie described her mistake: "We were fixing to do a rock and I thought, 'No—I'm going to take care of business first and then I'll get high.' When I get high, I don't pay attention to what I'm doing. So, it's my own stupid fault that I'm in jail."

A protocol was followed by professional prostitutes that they described as "get it on, get it off, get it down the road"—meaning take care of business first and get away from the scene. Professional prostitutes were always aware of the importance of maintaining control of the sexual encounter, especially the use of condoms. They reported that condoms were necessary if they wanted to continue their work. All of the prostitutes could describe the hazards of sexually transmitted diseases, including HIV infection, and they knew that condoms prevented these conditions. Even more importantly, the prostitutes believed they could control sexual encounters primarily by asking that men use condoms. They said that they valued their personal safety and health more than money or drugs. Trixie, a professional, described it this way: "I love myself. I'm the most important thing there is. I don't need your money. You can't pay me for my life. You can only pay me for what we're going to do right now. If you can't do it the way I want us to do it, we don't need to do it at all."

Sex and condom use

Women who described themselves as "prostitutes" were more likely to believe that they were at risk for diseases such as HIV infection. They would verbally acknowledge the need for condoms, but in the reality of street life, the use of condoms varied with the situation. If a woman engaged in sex on an occasional basis—"I am just going to do this for a little bit of money"— the activity might be viewed by society as prostitution, but the woman did not see herself as a "prostitute." Women with "friends on the side," women who sold sex on an occasional basis, and women who participated in social sex such as freaking and geaking were not seen as prostitutes. The participants said that women who were prostitutes "would sleep with anyone" or "do anything." Only three women in the sample admittedly met these self-defined criteria, even though others reported that they exchanged sex for money or drugs. Regardless of the nature of the sexual activity, the women reported that the use of condoms was not a routine practice. Most of the women could describe the awkwardness and discomfort they experienced when they had asked a man to use a condom. Table 1 shows the reasons women did not use condoms and illustrates how requesting condom use is transformed from a technically simple practice into a difficult task that is largely influenced, scheduled, and controlled by others.

Lack of comfort

Women said that they did not bring up the subject of condom use in their regular, established relationships because it would imply that they were questioning the man's integrity. Vicky described her reluctance to request condom use this way:

> Maybe it's the world that I come from, how I was raised or something. It's always the woman. If you say we should use a condom, there's a fight—first of all. Everything drops, like a dump truck, dumped on you. You're doing something wrong. It [asking about

Table 1. Reasons the women did not use condoms

Lack of comfort	*Lack of desire*	*Characteristics of partners*
Just don't talk about that kind of thing.	It's bad for business.	He's clean, not sleazy.
I was too young and didn't know about condoms.	Don't use one with my boyfriend.	He's good looking and honest.
He'll think I'm messing around with other men.	Don't care or I forget when I'm using drugs.	I trust him.
	It's not my responsibility to carry them.	
	I just don't have any use for them.	

condom use] always reflects on me, couldn't possibly be him. It's always me. His male ego. If push comes to shove, I wouldn't use condoms. Just forget it, because if you love each other and if anything happens, you don't mind.

Some women reported that when they first became sexually active, they did not know that condoms existed, much less how they were used. They said they were "too young"—that is, too inexperienced or unknowledgeable about how to interact with men. Even at present, they said they still felt awkward when talking about condoms or HIV disease with anyone.

Lack of desire

Women reported that they thought condoms were bad for business and social interactions. Taking the time to talk with a man about condoms and to negotiate for condom use during sexual encounters takes time in addition to social skills. Furthermore, the participants said that some men complained that they had decreased feelings with the use of condoms. If a woman wanted to use a condom during sex, the man would immediately be suspicious that she was a "prostitute" or that she "had VD [venereal disease]." If she asked a man to use a condom, the man would spread the rumor that she was sick. Why would she be using a condom? She must have something! These suspicions on the part of

both men and women had a destructive influence on personal relationships.

Who should actually provide the condom was another issue of concern. The women reported that professional prostitutes always carried condoms and that condoms were used by women who identified themselves as professional prostitutes. Other women, however, were reluctant to have condoms in their possession. Some men refused to purchase them, and most of the women said they dropped their request for condom use at the slightest resistance. Not insisting on a condom meant women could "ask for more," (ie, more money) for the sexual encounter.

Many women reported that they "dated" or "had friends on the side" most of the time. Maybe they even freaked and geaked, but these were not considered activities that put them at risk for HIV infection because they "weren't doing anything." When "boyfriends" were their sexual partners, women did not see any potential risk. Some women said that if they were heavily using drugs, it was easy for them to "forget" or not care about using condoms.

Characteristics of the partner

An important factor that influenced the use of condoms involved the characteristics of the intended sexual partner. Women reported that they relied on their ability to observe for cleanliness, illness, honesty, general appearance, and carriage, as well as other attributes. They were confident that they were not at risk for AIDS because they were selective about the personal characteristics of their partner. For example, trust and honesty were important when boyfriends and lovers were being assessed. When customers or "tricks" were evaluated, then personal appearance and cleanliness were the criteria to be considered. Except for the three women who acknowledged that they were professional prostitutes, the participants in this study did not see themselves at risk for HIV infection because they were not the kind of women who "had sex with men who were so out of control as to do anything." Men who were "out of control" were men who were "sleazy," not clean, or dishonest or who used drugs heavily.

One of the participants, an intravenous drug user, reported that she found it difficult to believe that she had tested seropositive for HIV infection. She said that she was not "sleazy"; she didn't "run in the streets" or "sleep with just anyone." She claimed that she had never shared needles. In fact, she believed that she really was not HIV positive; she thought that the drugs she had taken contained impurities that caused an "instability" in her system, and that made her test seropositive. She consistently maintained that she could not have HIV disease because she and the men in her life were "not the type."

DISCUSSION

This study described how a group of women in jail explained their behaviors related to drug use and sexual practices. All of the participants reported the use of crack cocaine and multiple sexual partners. However, the manner in which drugs were obtained and used as well as the kinds of sexual relationships they engaged in varied considerably among the women. Sex was used to obtain drugs and other favors. Women in this study came from a drug-oriented and chaotic environment; they had devised a variety of strategies to take care of themselves. They had learned that sex enabled them to participate in social activities, obtain money and drugs, and engage in intimacy. The women acknowledged

that risks were encountered when they engaged in sexual practices or used illegal drugs, and they might briefly consider these risks. However, in the reality of male-dominated street life, strategies that would ensure the use of condoms were difficult to implement without endangering relationships. These relationships were important to the women, because they had learned that sex enabled them to maintain intimate relationships with men who could help them financially or who could provide them with drugs. Most importantly, relationships with men provided women with a sense of emotional well-being. Asking a man to use a condom during sex would endanger the relationship, and it was obvious that "you don't go around askin' for trouble."

To the outsider, it may appear that women like those in this study live promiscuously with indiscriminate sexual encounters and widespread use of illegal drugs. Although sexual encounters and the use of drugs are common, this view is far too simplistic to explain the behavior of the women in this study. The use of drugs and sexual practices differed considerably according to the kinds of relationships women had with men. An important aspect of meaning for women in this study were relationships with men. It is around these different kinds of relationships that the women learned to organize their behavior and interpret their experiences.

IMPLICATIONS

Sexual practices and drug use were closely linked in this study of women at high risk for developing HIV disease. Sexual relationships and drug use provided women with opportunities for social interaction and intimate relationships that enhanced their self-esteem and sense of worth. Drug use and sexual practices, including the use of condoms, varied considerably according to the kinds of relationships engaged in by women. Professional prostitutes were willing to forgo establishing emotionally based relationships with men and expected only financial remuneration for sexual favors. In contrast, other women in the study valued the sense of being wanted and an intimate relationship with a member of the opposite sex. Maintaining such relationships and their positive benefits was the most important cultural theme in this research project. Until women like those who participated in this study can satisfy their emotional needs outside of the context of drugs and sex, efforts to encourage such women to use condoms and take other precautions against HIV infection will be relatively unsuccessful.

Furthermore, the findings supported the notion that the women underestimated the probability of HIV infection posed by their personal behaviors, because they did not view unprotected sex with multiple partners as risky. Instead, the use of condoms was influenced by the emotional overtones attributed to relationships, personal characteristics of sexual partners, and the assumption that women could detect their partners' risk behaviors.

● ● ●

The findings from this research support studies[30,31,33,37] that suggest personal empowerment may be an integral concept in working with drug-dependent or poor minority women. Indeed, it may be the first step in helping women negotiate condom use or instigate other positive behavioral changes. Multidimensional approaches that include educational programs that acknowledge client experiences, values, and contributions are necessary if empowerment is a goal of these programs. Integration of health and social programs that address the larger context and the effects of unequal power and economic bases as they relate to sexual issues must be incorporated in program designs. Emphasis should be placed on developing the skills related to negotiation for safer sex practices and rejection of the double standard that is so pervasive in the lives of these participants and other groups of women. Of critical importance, however, is that empowerment of women be viewed in the context of sociocultural, economic, and political considerations.

REFERENCES

1. Choi K, Coats TJ. Prevention of HIV infection. *AIDS*. 1994;8:1371–1389.

2. Becker MH, Joseph JG. AIDS and behavioral change to reduce risk: a review. *Am J Public Health*. 1988;78: 394–410.

3. Flaskerud JH, Rush CE. AIDS and traditional health beliefs and practices of black women. *Nurs Res*. 1989; 38:210–215.

4. Flaskerud JH, Nyamathi AM. Black and Latina women's AIDS-related knowledge, attitudes and practices. *Res Nurs Health*. 1989;12:339–346.

5. Jeffery RW. Risk behaviors and health: contrasting individual and population perspective. *Am Psychol*. 1989; 44:1194–1202.

6. Jemmott LS, Jemmott JB III. Applying the theory of reasoned action to AIDS risk behavior: condom use among black women. *Nurs Res*. 1991;40:228–233.

7. Ickovics JR, Morrill AC, Bern SE, Walsh U, Rodin J. Limited effects of HIV counseling and testing for women: a prospective study of behavioral and psychological consequences. *JAMA*. 1994;272:443–448.

8. Aggleton P, O'Reilly K, Slutkin G, Davies P. Risking everything? Risk behavior, behavior change, and AIDS. *Science*. 1994:265:341–345.

9. Des Jarlais D, Friedman S, Hopkins W. Risk reduction for the acquired immunodeficiency syndrome among intravenous drug users. *Ann Intern Med*. 1985;103:755–759.

10. Stall R, McKusick L, Wiley J, Coates T, Ostrow D. Alcohol and drug use during sexual activity and compliance with safe sex guidelines for AIDS: the AIDS behavioral research project. *Health Educ Q*. 1986;13: 359–371.

11. Grune JPC, Kaplan CD, Adriaans NFP. Needle sharing in the Netherlands: an ethnographic analysis. *Am J Public Health*. 1991;81:1602–1607.

12. DeHovitz JA, Kelly P, Feldman J, et al. Sexually transmitted diseases, sexual behavior and cocaine use in inner-city women. *Am J Epidemiol*. 1994;140:1125–1134.

13. Pivnick A, Jacobson A, Eric K, Doll L, Drucker E. AIDS, HIV infection and illicit drug use within inner-city families and social networks. *Am J Public Health*. 1994;84:271–274.

14. Centers for Disease Control. Update: acquired immuno-deficiency syndrome—United States, 1992. *MMWR*. 1993;42(28):547–557.

15. Centers for Disease Control. Additional recommendations to reduce sexual and drug abuse-related transmission of HTLV III/LAV. *MMWR*. 1986;35(10):152–156.

16. Centers for Disease Control. Antibody to human immunodeficiency virus in female prostitutes. *MMWR*. 1987;36(11):157–161.

17. Rosenberg MJ, Weiner JM. Prostitutes and AIDS: a health department priority? *Am J Public Health*. 1988;78:418–423.

18. Fullilove RE, Fullilove MT, Bowser P, Gross SA. Risk of sexually transmitted disease among black adolescent crack users in Oakland and San Francisco, Calif. *Sex Transm Dis*. 1990;263:851–855.

19. Booth RE, Waters JK, Chitwood DD. HIV risk-related sex behaviors among injecting drug users, crack smokers, and injection drug users who smoke crack. *Am J Public Health*. 1993;83:1144–1148.

20. Fullilove MT, Golden E, Fullilove RE, et al. Crack cocaine use and high-risk behaviors among sexually active black adolescents. *J Adolesc Health*. 1993;14:295–300.

21. Edlin BR, Irwin KL, Faruque S, et al. Intersecting epidemics—crack cocaine use and HIV infection among inner-city young adults. *N Engl J Med*. 1994;24:1422–1427.

22. Schilling R, El-Bassel N, Ivanoff A, Gilbert L, Su KH, Saffyer SM. Sexual risk behavior of incarcerated, drug-using women, 1992. *Public Health Rep*. 1994;109:539–547.

23. Leonard MA, Sacks JJ, Franks AL, Sikes K. The prevalence of human immunodeficiency virus, hepatitis B, and syphilis among female prostitutes in Atlanta. *J Med Assoc Ga*. 1988;77:162–167.

24. Guinan ME, Hardy A. Epidemiology of AIDS in women in the United States: 1982–1987. *JAMA*. 1988;257:2039–2042.

25. Melnick SL, Jeffery RW, Burke GL, et al. Changes in sexual behavior by young urban heterosexual adults in response to the AIDS epidemic. *Public Health Rep*. 1993;108:582–588.

26. Day S. Prostitute women and AIDS: anthropology. *AIDS*. 1988;2:421–428.

27. Campbell CA. Prostitution, AIDS, and preventive health behavior. *Soc Sci Med*. 1991;32:1367–1378.

28. Suffet F, Lifshitz M. Women addicts and the threat of AIDS. *Qual Health Res*. 1991;1:51–79.

29. Smeltzer SC, Whipple B. Women and HIV infection. *Image J Nurs Schol*. 1991;23:249–256.

30. Mondanaro J. Strategies for AIDS prevention: motivating health behavior in drug dependent women. *J Psychoactive Drugs*. 1987;19:143–149.

31. Weissman G. Promoting health behavior among women at risk for AIDS. *NIDA Notes*. 1988;(Winter):6–7.

32. Fullilove MT, Fullilove RE, Haynes K, Gross SA. Black women and AIDS prevention: a view towards understanding the gender rules. *J Sex Res*. 1990;27:47–64.

33. Harris RM, Kavanagh KH, Hetherington SE, Scott DE. Strategies for AIDS prevention. *Clin Nurs Res*. 1992;1:9–24.

34. Spradley JP. *The Ethnographic Interview*. New York, NY: Holt, Rinehart & Winston; 1979.

35. Spradley JP. *Participant Observation*. New York, NY: Holt, Rinehart & Winston; 1980.

36. Leininger M. Evaluation criteria and critique of qualitative research studies. In: Morse J, ed. *Critical Issues in Qualitative Research Methods*. Thousand Oaks, Calif: Sage; 1994.

37. Mondanaro J. *Chemically Dependent Women: Assessment and Treatment*. Lexington, Mass: D. C. Heath; 1989.

Beyond "True" and "False" Memories: Remembering and Recovery in the Survival of Childhood Sexual Abuse

Joanne M. Hall, RN, PhD
Assistant Professor

Lori L. Kondora, RN, CS, MS
Doctoral Candidate
University of Wisconsin–Madison School of
*   Nursing*
Madison, Wisconsin

According to the latest epidemiologic estimates, as many as one-fourth of all women in the United States were subjected to sexual abuse in childhood.[1] Adult women who were sexually abused as children often call themselves "survivors," not victims. They realize they were violated, not stricken by some illness. Yet trauma experienced in childhood can reverberate with aftereffects in adulthood that take a significant toll on health and happiness.[2] Recovery and rehabilitation are meaningful concepts in this context. "Recovery" has etymological roots that resonate with active processes of healing from childhood sexual abuse (CSA). *To recover* is to take back what was lost or stolen, to redeem or reclaim, to rediscover, and to be one's self again.[3] Recovery also implies self-protection and getting out of danger. "Rehabilitation" has its origin in language that relates to overcoming damage wrought by CSA. *To rehabilitate* means to dwell again (as in one's body),[4] to have, and to possess or hold.[3] CSA survivors struggle to grasp and keep their selves, their stories, and their futures from the grip of aftereffects of trauma. Both of these concepts and the processes they represent are interwoven with *memory*, which means a returning, a reclamation.[3]

At the time this work was conducted, the first author was supported by a National Research Service Award Individual Postdoctoral Fellowship grant F32NR06817 from the National Institute of Nursing Research, National Institutes of Health.

Source: Reprinted from J.M. Hall and L.L. Kondora, *Advances in Nursing Science,* Vol. 19, No. 4, pp. 37–54, © 1997, Aspen Publishers, Inc.

Adult women's delayed memories of CSA have stirred a controversy that places clients' credibility at stake. Questions about the truth or falsehood of remembering CSA are rife in the public media, in large part due to increasing numbers of adult women disclosing delayed memories of being sexually abused when they were children. A social movement has developed in response to these disclosures, attributing them to a "false memory syndrome." Proponents of this movement assert that adult CSA survivors' memories are "false" unless they meet legal criteria for rules of evidence. The movement's core is the False Memory Syndrome Foundation (FMSF), whose members lobbied unsuccessfully for the inclusion of "false memory syndrome" as a psychiatric diagnosis.

Caregivers, including psychiatrists, psychotherapists, nurses, psychologists, and counselors, have been accused by the FMSF of either naively accepting everything clients say as absolute historical fact or "planting" memories of abuse as explanation for current life difficulties. Inexperienced caregivers may have initially misunderstood some of the basic dynamics of memory and applied suggestive methods such as hypnosis to retrieve memories. These practices have been critiqued, and more educational opportunities are now available for caregivers to learn safe ways to support clients as they explore life events, without using suggestive approaches.

To be of assistance to survivors of CSA as they recover and rehabilitate, nurses need to understand the historical and political roots of this controversy and to be familiar with the empirical knowledgebase that exists about traumatic memory. It is essential that nursing develop its own knowledge and practices concerning CSA survivors and clarity about our role as witnesses to the healing process.[5]

This article is a critical feminist analysis of the topic. Its purposes are to provide a historical context for the current debate about "true" and "false" CSA memories; to discuss selected literature about conventional understandings of memory and their relevance to this debate; to present an integrative, phenomenological approach to memory in the recovery and rehabilitation of women CSA survivors; and to use the insights gained to draw conclusions from a nursing perspective about the authenticity of delayed CSA memories. Because of cultural diversity and differences in gender socialization, issues discussed here should not be considered inclusive of experiences of male CSA survivors, and they should not be generalized as prescriptive at the level of specific individual cases.

Toni Morrison provided an eloquent image of remembering and a metaphorical anchor for this analysis:

> . . . the act of imagination is bound up with memory. You know, they straightened out the Mississippi River in places, to make room for houses and livable acreage. Occasionally the river floods these places. "Floods" is the word they use, but in fact it is not flooding; it is remembering. Remembering where it used to be. All water has perfect memory and is forever trying to get back to where it was. . . . remembering where we were, what valley we ran through, what the banks were like, the light that was there and the route back to our original place. It is emotional memory—what the nerves and the skin remember as well as how it appeared. And a rush of imagination is our "flooding."[6(p305)]

CYCLES OF DISCLOSURE AND REPUDIATION

During periods of increased visibility of sexual abuse of children, society as a whole tends to deny it because its existence fractures cultural values about family.[7] From a historical perspective, the current controversy about the truth or falsehood of CSA memories is one in a series of societal repudiations of the existence and extent of CSA, especially incest.[2,8,9] In the majority of publicized discussions of "false memory syndrome," it is the delayed memories of women that are being challenged, suggesting that at the heart of this controversy are societal gender conflicts.

Turn of the century

Childhood sexual abuse first came to be viewed as potentially harmful to victims in the late 1800s. Pierre Janet[10] studied and treated women diagnosed with "hysteria," systematically identifying this disorder to be a result of dissociation in response to overwhelming traumatic experience. According to Janet, people make meaning of nontraumatic experiences and voluntarily "store" them in a singular, conscious memory schema. Traumatic experiences that do not fit this existing schema are involuntarily separated from conscious awareness as fragments. Unintegrated traumatic memory fragments manifest as "pathological automatisms" that provide clues to the core trauma. Janet viewed memory as including a creative element, rather than being simply a static recording of events.[11] He advocated clients' journaling of personal stories, hypnosis, reframing of experiences, and therapeutic support as ways to gain access to the separated fragments of experience.[8,11]

At about the same time, Sigmund Freud and Joseph Breuer studied the effects of traumatic memories in women diagnosed with "hysteria." They too posited a "splitting-off" of traumatic experience into the unconscious. They advocated "abreaction," or bringing into consciousness the unconscious traumatic events, and "catharsis," or releasing of associated affective tensions.[12] In 1896, Freud published *The Aetiology of Hysteria*. Based on interviews with women clients, he theorized that sexual abuse, usually perpetrated by fathers, was the root cause of hysteria.[8,13] Having witnessed hundreds of autopsies in Paris, Freud was well aware not only of the pervasiveness of sexual abuse of children, but also of the frequency of subsequent murders of abused children by their perpetrators. In 1905, however, under pressure from colleagues, Freud recanted his trauma-based theory. He offered a new etiology for the symptoms of "hysteria," suggesting that women were

fantasizing rather than remembering. He posited female children's desire for sexual activity with their fathers as a universal stage of psychosexual development. This theory defined thinking about sexual relations between parents and children for the next 60 years.[13] Reification of this theory about female children's "incestuous wishes" effectively silenced the voices of women who claimed to have been sexually abused in childhood, strengthened Freud's place in medical circles, and provided Western society a "scientific" alternative to acknowledging the prevalence of CSA.

Conflicting views of "hysteria" were left to obscurity. For instance, Freud's colleague Sandor Ferenczi was soundly discredited by the psychoanalytic community, in part because of his persistent promotion of the childhood trauma–based theory. Ferenczi's belief in his women patients' stories of abuse and his more nurturant clinical methods contrasted sharply with the male-dominated subculture of psychiatry of the period.[14] Similarly, Pierre Janet's work was overlooked and only recently has been resurrected in scientific circles as valuable in explaining processes by which traumatic memories are kept from conscious awareness.

Postwar years

Traumatic remembering was briefly explored in the 1930s and 1940s. These studies were confined to "shell shock" in survivors of World War I,[15,16] initially diagnosed as "gross stress reaction."[17] Rare studies about CSA at this time either minimized abuse or focused on mothers as deficient or even as facilitators of the child's abuse by the male partner.[18–21] In the post–World War II period, American psychoanalysts emphasized the role of the man as breadwinner, the place of women in the home, and the nuclear family as sacrosanct. In defining "normalcy," they applied Freudian principles of psychosexual development even more stringently than Freud had. They considered reports of CSA to be rooted in fantasy and associated with homosexuality.[22–24] Preoccupied with "deviance," these psychoanalysts exerted powerful influence on government and social policies and opposed interventions that might threaten the constricted roles of girls and women within the family unit.[25]

Current developments

The civil rights movement of the 1960s and the women's movement of the 1970s fostered a climate in which women could break the silence about violence against women and children, eventually even within scientific circles.[26] As more women entered science and academia, the pervasiveness of rape, spousal battering, and sexual harassment was documented through research. The establishment of women's studies programs catalyzed many of these efforts. At the grassroots level, women organized freestanding rape crisis, domestic violence, and child abuse services. In 1980 prevention of CSA became part of the national agenda for health.[27] With the Reagan era of the mid- to late 1980s, however, cutbacks were made in maternal and child health and welfare benefits.[28]

Research on posttraumatic remembering mushroomed in the late 1970s and 1980s due to the activism of Vietnam veterans.[29,30] A posttraumatic stress syndrome involving memory changes was legitimized as a psychiatric diagnosis for aftereffects suffered by combat survivors.[2] Over time and with the support of empirical evidence, this diagnosis has also been applied to women's and children's sexual trauma. The initial studies specifically focusing on CSA were descriptive of immediate childhood experiences.[31–35] These studies established that whether intrafamilial or extrafamilial, CSA nearly always occurs in multiproblem families.[36,37]

By the early 1980s the scope of research broadened to include the aftereffects of CSA in adult survivors. CSA aftereffects were found to vary widely depending on the type, intensity, and duration of abuse; the child's age at onset; the number of perpetrators and their relationship to the child; the use of force or threat; the occurrence of disclosure; and the role of the child within the family.[38–40] Documented aftereffects include depression, suicidality, low self-esteem, substance abuse, somaticization, dissociative problems, intrusive memories, affective numbness, sleep disturbances, distortions in body image, anxiety, phobias, eating disturbances, employment problems, blocks to intimacy and sexual expression, parenting difficulties, and increased potential for revictimization in adulthood.[8,41–48]

In addition to the development of an empirical knowledgebase about survival of CSA, recent years have seen a growing self-help consumer movement. Many mutual help groups and self-help books directed to CSA survivors offer a nonpathologizing, wellness-oriented view of healing from sexual abuse.[49–51] Media attention has also turned a public eye on CSA. Radio and television programs have frequently featured celebrity survivors, panels of perpetrators, families of survivors, and professional CSA experts. Increasing numbers of criminal and civil cases have also made CSA more visible, yet also contribute to public skepticism about it.[52–54] In the highly publicized 1984 case in Jordan, Minn, allegations were made that clandestine rings of adults sexually abused dozens of children in a small community.[55] Twenty-four adults were charged with sexual crimes. The case was beset with legal errors, claims of corruption, and improperly conducted interviews. Nearly all the defendants were exonerated; the only person convicted was a prior sex offender. During this case, a group called Victims of Child Abuse Laws (VOCAL) was organized by people accused of being sexual abuse perpetrators and their supporters.[55]

In 1992 parents accused of abuse by their adult children formed the FMSF.[56] This organization offers support, including legal fees, to family members accused of CSA. According to the FMSF, increasing reports of CSA have occurred because unethical psychotherapists and psychiatrists frequently "plant" false memories of abuse in their clients' minds to reap the financial benefits of treating consequent distress.[55–57] Concern has also been raised by the FMSF that therapists' "digging up" past trauma may be of more harm than good to women clients as well as to alleged perpetrators.[58] Such arguments contrast sharply: Is the problem "planting" memories or "digging them up?" One argument presumes no trauma occurred, the other presumes it occurred but should not be discussed.

Most scientists investigating traumatic memory doubt that memories of abuse could be "planted." In fact, CSA survivors would rather not believe that they had been so betrayed, especially by a family member. Furthermore, caregivers who work closely with traumatized individuals battle the temptation to suppress survivors' stories of abuse because such material tends to exhaust their own sense of efficacy, creativity, and hope.[8] Results of research about adult women who had delayed recall of CSA showed that 64% had some degree of amnesia regarding the trauma, but in the majority of cases, corroboration was available to verify that abuse had occurred.[59] In another study of 129 women with documented histories of CSA, 38% did not recall the abuse that had been reported and verified decades earlier. This lack of recall was especially likely among those abused at younger ages and among those whose perpetrators were known to them.[60] In fact, a body of empirical evidence indicates that it is common for abused children to reach adulthood without conscious awareness of the trauma.[2,8,40,61] Recall of childhood trauma tends to be triggered in adulthood by some reminder; it might be violence in a domestic relationship, an emotional crisis, or a role transition like becoming a parent.[8,62]

Media coverage; the organization of feminist, self-help, mutual help, and professional efforts to support CSA survivors' recoveries; development of an entire field of scientific study about the traumatic stress of surviving CSA; and the reactions against these efforts attest to the importance of understanding the dynamics of delayed CSA memories. Those who propose a "false memory syndrome" hold simplistic assumptions about human memory as technical and automatic: memory as the chronological recording and filing of detailed information. They believe that stored memories can be retrieved at will, regardless of their affective content and the

interpersonal and environmental conditions in which past events occurred. These assumptions are consistent with Western, positivist ideologies about the body as mechanical, time as linear, knowledge as apolitical, and reality as unidimensional. There is a need to describe memory in other ways, if its role in recovery and rehabilitation is to be understood. If memory is not mechanical, then what other understandings might we have of it?

EXTANT APPROACHES TO UNDERSTANDING MEMORY

Approaches to understanding memory are driven by particular disciplinary concerns and opportunities for exploration. Advocates of learning theory describe perception, processing, storage, and retrieval of information. Sports psychologists explore how the muscles, brain, and nerves can be trained to "remember" correct movements and maximize performance. Neurologists' observations of people with head injuries indicate that there are separate storage and retrieval functions of areas of the brain. Researchers interested in the effects of mood and drug-induced conditions suggest that memory is state dependent; memory stored while a person is in one state of mind will be most easily retrieved when that person is again in the same mood or drug-induced state.[63–65] Forensic psychologists study how accurately human perceptions can be preserved and articulated in a courtroom.[66,67] Developmentalists differentiate children's memory processes from those of adults, tracking changes at specific ages.[68–70] Those focused on the nature of the self who explore narrative and autobiographical memory posit that knowing one's own history is central to personhood.[71,72] Feminists explore gendered aspects of memory through studies of the mundane, everyday workings of memory in natural contexts.[73,74]

In general, research has shown that "normal" (presumably nontraumatized) people cannot reliably remember the details of their experiences from as recently as the previous week.[74] Yet in the case of courtroom battles about CSA, both children and adult survivors of sexual abuse are expected to recall vivid details of past events that occurred in the contexts of terror, pain, confusion, emotional abandonment, and secrecy.[75] Most relevant in exploring the basis of CSA memories are studies of trauma-associated remembering. Such disparate experiences as bereavement, combat stress, Holocaust events, and inescapable negative stimuli have been rich sources for cognitive explanations of traumatic remembering, illuminating facets of CSA remembering.

Horowitz[76] studied patterns of bereaved people. He developed an information processing model positing that human cognition has a tendency toward completion. Individuals strive to assimilate new information into existing cognitive schemata. Traumatic information is "unthinkable," so it does not fit into existing networks. This results in an "intrusion–numbing" cycle. Memory of trauma intrudes on cognitive functioning in such forms as dreams, uncontrollable imagery, and flashbacks. The numbing consists of warding off the negative reality, in this case loss, to protect overall psychological integrity and function.[76,77] This alternating pattern of intrusion and numbing has also been noted in other posttraumatic situations.[78]

In working extensively with survivors of combat, Lifton[79] observed that people are active in constructing their own reality based on their perceptions of life experiences. Nontraumatized people feel a connectedness with the world about them, a fluidity and wholeness, the result of what Lifton termed "psychoformative" processes. When a person is traumatized, the psychoformative processes are disrupted. Psychological numbing, fragmentation of the self, and a generalized loss of self-structure occur.[79,80] Others have agreed with this position, describing trauma as having the potential to "collapse the self along all referential planes."[81] A reorganization of the self is then required to restore a strand of continuity and an impression of wholeness. Lifton's[82] later work expanded his theory, focusing on how some traumatized people con-

sciously use their capacity to "fragment" and reorganize as a form of resilience. This changing of the "self-shape" is useful as long as it does not lead to severe "rootlessness."

Langer[83] explored survivors' experiences of the Holocaust. In his view, traumatic memories constitute "meaningless" pieces of an isolated reality; they cannot be shared with others because almost any audience is resistant and will not likely understand. Auschwitz survivors told of their concentration camp experiences, including loss of the ability to fantasize about the future and to imagine an outside world. They recalled impossible forced choices (eg, saving one's own life versus that of a child or spouse) and a routinization of terror. These experiences contrasted sharply with the pre- and postcamp self-image and experiences, requiring a "doubling" of the self. In the posttrauma period one can attribute the horrible situations as having happened to "someone else," the "Auschwitz self." This prevents the constant intrusion of traumatic memories into current daily life (although one cannot completely maintain this "walling off" of the horror from consciousness). Langer eloquently described the timeless quality of traumatic memory: "There is no need to revive what has never died. . . . Holocaust memory is an insomniac faculty whose mental eyes have never slept."[83(pxv)]

From laboratory experiments on both animals and humans, Seligman and associates[84–86] proposed the model of learned helplessness to explain how memory works in the context of unpredictable, traumatic incidents. This model holds that individuals subjected to uncontrollable, repeated trauma develop images of themselves as virtually powerless. A deep sense of futility is internalized after numerous unsuccessful attempts to avoid the trauma and remains even after the threat has passed. Applying this notion to humans, people are believed to see the world as a threatening and inhospitable place and thus experience depression, withdrawal, anxiety, and chronic fear.

These cognitive theories illustrate what Morrison[6] called "flooding." They describe the pressure and overflow that trauma forces on the individual psyche. They offer an understanding beyond the mechanical images of memory and point to the centrality that trauma can take in an individual's life.

A PHENOMENOLOGICAL UNDERSTANDING OF MEMORY AND CSA

Much that occurs in daily life is so mundane that people do not remember it in detail because the events lack immediate significance. At the other extreme, experiences like CSA may be so terrorizing as to be wholly or partially amputated from awareness. Memories are always reconstructive to some extent. Relationships between one's self, environment, and significant others are part of a larger narrative process in which memory allows people to discover and return to important places in life where there is incompleteness to be resolved. The resolution of this incompleteness is what Morrison compared to water's "perfect memory." Her metaphor intimates that a phenomenological understanding of memory and its relationship to experience may shed new light on the debate about "false memories." Perfect memory, in the case of the lived experience of remembering CSA, refers to the depth and power of memory as it holds and reveals essential aspects of experience, rather than mechanical accuracy of detail. Memory works "perfectly," that is, according to its own nature and purpose. It is a means of recovery—taking back what was lost or stolen—and of rehabilitation—dwelling again in the self. Phenomenological research with women CSA survivors points to the centrality of remembering in the healing process.[87,88]

In his phenomenological study of memory, Casey[89] advocated a broader understanding of remembering. Though not writing exclusively about traumatic memory, he succeeded in capturing aspects of it that are useful for understanding how authenticity of CSA memories may differ from evidentiary proof. Casey's concepts are outlined in the following sections by

applying them to circumstances of surviving CSA. As Casey said, memory is difficult to study because we are already "in the thick of it."[89(pix)] He viewed memory as living not only in the cognitive structures of the brain, but also in the body and the world. Noting that most studies of remembering involve intentional memory, or mental representation that resides in the mind, he devoted much of his effort to examining remembering that is other than a mental act.

Mnemonic modes

Casey[89] described three mnemonic modes: reminding, reminiscing, and recognition. Each of these aspects of remembering has a connectedness outside the mind, linking people to their environments.

Reminding

Reminding requires not only mental receptiveness, but also some environmental object that catches one's attention. Reminders are external objects, conditions, and interpersonal discourses that evoke internal counterprocesses, unifying fragments of experience. For women who have survived CSA but have not remembered it, reminding is the process by which their present environments draw them inward toward images of past trauma. A triggering event such as an impending or actual separation, the birth of a child, or an abusive partnership may be a reminder that pulls one's awareness toward the earlier trauma of CSA.[62] Although this conjoining of past and present is unifying, it is usually painful and disorienting, not only in terms of inner life, but also in how the environment appears to the survivor. Suddenly certain aspects of the present environment take on the terrifying aura of the CSA experience. Words such as "uncle" or "father," if they were the perpetrators, may send the survivor into a reverie of internal imagery and a reexperiencing of the sexual trauma. A darkened room may become a dangerous war zone rather than a nice place to sleep.

Present reminders approximate characteristics of past memories; they do not correspond exactly to details of actual traumatic events. As Casey[89] pointed out, there is no way cleanly to sever knowledge of the past from the influence of the reminding present. This should not be interpreted as evidence that delayed memory is unauthentic. On the contrary, when one's current reality can be "connected" with patterns of the past that have not before been accessible, there is a sense of completion, of wholeness. In the case of CSA memories, this process of integration may entail walking again through "buried" fear, rage, and loss. This is a kind of recovery or regaining, a way to reinhabit lost territory. The survivor may need to build new relationships between her self and aspects of her present environment so that reminders lose their charge, lose their power to obstruct life's joys.

Reminiscing

Reminiscing is an engaged, conscious talking out of what is being remembered in order to understand it more intimately. It is a transformative reentering of past environments and situations, a reliving that may be highly introspective or very public. It is most powerful when it is shared with others and is fully concretized in language. Reminiscing is not fictionalization. Telling the story of a past experience, although always an interpretation of "actual events," is still bound to concrete environments and events in the past and derives its credibility from the process of narration itself.[72]

Narrative is essentially the way we exist to ourselves and others in a temporal sense. To be unaware of having been sexually abused in childhood means the loss, the amputation, of some part of the storied self. Survivors do not merely "subtract" the traumatic images from their narrative as one clips articles from a newspaper. Major alterations in the life narrative must occur for CSA survivors who cannot access trauma memories. Disturbing questions arise about the whole self: Who am I? What was my family like? What have I experienced? How did I feel about it? Why can I not recall anything about my life from the age of four to eight? Why do I fear closed doors? Where is my life going? Lacking continuity of childhood memories,

some women survivors of CSA may have creatively woven together the bits of story they do have, sealing off knowledge of what occurred in the gaps. Lacking access to intense, negative past events, survivors may instead carry "mythicized," idealized versions of their pasts, often reinforced by other family members' denial, concealment, or lack of knowledge of the abuse.

A serious outcome of losing one's story is the tendency of some CSA survivors to reenact dynamics of past trauma in the present through unconscious susceptibility to battering relationships, injury, survival sex, or self-harm.[2,8,90] It is as though these survivors do not have access to words or are still (consciously or unconsciously) terrorized by the perpetrator's threats that "telling," or even recalling, are dangerous. Recovery through narrating is taking back one's story by "talking back" to one's perpetrators.[91]

Repetition of an idealized, contracted narrative may be reassuring and consistent to both teller and listener, giving the appearance of "accuracy." Yet it may be a means of burying CSA trauma. This would be the antithesis of reminiscing. Reminiscing, whether it occurs in psychotherapy or over coffee with a friend, implies openness to new words and new interpretations, to entering the mood of the story, to intimate engagement with the characters and the plot. It is in this process that recovery in the sense of discovering more about the past becomes possible for the CSA survivor. Thus, it is not necessarily the story that is always told in the same way, with the same details, that is most "credible" or authentic. In reminiscing, the CSA survivor reconnects the self and the past by capturing with each retelling new meanings and greater insights about the impact of traumatic events.

Reminiscing is healing in still another way. The future is inextricably linked to the past, and for those who cannot recall much of their past, there is often a corresponding inability to anticipate or plan for the time ahead. Locked in the present, CSA survivors may be unable to dream of a future for themselves because of its inescapable contiguousness with an "unspeakable" past. Telling the story releases one from these constraints.

Recognition

Recognition makes deeper aspects of one's experience accessible. Recognition merges the perceived with the remembered, casting a new light. By focusing on the object and exposing its shadow, the background against which it is contrasted, recognition lends insight. Recognition is thus enhanced by context. A matrix of intertwined factors converge, creating a situation that clarifies, and makes the recognizer more confident of her remembered knowledge. Recognition always retains a sense of betweenness, bordering on the activities of imagination, perception, cognition, and feeling. Through trusting one's dreams and imagination, for example, patterns of experience can be given more specific meaning. Sometimes recognition occurs as a sudden flash of awareness and certainty. Generally, it occurs more slowly and may never be complete or resolute. Recognition might be better described as increasing the sure-footedness of remembering.

Recognition is how current remembering experiences of CSA survivors conjoin imagery and perception. Recognition is a mediative process that allows access to the past without the necessity of "exact recall." For instance, the CSA survivor can recognize a core aspect of her abuse by exploring the void, what she did not feel, did not see, did not receive as a child. Likewise, in recognizing and naming what is familiar in past patterns, the present is accessible in a new way. Recognition is linked to the environment; it permits deviation and exploration of new territory by acting as an anchor to the familiar from which new streams of experience can be explored. Recognition is not a stamp of proof about the past, but rather represents movement, rehabilitation, in which the survivor begins to make sense of present perceptions in the light of something familiar in the past, a violation of the self. She is then empowered to draw distinctions consciously between powerful past memories and current environmental realities that seem similar, but no longer require her to fear, mistrust, isolate, and bear shame. Recognition decreases revictimization because exploitive dynamics in the present are more likely to be sensed consciously and avoided.

Types of memory

Casey[89] described three types of memory—body memory, place memory, and commemoration. Although indebted to the mind, these three types of memory provide a clearer image of memory as a person–environment phenomenon.

Body memory

Body memory, according to Casey,[89] is intrinsic to the flesh—a primary process of unconscious habituation, a physically centered "holding" of what is familiar to individuals in the world. The past is thus actively integrated into present embodied experiences, allowing for a recovery and reinhabiting of the body. Body memory is conceptually different from "mental unconsciousness." *Body memory* refers to actual traces of experience carried in physical sensation and form. Body memory involves regulation and familiarization that orient one to the environment. It also involves reorientation, rehabituation to the changing "lay of the land." One's body is unsettled and resettled in as one senses and moves within the changing environment.

In considering body memory, Casey[89] addressed traumatic memory separately. In traumatic memory, the fluidity between bodily being and the world around it is not merely unsettled, but broken. A part or parts of the body are focused on and marked in time, and their usual linkage with the environment is severed. Fragmentation and constriction occur in the body, accompanied by intense dread, pain, or numbing shock. Trauma imagery and experience are carried, whether consciously or not, with great poignancy. Sometimes this poignancy becomes positive, as might occur in the case of remembering the pain of a fractured bone that has healed. But severe, unresolved physical and psychic trauma retains a threatening, ghastly aura. One way to keep such horror from conscious awareness is to somaticize it, to contain or channel it into a specific body area. This kind of traumatic memory requires more than just rehabituation and resettlement, because the process of experience itself has become disjointed and disabling, perpetuating constrained, painful life processes from the past.

There is growing evidence to support the idea that some survivors channel memories within the body, contributing to the development of a wide variety of systemic illnesses, some of which have ambiguous symptom patterns.[92] Chronic pelvic pain has been correlated with higher levels of dissociation as well as greater incidence of CSA in women.[93] Eating disorders and increased incidence and severity of substance misuse are also associated with a history of CSA.[44,45,94-96] These findings suggest that physiologic processes are altered within the individual to turn away from traumatic symbols and associated painful effects.[2] Body image research shows that some survivors visualize their current body features as those of the developmental period preceding the onset of abuse, thereby psychically disconnecting the present body experience from the trauma.[97] Some CSA survivors do self-cutting to interrupt body memories, to "let out" emotional responses to trauma, and to stop the disintegrating physico-psychic feelings that can accompany memories of CSA.[8,98] These self-harm behaviors have led to confusion because caregivers tend to focus on these behaviors, rather than seeing the whole picture of how the behaviors relate to past trauma.

Body image may be so damaged in CSA survivors as to obliterate boundaries between self and others. Not only is there the experience that boundaries have been crossed and the self made "foreign" to itself, but also the sense that such boundaries "never existed."[99] From this perspective, the survivor's body memories become entangled with the intrapersonal conflicts and sensory impact of the perpetrator's body. Casey's[89] explanation of immersion in bodily experience helps to clarify how difficult it may be for survivors of very invasive early childhood trauma to become conscious and verbally articulate about it.

Body memories are no less significant than visual, intellectual knowledge of the abuse experience. If we can believe that very early experiences with fire establish in children a strong bodily response of withdrawal from the flame, it should not be difficult to imagine that reminders of being raped as a child would set off deep, but perhaps not as immediately interpretable, traces of memory within the CSA survivor's body. Sometimes body memories of CSA gradually develop into clearer images that can be verbalized. Sensory, cognitive, and developmental differences in children's CSA experiences may mean that not all body memories can eventually be translated into visual and verbal images.[100] In Casey's[89] view, however, verbalization is not necessary to authenticate these memories.

Place memory

Individuals' memories of what they experience are place-specific, an aspect of memory that has often been overshadowed by preoccupation with time. By *place* is meant the boundaries of experience, held fast and contained. Body memory is thought to be coterminus with place memory. In Casey's words, "my body not only takes me into places; it habituates me to their peculiarities and helps me to remember them vividly."[89(p180)] Place—that is, retrospectively known environmental reality—is differentiated from the concept of *site*, defined as a locus with features that change through time. Place is a constant image kept alive through time by the reality of the living body. Because of the body's roles in containing past places and in taking us to "old haunts," we can be transported back to the physical, interpersonal environments we recall. Place therefore serves as a shelter, a unifying force, drawing and holding many memories together. Place also refers to the trail of clues that we envision and traverse to reach a past destination that holds a core meaning for us, even if the meaning is very painful and unacceptable. The multiple pathways of place, according to Casey,[89] are remarkably similar to notions of memory as an integrative network, with the potential to reach a single destination via many roads.

The importance of place in memory can be seen in the experiences of many CSA survivors.[101] For some, separation from the actual site of the abuse (eg, the family house or the home town) may be needed to allow the discovery of the place of the abuse memories, wherein the meanings of the trauma converge and make sense. Conversely, returning to the site of abuse or visiting a similar locality may open a pathway to an experienced place in memory. The body reveals characteristics of the place through its remembrance of sights, sounds, touches, and smells. The rehabilitative aspect of place memory for CSA survivors is that on revisitation and reflection, the body can become a safe enclosure for what has been experienced as traumatic. Thus, place memory is no longer a prison, but a garden that has been tilled and sifted through and claimed as one's own territory, even if it is laden with thorns.

Commemoration

Casey[89] spoke of commemoration, the act of intensified remembering. He explained this type of memory as a "remembering through,"[89(p.221)] the conscious action of ritual "doing again." The words re-covery, re-membering, and re-habilitate all begin with the prefix that implies return, doing again. Commemoration signifies solemnity and seriousness, the importance and centrality of certain memories. It is a purposeful, transformative process, in which one participates with the past so as to bring about an ending, albeit an ongoing ending, to a memory. Commemoration is the antithesis of the repetition of abuse dynamics through retraumatization, because it is done with awareness and integrity. Casey spoke of consolidation and continuity of endings.

Examples of commemoration can be found in cases of CSA. Many survivors create for themselves some memorial symbol or process externalizing the meanings of their trauma experience, whether this be a journal, a work of art, a psychotherapeutic relationship,[102] a planned disclosure and confrontation of perpetrators,[8,103,104] or a symbolic image they carry with them.[105]

Some women plan rituals, including the burning of photographs or writings, as a means of coming to terms with the reality of abuse while also stepping away from its power over them into a new phase of life.[49,106,107] This is the healing aspect of commemoration, where past, present, and future are gathered and felt as a whole. Commemoration is a conscious choice to remember what one would rather forget, but to do so in a self-determined, self-defined manner.

Thick autonomy of memory

Casey[89] completed his phenomenological analysis of memory by writing about "the thick autonomy of memory." The term "thick" here means "not easily penetrable by the direct light of consciousness; resistant to conceptual understanding; sedimented in layers; and having 'historical depth.'"[89(p265)] Again, emphasis is on memory as immersion in the temporal, meaningful environment rather than on memory as confinement of information within the person. Casey described memory as already everywhere: "Memory is . . . more porous than enframing."[89(p310)] The mind does not capture memories by internalizing exact replicas of experienced events. Rather, people find themselves surrounded by layers of meaning, awareness, and reinterpretation that are affected by social and cultural constructions. In other words, individuals are not in command of memory as an internal store of facts.

Surviving CSA provides a very cogent example of the thick autonomy of memory. For the survivor, the depth and impenetrability of traumatic memories are compounded by associated intense effects, the extremes of shock and numbing, and the unacceptability of betrayal by trusted caretakers involved in the abuse. For most survivors, remembering takes an even more "autonomous" journey within their lives, because the "thick" shame and secrecy about CSA make it an intensely privatized experience. Its subsequent unfolding in memories reflects the diversity of privatized experience and the sense that no outsider can truly know how it felt.

The environmental silence about CSA,[103] coupled with the internalized sense of shame associated with it,[108] are person–environment barriers to remembering the sexual trauma. Shame means there is the threat of intolerable exposure. In desiring not to be seen, the survivor's connection with others is stunted. The individual frequently averts her eyes from the world around her and searches within herself for the "cause" of her shame. She may even become ashamed of being ashamed.[108] The morass of shame in which CSA survivors often become entangled contributes to layers of hiddenness of the abuse itself. Even in the therapeutic relationship, both conscious and unconscious shame-related feelings of vulnerability and exposure can be incredibly intense for the CSA survivor. To use Casey's[89] terms, such memories are deeply held under layers of partial awarenesses and less-threatening beliefs. This protects one against feeling out of control in one's body and out of control in one's social and sexual relating.

The notion of memory as "autonomous" illuminates the pattern of delayed recall of CSA. The core experiences of deep violation of soul and body emerge in the synchrony of the survivor's readiness and the safety of the environment. The telling cannot happen, cannot override the effects of shame, until there is a listener and a sheltering, nonjudgmental place for the story to be told. This is the role of nursing in recovery and rehabilitation, to listen to what has heretofore been "unspeakable." The thick autonomy of memory, as explained by Casey,[89] also accounts for why CSA memories do not always emerge all at once, but often as intrusions, in layers that are fitted together gradually over time.

•   •   •

Recovery and rehabilitation from CSA are complex individual and social processes with which nurses need to be familiar. U.S. society is in the midst of a controversy about delayed recall of CSA memories, but such contention is not new. Studies of memory have revealed many of its aspects, but there has been little synthesis of the findings across lines of research. General models of memory fall short in explaining holistically the experiences of severely traumatized people. Using cognitive models of trauma effects, one might view traumatic memories as incongruent with prior mental schemata, interruptive of psychoformative processes, dividing of self-concepts, and consequential in the development of learned helplessness, shedding light on the internal experiences of memory as it might be experienced by CSA survivors. Casey's[89] phenomenological view of remembering reveals subtle subconcepts that resonate with the recovery and rehabilitation processes of CSA survivors.

What does the exploration of delayed memories of CSA within Casey's[89] phenomenological perspective contribute to the debate about "false memory syndrome"? There are two quite separate questions at the root of this debate. One is the question of fact-finding about past events in the case of memories of childhood sexual abuse. That is, how can we best determine, for legal purposes, what actually occurred in the past when allegations of abuse result from delayed recall of CSA? The other question is about the role of remembering in the survival, healing, and empowerment of CSA survivors. Nursing's role is most clearly situated in the latter aspect of CSA remembering.[5]

In terms of fact-finding, there are limits to establishing the details and actuality of any past event. An oversimplified view of memory, unsupported by the weight of both empirical and experiential studies, is not helpful in clarifying the actuality of past events. A phenomenological perspective on memory coupled with a political analysis of power disparities between men and women, between adults and children, can account for many of the queries made by proponents of a "false memory syndrome": Why was there a delay in telling? Why might the memories have emerged after a triggering event, or within a therapeutic relationship? How has the CSA survivor's leaving the site of her abuse, or returning to it, somehow contributed to the recall of her traumatization? Why might visual or verbally detailed accounts of these events be inaccessible to a survivor? What is the CSA survivor's purpose in confronting the perpetrators of the abuse? Casey's[89] concepts and a feminist lens offer bases for understanding apparent inconsistencies in the process of remembering CSA without losing sight of the essential authenticity of the memories.

The role of memory in recovery and rehabilitation is salient for CSA survivors. A phenomenological perspective like Casey's[89] can guide nurses in working with CSA survivors who are confronting the complexities of remembering childhood trauma. It guards against what Friedman called "our susceptibility to the chronological illusion"[109(p60)] of autobiographical memory. Processes such as reminding, reminiscing, and recognition reflect the patterns many survivors manifest, although there is great variability among them, presumably because CSA is a very privatized experience. Nurses can contribute to the healing and empowerment of these women by avoiding pathologization of creative, protective strategies women have developed to survive and by creating safe places for narrating about abuse.

Breaking the silence in adulthood about sexual abuse that occurred in childhood has awakened new awarenesses of what it means to remember and of what remembering is not. Remembering is not a singular process for the purpose of documenting facts. Realizing the complexity of remembering is not an impediment to finding the "truth" about CSA. Nor is acknowledging the value and purposes of remembering as a recovery process a reason to reject delayed memories as inherently inaccurate, exaggerated, or unauthentic. We need not create yet another mask to cover the ugly face of CSA, nor another barrier to survivors speaking of it.

If children were allowed opportunities to report abuse when it was occurring and guaranteed safe remedies, there would be far fewer cases of "delayed memory" in adulthood. As it is, many children who disclose are met with disbelief, more abuse, or family disintegration, all of which they may internalize as "their fault." Societal patterns of ineffective and damaging responses to the abuse of children must change. Many adult survivors despair of the time, often years, it takes for them to remember and heal from CSA. Furthermore, remembering is not all that is needed for recovery in the survival of CSA. Trustworthy, safe support for developing a stronger, cognizant, empowered self must accompany the memory work.

Toni Morrison's[6] image of the river "remembering" is compatible with Casey's[89] exploration of memory from a phenomenological perspective. Like the waters of the river, we as people have "perfect memory." The idea of perfection implies that there are no real mistakes; remembering is a living process for which there is no single path toward the "truth." Remembering moves and completes our being. It heals us, connecting us with the world around us in time and space. Particularly in the case of delayed recall of CSA, we cannot avoid the complexity of remembering, its political and relational ramifications, and its authenticity as an empowering phenomenon.

REFERENCES

1. Finkelhor D, Hotaling G, Lewis I, Smith C. Sexual abuse in a national survey of adult men and women: prevalence, characteristics and risk factors. *Child Abuse Neglect.* 1990;14(1):19–28.

2. van der Kolk BA, McFarlane AC, Weisaeth L, eds. *Traumatic Stress: The Effects of Overwhelming Experience on Mind, Body and Society.* New York, NY: Guilford Press; 1996.

3. Partridge E. *Origins: A Short Etymological Dictionary of Modern English.* New York, NY: Greenwich House; 1983.

4. Draucker CB. The healing process of female adult incest survivors: constructing a personal residence. *Image. J Nurs Schol.* 1992;24(1):4–8.

5. Hall JM. Delayed recall of childhood sexual abuse: psychiatric nursing's responsibilities to clients. *Arch Psychiatr Nurs.* 1996;10:342–346.

6. Morrison T. The site of memory. In: Ferguson R, Gever M, Minh-ha T, West C, eds. *Out There: Marginalization and Contemporary Cultures.* Cambridge, Mass: MIT Press; 1990.

7. Summit R. Hidden victims, hidden pain: societal avoidance of child sexual abuse. In: Wyatt G, Powell G, eds. *Lasting Effects of Child Sexual Abuse*. Newbury Park, Calif: Sage; 1988.

8. Herman J. *Trauma and Recovery*. New York, NY: Basic Books; 1992.

9. Olafson E, Corwin D, Summit R. Modern history of child sexual abuse awareness: cycles of discovery and suppression. *Child Abuse Neglect*. 1993;17:7–24.

10. Janet P. *L'automisme psychologique: Essai de psychologie experimental sur les formes inferieures de l'activité humaine*. Paris, France: Alcan; 1889.

11. van der Kolk B, van der Hart O. Pierre Janet and the breakdown of adaptation in psychological trauma. *Am J Psychiatry*. 1989;146:1530–1540.

12. Breuer J, Freud S; Strachey J, Trans. *Studies on Hysteria* (Standard ed, Vol. 2) London, England: Hogarth Press; 1895/1955.

13. Masson J. Freud and the seduction theory. *Atlantic Monthly*. 1984;Feb:33–60.

14. Dupont J, ed; Balint M, Jackson N, Trans. *The Clinical Diary of Sandor Ferenczi*. Cambridge, Mass: Harvard University Press; 1988.

15. Grinker R, Spiegel J. *Men Under Stress*. New York, NY: McGraw-Hill; 1945.

16. Kardiner A. *The Traumatic Neuroses of War*. New York, NY: Hoeber; 1941.

17. American Psychiatric Association. *Diagnostic and Statistical Manual of Mental Disorders*. Washington, DC: APA; 1952.

18. Kaufman I, Peck A, Tagiuri W. The family constellation and overt incestuous relations between father and daughter. *Am J Orthopsychiatry*. 1954;24:266–279.

19. Kinsey A, Pomeroy W, Martin C, Gebhard P. *Sexual Behavior in the Human Female*. Philadelphia, Pa: W.B. Saunders; 1953.

20. Rush F. *The Best Kept Secret: Sexual Abuse of Children*. New York, NY: McGraw-Hill; 1980.

21. Weinberg K. *Incest Behavior*. New York, NY: Citadel; 1955.

22. Chideckel M. *Female Sexual Perversion: The Sexually Aberrated Woman as She Is*. New York, NY: Eugenics; 1935.

23. Socarides CW. *The Overt Male Homosexual*. New York, NY: Grune & Stratton; 1968.

24. Stekel W. *The Homosexual Neurosis*. New York, NY: Emerson; 1946.

25. Stevens PE, Hall JM. A critical historical analysis of the medical construction of lesbianism. *Int J Health Services*. 1991;21:291–307.

26. Herman J, Hirschman L. *Father–Daughter Incest*. Cambridge, Mass: Harvard University Press; 1981.

27. U.S. Dept of Health and Human Services. *Promoting Health/Preventing Disease*. Washington, DC: Government Printing Office; 1980.

28. Plotnick RD. Changes in poverty, income inequality, and the standard of living in the United States during the Reagan years. *Int J Health Services*. 1993;23:347–358.

29. Stretch R. Post-traumatic stress disorder among Vietnam and Vietnam-era veterans. In: Figley C, ed. *Trauma and Its Wake: Traumatic Stress Theory, Research and Intervention*. New York, NY: Brunner/Mazel; 1986.

30. Trimble M. Post-traumatic stress disorder: history of a concept. In: Figley C, ed. *Trauma and Its Wake: Traumatic Stress Theory, Research and Intervention*. New York, NY: Brunner/Mazel; 1986.

31. Benward J, Densen-Gerber J. Incest as a causative factor in antisocial behavior: an exploratory study. *Contemp Drug Problems*. 1975;4:323–340.

32. Butler J. *Conspiracy of Silence: The Trauma of Incest*. San Francisco, Calif: New Glide; 1978.

33. Finkelhor D. *Sexually Victimized Children*. New York, NY: Free Press; 1979.

34. Jaffe A, Dynneson L, Ten-Bensel R. Sexual abuse: an epidemiological study. *Am J Dis Children*. 1975;129:689–692.

35. Meiselman K. *Incest*. San Francisco, Calif: Jossey-Bass; 1978.

36. Briere J, Elliott DM. Sexual abuse, family environment, and psychological symptoms: on the validity of statistical control. *J Couns Clin Psychol*. 1993;61:284–288.

37. Mullen PE. Child sexual abuse and adult mental health: the development of disorder. *J Interpersonal Violence*. 1993;8:428–432.

38. Browne A, Finkelhor D. Impact of child sexual abuse: a review. *Psychol Bull*. 1986;99:21–27.

39. Downs WR. Developmental considerations for the effects of childhood sexual abuse. *J Interpersonal Violence*. 1993;8:331–345.

40. Schetky DH. A review of the literature on the long term effects of childhood sexual abuse. In: Kluft RP, ed. *Incest-Related Syndromes of Adult Psychopathology*. Washington, DC: American Psychiatric Press; 1990.

41. Briere J, Runtz M. Differential adult symptomatology associated with three types of child abuse histories. *Child Abuse Neglect*. 1990;14:357–364.

42. Briere J, Runtz M. Childhood sexual abuse: implications for psychological assessment. *J Interpersonal Violence*. 1993;8:312–330.

43. Fry R. Adult physical illness and childhood sexual abuse. *J Psychosom Res*. 1993;37:89–103.

44. Hall JM. The pervasive effects of childhood sexual abuse in lesbians' recovery from alcohol problems. *Substance Use Misuse*. 1996;31:225–239.

45. Hurley DL. Women, alcohol, and incest: an analytical review. *J Stud Alcohol.* 1991;52:253–268.

46. Kluft RP, ed. *Incest-Related Syndromes of Adult Psychopathology.* Washington, DC: American Psychiatric Press; 1990.

47. Putnam FW. Disturbances of "self" in victims of child sexual abuse. In: Kluft RP, ed. *Incest-Related Syndromes of Adult Psychopathology.* Washington, DC: American Psychiatric Press; 1990.

48. Shengold L. *Soul Murder: The Effects of Childhood Abuse and Deprivation.* New Haven, Conn: Yale University Press; 1989.

49. Bass E, Davis L. *The Courage to Heal: A Guide for Women Survivors of Child Sexual Abuse.* New York, NY: Perennial Library; 1986.

50. Lew M. *Victims No Longer: Men Recovering from Incest and Other Sexual Child Abuse.* New York, NY: HarperCollins; 1990.

51. Maltz W. *The Sexual Healing Journey: A Guide for Survivors of Sexual Abuse.* New York, NY: HarperCollins; 1991.

52. Goleman D. Childhood trauma: memory or invention? *New York Times,* 1992;July 21:B1,B8.

53. Horn M. Memories lost and found. *U.S. News World Rep.* 1993;Nov. 29:52–63.

54. Toufexis A. When can memories be trusted? *Time.* 1991;Oct 28:86–88.

55. Hechler D. *The Battle and the Backlash: The Child Sexual Abuse War.* Lexington, Mass: Lexington Books; 1988.

56. False Memory Syndrome Foundation. *Basic Information Packet.* Philadelphia, Pa: FMSF; 1993.

57. Lego S. Repressed memory and false memory. *Arch Psychiatr Nurs.* 1996;10:110–115.

58. Loftus E, Garry M, Feldman J. Forgetting sexual trauma: what does it mean when 38% forget? *J Consult Clin Psychol.* 1994;16:1177–1181.

59. Herman J, Schatzow E. Recovery and verification of memories of childhood sexual trauma. *Psychoanal Psychol.* 1987;4(1):1–14.

60. Williams LM. Recall of childhood trauma: a prospective study of women's memories of child sexual abuse. *J Consult Clinical Psychol.* 1994;62:1167–1176.

61. Briere J. *Child Abuse Trauma: Theory and Treatment of the Lasting Effects.* Newbury Park, Calif: Sage; 1992.

62. Kinzl J, Biebl W. Long-term effects of incest: life events triggering mental disorders in female patients with sexual abuse in childhood. *Child Abuse Neglect.* 1992;16:567–573.

63. Bower GH. Mood and memory. *Am Psychol.* 1981; 36:129–148.

64. Eich JE. The cue-dependent nature of state-dependent retrieval. *Mem Cognition.* 1980;8:157–173.

65. Ho BT, Richards DW III, Chute DL. *Drug Discrimination and State Dependent Learning.* New York, NY: Academic Press; 1978.

66. Gudjonsson G. *The Psychology of Interrogations, Confessions and Testimony.* Chichester, England: Wiley; 1992.

67. Loftus E. The reality of repressed memories. *Am Psychol.* 1993;48:518–537.

68. Jennings AG, Armsworth MW. Ego development in women with histories of sexual abuse. *Child Abuse Neglect.* 1992;16:553–565.

69. Rutter M. Meyerian psychobiology, personality development and the role of life experiences. *Am J Psychiatry.* 1986;143:1077–1087.

70. Winnicott DW. *Playing and Reality.* New York, NY: Basic Books; 1971.

71. Barclay CR, Smith TS. Autobiographical remembering and self-composing. *Int J Pers Construct Psychology.* 1993;6:231–251.

72. Freeman M. *Rewriting the Self: History, Memory, Narrative.* New York, NY: Routledge; 1993.

73. Crawford J, Kippax S, Onyx J, Gault U, Benton P. *Emotion and Gender: Constructing Meaning from Memory.* Newbury Park, Calif: Sage; 1992.

74. Neisser U, ed. *Memory Observed: Remembering in Natural Contexts.* San Francisco, Calif: Freeman; 1982.

75. Wylie M. The shadow of a doubt. *Fam Therapy Networker.* 1993;17(5):18–29.

76. Horowitz M. Psychological response to serious life events. In: Hamilton V, Warburton D, eds. *Human Stress and Cognition.* New York, NY: Wiley; 1979.

77. Horowitz M. *Stress Response Syndromes.* New York, NY: Jason Aronson; 1979.

78. McFarlane AC. Avoidance and intrusion in posttraumatic stress disorder. *J Nerv Ment Dis.* 1992;180:439–445.

79. Lifton R. *The Broken Connection.* New York, NY: Basic Books; 1983.

80. Lifton R, Olson E. The human meaning of total disaster—the Buffalo Creek experience. *Psychiatry.* 1976; 39:1–18.

81. Benyakar M, Kutz I, Dasberg H, Stern M. The collapse of a structure: a structural approach to trauma. *J Traumatic Stress.* 1989;2:431–449.

82. Lifton R. *The Protean Self: Human Resilience in an Age of Fragmentation.* New York, NY: Basic Books; 1993.

83. Langer L. *Holocaust Testimonies: The Ruins of Memory.* New Haven, Conn: Yale University Press; 1991.

84. Abramson L, Seligman M, Teasdale J. Learned helplessness in humans: critique and reformulation. *J Abnorm Psychol.* 1978;87:49–74.

85. Peterson C, Seligman M. Learned helplessness and victimization. *J Social Issues.* 1983;2:103–116.

86. Seligman M. *Helplessness: On Depression, Development, and Death.* San Francisco, Calif: Freeman; 1975.

87. Kondora LL. A Heideggerian hermeneutical analysis of survivors of incest. *Image: J Nurs Schol.* 1993;25: 11–16.

88. Kondora LL. Living the coming of memories: an interpretive phenomenological study of surviving childhood sexual abuse. *Health Care Women Int.* 1995; 16(1):21–30.

89. Casey E. *Remembering: A Phenomenological Study.* Bloomington, Ind: Indiana University Press; 1987.

90. van der Kolk BA. *Psychological Trauma.* Washington, DC: American Psychiatric Press; 1987.

91. Hall JM, Stevens PE, Meleis AI. Marginalization: a guiding concept for valuing diversity in nursing knowledge development. *ANS.* 1994;16(4):23–41.

92. Lechner ME, Vogel ME, Garcia-Shelton LM, Leichter JL, Steibel KL. Self-reported medical problems of adult female survivors of childhood sexual abuse. *J Fam Pract.* 1993;36:633–638.

93. Walker EA, Katon WJ, Neraas K, Jemelka RP, Massoth D. Dissociation in women with chronic pain. *Am J Psychiatry.* 1992;149:534–537.

94. Abramson EE, Lucido GM. Childhood sexual experiences and bulimia. *Addictive Behav.* 1991;16:529–532.

95. Williams HJ, Wagner H, Calam RM. Eating attitudes of survivors of unwanted sexual experiences. *Br J Psychol.* 1992;31:203–206.

96. Wonderlich SA, Wilsnack RW, Wilsnack SC, Harris TR. Childhood sexual abuse and bulimic behavior in a nationally representative sample. *Am J Public Health.* 1996;86:1082–1086.

97. Simonds SL. Sexual abuse and body image: approaches and implications for treatment. *Arts Psychotherapy.* 1992;19:289–293.

98. Greenspan GS, Samuel SE. Self-cutting after rape. *Am J Psychiatry.* 1989;146:789–790.

99. Young L. Sexual abuse and the problem of embodiment. *Child Abuse Neglect.* 1992;16:89–100.

100. Johnson EK, Howell RJ. Memory processes in children: implications for investigations of alleged child sexual abuse. *Bull Am Acad Psychiatry Law.* 1993; 21:213–226.

101. Hall JM. Geography of childhood sexual abuse: women's narratives of their childhood environments. *ANS.* 1996;18:29–47.

102. Johnson DR. The role of the creative arts therapies in the diagnosis and treatment of psychological trauma. *Arts Psychotherapy.* 1987;14:7–13.

103. Barringer CE. The survivor's voice: breaking the incest taboo. *National Women's Stud Assoc J.* 1992;4:4–22.

104. Sauzier M. Disclosure of child sexual abuse: for better or for worse. *Psychiatr Clin North Am.* 1989;12:455–469.

105. Waites EA. *Trauma and Survival: Post-Traumatic Stress and Dissociative Disorders in Women.* New York, NY: Norton; 1993.

106. Imber-Black E. *Rituals in Families and Family Therapy.* New York, NY: Norton; 1988.

107. Wisechild LM. *The Obsidian Mirror: An Adult Healing from Incest.* Seattle, Wash: Seal Press; 1988.

108. Nathonson DL. Understanding what is hidden: shame in sexual abuse. *Psychiatr Clin North Am.* 1989;12: 381–388.

109. Friedman WJ. Memory for the time of past events. *Psychol Bull.* 1993;113:44–66.

Unit V

Selected Holistic Nursing Interventions

I was euphoric when I stood back and viewed the variety of holistic nursing interventions that had been selected for this unit (i.e., relaxation techniques, imagery, music therapy, therapeutic touch, and massage). The articles range from superb literature reviews and research investigations to practical recommendations and experiences for implementing holistic therapies in clinical practice. These articles represent the sights and sounds of a change in nursing practice.

Although the interventions in this unit are used for a variety of clients with assorted problems that will produce a range of different outcomes, all of these interventions have several common goals. They all have the potential to achieve the relaxation response, reduce anxiety and stress, and promote healing and wholeness. In effect, these interventions provide multiple paths capable of reaching a single destination. Thus, as nurses, we have the luxury of options based on our skills as well as what we judge would help clients. Our clients, in turn, have the luxury of options based on their preferences, beliefs, and attitudes. Both practitioner skill and client preference must be delicately balanced in selecting the appropriate interventions. Some clients, for example, may fear the cultic overtones associated with meditation, others may doubt their imagery skills, and some may not wish to be touched. With a range of options with common endpoints available to both nurse and client, however, the feasibility of achieving maximum, therapeutic patient outcomes is enhanced.

Several of the clinical and research articles in this section focus on the effects of holistic interventions on clients who are in high stress situations (those undergoing cardiac catheterizations [Warner et al.] or magnetic resonance imaging [Thompson and Coppens]), those who are in pain (Schorr) or bereaved (Quinn and Strelkauskas), or those who are in critical care units for cancer (Johnston and Rohaly-Davis) or heart disease (Steckel and King). It has been postulated by several researchers that the effectiveness of holistic interventions can be evaluated best under high stress and illness conditions.

For those readers interested in determining the efficacy of holistic interventions, the comprehensive review articles in this unit will be valuable. Researchers, too, will be interested in the methodology and outcome variables of the 38 studies critiqued (with summary tables) that investigated the effects of relaxation (Mandle et al.) as well as the extensive literature review on the effects of therapeutic touch on stress, anxiety, pain, wound healing, and psychoneuroimmunology (Mulloney and Wells-Federman). It is important to note that most of these studies have been conducted on adults. Because the results cannot be generalized to children, the possibilities for investigating the effects of these techniques on children offer a plethora of research ideas for interested researchers. The clinical article and literature review on massage for infants (Schneider) provides a psychophysiologic roadmap for researching such holistic interventions with infants and children.

Several of the authors in this unit discuss the methodological inconsistencies used in researching various holistic therapies. Such problems lead to difficulty in evaluating the validity and reliability of the research findings and in accurately assessing the clinical efficacy of the intervention. I will add my own reflections on this problem. Many studies measuring the effectiveness of holistic interventions evaluate one or several psychophysiologic endpoints of relaxation. Relaxation, however, is a learned response that is a function of practice. Thus, to achieve therapeutic outcomes and detect significant differences between groups, it is not only appropriate but logical to design a study that would ensure repeated exposure to the intervention so that the "best shot" approach at determining differences between groups could be evaluated based on the cumulative effect of the intervention. Thus, studies that use a "one shot," one-time exposure to the intervention, in my observation, often are doomed because they have ignored a basic premise of relaxation (i.e., practice makes perfect).

Moreover, using multiple outcome variables to evaluate interventions that have the ability to affect the body-mind-spirit also is prudent in designing a "best shot" study. Measuring psychologic, physiologic, and hematologic outcomes along with rich, subject client evaluations obtained by qualitative methods broaden one's chances of finding differences and relationships among the outcomes. Quinn and Strelkauskas' research on therapeutic touch is an exemplary study that investigated the effects of multiple sessions using multiple outcomes including time perception, perceived effectiveness of treatment, psychologic outcomes, and a variety of immunologic measures. In addition, these researchers also included another unprecedented perspective—that of measuring these multiple outcomes in both the client and the practitioner to determine the pattern among and the relationship between client and nurse. The principle underlying this line of investigation reflects the understanding that the researcher does not stand apart from the research or the research subject. As researchers, we become an integral part of the experiment. Our participation affects us and the results we obtain. This line of investigation must be encouraged in future studies.

The articles and research contained in this unit illustrate the widespread range of holistic, independent nursing interventions that are being integrated into clinical practice. They serve to validate who we are and what we do in making a difference in the lives of our clients and families.

The Efficacy of Relaxation Response Interventions with Adult Patients: A Review of the Literature

Carol Lynn Mandle, PhD, RN
Associate Professor
Boston College School of Nursing
Associate for Research and Consultation
Beth Israel Hospital
Codirector
Behavioral Medicine General Programs
Division of Behavioral Medicine
Deaconess Hospital
Scientist
Mind/Body Medical Institute
Harvard Medical School

Sue C. Jacobs, PhD
Associate Professor and Director of PhD
*   Counseling Psychology Training Program*
Department of Counseling
University of North Dakota
Grand Forks, North Dakota

Patricia Martin Arcari, PhD(C), RN
Codirector
Behavioral Medicine General Programs
Division of Behavioral Medicine
Deaconess Hospital

Alice D. Domar, PhD
Staff Psychologist
Division of Behavioral Medicine
Deaconess Hospital
Senior Scientist
Mind/Body Medical Institute
Assistant Professor in Medicine
Harvard Medical School
Boston, Massachusetts

Source: Reprinted from C.L. Mandle, S.C. Jacobs, P.M. Arcari, A.D. Domar, *The Journal of Cardiovascular Nursing,* Vol. 10, No. 3, pp. 4–26, © 1996, Aspen Publishers, Inc.

Many medical syndromes are caused or exacerbated by stress. These include but are not limited to hypertension,[1] coronary artery disease,[2] sudden cardiac death,[3] pain,[4,5] dermatologic disorders,[6] brain cell death,[7] infertility,[8] and premenstrual syndrome.[9]

Stress contributes to the development and intensification of clinical syndromes and also may complicate patients' progress through diagnostic and therapeutic procedures. Stress can either lead to a harmful pattern of avoiding medical procedures[10] or actually affect a patient's status during procedures by increasing vital signs, causing the need for higher doses of analgesics, tranquilizers, and anesthetics and increasing intraoperative complications.[11–13] Stress also may complicate the operative recovery period by increasing the need for medication and length of hospital stay.[10,14–16]

The fight or flight stress response, manifested by such physiologic reactions as dilation of the pupils and increased blood pressure, respiratory rate, and motor excitability,[17] results from stimulation of the sympathetic nervous system. The relaxation response described by Benson[18] as the physiologic counterpart of the fight or flight response has been found to be an effective, innate protective mechanism against stressful stimuli. By eliciting the relaxation response—marked by a decrease in pulse, respiratory rate, blood pressure, and metabolism—the harmful effects of stress can be lessened through changes in the autonomic, endocrine, immune, and neuropeptide systems.

Supported in part by NIMH Grant #MH45591 and the Sherman/Warburg Fellowships.

THE RELAXATION RESPONSE: RESEARCH IN PHYSIOLOGIC AND SPIRITUAL EFFECTS

The relaxation response is the physiologic opposite of the fight or flight response first described by Cannon in 1914. In his classic experiments, Cannon removed the adrenal glands from cats and extracted a substance (now known as epinephrine/norepinephrine or adrenaline/noradrenaline) and injected it into other cats. The cats receiving these catecholamines all developed increased blood pressure, heart rates, and breathing rates.[17] In 1943 Hess and Brugger elicited this same fight or flight response by electrically stimulating areas within the hypothalamus of cats' brains. When they stimulated areas of the anterior hypothalamus, however, Hess and Brugger elicited a hypoarousal state that he described as the trophotropic syndromes. They theorized that this response functioned as a protective mechanism against excessive stress, countering the potentially harmful effects of the fight or flight stress response.[18, 19]

The specific physiologic and behavioral changes associated with Hess and Brugger's trophotropic syndrome have been found to be reproducible through a variety of meditative practices. Although meditation has been a vital component of human life throughout recorded history, the studies of yogis[20–23] and of Zen masters[24–26] were the first scientific studies of meditation and prayer. Interest in these investigations was developed further with studies describing the hypometabolic, physiologic responses to meditation.[27–29] A review of the subsequent literature on meditation found 962 studies.[30] These scientific investigations have complemented the historic insights of many religions and traditions.

The relaxation response has been further defined as "a set of integrated physiological changes that are elicited when a subject assumes a relaxed position within a quiet environment, with the mental repetition of a word, sound, phrase or prayer," and the adoption of a passive attitude.[31(p.27)]

Studies have shown that the relaxation response is elicited through a variety of techniques in addition to meditation such as imagery, hypnosis, autogenic training, and progressive muscle relaxation.[32–38] These techniques share what are believed to be the essential ingredients of the relaxation response—a repetitive mental focus and the adoption of a passive attitude.

The physiologic alterations of the relaxation response are consistent with decreased sympathetic nervous system activity including decreased oxygen consumption and increased carbon dioxide elimination, heart rate, respiratory rate, blood pressure, minute ventilation, muscle tones, arterial blood lactate, skin resistance, and alpha brain activity.[35] These changes contrast with the physiologic manifestations of sitting quietly[35,37,38] or sleeping.[28]

Nursing theory, research, and practice typically view patients in terms of wholeness of mind, body, and spirit and the relationship of these dimensions to the environment. Because no part of the patient exists in isolation and each is influenced by the other, the physiologies of the relaxation and stress responses can affect the cognitive, emotional, social, spiritual, and behavioral well-being of the patient through the activities of the autonomic nervous, musculoskeletal, and psychoneuroendocrine systems. Understanding these principles forms the foundation of many nursing activities in practice and research.[39–41]

METHODOLOGY OF REVIEWING THE LITERATURE

Selected computer searches (QUEST and Silver Platter) of the literature were conducted using the terms stress, anxiety, pain, hypertension, and relaxation. In evaluating these studies the authors examined the focus, sample, study site, design, measures, and outcomes. Thirty-seven studies fit the criteria for inclusion. The results of these examinations are in the Appendix.

FOCUS

The efficacy of the relaxation response has been demonstrated with a wide variety of adult patient populations. These include the following: cardiac,[42–45] abdominal–perineal,[46–51] orthopedic,[52] dental surgery,[53–55] cardiac and femoral angiography,[56,57] sigmoidoscopy,[13] coronary risk factors,[58] presumptive myocardial infarction,[59] cardiac rehabilitation,[60] premature ventricular contractions in patients with mild ischemic heart disease,[61] moderate hypertension,[62–67] rheumatoid arthritis,[68] chronic pain,[69–71] chronic asthma and obstructive lung disease,[72,73] mechanical ventilation weaning,[74] infertility,[75] and premenstrual syndrome.[76]

SAMPLES AND SITES

Sample sizes of the studies ranged from one case study[54] to 112 subjects.[65] All of the patients were adults, but specific ages were not specified on all of the studies. Both genders and a variety of demographic characteristics were represented. The clinical settings of the investigations included clinics, hospitals, nursing homes, and dentists' offices.

FINDINGS

A number of studies have not demonstrated the efficacy of the relaxation response. For example, several investigations[77–79] failed to demonstrate significant reduction in either systolic or diastolic blood pressures. A study of 60 orthopedic surgery patients[80] failed to demonstrate the effectiveness of listening to a 20-minute relaxation and procedural information tape the evening before orthopedic surgery versus a control group that listened to a hospital orientation audiotape. A major deficiency in this study was inconsistent data collection throughout the data collection period, which occurred up to 3 months after the surgery.

Similarly, Perri and Perri[81] investigated the effectiveness of preoperatively taught and practiced progressive muscle relaxation in postoperative pain and analgesic use in a study of 26 vaginal hysterectomy patients. There were no significant differences in the pain measures between the treatment group and the control group. The authors themselves questioned whether the patients actually practiced progressive muscle relaxation and whether the staff encouraged relaxation versus the use of routine analgesics.

Domar et al[82] investigated the effectiveness of preoperative, regular elicitation of the relaxation response by 21 patients in a study of 49 patients undergoing surgical excision of skin cancer. Although subjective reports of stress associated with surgery were altered, there were no significant differences in the psychologic or physical measures of anxiety or pain. However, none of the patients in the study demonstrated increased anxiety or blood pressure preoperatively, thus limiting the ability to show demonstrable differences between the two groups. The researchers also suggested that a more anxiety-provoking procedure might have led to increased compliance and significant effects.

In contrast, many studies have demonstrated the efficacy of relaxation response interventions on reducing clinical signs and symptoms. Many subjective and objective outcomes have been gained from a variety of relaxation response interventions. Improvements have been most consistently displayed by patients with mild or moderate hypertension. Also, there have been fairly consistent alleviations of headache, insomnia, pain, and anxiety. Differences have been more consistently demonstrated for medical than for surgical patients. These observations and recommendations are supported in a meta-analysis of the effects of relaxation training, although the reviewed investigations were not specifically identified.[83] Because of the small number of studies on some clinical problems, these generalizations need stronger validation through future investigations.

CRITIQUE

It was difficult to evaluate the reliability and validity of the research because of variations within and across studies. There was great variation in populations, stressors, interventions, and procedures, as well as outcome measures. Thirteen of the studies did not use randomization.

Dependent variables included standardized tests, self and clinical ratings of mood and pain, insomnia, analgesics requested, analgesics given, length of hospitalization, temperature, heart rate, diastolic and systolic blood pressure, degree of urinary retention, palmar sweat indices, and biochemical measures.[83] Interventions studied included Jacobson's progressive muscle relaxation,[32] rhythmic breathing, imagery, autogenic training, hypnosis, transcendental meditation, yoga, and Zen, all of which contain the key elements of the relaxation response: having a passive attitude and focusing on a word or phrase.[18,27,29] Few of the investigators have done more than one study on relaxation response interventions. The lack of research programs in this area limits the expansion of intial explorations. In addition, replications are limited by inadequate descriptions of the interventions and teaching processes, which appear to vary widely from one study to another.

The failure to use standardized procedures is further compounded by small sample designs, differing populations, confounding variables, and methodologic problems, all of which limit the generalizability of findings toward developing future research and practice. Control groups were often inadequate or nonexistent. Many investigations did not adequately control for observer bias. Within many studies there were a combination of various diagnostic or therapeutic procedures with different meanings, processes, and outcomes for the patients (eg, cholecystectomies and hysterectomies).

Data analysis was deficient in many studies. Basic statistical analyses frequently were not used (ie, mean comparisons of groups without t tests or analysis of variance). Frequently, quantification of results (eg, means and standard deviations) were not described. At times it appeared that "significant results" may actually have been a regression to the mean.

RECOMMENDATIONS FOR FUTURE RESEARCH ON RELAXATION RESPONSE INTERVENTIONS

To assess the clinical efficacy of the relaxation response accurately, these methodologic deficiencies must be rectified. More investigations should be repeated using larger and comparable populations and psychometrically sound data analysis techniques. Confounding variables, such as mixed procedures, must be eliminated. Greater control of variations in the characteristics of populations, stressors, interventions, and procedures is necessary. The specific components of the relaxation response require increased identification within each study to optimize the recognition of the actual elicitation of the relaxation response. Compliance and actual elicitation of the relaxation response warrant clear inclusion in future research.

Specific details about the relaxation response interventions and teaching processes need to be clearly documented in research reports. More attention should be given to the teaching strategies (eg, individual versus group teaching). This is particularly important given the current cost-effectiveness concerns of health care.

Future research on relaxation response interventions must include rigorously structured experimental investigations that use tight controls to validate outcomes brought about by relaxation techniques. Emphasis is needed on the relationship between changes in psychophysiologic and behavioral measurements and on specific interventions to determine which produces the most effective outcomes.

RECOMMENDATIONS FOR CLINICAL USE OF RELAXATION RESPONSE INTERVENTIONS

In spite of these methodologic flaws, relaxation response interventions have been shown to promote health and alleviate a variety of symptoms manifested by adult patients, specifically within the cardiovascular population. Although this review has highlighted some of the flaws in selected research studies on relaxation response, the overall quality of investigations is improving and the benefits of the relaxation response continue to be documented by much needed scientifically conducted investigations.

Nurses guide people to be more aware of connections between their minds and the environment, as well as the mind–body interactions. In addition to benefiting from physiologic, psychologic, and behavioral changes, people can focus attention more easily and appraise reality in a more conscious way after eliciting the relaxation response. These benefits can be helpful in managing acute problems such as anxiety and pain during hospitalization. Patients can then begin to replace ways of thinking and behaving that have not served them well with new, more positive health-promoting ones.[18,84–88] Such thinking allows for an openness to new possibilities and the possibility of changing behaviors to promote health and facilitate adjustments to illness.[40] Regardless of the approach, the end result is a movement of the person toward balance and healing.[39] A variety of relaxation response interventions have been used by nurses to maximize the health of diverse patient populations across the health spectrum and in a variety of practice settings. This plethora of approaches is a double-edge sword. Although opportunities for using relaxation strategies are numerous, the lack of specificity of definitions creates a risk for inappropriate or ineffective applications in nursing practice.

With each patient the nurse determines the most appropriate health goals and related relaxation response interventions and, subsequently, whether the desired outcomes were achieved. Patient assessment as well as outcome research on the efficacy of relaxation response interventions will guide future nursing practice.

REFERENCES

1. Julius S, Cottier C. Behavior and hypertension. In: Dembroski T, Schmidt T, eds. *Behavioral Bases of Coronary Heart Disease*. Basel, Switzerland: Karger; 1983.

2. Clarkson T, Mancusk S, Kaplan J. Potential role of cardiovascular reactivity in atherogenesis. In: Matthews K, Weiss S, Detre T, et al., eds. *Handbook of Stress, Reactivity, and Cardiovascular Disease*. New York, NY: Wiley; 1986.

3. Lawn B, Verrier R, Rabinowitz S. Neural and psychologic mechanisms and the problem of sudden cardiac death. *Am J Cardiol*. 1987;39:890–902.

4. Turk D, Meichenbam D. A cognitive-behavioral approach to pain management. In: Wall P, Melzack R, eds. *Textbook of Pain*. Edinburgh, Scotland: Churchill-Livingstone; 1984.

5. Melzack R, Wall P. Psychophysiology of pain. *Int Anesthesiol Clin*. 1970;8:3–34.

6. Fava G, Perino G, Santumastaso P, Fornasa C. Life events and psychological distress in dermatologic disorders: psoriasis, chronic urticaria, and fungal infections. In: Miller T, ed. *Stressful Life Events*. Madison, Wis: International Universities Press; 1989.

7. Roberts S, Barnes D. The brain drain in stress. *J NIH Res*. 1990;2:70–71.

8. Seibel M, Taymor M. Emotional aspects of infertility. *Fertil Steril*. 1982;37:137.

9. Woods N, Most A, Longenecker G. Major life events, daily stressors, and premenstrual symptoms. *Nurs Res*. 1985;34:263–267.

10. Rogers M, Reich P. Psychological intervention with surgical patients: evaluation outcome. *Adv Psychosom Med*. 1986;15:23–50.

11. Williams J, Jones J, Workhaven M, Williams B. The psychological control of preoperative anxiety. *Psychophysiology*. 1975;12:50–54.

12. Kendall P, William L, Pechacek T, Graham L, Shisslak D, Herzoff N. Cognitive-behavioral and patient education interventions in cardiac catheterization procedures: the Palo Alto medical psychology project. *J Consult Clin Psychol*. 1979;47:49–58.

13. Kaplan R, Atkins C, Lenhard L. Coping with a stressful sigmoidoscopy: evaluation of cognitive and relaxation preparations. *J Behav Med*. 1982;5:67–82.

14. Spielberger C, Auerbach S, Wadsworth A, Dunn T, Taulbee E. Emotional reactions to surgery. *J Consult Clin Psycol*. 1973;40:33–38.

15. Ray C, Fitzgibbon G. Stress arousal and coping with surgery. *Psychol Med*. 1981;11:741–746.

16. Mumford E, Schlessinger H, Glass G. The effects of psychological intervention on recovery from surgery and heart attacks: an analysis of the literature. *Am J Public Health*. 1982;72(2):141–151.

17. Cannon W. The emergency function of the adrenal medulla in pain and the major emotions. *Am J Physiol*. 1914;33:356–372.

18. Benson H. *Beyond the Relaxation Response*. New York, NY: Time Books; 1984.

19. Hess WR, Brugger M. *Das Subkortikale Zentrum der Affektiven Abwehrreoktiow Helv Physiol Pharmacol Acta*. 1943;1:33–52.

20. Bagchi BK, Wenger MA. Electrophysiological correlation of some yoga exercises. *Electroencephalogr Clin Neurophysiol*. 1957;7:132–149.

21. Anard BK, Ckhina GS, Singh B. Some aspects of electroencephalographic studies in yogis. *Electroencephalogr Clin Neurophysiol.* 1961;13:452–456.

22. Wenger MA, Bagchi BK. Studies of autonomic functions in practitioners of yoga in India. *Behav Sci.* 1961;6:312–323.

23. Wenger M, Bagchi B, Anand B. "Voluntary" heart and pulse control by yoga methods. *Int J Parapsychol.* 1963;5:25–41.

24. Kasamatsu A, Hirdi T, Ando N. EEG responses to click stimulation in Zen meditation. *Proc Jpn EEG Soc.* 1962;6:77–78.

25. Hirdi T. Electroencephalographic study on the Zen Meditation (Zazen): EEG changes during the concentrated relaxation. *Psychiatr Neurol Jpn.* 1960;62:76–105.

26. Hirdi T, Izawa S, Koga E. EEG & Zen Buddhism: EEG changes in the course of meditation. *Electroencephalogr Clin Neurophysiol.* 1959;55(suppl 18):52–53.

27. Wallace RK. Physiologic effects of transcendental meditation. *Science.* 1970;167:1,751–1,754.

28. Wallace R, Benson H. The physiology of meditation. *Sci Am.* 1972;226:84–90.

29. Wallace RK, Benson H, Wilson AF. A wakeful hypometabolic physiologic state. *Am J Physiol.* 1971;221:795–799.

30. Wallace RK, Benson H, Donovan S. *Contemporary Meditation Research.* San Francisco, Calif: The Esalen Institute Transformation Project; 1985.

31. Lehmann JW, Benson H. Nonpharmacologic therapy of blood pressure. *Gen Hosp Psychiatry.* 1982;4:27–32.

32. Jacobson E. *Progressive Relaxation.* Chicago, Ill: University of Chicago Press; 1938.

33. Luthe W. *Autogenic Therapy.* New York, NY: Grune & Stratton; 1969.

34. Luthe W. Autogenic therapy and excerpts on application to cardiovascular disorders and hypercholesterolemia. In: *Biofeedback and Self Control.* New York, NY: Aldine-Atherton; 1972.

35. Benson H, Beary J, Carol M. The relaxation response. *Psychiatry.* 1974;37:37–46.

36. Snyder M. Relaxation. *Annu Rev Nurs Res.* 1988;6:111–129.

37. Beary J, Benson H. A simple psychophysiologic technique which elicits the hypometabolic changes of the relaxation response. *Psychosom Med.* 1974;36:115–120.

38. Benson H. *The Relaxation Response.* New York, NY: Avon Books; 1975.

39. Kolkmeier LG. Relaxation: opening the door to change. In: Dossey BN, Keegan L, Guzzetta CE, Kolkmeier LG, eds. *Holistic Nursing: A Handbook for Practice.* 2nd ed. Gaithersburg, MD: Aspen Publishers; 1995.

40. Wells-Federman CL, Stuart EM, Deckro JP, Mandle CL, Baim M, Medich C. The mind-body connection: the psychophysiology of many traditional nursing interventions. *Clin Nurs Spec.* 1995;9(1):59–66.

41. Benson H. The relaxation response and the treatment of anxiety. In: Grinspoon L, ed. *Psychiatry Update.* Vol 111. American Psychiatric Press; 1984.

42. Aiken L, Henrichs T. Systematic relaxation as a nursing intervention technique with open heart surgery patients. *Nurs Res.* 1971;20:212–217.

43. Aiken L. Systematic relaxation to reduce postoperative stress. *Can Nurs.* 1972;68:38–42.

44. Miller KM, Perry PA. Relaxation techniques and postoperative pain in patients undergoing cardiac surgery. *Heart Lung.* 1990;19(2):136–146.

45. Leserman J, Stuart EM, Mamish ME, Benson H. The efficacy of the relaxation response in preparing for cardiac surgery. *Behav Med.* 1989;15:111–117.

46. Flaherty G, Fitzpatrick J. Relaxation technique to increase comfort level of postoperative patients: a preliminary study. *Nurs Res.* 1978;27:352–355.

47. Lorenzi EA. Relaxation: episiotomy incisional pain and overall discomfort. *J Adv Nurs.* 1991;16(6):701–709.

48. Wilson J. Behavioral preparation for surgery: benefit or harm? *J Behav Med.* 1981;4:79–102.

49. Wells N. The effect of relaxation on postoperative muscle tension and pain. *Nurs Res.* 1982;31:236–238.

50. Mogan J. Using relaxation to manage postoperative muscle tension and pain. *Can Nurs.* 1984;80:15.

51. Wells J, Howard G, Nowlin W, Vargas M. Presurgical anxiety and postsurgical pain and adjustment: effects of stress inoculation procedure. *J Consult Clin Psychol.* 1986;57:831–835.

52. Ceccio C. Postoperative pain relief through relaxation in elderly patients with fractured hips. *Orthop Nurs.* 1984;3:11–19.

53. McAdmond D, Davidson P, Kovitz M. A comparison of the effects of hypnosis and relaxation training on stress reactions in a dental situation. *Am J Clin Hypn.* 1971;3:233–242.

54. Palmer D. Inspired analgesia through transcendental meditation. *NZ Dent J.* 1980; 76:61–64.

55. Corah N, Gale E, Illig S. Psychological stress reduction during dental surgery. *J Dent Res.* 1979;58:1,347–1,351.

56. Mandle CL, Domar A, Harrington D, et al. Relaxation response in femoral angiography. *Radiology.* 1990;174:737–739.

57. Warner CD, Peebles BU, Miller J, Reed R, Rodriquez S, Martin-Lewis E. The effectiveness of teaching a relaxation technique to patients undergoing elective cardiac catheterization. *J Cardiovasc Nurs.* 1992;6(2):66–75.

58. Carson M, Hathaway M, Tuohey J. The effect of a relaxation technique on coronary risk factors. *Behav Med.* 1988;14:71–77.

59. Guzzetta C. Effects of relaxation and music therapy on patients in a coronary care unit with presumptive acute myocardial infarction. *Heart Lung.* 1989;18:609–616.

60. Munro B, Creamer A, Haggerty M, Cooper F. Effect of relaxation therapy on post-myocardial infarction patients' rehabilitation. *Nurs Res.* 1988;37:231–235.

61. Benson H, Alexander S, Feldman C. Decreased premature ventricular contractions through the use of the relaxation response in patients with stable ischemic heart disease. *Lancet.* 1975;2:380–382.

62. Benson H. Systemic hypertension and the relaxation response. *N Eng J Med.* 1977;296(20):1,152–1,156.

63. Pender N. Effects of progressive muscle relaxation on anxiety and health locus of control among hypertensive adults. *Res Nurs Health.* 1985;8:67–72.

64. Stuart E, Caudill M, Leserman J, Darrington C, Friedman R, Benson H. Nonpharmacologic treatment of hypertension: a multiple-risk-factor approach. *J Cardiovasc Nurs.* 1987;1:1–14.

65. Patel C, Marmot M. Can general practitioners use training in relaxation and management of stress to reduce mild hypertension? *Br Med J.* 1988;296:21–24.

66. Lesko W, Summerfield L. The effectiveness of biofeedback on home relaxation training on reduction of borderline hypertension. *Health Ed.* 1988;19:19–23.

67. Leserman J, Stuart EM, Mamish ME, et al. Nonpharmacologic intervention for hypertension: long-term follow-up. *J Cardiopul Rehabil.* 1989;9:316–324.

68. Bradley LA, Turner RA, Young LD, Agudelo CA, Anderson KO, McDaniel LK. Effects of psychological therapy on pain behavior of rheumatoid arthritis patients. *Arthritis Rheum.* 1987;30:1,105–1,114.

69. Arena J, Hightower N, Chong G. Relaxation therapy for tension headache in the elderly: a prospective study. *Psychol Aging.* 1988;3:96–98.

70. Kabat-Zinn J, Lipworth L, Burney R. The clinical use of mindfulness meditation for the self-regulation of chronic pain. *J Behav Med.* 1985;8:163–190.

71. Strong J. Relaxation training and chronic pain. *Br J Occup Ther.* 1991;54(6):216–218.

72. Gift AG, Moore T, Soekew K. Relaxation to reduce dyspnea and anxiety in COPD patients. *Nurs Res.* 1992; 41(4):242–246.

73. Renfroe K. Effect of progressive relaxation on dyspnea and state anxiety in patients with chronic obstructive pulmonary disease. *Heart Lung.* 1988;17:408–413.

74. Holliday J, Hyers T. Reduction of weaning time from mechanical ventilation using tidal volume and relaxation biofeedback. *Am Rev Respir Dis.* 1990;141:1,214–1,220.

75. Domar A, Seibel M, Benson H. The mind/body program for infertility: a new behavioral treatment approach for women with infertility. *Fertil Steril.* 1990;53:246–249.

76. Goodale IL, Domar A, Benson H. Alleviation of premenstrual syndrome symptoms with the relaxation response. *Obstet Gynecol.* 1990;75:649–655.

77. Alexander C, Chandler H, Langer E, Newman R, Davies J. Transcendental meditation, mindfulness and longevity: an experimental study with the elderly. *J Pers Soc Psychol.* 1989;57:950–964.

78. Peters R, Benson H, Peters J. Daily relaxation response breaks in a working population:2. blood pressure. *Am J Public Health.* 1977;67:954–959.

79. Lehmann J, Benson H. The nonpharmacologic treatment of hypertension. In: Genest J, Kucher O, Hamet P, Cantin M, eds. *Hypertension.* 3rd ed. New York, NY: McGraw Hill; 1983:1,238–1,245.

80. Field P. Effects of tape-recorded hypnotic preparation for surgery. *J Clin Exp Hypn.* 1974;22:54–61.

81. Perri K, Perri M. Use of relaxation training to reduce pain following vaginal hysterectomy. *Percep Mot Skill.* 1979;48:478.

82. Domar AD, Noe JM, Benson H. The preoperative use of the relaxation response with ambulatory surgery patients. *J Hum Stress.* 1987;13:101–107.

83. Hyman R, Feldman H, Harris R, Levin R, Malloy G. The effects of relaxation training on clinical symptoms: a meta-analysis. *Nurs Res.* 1989;38:216–220.

84. King K. Measurement of coping strategies, concerns, and emotional response in patients undergoing coronary artery bypass grafting. *Heart Lung.* 1985;14:579–586.

85. Reading A. The short-term effects of psychological preparation for surgery. *Soc Sci Med.* 1979;13A:641–654.

86. Benson H. *Your Maximum Mind.* New York, NY: Times Books; 1987.

87. Benson H, Stuart E, eds. *The Wellness Book: A Comprehensive Guide to Maintaining Health and Treating Stress-Related Illness.* New York, NY: Simon & Schuster; 1993.

88. Stuart E, Deckro JP, Mandle CL. Spirituality in health and healing: a clinical program. *Holist Nurs Prac.* 1989;3(3):35–46.

Summary of Studies Using Relaxation-Response Interventions

Authors	Date	Issues	Site	Sample size	Random	Instruments and clinical evaluations	Interventions	Significant relaxation results:
Aiken Henrichs	1971	Cardiac surgery	Hospital	30	No	MMPI	1. Relaxation audiotape with nurse supervision 3–5 days preoperatively 2. Control	Relaxation: 1. Less time on cardiopulmonary bypass 2. Fewer units of blood during surgery
McAmmond Davidson Kovitz	1971	Dental	Office	27	Yes	1. Pressure algometer pain tolerance test 2. STAI (Spielberger, 1970)	1. Relaxation audiotape 2. Control	Relaxation: More effective pain reduction than hypnosis or control
Aiken	1972	Cardiac surgery	Hospital	30	No	None	1. Nurse-taught relaxation 3–4 days preoperatively 2. Control	Relaxation: 1. Lower duration of hypothermia 2. Decreased cardiopulmonary bypass time 3. Decreased anesthesia time 4. Fewer units of blood during surgery
Benson Alexander Feldman	1975	PVCs in patients with stable ischemic heart disease	Clinic Home	11	No	Pre-post Holter monitoring	4 weeks of practicing relaxation response	Reduced frequency of PVCs documented in 8 of 11 patients, especially during sleeping
Palmer	1976	Dental surgery	Office	1	No	Clinical evaluations	Case report of patient using transcendental meditation during 2 dental surgeries	No operative or postoperative analgesia Uneventful recoveries

continues

Continued

Authors	Date	Issues	Site	Sample size	Random	Instruments and clinical evaluations	Interventions	Significant relaxation results:
Benson	1977	Hypertension	Clinic	86	No	Clinical evaluations	Experimental study using transcendental meditation, 6-week control (weekly evaluations) 5 to 6 month experimental evaluations (biweekly evaluations)	Reduced systolic and diastolic blood pressure during control period, return of high levels of blood pressure within 4 weeks postcontrol
Flaherty Fitzpatrick	1978	Post surgery (Cholecystectomy, herniorrhaphy, hemorrhordectormy)	Hospital	42	No	Johnson Pain and Distress Scales (1972, 1973)	2 groups: 1. Jaw relaxation technique 2. Control	Less incisional pain, body distress, analgesic consumption, and respiratory rate
Corah Gale Illig	1979	Dental surgery	Office	80	Yes	1. Corah Dental Anxiety Scale 2. Rotter Locus of Control Scale 3. Need for Social Approval Scale 4. 7-point Discomfort Scale (self-rating)	Four groups with two visits: 1. Relaxation progressive muscle relaxation audiotape 2. Control 3. Perceived control (light & buzzer) 4. Active distraction (videogame)	Relaxation and active distraction Patients experience less discomfort

Author	Year	Condition	Setting	N		Measures	Conditions	Results
Wilson	1980	Post surgery (cholecystectomy, abdominal hysterectomy)	Hospital	70	Yes	1. Questionnaire measures of fear, mood, social support, coping style (self-rating) 2. 6-point recovery inventory (self-rating) 3. 10-point pain-distress inventory (self-rating)	1. Relaxation audiotape used pre- and postoperatively 2. Information 3. Information and relaxation 4. Control	Relaxation Reduced hospital stay, pain, use of analgesics and increased strength, energy, and postoperative epinephrine levels Less frightened patients benefited more than very frightened
Ceccio	1984	Orthopedic surgery (surgical repair of fractured hip)	Hospital	20	Yes	Johnson Pain-Distress Rating Scale (1973)	Two groups: 1. Relaxation (Jacobson) 2. Control	Relaxation: Lower self-reports of pain and distress and lower use of analgesics
Mogan	1984	Abdominal surgery		100	Yes	Johnson Pain-Distress Rating Scale (1973)	Two groups: 1. Relaxation written instructions (teaching by nurse and practice preoperatively) 2. Control	Relaxation: Less distress by painful sensations (hysterectomy patients benefited more than cholecystectomy patients)
Pender	1985	Hypertension	Clinic	44	Yes	1. STAI (Spielberger, 1983) 2. Multidimensional Health Locus of Control Scales	Two groups: 1. Relaxation (progressive muscle relaxation) 2. Control	Relaxation: Less anxiety and higher in beliefs in personal control of health and lower in beliefs that chance or luck affected health outcomes

continues

Continued

Authors	Date	Issues	Site	Sample size	Random	Instruments and clinical evaluations	Interventions	Significant relaxation results:
Kaplan Atkins Lenhard	1980	Sigmoidoscopy	Clinic	66	Yes	1. Lafayette Instruments Heart Rate Monitor 2. Recorded verbalizations by trained observers 3. Therapist and self-anxiety ratings 4. Questionnaire (discomfort and sensitivity)	Three groups: 1. Self-instruction 2. Relaxation (progressive muscle relaxation supervised and deep breathing) 3. Control	Relaxation: Made fewer requests to stop exam and rated themselves as less anxious
Wells	1982	Cholecystectomy (postoperative muscle pain and tension)	Hospital	12	Yes	Pre and Posttest 1. Abdominal muscle tension (surface EMG) 2. Self-report of sensory and distress ratings 3. Johnson Pain-Distress Rating Scale (1973)	Two groups: 1. Relaxation (Jacobson progressive muscle relaxation and Beary breathing) 4 days preoperative practice with nurse 2. Control	Relaxation: Lower self-reports of pain and distress and lower use of analgesics
Wells Howard Nowlin Vargas	1986	Elective surgery (abdominal)	Hospital	24	Yes	STAI (Spielberger, 1970) Hospital Anxiety Scale (Lucente & Fleck, 1972) Pain Visual Analog Scale (Keefe, Brown, Scott, & Ziesat, 1982)	Control: Standard hospital preparatory instructions Experimental: 1. Standard hospital preparatory instructions 2. Stress inoculation training 3. Skill acquisitions	Experimental: Less presurgical anxiety (STAI) Less postsurgical anxiety (HAS) More positive nurse ratings of patient adjustment to hospitalizations

| Bradley Turner Young Aqudelo Anderson McDaniel | 1987 | Rheumatoid arthritis | Clinic | 53 | Yes | a. Monitoring cognitive and physical cues for stress reactions
b. Deep breathing
c. General passive muscle relaxation
d. Imaging
e. Coping self-statements
f. Instructions for rehearsing the procedure

Three groups:
1. Psychologic support (5 sessions including relaxation training)
2. Social support
3. Control | 1. STAI (Spielberger, 1983)
2. Depression Adjective Checklist
3. 10-cm Visual Analog Scale ratings of pain intensity and unpleasantness
4. Health Locus of Control
5. Arthritis Helplessness Index
6. Video recorded pain behaviors
7. Physiologic measures
8. Rheumatoid Activity Index | Less pain intensity (PVAS)
Lower use of analgesics as rated by physicians

Psychologic:
Reduced pain behavior disease activity and trait anxiety at posttreatment and 6-month follow up |

continues

Continued

Authors	Date	Issues	Site	Sample size	Random	Instruments and clinical evaluations	Interventions	Significant relaxation results:
Stuart Caudill Leserman Darrington Friedman Benson	1987	Hypertension	Clinic	98	No		11-session program Cardiovascular risk factors, relaxation response, self-monitoring, goal setting nutrition, exercise, stress management	Decreased and clinical systolic and diastolic blood pressures and anti-hypertensive medications
Lesko Summerfield	1988	Hypertension (borderline)	Clinic	112	Yes		7-week treatments 7 groups: 1. Biofeedback 2. Relaxation 3. Exercise and nutrition 4. Biofeedback and relaxation 5. Biofeedback and exercise/nutrition 6. Biofeedback, relaxation with exercise/nutrition 7. Relaxation and exercise/nutrition (relaxation = 30 min audiotape/ each day)	1. Significant subject losses in groups with exercise 2. Reduced diastolic and systolic blood pressure in both relaxation and relaxation and biofeedback groups 3. Reduced diastolic blood pressure in biofeedback group

Arena Hightower Chong	1988	Chronic headache (tension)	Clinic	10	No	Headache Index (intensity and duration)	8-week PMR— relaxation therapy	At 3 months posttreatment: 1. Reduced headache activity, analgesic use, prophylactic drug use 2. Improved headache-free days peak headache rating
Patel Marmot	1988	Hypertension	Clinic	103	Yes	None	Three groups: 1. Regular medical surveillance 2. Placebo medication 3. 8-session program a. Relaxation b. Response training c. Stress management d. Coping strategies e. Social support f. Coronary-prone personality	Relaxation: Decreased systolic and diastolic blood pressures 1 year postprogram
Leserman Stuart Mamish Deckro Beckman Friedman Benson	1989	Hypertension	Clinic	54	No		3-year follow up (following 11-session program)	At 3 years follow up (following 11-session program) 94% reporting eliciting relaxation response at least 2 times/week Significant reductions in home and clinic blood pressure

continues

Continued

Authors	Date	Issues	Site	Sample size	Random	Instruments and clinical evaluations	Interventions	Significant relaxation results:
Leserman Stuart Mamish Benson	1989	Cardiac surgery	Hospital	27	Yes	1. California Profile of Mood States	Two groups: 1. Relaxation response pre- and postoperatively 2. Control	Relaxation: Lower incidence postoperative supraventricular tachycardia and greater decreases in psychologic tension and anger
Renfroe	1988	COPD Anxiety Dyspnea	Clinic	20	Yes	STAI (Spielberger, 1983) 20-cm Visual Analog Scale for dyspnea	Two groups: 1. 4 weeks of weekly sessions and daily practice of PMR audiotape 2. Control	Relaxation reductions in 1. Dyspnea and anxiety during each session 2. Respiratory rates
Munro Creamer Haggerty Cooper	1988	Cardiac rehabilitation (postmyocardial infarction)	Clinic	57	Yes	Sickness Impact Profile Jenkins Activity Survey (Type A behavior pattern)	Two groups: 1. Relaxation 20 min audiotape 2 times/day 2. Control (both groups in 12-week usual cardiac rehabilitation program)	Relaxation: Reduced diastolic blood pressure (1st week through 3-month follow up)

Author	Year	Condition	Setting	N		Measures	Design	Results
Carson Hathaway Tuohey	1988	Coronary risk factors	Clinic	16	Yes	STAI Self-reports of diet compliance	Two groups for 8 weeks: 1. Relaxation 2 times/daily 30 min and audiotape Both groups on American Heart Association, Phase II, low-cholesterol diet and weight reduction and coronary risk management classes	Relaxation: 1. Reduced systolic blood pressure 2. Reduced low-density lipoprotein cholesterol 3. Correlations systolic blood pressure reduction and report of diet compliance
Guzzetta	1989	Myocardial infarction (pre-sumptive, acute)	Hospital coronary care unit	80	Yes	Clinical evaluations Patient self-report	Three groups: 1. Relaxation response (PMR and meditation) 2. Music with PMR 3. Control (three 20-min guided sessions over 2-day period)	Relaxation and music groups 1. Reduced apical pulses 2. Increased peripheral temperatures 3. Reduced incidence of cardiac complications (persistent chest pain, cardiac arrest, congestive heart failure, pericarditis)

continues

Continued

Authors	Date	Issues	Site	Sample size	Random	Instruments and clinical evaluations	Interventions	Significant relaxation results:
Alexander Chandler Langer Newman Davies	1989	Aging	Nursing homes	73	Yes	1. Dementia screening test 2. Associate Learning Subtest, DST (Wechsler Memory Scale) 3. Word Fluency Subtest, DST (Multilingual Aphasia Examination) 4. Overlearned Verbal Task 5. Stroop Color-Work Interference Test 6. Objective Uses Test 7. STAI (Spielberger, 1983) 8. Self-Rating Depression Scale 9. Internal Locus of Control Scale 10. Self-reports 11. Nursing home staff reports	1. Control 2. Transcendental meditation program 3. Mindfulness training program 4. Relaxation program	Transcendental meditation group improved most, followed by mindfulness training on • paired associate learning • cognitive flexibility • mental health • decreased systolic • behavioral flexibility • treatment efficacy
Mandle Domar Harrington Leserman Bozadjian Friedman Benson	1990	Anxiety and pain	Angiography procedure room	45	Yes	Spielberger STAI McGill-Melzack Pain Inventory	Three groups: 1. Control 2. Music audiotape 3. Relaxation response audiotape	Relaxation-response group Significant decrease in patient and nurse perceived anxiety and pain and medication request and usage

Author	Year	Condition	Setting	N	Randomized	Measures	Design	Results
Holliday Hyers	1990	Mechanical ventilation weaning	Hospital intensive care unit	40	No	1. Respitrace (breathing patterns and EMG measurements) 2. Patient self-reports of anxiety	Two groups: 1. Relaxation-biofeedback 2. Control: attention with reassurance (matched APACHE II scores) (cardio-vascular, respiratory, renal, and neurologic function)	Relaxation: 1. Reduced mean ventilation days 2. Increased baseline tidal volume (diaphragm EMG) 3. Reduced anxiety
Kabat-Zinn Lipworth Burney	1985	Chronic pain (varied sites)	Clinic	90	No	1. McGill-Melzack Pain Rating Index (1975) 2. Body Parts Problem Assessment Scale 3. Table of Levels of Inference (effect of pain on activities of daily living) 4. Body Pain Map (changes in pain, distribution, intensity, and frequency) 5. Medically oriented symptom checklist 6. Profile of mood states 7. SCL-90-R 8. Summary outcome questionnaire	Two groups: 1. Experimental 10-week stress reduction and relaxation program 45 min/day mindfulness meditation 6 days/week 2. Control: tradi-tional treatment in pain clinic (transcutaneous electrical nerve stimulation, physical therapy, analgesics, antidepressants, and nerve blocks)	At the end of program: Experimental patients A. Reduced measures of 1. Present-moment pain 2. Negative body image 3. Inhibition of activity by pain, symptoms, mood disturbances, and psychologic symptomatology (including anxiety and depression) 4. Pain-related drug use B. Increased self-esteem At 15-month follow up: A. All measures main-tained except pre-sent-moment pain B. High compliance with mindfulness meditation

continues

Continued

Authors	Date	Issues	Site	Sample size	Random	Instruments and clinical evaluations	Interventions	Significant relaxation results:
Miller Perry	1990	Cardiac surgery	Hospital	29	No	Visual Analog Scale for pain Vertical pain descriptors scale	1. Relaxation response training 2. Control	Relaxation: Decreased vital signs Decreased self-report and Visual Analog Scale ratings of pain
Gift Moore Soekew	1992	COPD	Clinic	26	Yes	None	1. Relaxation response audiotape 2. Control	Relaxation: Decreased dyspnea, anxiety and airway obstruction
Warner Peebles Miller Reed Rodriquez Martin-Lewis	1992	Cardiac catheterization	Cardiac catheterization laboratory	40	Yes	STAI	1. Progressive muscle relaxation and meditation 2. Control	Relaxation: Decreased STAI scores and diazepam use
Strong	1991	Chronic low back pain	Clinic	21	No	McGill Pain Questionnaire	Relaxation response training	Relaxation: Decreased present pain intensity, number of words chosen, pain rating index total, and pain rating index sensory, affective, and evaluative
Lorenzi	1991	Episiotomy incisional pain	Hospital	40	No		1. Relaxation response training 2. Control	Relaxation: A general trend for decreased pain

Author	Year	Condition	Setting	N	Randomized	Measures	Intervention	Results
Domar Seibel Benson	1990	Infertility	Clinic	54	No	Pre-post: Profile of Mood Scale Spielberger STAI Speilberger Anger Expression Scale	10-week program: Relaxation response teaching Stress management Exercise Nutrition Group support	Significant decreases in depression/ dejection, tension/ anxiety, and fatigue/inertia; Increases in vigor/ activity; Subjective reports of feeling of control, security, well-being, and self-esteem; 18(34%) of partici- pants conceived within 6 months of completing program (vs national rates of 18%)

APACHE II = acute physiology and chronic health evaluation; COPD = chronic obstructive pulmonary disease; DST = dementia screening test; EMG = electromyogram; HAS = Hospital Anxiety Scale; MMPI = Minnesota Multi-phase Personality Inventory; PVAS = Pain Visual Analog Scale; PVC = premature ventricular contraction; PMR = progressive muscle relaxation; STAI = State-Trait Anxiety Inventory

The Effectiveness of Teaching a Relaxation Technique to Patients Undergoing Elective Cardiac Catheterization

Christi Deaton Warner, MN, RN, CCRN
Clinical Nurse Coordinator
Crawford Long Hospital of Emory University

Belinda Utley Peebles, MN, RN, CCRN
Nurse Coordinator
Crawford Long Hospital of Emory University

Joni Miller, RN
Clinical Nurse, Cardiology
Emory Clinic

Roberta Reed, BSN, RN
Clinical Nurse, Cardiology
Emory Clinic

Sherry Rodriquez, BBA/BHA, RN
Technical Director, Cardiac Catheterization
    Laboratory
Crawford Long Hospital of Emory University

Evelyn Martin-Lewis, MSN, RN
Data Coordinator, Cardiac Data Bank
Crawford Long Hospital of Emory University
Atlanta, Georgia

Patients admitted to the hospital cope with many situations that may be perceived as threatening. One of these is cardiac catheterization (CC). The medical procedure of CC has been identified as an extremely stressful experience.[1–3] The anxiety experienced is related in part to the new situation, lack of knowledge of what to expect, and thoughts of discomfort that may be associated with the procedure. A patient's anxiety and ability to cope with anxiety may influence his or her physiologic responses, such as respiratory rate, heart rate, blood pressure, myocardial oxygen consumption, and plasma concentrations of epinephrine and norepinephrine.[4–6] Physiologic and psychological responses to the CC may increase the length of the procedure and the amount of sedating medication that is given to the patient during CC.

Nurses should assess the patient's level of anxiety and coping ability prior to CC and should intervene to decrease anxiety and provide the patient with better coping skills. Nurses can teach patients relaxation techniques to enhance their coping skills. The purpose of this study was to determine if practicing a particular relaxation technique (RT) before and during CC would affect the patient's level of anxiety, the variability in vital signs (ie, fluctuations in heart rate and blood pressure dur-

Source: Reprinted from C.D. Warner, B.U. Peebles, J. Miller, R. Reed, S. Rodriquez, E. Martin-Lewis, *The Journal of Cardiovascular Nursing,* Vol. 6, No. 2, pp. 66–75, © 1992, Aspen Publishers, Inc.

The authors acknowledge the assistance of Shirley Carey, RN, PhD, Carol Bush, RN, PhD, the staff of the Cardiac Catheterization Lab, Douglas Morris, MD, Henry Liberman, MD, and Louis Battey, MD.

ing CC), the length of procedure, and the amount of sedation required during CC.

BACKGROUND

Relaxation therapy has gained acceptance as an effective adjunct or therapeutic alternative for a wide range of disorders. RTs affect various physiologic and psychological variables: for example, they

- decrease blood pressure in hypertensive patients[7–11]
- decrease premature ventricular contractions in patients with ischemic heart disease[12]
- reduce anxiety about public speaking,[13] and
- control stress-induced reactivity[14]

RTs are within the realm of nursing interventions and have been used by nurses in treating many different human responses. An effective lowering of apical heart rates and a raising of peripheral temperatures were found when patients admitted with a presumptive diagnosis of acute myocardial infarction participated in Benson's RT (a sequence of relaxation of major muscle groups combined with coupled exhalation word repetition) or music therapy.[15] In a cardiac rehabilitation program, practicing Benson's RT had a significant effect on diastolic blood pressure irrespective of a patient's behavioral style.[16] A reduction in dyspnea and anxiety was demonstrated in patients with chronic obstructive pulmonary disease who used progressive muscle relaxation (PMR).[17] The RTs used by these patients included guided imagery and PMR. However, PMR, while used widely since it was first described in the 1930s, has the potential to induce the Valsalva response. In a study of 60 healthy adult volunteers practicing PMR, 43% exhibited the Valsalva response, consisting of changes in blood pressure, pulse pressure, heart rate, cardiac stroke volume, and peripheral vascular resistance.[18] These changes occur when an individual exhales against resistance. The Valsalva response has potentially deleterious effects on the compromised cardiovascular system of cardiac patients and may precipitate

dysrhythmias or angina. A second study[19] of the Valsalva response during the tense-and-relax cycles of PMR indicated that controlling the breathing pattern and decreasing the tensing time may limit its occurrence. In that study, only 18% of the sample exhibited the Valsalva response in one or more of the tense-and-relax cycles.

Other studies focused on levels of anxiety,[20] postoperative discomfort,[21–23] and the distress accompanying adversive procedures.[24] A recent study[25] found that patients undergoing cholecystectomy who listened to an audiotape series on relaxation with guided imagery demonstrated significantly less state anxiety, lower cortisol levels the day after surgery, and less surgical wound erythema than did the control group.

RTs were evaluated in two studies of patients undergoing CC. The effects on 15 patients of training to relax-by-letting-go while undergoing CC were evaluated.[26] The relaxation group in this study did not report having less distress or anxiety than the control group before or during CC. In another study,[27] a group of 10 patients trained in Benson's RT before CC demonstrated significant differences in respiratory rate from the control group. Although the differences were not statistically significant, clinically significant differences in blood pressure and state anxiety were demonstrated in the groups, with the experimental group having lower systolic and diastolic blood pressures and lower mean state anxiety scores.

The benefits of relaxation therapy seem to lie in its effect on the sympathetic nervous system. An integrated hypothalamic response called the "relaxation response"[28] seems to result in generally decreased sympathetic nervous system activity and perhaps in increased parasympathetic activity. This response is opposite to the stress response or the "fight-or-flight" reaction. The relaxation response may be elicited by a technique made up of four basic elements:

1. a mental device to prevent distracting thoughts
2. a passive attitude

3. a decrease in muscle tonus, and
4. a quiet environment[29]

With elicitation of the relaxation response, decreases in oxygen consumption, carbon dioxide elimination, heart rate, respiratory rate, minute ventilation, and arterial blood lactate occur. One researcher advocates the playing of certain types of music to potentiate the hypometabolic counterarousal state.[30]

Given the documentation of the relaxation response's effect on the sympathetic nervous system, and the anxiety of patients with cardiovascular disease undergoing CC, this study was undertaken to evaluate the effects of RT on a larger group of patients scheduled for elective catheterization. Four hypotheses were tested:

1. Patients who practiced RT would demonstrate less anxiety as measured by the State-Trait Anxiety Inventory (STAI) than patients who did not practice this technique.
2. Patients who practiced RT would demonstrate less variability in vital signs (fluctuation in respiration, heart rate, and blood pressure) than patients who did not practice this technique.
3. Patients who practiced RT would have shorter procedure times than patients who did not practice this technique; and
4. Patients who practiced RT would require less sedation than patients who did not practice this technique.

METHOD

Data were collected prospectively over a 3-month period. A nonrandomized pretest posttest design with random assignment to groups was used in the study. Permission to conduct the study was approved by the Human Investigations Committee before the data were collected.

Sample

The target population included patients admitted to the cardiology service of a large, metropolitan, university-associated hospital for di-agnostic CC. Exclusion criteria were outpatient CC, previous CC, acute myocardial infarction less than 72 hours before CC, history of psychological problems (especially hallucinations), routine use of narcotics, routine use of anti-anxiety medications, and current use of vasoactive intravenous (IV) medications. The nonrandom sample consisted of 40 subjects. The experimental group consisted of 10 men and 10 women and the control group of 13 men and seven women. The subjects ranged in age from 30 years to 80 years, with a mean age of 59.5 years. There were no significant differences between the two groups in medical history or the duration and severity of cardiovascular disease. No concomitant disorders that would influence the results of the study (eg, peripheral vascular disease, which would make arterial cannulation difficult) were noted in either group.

Instruments

The questionnaire used to measure anxiety was the STAI,[31] which consists of separate self-reporting scales for measuring state and trait anxiety. The S-anxiety scale (STAI Form-4-1) has 20 statements that evaluate the current state of anxiety, or how respondents feel "right now, at this moment." This scale has been found to be a sensitive indicator of changes in transitory anxiety experienced by clients participating in counseling and psychotherapy. The scale has also been used to assess the level of anxiety induced by stressful experimental procedures and unavoidable life stressors, such as eminent surgery, dental treatment, job interviews, and important school tests. The stability coefficients for the S-anxiety scale ranged from 0.16 to 0.62. The S-anxiety coefficient alphas were primarily above 0.90 for the samples of working adults, students, and military recruits.

The T-anxiety scale (STAI Form-4-2) consists of 20 statements that assess how respondents generally feel, or their characteristic trait of anxiety. Test-retest reliability correlations for the T-anxiety scale ranged from 0.73 to 0.86. Alpha reliability coefficients for the T-anxiety scale given under stress conditions were between 0.89 and 0.94. Spielberger[31] provided data to support concurrent, convergent, divergent, and construct validity of the STAI scales.

Data collection

Once a patient's eligibility was established, a staff nurse acted as an intermediary, approaching the patient for verbal agreement to talk with one of the investigators. Informed consent was obtained by one of the six investigators the evening prior to CC, and then subjects completed the STAI. Randomization was accomplished by a computer-generated series of random-sequence envelopes assigning each subject to either the control or experimental groups. Subjects in the experimental group were taught a simple RT made up of the four basic elements as postulated by Benson.[10,12,28,29] First, a sign indicating that the patient was not to be disturbed was placed on the door (quiet environment). Second, the patient (and family member if present) was instructed to assume a comfortable position. Third, the patient was taken through a sequence of relaxing the major muscle groups, starting with the feet and working upward (relaxed muscle tonus). And, fourth, the patient was instructed to allow relaxation to happen, not to try to force it (passive attitude). Once verbal instruction of relaxation was completed, the patient was asked to become aware of his or her breathing. With each exhalation, the patient was taught to repeat a word silently, either a word that was value-neutral or a word that had some meaning to the patient. This word, repeated with each exhalation, became the mental device that blocked distracting thoughts. If distraction occurred, the patient was instructed to go back to being aware of his or her breathing and silently repeating the word. A period of silence of approximately 10 minutes then followed, so that the patient could practice the technique. Teaching of the RT was done by written instruction and audiotape to minimize variability among the investigators. Subjects were asked to practice the technique three times: during the initial instruction, in the morning prior to CC, and during

CC. For the control group, the procedure of filling out the questionnaire and interacting with the investigators served to some degree as a placebo and functioned to minimize the effects of one group's receiving more attention than the other. Both groups received the same nursing care, including precatheterization teaching by the primary nurse.

Data on blood pressure, heart rate, and respiratory rate were collected on admission, immediately before CC, during the catheterization while the artery was being cannulated, and immediately after CC. A record was maintained of all anti-anxiety medications the subject received before and during CC, as well as of total procedure time. Subjects in the experimental group were reminded before the procedure to practice RT during CC, but they were not prompted during CC. Subjects completed the S-anxiety scale of the STAI shortly after CC. If a subject was unable to read or to see the questions because of his or her position or vision, the STAI was read to that subject by an investigator.

RESULTS

Level of anxiety, variability in vital signs, length of procedure time, and amount of sedation requested and received during CC were compared for the experimental and control groups using analysis of variance, multivariate analysis of variance, and *t* tests.

The first hypothesis was that there would be a difference between the state anxiety levels in the two groups, as evidenced by the STAI. No difference in trait anxiety scores was found for the two groups, which indicates that the groups were homogeneous with respect to their level of characteristic anxiety. No significant difference was found for the two groups in state anxiety scores, before or after CC (Table 1). However, a significant difference between the pre-CC and post-CC state anxiety scores was noted in the experimental group; state anxiety scores decreased from 39.1 before CC to 31.39 after CC ($p < 0.05$). The change in the scores of the control group before and after CC was not significant.

Table 1. State-Trait Anxiety Inventory (STAI) scores

STAI	Control	Experi-mental	p values
Trait	38.84	33.47	NS*
Pre-CC† state	43.50	39.10	NS
Post-CC state	39.33	31.39	NS

*Not significant
†Cardiac catherization

The second hypothesis was that there would be less variability in the vital signs of the experimental group than the control group. Significant differences between groups were not found in baseline or pre-CC vital signs. This trend continued throughout the CC procedure, in that no significant differences between or within the groups were found in vital signs.

The third hypothesis was that there would be a difference between the two groups in procedure time, but this was not supported. Procedure times were not significantly different in the two groups (experimental, 33.6 minutes; control, 29.3 minutes).

The fourth hypothesis was that differences would be noted in the amount of sedation required by the two groups. IV diazepam is routinely given in this CC lab, and this procedure continued according to the following schedule: subjects weighing < 120 lb were given 3 mg; those weighing 121 to 180 lb were given 4 mg; and those weighing > 180 lb were given 5 mg. Additional diazepam was given if requested by the patient or if the CC nurse or physician felt that the patient needed it. Patients were instructed prior to the procedure that they could ask for additional medication. The mean amounts of diazepam required by the control and experimental groups are shown in Table 2: the experimental group received significantly less than the control group. Weight did not influence this finding, as the mean weight in the control group was less than that in the experimental group (166 lb vs 174 lb).

DISCUSSION

In the review of the literature, an inconsistency was noted in the research findings on the capacity of relaxation training to reduce anxiety. Previous researchers[17,20,24] noted decreases in anxiety when RTs were used by patients during a variety of medical interventions. Investigators studying patients undergoing CC,[26,27] however, did not find statistically less anxiety in the relaxation group than in the control group. The lack of statistically significant differences in the state anxiety scores of the two groups in this study supports the findings of these two previous studies. The finding that post-CC state anxiety scores were lower in both groups may be related to the fact that all patients felt relieved when the procedure was completed. Moreover, some patients from both groups had already been informed of the results of their CC (usually when test results were negative) before they completed their second state anxiety questionnaire. However, a significant decrease in scores after CC was noted in the experimental group; the decrease in the control group was not significant. This finding suggests that the experimental group experienced a greater reduction in anxiety after CC beyond that associated with relief that the procedure was complete, and perhaps this greater reduction was due to RT.

No significant differences in heart rate or blood pressure were found. This finding may be related to the cardiac medications that these ischemic cardiac patients were taking, as medications affecting heart rate and blood pressure were not controlled for in this study. No differ-

---

Table 2. Diazepam given

	Mean diazepam (mg)	Men	Women
Control	5.05	4.69	5.71
Experimental	3.95	4.10	3.90
p value	<0.05		
Mean		4.39	4.64

ence in respiratory rate was found, which differs from the findings of Frenn and associates,[27] who documented a significant difference in the respiratory rates in groups of CC patients.

This study demonstrated a decrease in the amount of sedation required by patients practicing RT. This finding is clinically significant, as it would decrease both recovery time and the risk of complications of sedation. As noted, the control group required more diazepam than the experimental group. Five patients in the control group received additional diazepam: three because of complications during CC, one because of the delay of an unplanned interruption in the procedure, and one by the patient's own request. No patients in the experimental group requested additional medication. A difference in sedation requirements was also noted for men and women. The mean dose of diazepam for the entire sample of women was 4.64 mg and that for men was 4.39 mg, despite the generally greater mean weight of the men.

This study did not demonstrate any differences in the variability of vital signs in the two groups. However, this finding could be influenced by the types of cardiovascular drugs taken by the subjects. In future studies, cardiovascular medications received prior to CC should be controlled to allow a more accurate assessment of blood pressure and heart rate effects.

The use of an RT did not decrease procedure time in this study. This finding could be related to the experience of the CC team or the relatively low acuity of the subjects. Subjects were excluded if they were taking IV vasoactive medications or had had a myocardial infarction in the previous 72 hours.

Limitations of this study include the fact that state anxiety was measured before the subjects were taught RT and after they had undergone CC; measuring anxiety before CC only might have been a more sensitive measure of the RT's effect on anxiety. Further, the time of completion of the second questionnaire was somewhat variable, ranging from immediately after catheterization to a few hours later in the patient's hospital room. This variability in timing makes it diffi-

cult to draw firm conclusions about the efficacy of RT in reducing anxiety. This study could also be redesigned so that no diazepam or other sedating medication is given in the catheterization laboratory unless the patient requests it.

Although this study did not demonstrate a significant difference in the anxiety scores of the two groups, further study is required before a definitive statement can be made. A research tool more suited to assessing anxiety in this particular situation should be used, and different timing of the administration of the second state anxiety test would be advisable. Patients may need more practice to become comfortable with using RT in a threatening situation. However, 70% of the experimental group in this study reported practicing the RT during CC, which suggests that it is easily learned and practiced with minimal time and instruction.

This particular patient sample was hospitalized prior to CC, but an increasing number of patients are undergoing CC on an outpatient basis and are seen by the nurse before the procedure for only a brief time. That limited time frame makes teaching an RT more challenging. The technique proposed by Benson is easily taught in only a few minutes, and patients could practice it during their preparation for CC or while waiting for the procedure to begin. The ability to evoke the relaxation response improves with practice, but there is evidence that benefits may begin immediately.

In Guzzetta's study,[15] peripheral temperatures (a sensitive measure of psychophysiologic relaxation) increased significantly in patients in the relaxation and music groups after each session, including the first, without a cumulative effect over time. Benson indicated in a conversation (April 1988) that benefits begin with the first session. Other studies demonstrate the effectiveness of teaching RT immediately prior to a procedure. Mandle[32] enrolled 35 patients into one of three groups immediately before a scheduled femoral arteriogram. One group was taught to evoke the relaxation response, one group listened to taped music during the procedure, and one group served as a control. The relaxation group had significantly less anxiety, pain, and medication use than either the music or control groups. These findings need to be validated in patients undergoing outpatient CC.

Further research is warranted regarding therapy such as RTs, so that patients can attempt to maintain control during stressful events. Further study of the effects of practicing RT during CC and other diagnostic procedures is needed. Patient completion of the state anxiety test just before, rather than after, CC might yield a truer picture of the effects of RT on the patient's anxiety level.

NURSING IMPLICATIONS

The RT used in this study was easily taught in only a few minutes and was well received by patients. Most patients appreciated having the opportunity to learn an RT. Patients who were randomized to the control group (no RT) expressed disappointment that they would not be taught the RT. The RT subjects enjoyed the one-on-one teaching sessions and thought RT assisted them in relaxing during CC, and they intended to continue to practice the technique after their return home. Patients were judged to be performing RT correctly after only brief instruction by the investigators. Learning the technique was not dependent upon the patient's being able to read.

Nurses should look for creative ways to communicate with patients prior to their outpatient admissions. Nurses in the CC lab could coach patients in an RT as part of their practice. Patients might be taught at the cardiologist's office when their CC procedure is scheduled or when they come in for preadmission testing. Alternatively, pre-CC instruction may be provided over the telephone and/or through written materials, with follow-up teaching the morning of the procedure. Providing an intervention such as relaxation not only is beneficial to patients, but also emphasizes the independent role of the nurse.

For patients who are hospitalized, staff nurses can include RT in their usual CC preparation and teaching. The investigators found that taped instructions were useful for teaching patients the RT. The use of a tape would also decrease the amount of time required of the staff nurse in teaching the patient.

In summary, RTs are useful tools, and they can be easily incorporated into the overall nursing care of the patient. These techniques are independent nursing interventions that can be taught to patients undergoing perceived stressful procedures and can even be taught routinely during hospitalization.

REFERENCES

1. Finesilver C. Preparation of adult patients for cardiac catheterization and coronary cineangiography. *Int J Nurs Stud.* 1978;15:211–221.

2. Holcomb BJ. *Exploring a Cardiac Catheterization.* Detroit, Mich; Wayne State University; 1978. Thesis.

3. Rice VH. *Effects of Need for Personal Control and Information of Strains Associated with a Threatening Event (Cardiac Catheterization). Dissertation Abstracts International* 1982.

4. Bassam M, Marcus H, Ganz W. The effect of mild to moderate mental stress on coronary hemodynamics in patients with coronary artery disease. *Circulation.* 1980;5:933–935.

5. Turton MB, Deegan T, Coulshed N. Plasma catecholamine levels and cardiac rhythm before and after cardiac catheterization. *Br Heart J.* 1977;39:1307–1311.

6. Burch GE, Giles T. Aspects of the influence of psychic stress on angina pectoris. *Am J Cardiol.* 1973;31:108–109.

7. Lesko WA, Summerfield LM. The effectiveness of biofeedback and home relaxation training on reduction of borderline hypertension. *Health Educ.* 1988;19(5):19–22.

8. Agras WS. Relaxation therapy in hypertension. *Hosp Pract.* 1983;129–137.

9. Patel C, Marmot M, Terry D. Controlled trial of biofeedback-aided behavioural methods in reducing mild hypertension. *Br Med J.* 1981;282:2005–2008.

10. Benson H, Marzetta B, Rossner B. Decreased blood pressure associated with the regular elicitation of the relaxation response: A study of hypertensive subjects. *Stress and the Heart.* Mount Kisco, NY: Futura, 1974.

11. Shoemaker J, Tasto D. The effects of muscle relaxation on blood pressure of essential hypertensives. *Behav Res Ther.* 1975;13:29–43.

12. Benson H, Alexander S, Feldman C. Decreased premature ventricular contractions through use of the relaxation response in patients with stable ischemic heart-disease. *Lancet.* 1975;2:380–382.

13. Goldfried M, Trier C. Effectiveness of relaxation as an active coping skill. *J Abnorm Psychol.* 1974;83:348–355.

14. Eliot R, Morales-Ballejo H, Longfellow L, Baker D, Sawyer T, Requa R. The control of stress-induced reactivity by nonpharmacologic techniques: A pilot study. *Qual Life Cardiovasc Care.* 1987;3:87–93.

15. Guzzetta C. Effects of relaxation and music therapy on patients in a coronary care unit with presumptive acute myocardial infarction. *Heart Lung.* 1989;18:609–616.

16. Munro BH, Creamer AM, Haggerty MR, Cooper FS. Effect of relaxation therapy on post-myocardial infarction patients' rehabilitation. *Nurs Res.* 1988;38:231–235.

17. Renfroe K. Effect of progressive relaxation of dyspnea and state anxiety in patients with chronic obstructive pulmonary disease. *Heart Lung.* 1988;17:408–413.

18. Herman J. The effect of progressive relaxation on Valsalva response in healthy adults. *Res Nurs Health.* 1987;10:171–176.

19. Herman J. Valsalva response during progressive relaxation: An extension study. *Scholarly Inquiry for Nursing Practice: An International Journal.* 1989;3:217–226.

20. Pender N. Effects of progressive muscle relaxation training on anxiety and health locus of control among hypertensive adults. *Res Nurs Health.* 1985;8:67–72.

21. Horowitz BF, Fitzpatrick JJ, Flahrety GG. Relaxation techniques for pain relief after open heart surgery. *Dimens Crit Care Nurs.* 1984;3:364–371.

22. Wells N. The effect of relaxation on postoperative muscle tension and pain. *Nurs Res.* 1982;31:236–238.

23. Flaherty G, Fitzpatrick J. Relaxation technique to increase comfort level of postoperative patients. *Nurs Res.* 1978;27:352–355.

24. Donovan M. Relaxation with guided imagery: A useful technique. *Cancer Nurs.* 1980;3(1):27–32.

25. Holden-Lund C. Effects of relaxation with guided imagery on surgical stress and wound healing. *Res Nurs Health.* 1988;11:235–244.

26. Rice V, Caldwell M, Butler S, Robinson J. Relaxation training and response to cardiac catheterization: A pilot study. *Nurs Res.* 1986;35:39–43.

27. Frenn M, Fehring R, Kartes S. Reducing the stress of cardiac catheterization by teaching relaxation. *Dimens Crit Care Nurs.* 1986;5:108–116.

28. Benson H, Beary J, Carol M. The relaxation response. *Psychiatry.* 1974;37:37–45.

29. Beary J, Benson H. A simple psychophysiological technique which elicits the hypometabolic changes of the relaxation response. *Psychosom Med.* 1974;36:115–120.

30. Fried R. Integrating music in breathing training and relaxation: II. Applications. *Biofeedback Self Regul.* 1990;15:171–177.

31. Spielberger CD. *State-Trait Anxiety Inventory.* Palo Alto, Calif: Consulting Psychologists Press; 1983.

32. Mandle CL. *The Use of the Relaxation Response With Patients During Femoral Arteriograms.* Boston, Mass: Boston College; 1988. Dissertation.

The Effects of Guided Imagery on Anxiety Levels and Movement of Clients Undergoing Magnetic Resonance Imaging

Maureen Bryan Thompson, MS, RNC
Family Nurse Practitioner
Newburyport, Massachusetts

Nina M. Coppens, PhD, RN
Professor, Department of Nursing
University of Massachusetts Lowell
Lowell, Massachusetts

Magnetic resonance imaging (MRI) has become an increasingly popular tool for clinical diagnosis. The MRI works by aligning the atomic spins of molecules that make up the human body and then applying a radio frequency field that rotates the spin of the body's atoms away from their equilibrium alignment.[1] The process results in an emission of energy from body tissues, which exposes a photographic plate. This energy allows for detailed images of anatomy and pathology.

Although the procedure is not physically painful, the person undergoing MRI is required to be completely still for 30 minutes or for as much as 2 hours while enclosed in a dark tomblike structure with little space surrounding the body. This experience has been described as being similar to lying in a coffin or being in a mechanical monster.[2] Not surprisingly, anxiety has been noted in people both in anticipation of and during the MRI.[3–5] The constraint of lying still in a confining space has been suggested as one reason for increased anxiety levels.[3–5] Because MRI is very sensitive to motion, it is essential that clients do not move. This movement may necessitate longer scan time or a repeat of the entire procedure.[6]

This research was conducted while the first author was a master's student in the Family and Community Health Nursing Program. The research was supported in part by a University Graduate Student Research Award.

Source: Reprinted from M.B. Thompson and N.M. Coppens, *Holistic Nursing Practice,* Vol. 8, No. 2, pp. 59–69, © 1994, Aspen Publishers, Inc.

Clients have identified their preparation for the MRI experience as absent, incomplete, or misleading.[5] Even without instruction from the health care provider on techniques that could be used during MRI, clients have reported their use of relaxation and visualization of pleasant images in an attempt to cope with the experience.[5] These actions by clients are similar to guided imagery, which has been used as a therapeutic intervention by nurses, other health professionals, and lay people for purposes of relaxation and anxiety reduction.[7] This holistic, noninvasive intervention enables the client to produce a relaxation response by concentrating on a pleasant scene or image. The purpose of this study was to determine the effects of guided imagery on anxiety levels and on movement of clients undergoing MRI.

THEORETICAL FRAMEWORK

Rogers' Science of Unitary Human Beings is proposed as an explanation for the anxiety response to the MRI experience and the therapeutic effects of guided imagery. This holistic world view presents person and environment as irreducible, pandimensional energy fields that are integral with each other while mutually changing with each other.[8] The MRI is an aspect of the environmental field and may create disorganization resulting in a state of disharmony manifested by clients as anxiety. The disharmony created by the enclosed space of the MRI scanner and clients' tendency to reestablish a harmonious pattern may also increase clients' need to change. It is expected that this change is manifested in clients' use of physical movement in an attempt to reestablish their previous more pleasant experience outside the scanning device. By imposing a self-organized pattern through the use of guided imagery, the individual may establish a new more pleasant and peaceful rhythm to the person-environment integrality, thus reducing the amount of anxiety manifested and decreasing the need to move.

Barrett[9] has derived from Rogers' science a theory that focuses on power as the capacity of individuals to participate knowingly in the nature of change. This power is manifested through awareness, choices, freedom to act intentionally, and involvement in creating changes. By providing clients with guidance in the use of guided imagery during MRI, each of these components may be enhanced, thus promoting clients' harmony within the clinical setting.

HYPOTHESES

1. Those subjects who listen to the guided imagery/relaxation tape before their MRI and use guided imagery during their MRI have lower levels of state anxiety than those subjects who do not listen to the guided imagery/relaxation tape and do not use guided imagery during their MRI.
2. Those subjects who listen to the guided imagery/relaxation tape before their MRI and use guided imagery during their MRI are less likely to move during the MRI than those subjects who do not listen to the guided imagery/relaxation tape and do not use guided imagery during their MRI.

REVIEW OF LITERATURE

Brennan and associates[3] found that of 52 adult patients having an MRI, 18 (35%) reported feeling anxious. One-third of the patients who experienced anxiety reported being extremely anxious, and 2% of the total MRI patients needed to have the procedure terminated prematurely. They did not find associations between reported anxiety and age, sex, race, or site of the scan. Another investigation, based on interviews with 26 patients, revealed that 65% had experienced anxiety associated with the MRI.[5] Other researchers have also identified severe psychological reactions to MRI, including long-term claustrophobia.[4,10] These findings indicate that the person undergoing MRI may be at psychological risk, thereby providing support for the need to study therapeutic interventions that may help alleviate anxiety symptoms in those undergoing MRI.

Guided imagery along with relaxation has been found to be an effective intervention in reducing anxiety in a variety of situations. Both graduate[11] and undergraduate[12] nursing students have been able to lower their anxiety through guided imagery. This technique has also been effective among severely burned patients before and after wound treatment[13] and among surgical patients following cholecystectomy.[14] In both of these clinical studies, the experimental group had lower anxiety scores than did the control group.

Only one investigation was identified that specifically examined the effect of guided imagery in reducing clients' anxiety during MRI. Quirk and associates[15] compared the effectiveness of three anxiety-reducing interventions: (1) information about the MRI experience (n = 16), (2) information plus counseling that provided a description of relaxation strategies including visualization (n = 18), and (3) information plus doing a relaxation exercise that included the creation of a visual image of a stroll through a flower garden (n = 16). Although the authors never specified that any of the groups were actually directed to use guided imagery during the MRI, subjects in the second group were told that the described strategies might be useful in managing potential anxiety during the examination, and the third group was told that the exercise they participated in can be recreated at any time without the use of the tape. As with previously cited studies, these researchers used the state portion of the Spielberger State-Trait Anxiety Inventory (STAI) to measure anxiety levels. The questionnaire was completed before they began the intervention, before the MRI, and again immediately following the MRI. On the post questionnaire they were told to report their anxiety during the scan. Those who received "information only" had a significant increase in their anxiety levels from pre-MRI to post-MRI, and those in the other two groups did not have statistically significant changes. However, based on repeated measures analysis of variance (ANOVA), there was a significant interaction between intervention group and time. Those receiving the relaxation plus guided-imagery exercise showed a decrease in anxiety compared to the other two groups. Although this finding supports the use of a guided-imagery exercise before the MRI experience, the report did not specify whether any of the three groups had actually used guided imagery during the MRI experience.

There were no studies located that measured clients' movement during MRI. Butcher and Parker's[16] research, also based on Rogers' science, studied the effects of guided imagery in relation to volunteer staff members' subjective feelings of motion. Explanations suggested for the lack of differences between the experimental and control groups' scores on the Human Field Motion Tool were that the participants may have returned to their normal state by the time they completed the tool, the terminology in the tool may have been confusing, and the subjects had no previous experience with guided imagery.[16] In contrast to their study, our investigation examined reports of actual movement.

With the exception of King's[11] study in which graduate students selected their own image, all of the investigations presented in this review used predetermined guided-imagery scenes. In our investigation, the guided imagery was self-directed by the clients. The primary reason for this self-directness was to encourage the clients' having a sense of power while experiencing a positive mutual process with the environment. A flowing river may be pleasant for one person; however, it may produce the opposite reaction for another person. Second, during the MRI scan, there is a great deal of banging noise, which could interfere with the listening to a guided-imagery tape.

METHODS

An experimental design was used to test the two hypotheses. Randomization of subjects was accomplished by random assignment of days so that subjects scheduled for an MRI on a given day were assigned to either the control or experimental group.

Subjects

The 41 subjects involved in the testing of the hypotheses, 20 in the experimental group and 21 in the control group, met the study's criteria for inclusion. These criteria were that those in the experimental group actually used guided imagery during the MRI, those in the control group did not use guided imagery during the MRI, the MRI scan was completed, and there were no missing data on the measures of anxiety. The subjects were 26 women and 15 men scheduled for a nonemergency MRI at one of two community hospitals in New Hampshire. Both hospitals used the same traveling MRI unit. The age range of the subjects in the experimental group was 22 to 80 years (M = 52, SD = 17) and in the control group was 18 to 79 years (M = 42, SD = 14). A comparison for age differences between the two groups found those in the experimental group to be significantly older ($t = 2.15, df = 37, p = 0.04$, missing information on one person from each group). Comparison of the demographic data between groups by chi-square analyses indicated that the groups were similar with respect to sex, marital status, previous MRI, chronic illness, use of medication, and prior use of relaxation techniques. The average time the subjects were in the MRI scanner was 1 hour. This was similar for the experimental and control groups.

Measures

Anxiety

The STAI was used to measure anxiety levels. It consists of two separate 20-item self-report scales. The trait portion measures the participants' anxiety level in general, whereas the state portion measures anxiety level at the current time. For each item subjects respond to a 4-point scale, ranging from "not at all" to "very much so." The total score for each scale can range from 20 to 80, with a higher score indicating higher anxiety. The trait scores were used to determine the effectiveness of randomization of subjects, and the state scores, to test the hypothesis. Holden-Lund[14] determined the Cronbach alpha of the items on the scales to range from 0.83 to 0.92. The concurrent validity of the scales has been established through correlation

with the Taylor Manifest Anxiety Scale (0.79 to 0.83) and the Institute for Personality and Ability Anxiety Scale (0.75 to 0.77).[17]

Movement during the MRI scan

As part of the routine MRI procedure, the subjects' arms were strapped to their bodies and they were told by the operator not to move. To determine movement during the scan, the MRI operators were asked to monitor the number of times the clients moved during the scan. The operator did not know to which group the subjects were assigned. It was decided on the third day of data collection to add clients' report of their movement. Following the MRI, the subjects were asked by the researcher how many times they moved during the scan. The data on movement were categorized into dichotomous variables: either the subject moved or did not move during the MRI. Subjects' and operators' judgments on movement were compared to estimate concurrent validity of the measures, and each measure was used to test the second hypothesis.

Procedure

Potential participants were called the night before their MRI by the first author. An explanation of the study was given, and they were invited to participate. Those assigned to be in the guided-imagery group were asked to come in 1 hour before their scheduled appointment, and those in the control group were asked to arrive one-half hour early. On arrival questions were answered and written consent and demographic data were obtained. To facilitate consistency, instructions and information were given and questionnaires were administered by the first author. Subjects were asked to complete the initial state anxiety scale and then the trait anxiety scale. The state portion was completed first because it is variable according to the person's present state as compared to the trait portion, which is more stable. All participants were then informed in general terms about the MRI procedure, what to expect, and what they were expected to do, which took 10 to 15 minutes. On the experimental days, the use of guided imagery as a relaxation technique was explained. This group was encouraged to use guided imagery during the MRI with the hope that the procedure would be more pleasant.

At this point the guided-imagery group was left alone to listen to the 10-minute guided-imagery/relaxation tape twice. The tape first brought the participants through 20 seconds of deep breathing and then through 3 minutes of concentrating on relaxing specific body parts. The final 6 minutes encouraged the participants to concentrate on a pleasant scene whether from the past or future. The tape emphasized that this place was safe and peaceful. The participants were encouraged to imagine the colors, sounds, smells, and feelings this place brought to them.

The control group followed the same procedure as the experimental group with the exclusion of discussing guided imagery and listening to the audio tape. Each group was asked to complete the state anxiety scale again before their MRI. The amount of time the participants had to wait before their MRI varied according to scheduling.

Once the MRI was completed, the participants were asked by the first author how many times they thought they moved during the scan. All subjects were then brought back into the waiting area and asked to complete the state anxiety scale for the third time and a brief questionnaire directed at describing their MRI experience as well as any relaxation techniques used during the scan.

RESULTS

The mean trait anxiety scores for the experimental ($M = 37$) and control ($M = 39$) groups were similar ($t = 0.63$, $df = 39$, $p = 0.53$). Scores on the state anxiety scale for the two groups during the three measurement times (initially, before MRI, and after MRI) are presented in Table 1. As with the mean trait anxiety scores, the initial state anxiety scores were similar for the experimental and control groups ($t = 0.40$, $df = 39$, $p = 0.69$), suggesting assignment to groups was random. The experimental group's mean state anxiety scores changed in the expected direction. After listening to the relaxation/guided-imagery tape, the experimental group had an 11.2 drop in their mean state anxiety score, whereas the control group had a drop of only 1.3 after the information session. Although the experimental group's mean state anxiety score was slightly higher following the MRI compared to their mean state score just before the MRI, it continued to be lower than their initial mean score and all three mean scores of the control group.

The distributions of state anxiety scores had a positive skew of 0.195, 0.538, and 0.930 for the three time periods, respectively, indicating more low than high scores, especially following the MRI experience. Log transformations were performed, and the skew in distribution for the last measure was reduced to 0.413. The transformed variables were used to test the first hypothesis.

Table 1. Initial, pre-MRI, and post-MRI state anxiety scores for the experimental guided-imagery group and the control group

State anxiety	Guided imagery (n = 20)			Control (n = 21)		
	Mean	SD	Range	Mean	SD	Range
Initial	40.2	13.0	20–64	38.6	13.0	20–62
Pre-MRI	29.0	10.3	20–51	37.3	11.9	20–60
Post-MRI	31.0	10.5	20–52	33.4	11.7	20–60

SD = standard deviation; MRI = magnetic resonance imaging.

A repeated measures ANOVA, with assigned group as the between-subjects factor and state anxiety scores across the three times as the between-trials factor, was conducted. This multivariate testing of the hypothesis found a significant interaction effect $(f = 15.8, df = 2,38, p < 0.001)$, which provided support for the research hypothesis. The two groups differed in their anxiety levels across time. The difference contrast within the $SPSS^x$ (Statistical Package for the Social Sciences) multivariate analysis of variance (MANOVA) repeated measures program was used to obtain univariate comparisons. The first comparison also substantiated that those subjects who listened to the relaxation/guided-imagery tape experienced a lower level of anxiety than did the control group before the MRI when compared to their initial scores $(t = 5.4, p < 0.001)$. When the combination of the initial state anxiety scores and the pre-MRI scores was contrasted to the scores obtained after the MRI, the significant interaction effect no longer existed $(t = 0.35, p = 0.72)$. This finding suggests that the strong difference in anxiety that existed between the experimental and control groups occurred following the instruction of guided imagery. Although the experimental group continued to have lower anxiety scores than the control group after the MRI, the difference and change across time were no longer statistically significant.

Because mean age was different between the two groups, and age was correlated with state anxiety scores $(n = 39)$ immediately before MRI $(r = -0.36, p < 0.05)$ and after MRI $(r = -0.34, p < 0.05)$, a second repeated measures ANOVA was conducted with age entered as a covariate. Age was not reported by one person in each group; therefore, this analysis was conducted on data from 39 subjects. The significant interaction effect again provided support for the research hypothesis $(f = 14.8, df = 2,36, p < 0.001)$. The univariate comparison between groups across the first and second time periods indicated a difference $(t = 5.1, p < 0.001)$. The level of anxiety was lower for the experimental group compared to the control group following the guided-imagery practice session and before the

MRI. The group scores for times one and two contrasted to scores obtained after the MRI did not achieve statistical significance $(t = 0.03, p = 0.98)$. The findings from this second repeated measures ANOVA with age entered as a covariate were essentially the same as the first analysis.

Correlation coefficients calculated between the trait and state anxiety scores revealed that for the control group, trait anxiety scores were significantly correlated $(p < 0.01)$ with each of the three measures of their state anxiety $(r = 0.57, 0.55,$ and $0.56,$ respectively). However, for the experimental group, trait anxiety was significantly correlated with the initial measure of their state anxiety $(r = 0.61)$ and not with scores from the later two time periods (after guided-imagery instruction, $r = 0.38,$ and following the MRI, $r = 0.21$). These findings suggest that a change occurred in the experimental group's situational specific anxiety response following the introduction of guided imagery in that it no longer correlated with their more general anxiety response.

The second hypothesis was concerned with client movement during the MRI scan. Subjects' report of movement was collected starting on the third day. Thus subject movement scores were based on $n = 15$ for the control group and $n = 16$ for the experimental group. In the control group, 9 subjects (60%) reported that they did not move during the MRI as compared to 15 (94%) in the guided-imagery group who reported that they did not move. For operator-reported movement, analysis was based on 21 in the control group and 19 in the experimental group; 13 subjects (62%) in the control group did not move compared to 17 (89%) in the experimental group. There was strong agreement between subject-reported movement and operator-reported movement $(\chi^2 = 19.9, df = 1, p = < 0.001)$. The guided-imagery group moved less frequently during the MRI than the control group based on subject-reported movement $(\chi^2 = 5.04, df = 1, p = 0.02)$ and operator report of movement $(\chi^2 = 4.04, df = 1, p = 0.04)$; therefore, support was provided for the second hypothesis. Age, although different between the two groups, was not correlated to reported movement by either subjects or operator; therefore, it was not considered in the testing of this hypothesis.

POTENTIAL SUBJECTS NOT INCLUDED IN THE TESTING OF THE HYPOTHESES

Of the 108 clients that were called the night before their MRI, 81 (75%) agreed to participate in the study. Of the 27 (25%) that refused, the most common reasons for refusal were time constraints (18, 67%) and disinterest (6, 22%). Although 81 clients agreed to participate, 19 (23%) did not because of late arrivals or schedule changes on the day of their MRI. Data from an additional 21 participants were excluded from the testing of the hypotheses because they did not meet the criteria for inclusion in the study. This included 11 clients originally in the control group who, on the post questionnaire, indicated that they had used guided imagery to relax during the MRI, 6 clients in the experimental group who reported that they did not use guided imagery to relax during the MRI, 3 clients who did not finish the MRI because of their reported claustrophobia, and 1 client who did not complete the post-MRI questionnaire.

Although they had done the guided-imagery exercise before the scan, clients gave several reasons for why they did not use guided imagery during the MRI. These reasons were that there was too much noise and it was too hard to concentrate, spaced out, unable to do it, did not believe it would help, and felt dizzy. Two of the clients who did not complete the scan were from the control group, and one was from the guided-imagery group. The client from the guided-imagery group completed 12 minutes of the MRI and indicated that she would not have been able to remain in the scanner at all if she was not prepared to use guided imagery. She also mentioned that she would have benefited from more guided-imagery practice time. Her anxiety scores were 54, 41, and 79, respectively. The client who did not complete the post-MRI questionnaire had been in the experimental group. She indicated that she was petrified the last time she had an MRI. This time she felt prepared

and everything was going well with her use of guided imagery during the MRI until she was pulled out, given an injection, and put back in the scanner. She had thought she was finished and was upset that she had not been told this would happen. She commented that she was too upset to complete the questionnaire, but she loved the tape and requested a copy because it was so helpful. Her initial state anxiety score had been 36 and the pre-MRI score, 21, thus providing support that the guided-imagery instruction had lowered her anxiety in preparation for the MRI.

DISCUSSION

The results of this study lend support to Rogers' Science of Unitary Human Beings. The comparatively high mean state scores on the initial measure taken after arrival suggest that subjects had formed an image of the MRI experience that reflected a state of disharmony. Following their use of the guided-imagery/relaxation tape, anxiety was lowered significantly for the experimental group before having the MRI but not for the control group who had only received information. Although the mean state anxiety score of the experimental group did not decrease further following the MRI, it did remain lower than that of the control group. These findings suggest that the use of guided imagery allows for patterning of the human and environmental energy fields from a disharmonious interchange to one that is more harmonious.

The results of our study are in agreement with those of others who have found a positive effect of guided imagery in lowering anxiety. The data also indicated that it is necessary to verify subjects' actual use of guided imagery during the MRI. Quirk and associates[15] did not report whether clients in any of their three groups had actually used guided imagery. Data from our investigation indicate that this cannot be assumed. Several clients were eliminated from the testing of the hypotheses based on their report that they had used guided imagery during their MRI even though they had not been given information on imagery techniques by the researcher or the MRI staff. Although fewer in number, some clients who were given guided-imagery information reported that they had not used this technique during the MRI. The actions of those who were originally in the control group suggest that clients may be using guided imagery in health care settings far more frequently than health professionals realize. Explanations given by clients who were provided with instruction on the technique but did not use guided imagery during the MRI revealed that some clients may need more instruction and practice in guided imagery than they were given as part of this study and that some clients, even with more instruction, may not find this technique useful.

Implications for practice

This study lends support for the use of guided imagery as a therapeutic intervention to reduce the risk of an adverse psychological response to MRI. Nurses can have a major role in introducing guided imagery to their clients. This holistic technique can be readily incorporated into the MRI experience. It could be presented to the client on the day of the MRI, as in our study. An alternative would be to run a guided-imagery session with individuals or groups before the day of the scan and encouraging clients to practice at home.

If frequency of movement during MRI is less likely to occur for those clients using guided imagery, this has clinical and economic implications. The number of unfinished and unclear scans may be reduced as well as the need to repeat the MRI. The cost of providing guided-imagery instruction is low; therefore, this type of intervention should be very cost effective.

Limitations

Even though the subject- and operator-reported frequency of movement were strongly correlated, the validity of these measures can be questioned. The operator could see only one end of the client through the viewing window and therefore could see only certain body movements. This operator was responsible for operation of the MRI and thus could not be constantly watching the client. Subject-reported movement should also be questioned

because the operator instructed the client not to move. Although these instructions were given to both groups, this expectation may have caused the subjects to be reluctant to reveal any movement to the researcher.

When interpreting this study's findings, the conditions of the MRI situation also need to be considered. The banging noise of the MRI as well as the many interruptions during the scans could interfere with the subjects' concentration in using guided imagery. These interruptions numbered anywhere from 5 to 15 times during the MRI and would often include dialogue with the subjects. The operator, in an attempt to reassure the clients, would ask how they were doing and would comment on how many sets of imaging were left and how long each set would be. These interruptions potentially played two roles. Being spoken to may bring the subjects out of the scene they were imaging. The operator would often call the subjects' attention to the physical constraints of the MRI, which may have affected anxiety level. The effect of operator interactions with clients during the scan needs to be tested in future research.

The subjects only had two 10-minute practice sessions of guided imagery before their scan. Guided imagery takes some degree of concentration, especially when one is in an unfamiliar and loud setting. A longer practice session may have contributed to a stronger effect for lowering anxiety and decreasing frequency of movement.

Future research

Although higher than those in the experimental group, the anxiety scores for the control group did show a decrease following the scan. Other researchers have also noted this decrease among clients who did not receive an intervention targeted at lowering anxiety.[5] This decrease could have been due to the situation having changed; the procedure was completed and the clients were no longer in the scanner. In future research clients could be asked to complete the anxiety scale according to how they felt during the MRI as done in the study by Quirk and associates.[15] However, state anxiety as measured by the Spielberger scale is based on how the person feels right now, at this moment. Different indexes of anxiety that may be more holistic in nature and sensitive in detecting changes across time are physiological measures (eg, blood pressure, pulse, respirations) and the Visual Analogue Scale (VAS).[18,19] The VAS is a line, usually 100 mm in length, with end anchors to indicate the extremes of the sensation. Subjects are asked to make an X on the line that depicts the amount of sensation they experienced.

As suggested previously, future research should examine potential differences in the effectiveness of guided imagery for those who receive instruction just before the MRI, as in our investigation, compared to those who receive training and practice before the day of the MRI. Also, an observer whose sole responsibility is to monitor clients' movement should be utilized to enhance the validity of this measure. Another indicator of the effect of movement closely linked to clinical and economic outcomes would be a comparison of the clarity of the experimental and control groups' MRI scans. These studies will further expand on the evaluation of guided imagery as a strategy that can be used to reduce clients' risk of psychological trauma and to promote positive outcomes.

REFERENCES

1. Jones J. Physics of the MR image: from the basic principles to image intensity and contrast. In: Partain C, Price R, Patton J, Kulkarni M, James A Jr, eds. *Magnetic Resonance Imaging, Vol II, Physical Principles and Instrumentation.* 2nd ed. Philadelphia, Penn: WB Saunders; 1988.

2. Notini E. Panic. *The Journal of the American Medical Association.* 1988;259(6):897.

3. Brennan S, Redd W, Jacobsen P, et al. Anxiety and panic during magnetic resonance scans. *Lancet.* 1988;2(8609):512.

4. Flaherty J, Hoskinson K. Emotional distress during magnetic resonance imaging. *New England Journal of Medicine.* 1989;320(7):467–468.

5. Quirk M, Letendre A, Ciottone R, Lingley J. Anxiety in patients undergoing MR imaging. *Radiology.* 1989;170:463–466.

6. Bajakian R. MRI vs. CT scanning for neurologic disorders. *Brigham and Women's Hospital Medical Update.* 1991;3(4):1–5.

7. Vines S. The therapeutics of guided imagery. *Holistic Nursing Practice.* 1988;2(3):34–44.

8. Rogers M. Nursing science and the space age. *Nursing Science Quarterly.* 1992;5(1):27–34.

9. Barrett E. Using Rogers' science of unitary human beings in nursing practice. *Nursing Science Quarterly.* 1988;1(2):50–51.

10. Fishbain D, Goldberg M, Labbe E, Zacher D, Steele-Rosomoff R, Rosomoff H. Long-term claustrophobia following magnetic resonance imaging. *American Journal of Psychiatry.* 1988;145(8):1038–1039.

11. King J. A holistic technique to lower anxiety: relaxation with guided imagery. *Journal of Holistic Nursing.* 1988;6(1):16–20.

12. Stephens R. Imagery: a treatment for nursing student anxiety. *Journal of Nursing Education.* 1992;31(7):314–320.

13. Achterberg J, Kenner C, Lawlis G. Severe burn injury: a comparison of relaxation, imagery and biofeedback for pain management. *Journal of Mental Imagery.* 1988;12(1):71–88.

14. Holden-Lund C. Effects of relaxation with guided imagery on surgical stress and wound healing. *Research in Nursing and Health.* 1988;11:235–244.

15. Quirk M, Letendre A, Ciottone R, Lingley J. Evaluation of three psychologic interventions to reduce anxiety during MR imaging. *Radiology.* 1989;173:759–762.

16. Butcher H, Parker N. Guided imagery within Rogers' science of unitary human beings: an experimental study. *Nursing Science Quarterly.* 1988;1(3):103–110.

17. Spielberger C. *Manual for the State–Trait Anxiety Inventory, STAI Form Y.* Palo Alto, Calif: Consulting Psychologist Press; 1983.

18. Gift A. Visual analogue scales: measurement of subjective phenomena. *Nursing Research.* 1989;38:286–288.

19. Wewers M, Lowe N. A critical review of visual analogue scales in the measurement of clinical phenomena. *Research in Nursing and Health.* 1990;13:227–236.

Music and Pattern Change in Chronic Pain

Julie Anderson Schorr, PhD
Associate Professor
Department of Nursing
Northern Michigan University
Marquette, Michigan

Music hath charms to soothe a savage breast, To soften rocks, or bend a knotted oak.[1(p240)]

—William Congreve

For both chronic pain and rheumatoid arthritis there is a connotation of failure to cure. Both terms suggest change in one's pattern of interaction with the environment, particularly in regard to ability for and freedom of physical movement. The quotation illustrates music's ability to influence the mutual process between people and their environment(s), suggesting movement beyond one's present shape, form, or way of being. Music's inherent relationships among temporal, spatial, and movement patterns reflect infinite potential for patterns of person–environment interaction, manifested through unitary, pandimensional musical experiences. The notion of music as a pandimensional phenomenon with inherent movement potential suggests possibilities for evolving patterns of person–environment interaction that may facilitate transformation of the "savage breast" and "knotted oak" of rheumatoid arthritis. Newman's[2,3] theory of health as expanding consciousness provides a framework for understanding music as a pandimensional phenomenon and vehicle for transformation.

Newman[3] postulates that consciousness is a manifestation of an evolving pattern of person–

Source: Reprinted from J.A. Schorr, *Advances in Nursing Science,* Vol. 15, No. 4, pp. 27–36, © 1993, Aspen Publishers, Inc.

The author thanks Cheryl Morekind, RN, MS, for data collection.

environment interaction. Consciousness is further defined as the informational capacity of the human being, ie, the ability to interact with the environment. According to Newman, consciousness includes the interconnectedness of the entire living system, subsuming cognitive and affective awareness, physiochemical maintenance, growth processes, and the immune system. Newman proposes that this pattern of information is part of a large, undivided pattern of an expanding universe. She further postulates that health and the evolving pattern of consciousness are one and the same, whereby a person is identified by his or her pattern. Each individual's pattern evolves through various permutations of order and disorder, ie, health and disease. The process is one of increasing complexity, with both health and disease manifestations of the evolving pattern.

Synthesizing Young's theory of human evolution, Newman[2] depicts expanding consciousness as beginning with potential consciousness (freedom) and moving through processes of binding in time and centering in space toward a turning point where choice occurs in relation to changes in movement. This turning point of choice/movement enables transcendence of the physical self toward decentering in infinite space and unbinding in timelessness toward an evolutionary ideal of real freedom/absolute consciousness. Thus, Newman is suggesting that people come into being from a state of potential consciousness, are bound in time, find identity in space, and through movement learn how things work and make choices that ultimately take them beyond space and time to a state of absolute consciousness.

Newman postulates that development of the physical self is necessarily binding in time and space and that movement provides a means of controlling one's environment. She suggests that as physical disability engenders restriction in body movement, losses of freedom become more apparent. As such, the restrictions in movement/space/time force an awareness that extends beyond the physical self. Newman proposes that such awareness occurs when patterns of interaction that worked in the past are no longer effective. Thus in order to survive, the person seeks new and different answers, reflecting a limitation of self that concurrently becomes a process of inner growth, a transformation.[2]

Building on Newman's postulates and incorporating the notions of Prigogine,[4,5] the process of transformation, or consciousness, can be conceptualized as a dissipative structure.[6] Consciousness, or the process of transformation, may be considered a primary manifestation of the underlying pattern of the human field, incorporating patterns of time, space, and motion. Time and space are viewed as equivalent phenomena as are motion and perception. Time and space are experienced through motion and perception. Consciousness, or transformation, reflects patterning among time, space, and motion and is manifested through the individual's mutual process with the environment. Manifest patterns reflect the underlying dissipative structure of consciousness, which changes as perturbations occur within the relationships among temporal, spatial, and motion patterns. Space within consciousness expands with new experiences and knowledge. This expansion generates energy flow, which is manifested through perturbations and the extension of space into time as knowledge and experiences are synthesized. Motion and perception, as equivalent phenomena, reflect awareness of changes in patterns of time and space. Thus, as knowledge and experiences are synthesized, perturbations may be experienced as alterations in thinking, disturbances in space–time sense, changes in body image, distortions of perception, changes in meaning or significance, a sense of the ineffable, feelings of rejuvenation, and hypersuggestibility.[7,8] A sudden reorganization occurs as the informational capacity of the individual increases in complexity and increasingly diverse patterns of behavior emerge. As the complexity of the dissipative structure increases, energy consumption increases. Perturbations that occur are stronger, thus the fragility of the dissipative structure of consciousness increases. As higher order forms of energy in the form of information occur within the mutual process between person and environment, higher order dissipative structures of consciousness or transformations emerge, and the complexity and diversity of time, space, and motion patterns increase. The individual experiences expanding consciousness, patterns of behavior change, and awareness of the pandimensional nature of life emerges.[6]

Within this framework, changes in time–space–motion patterns, ie, patterned environmental resonance, may precipitate a shift in consciousness, a transformation. Perturbations or disruptions in movement patterns may be expressed through changes in manifest patterns of consciousness. Thus, imposed perturbations or disruptions in patterns of movement via exposure to patterned environmental resonance may be reflected by changes in indicators to consciousness, including perceptual phenomena such as the experience of pain.

Newman[3] suggests that recognition of the pattern of a perceptual or movement phenomenon and its action potential provides the framework for nursing practice. Pattern recognition is proposed as essential to the process of evolving to higher levels of consciousness. When it occurs, it makes explicit the possibilities for action. Nursing facilitates this pattern recognition process by rhythmic connecting with people in an authentic way for the purpose of illuminating the pattern and discovering the new rules of a higher level of consciousness.

The experience of chronic pain and its associated restriction of physical movement by people with rheumatoid arthritis illuminates the tenets of the theory. Recognition of an inevitable pattern of intractable pain over the course of one's life may be viewed as a key to higher levels of consciousness rather than as an inability to eliminate a disease process and pain. Realization and integration of the fact that chronic pain is a manifestation of the disease may illuminate the possibilities for action. As Newman states, "It is like the difference between being in the dark and turning on the light: when the light comes on, one can see the possibilities for movement."[3(p40)] Thus, the pain pattern of rheumatoid arthritis

may be viewed as an evolving pattern of the whole, with action potentials to be uncovered.

The use of patterned environmental resonance in the form of music may provide an avenue toward uncovering action potentials within the pain patterns of individuals with rheumatoid arthritis. In a study comparing the effects of quiet ambient sounds and harmonic sounds of music on the perception of rest, Smith[9] found that patterned environmental resonance using varied harmonic sounds significantly increased the perception of restedness. A relaxation response to the use of sedative or patterned music has also been described. This relaxation response includes decreases in heart and respiratory rate, muscle relaxation, sleep, decreased oxygen consumption, lowered metabolic rates, and a reduction in circulating corticosteroids.[10–14] In addition, psychophysiologic processes, including endorphin release, autogenic conditioning and distraction, may be activated by patterned environmental resonance.[15–19] Thus, the literature supports the notion that music may facilitate movement through various permutations of order and disorder (health and disease) manifested via changes in consciousness and perception of pain.

Gaston[11] describes sedative music as characterized by a regular rhythm, predictable dynamics, harmonic consonance, and recognizable vocal and instrumental timbre. As such, sedative music may be conceptualized as patterned environmental resonance, amenable to the pattern recognition process described by Newman.[3] Music, therefore, may provide the "light" that enables the person with rheumatoid arthritis to see the "possibilities for movement" beyond the personal restrictions in physical movement.[3] Music may also provide a means through which nurses might rhythmically connect with people in an authentic way, thereby illuminating the pattern of pain and assisting in the discovery of new rules for movement (ie, action potentials) beyond physical movement. In turn, the discovery of new action potentials facilitates movement to higher levels of consciousness, ie, evolving patterns of person–environment interaction, transformations.

BACKGROUND

The literature is replete with studies of pain, the pain experience, and nursing interventions designed to relieve pain.[15,20–31] The theme that emerges from these studies reflects a conceptualization of pain as an overwhelmingly negative human experience. Chronic pain in particular is characterized as failure by both health care providers and by "victims."

The effects of patterned environmental sound (ie, music) on physiologic and emotional responses to various human experiences have been investigated in several studies. Updike[32] explored the physiologic and psychologic effects of music therapy as a holistic nursing intervention. In critically ill intensive care unit (ICU) patients, Updike reported significant reductions in systolic blood pressure, mean arterial pressure, and the double product index after listening to taped music selections. In addition, patients' moods shifted significantly in the direction of a more desirable state of well-being, with significant reductions in anxiety and depression, and a diminished pain experience. Frank[33] and Cook[34] reported reductions in nausea and vomiting following music therapy among cancer patients undergoing chemotherapy. These authors suggest that music therapy may be an effective potentiator with antiemetic agents. Studies by Smith and Morris,[35] Peretti and Zweifel,[36] and Moss[37] report conflicting results regarding the effects of various types of music on anxiety. However, Peretti and Zweifel suggest that the subjects' preferences regarding type of music used rather than arbitrary labeling by the investigator as to type (sedative or stimulative) is a significant factor. In addition, Davis-Rollans and Cunningham[38] reported a significant decrease in heart rate and an improvement in mood state among cardiac patients in response to classical music.

Thus, the literature supports the notion that music as patterned environmental resonance influences the interconnectedness of the entire living system, subsuming cognitive and affective awareness, physiochemical maintenance, growth processes, and the immune system; ie, the consciousness of the human being, the ability of a person to interact with the environment.[3]

PURPOSE

The purpose of this exploratory study, therefore, was to investigate the use of music as a unitary–transformative means of altering the perception of chronic pain among women with rheumatoid arthritis within the context of Newman's model of health as expanding consciousness. It was hypothesized that the pain perception threshold would increase with the use of music as a unitary–transformative nursing intervention.

METHODS

Subjects

The sample for this repeated measures investigation consisted of 30 female volunteers who had been diagnosed with rheumatoid arthritis for a minimum of 6 months. Subjects were solicited from the practices of private physicians in a medium-sized city in the western United States, were able to read and speak English, and were capable of giving informed consent.

Instruments

The McGill Pain Questionnaire[39] (MPQ) was used to measure subjects' perceived pain thresholds. The MPQ provides information regarding the human pain experience through the use of descriptions of the present pain pattern and the present pain index. The MPQ asks subjects "What does your pain feel like now?" and consists of 78 words, each assigned a numerical value from one to five, that are sensory, affective, or evaluative in nature. The MPQ was designed to provide quantitative measures of the human pain experience. It generates several pain rating indices based on two types of numerical values that may be assigned to each word descriptor, the number of words chosen to describe the present pain experience, and the present pain intensity based on a 1 to 5 scale. Specifically, the Pain Rating Index, based on subjects' mean scale values consisting of the total words chosen in a given category (sensory, affective, evaluative) or in all categories, is designated as the Pain Rating Intensity scale (PRI[s]). The Pain Rating Index, based on the rank value of the words chosen, is designated as the Pain Rating Intensity–Rank (PRI[R]). The Number of Words Chosen (NWC) represents the sum of all words selected by the subjects as descriptive of their pain experience. The final measure generated is the Present Pain Intensity (PPI), which is based on a 1 to 5 intensity scale. The PPI is recorded as a number from one to five in which each number is associated with the following words: 1 = mild, 2 = discomforting, 3 = distressing, 4 = horrible, 5 = excruciating. According to McGuire,[20] extensive research and a multitude of pain measurement instruments support the MPQ as both a reliable and valid indicator of clinical pain. For the purpose of this study, the PPI was used to determine that subjects were experiencing some degree of pain. The PRI(R) and the NWC were utilized for analysis since these scores presented a more synthesized or unitary view of the overall pain experience.

Procedure

Following human subjects' approval, names of potential volunteers who met the preestablished criteria for inclusion in the study were solicited from collaborating physicians. Following referral from physicians, prospective subjects were contacted by telephone to request their participation in the research study. During the telephone interview, the potential subject was asked to identify temporal pain patterns (Can you tell me when you usually experience pain?) so that an appointment could be scheduled during a peak pain period. If the subject agreed to participate in the study, an interview date and time were scheduled. All interviews took place in the subjects' homes at their convenience. Each potential subject was asked to identify her favorite type of music and whether she had a cassette tape that could be used during the

intervention. If each subject had a tape with her favorite music, it was used during the intervention. If she did not, a cassette tape of the type of music preferred by the subject was provided by the researcher for use during the intervention.

Informed consent was obtained at the beginning of the scheduled interview, and subjects completed both demographic information and the MPQ, including the PPI. Subjects were then directed to begin playing the music using a small portable cassette player, to set the volume to a preferred level, and to assume as comfortable a position as possible. Subjects listened to the music for an uninterrupted period of 20 minutes, at which point they were directed to complete the MPQ (What does your pain feel like now?) again. Following completion of the second MPQ, the music was terminated. Subjects completed the MPQ again in 2 hours.

Analysis of the data

Demographic characteristics of the sample are presented in Table 1. Unless otherwise noted, n = 30. Information describing the extent to which the interview occurred during peak pain periods is presented in Table 1 (choice of single word to describe pain right now, at its worst, at its least). Descriptive statistics are presented in Table 2.

Data were analyzed using repeated measures analysis of variance for each variable. While the underlying particulate assumptions of quantitative methods may appear incongruent with the underlying unitary assumptions of the theoretical model in this study, repeated measures analysis of variance (ANOVA), with its focus on comparing differences within subjects as opposed to differences between subjects, was viewed as useful in answering the question posed in this exploratory investigation. Paired *t*-tests were selected as the method of choice for post hoc analysis of the differences between pairs of means at the various treatment levels for each variable. With a repeated measures design, the means are highly correlated and the variance among means is homogeneous. Thus, the paired

Table 1. Demographic characteristics (n = 30)

Category	Frequency	Category	Frequency
Age (years)		Occasional need to stop all	
31–40	2	work due to pain	
41–50	2	Yes	23
51–60	12	No	7
61–81	14	Frequency of need to stop all	
		work due to pain	
Years of pain		Daily	14
1–5	4	Weekly	11
6–10	7	Monthly	5
11–15	6		
16–35	13	*Pain description*	
		Choice of word group to	
Ethnic background		describe pain	
White	27	Continuous, steady, constant	16
Hispanic	1	Rhythmic, periodic,	
Native American	2	intermittent	13
		Brief, momentary, transient	1
Marital status		Choice of single word to describe	
Not married	2	Pain right now	
Married	21	Mild	9
Divorced/separated	2	Discomforting	11
Widowed	5	Distressing	6
		Horrible	3
Number of children		Excruciating	1
None	5	Pain at its worst	
1–2	9	Mild	0
3–5	15	Discomforting	0
6 or more	1	Distressing	5
		Horrible	5
Pain and work/activity pattern		Excruciating	20
Type of work		Pain at its least	
Housewife	21	Mild	21
Office	4	Discomforting	8
Service	2	Distressing	1
Professional	3	Horrible	0
Ability to work outside of home		Excruciating	0
Able	9		
Unable	21		

t-test approach, considered to be more powerful under such circumstances, was utilized in favor of the Tukey or Scheffe, since the latter approaches are more appropriately used with independent means. Hotelling's T² may have been an appropriate method had there been two or more variables in the repeated measures design. Since each variable in this study was examined individually, this method was also considered to be not appropriate. Given the high level of significance obtained for each variable in this study, the possibility of Type I error associated with the use of multiple *t*-tests is minimized.

Repeated measures ANOVA regarding the PRI(R) yielded an F of 32.67, which was significant at the <0.001 level. Paired *t*-tests indicated significant differences between the PRI(R) at premusic and during music, between the PRI(R)

Table 2. Descriptive statistics (n = 30)

	Mean	SE*
PRI(R)*		
Premusic	24.87	2.23
During music	9.93	1.52
Postmusic	16.67	2.44
NWC*		
Premusic	11.27	.77
During music	5.93	.84
Postmusic	8.23	.96

*PRI(R) = Pain Rating Intensity–Rank; SE = standard error of mean; NWC = Number of Words Chosen.

at premusic and postmusic, and between the PRI(R) during music and postmusic. Specific results are presented in Table 3.

Repeated measures ANOVA regarding the NWC yielded an F of 18.23, which was significant at the <0.001 level. Paired *t*-tests indicated significant differences between the NWC at premusic and during music, between the NWC at premusic and postmusic, and between the NWC during music and postmusic. Specific results are presented in Table 4.

DISCUSSION

Results of the study indicate that the pain perception threshold increased while subjects lis-

tened to music for a period of time following the intervention. In this study, it appears that patterned environmental resonance may have enabled subjects to move beyond their pain, at least for the duration of the intervention experience. These results are congruent with those of McDonald,[40] who examined the relationship between visible light waves and the experience of pain among women, ages 40 to 60 years, with rheumatoid arthritis. McDonald reported that subjects exposed to shorter, higher frequency waves (blue light) were more likely to experience a reduction in pain than women exposed to either longer, lower frequency waves (red light) or a control condition of ambient light. In addition, McDonald's results indicated that the longer the exposure to blue light, the progressively greater the reduction in pain.

The interventions used in the present study and in McDonald's study both reflect the notion of energy as wavelength and the influence of the frequency of that wavelength on the human experience of pain. Subjects in both studies were women, primarily between 40 and 60 years of age, who were experiencing pain patterns associated with rheumatoid arthritis. Capra[41] postulates that wavelength and its frequency define a particle's state of motion. Ference[42] extends Capra's postulate to the human energy field and suggests that frequency of environmental energy waves (ie, visible light waves and sound waves)

Table 3. Pain Rating Intensity–Rank [PRI(R)]

	Paired t-tests	
Level	t	P
Premusic During music	9.09	0.000
Premusic Postmusic	4.08	0.000
During music Postmusic	3.47	<0.01

Repeated measures ANOVA: F = 32.67, P<0.001.

Table 4. Number of Words Chosen (NWC)

	Paired t-tests	
Level	t	P
Premusic During music	8.50	0.000
Premusic Postmusic	4.06	0.000
During music Postmusic	2.99	<0.01

Repeated measures ANOVA: F = 18.23, P<0.001.

may transform the pattern of that human field. The interventions used in both studies may be construed as unitary–transformative in nature, reflecting the notion of patterned environmental resonance and its ability to transform the pattern of the person. It appears that patterned environmental resonance may increase the motion within the current dissipative structure, in this instance of pain, thereby precipitating a transformation of the pattern toward one of comfort and the emergence of diverse knowledge and experiences (ie, action potentials) not previously accessible. Ference[42] theorizes that human field motion is the essential dimension of transformation, proposing relationships among humor, imagery, sound frequency, breathing, and field touch. Congruent with the theoretical underpinnings of this study, Ference suggests that change occurs as human field motion increases, thereby transforming the pattern of the person and the mutual process between the person and the environment, with movement from a pattern of pain toward a pattern of comfort.

As such, the results of this exploratory study generate preliminary support for the use of music as a pain management or healing strategy for women with rheumatoid arthritis and for the theoretical constructs proposed by Newman.[3] However, further study is necessary to explicate Newman's theory of health more fully as expanding consciousness and the model of consciousness as a dissipative structure. Specification and utilization of unitary measurements for unitary, pandimensional, transformative phenomena are critical. Inclusion of the Human Field Motion Tool[43] might have strengthened the study by providing a unitary measure of the underlying motion of the human energy field and any changes in that motion. In addition, one 20-minute period of listening to music, while associated with reduction in the experience of pain, is likely not sufficient to engender a transformation. Future studies might consider a longitudinal approach so that both pain pattern change and human field motion change might be explicated. Additional measures of the human pain experience that may be integrative or unitary in nature, such as visual analogue scales or auditory analogue approaches such as auditory sensory matching, should also be considered for further investigation into strategies with the potential to facilitate moving beyond one's present shape, form, or way of being, ie, to transform, to heal, "to soothe a savage breast, to soften rocks, or bend a knotted oak."[1(p240)]

REFERENCES

1. Congreve W. The mourning bride, I,1. In: Davidoff H, ed. *The Pocket Book of Quotations.* New York, NY: Pocket Books; 1952.

2. Newman MA. *Health as Expanding Consciousness.* St. Louis, Mo: Mosby; 1986.

3. Newman MA. Newman's theory of health as praxis. *Nurs Sci Q.* 1990;3(1):37–41.

4. Prigogine I. Time, structure and fluctuation. *Science.* 1978;201:777–785.

5. Prigogine I. *Order Out of Chaos.* New York, NY: Bantam Books; 1984.

6. Schorr JA, Schroeder CA. Consciousness as a dissipative structure: an extension of the Newman model. *Nurs Sci Q.* 1989;2(4):183–193.

7. Ludwig AM. Altered states of consciousness. In: Tart CT, ed. *Altered States of Consciousness.* New York, NY: Wiley; 1969.

8. Tart CT. *States of Consciousness.* New York, NY: EP Dutton; 1975.

9. Smith MJ. Human–environment process: a test of Rogers' principle of integrality. *ANS.* 1986;9(1):21–28.

10. Bonny HL. *The Role of Taped Music Program in the Guided Imagery in Music (GIM) Process.* Baltimore, Md: ICM Press; 1978.

11. Gaston ET. Dynamic factors in mood change. *Music Educators J.* 1951;37:43–44.

12. Benson HL. *The Relaxation Response.* New York, NY: Avon Books; 1975.

13. Jacobson HL. A study of the effects of sedative music on the tension, anxiety, and pain experienced by mental patients during dental procedures. Lawrence, Kan: University of Kansas; 1976. Thesis.

14. Rider MS, Floyd JW, Kirkpatrick J. Effect of music, imagery and relaxation on adrenal corticosteroids and

reentrainment of circadian rhythms. *J Music Therapy.* 1985;22(1):48–58.

15. Gardner W, Licklider JCR, Weisz AZ. Suppression of pain by sound. *Science.* 1960;132:32–33.

16. Goldstein A. Opioid peptides (endorphins) in pituitary and brain. *Science.* 1976;193:42–58.

17. Goldstein A. Thrills in response to music and other stimuli. *Physiol Psychol.* 1980;8:1.

18. Clark ME, McCorkle RR, Williams S. Music therapy assisted labor and delivery. *J Music Therapy.* 1981;18: 88–100.

19. Chandler C. Hypoanesthesia and analgesia. *J Am Assoc Nurse Anesth.* June 1980;241–247.

20. McGuire DB. The measurement of clinical pain. *Nurs Res.* 1984;33(3):152–156.

21. Turner JA, Chapman CR. Psychological interventions for chronic pain: a critical review/relaxation training and biofeedback. *Pain.* 1982;12(1):1–21.

22. Wolfe DE. Pain rehabilitation and music therapy. *J Music Therapy.* 1978;14(4):162–178.

23. Rider MS. Entrainment mechanisms involved in pain reduction, muscle relaxation, and music-mediated imagery. *J Music Therapy.* 1985;22(4):183–192.

24. Kim S. Pain: theory, research and nursing practice. *ANS.* 1980;2(2):43–59.

25. Johnson J, Rice V. Components of pain: sensory and distress. *Nurs Res.* 1974;23:203–209.

26. Huhman M. Endogenous opiates and pain. *ANS.* 1982;4(4):62–71.

27. Fordyce WE, Lansky K, Calsyn DA, Shelton JL, Stolov WC, and Rock DL. Pain measurement and pain behavior. *Pain.* 1984;18:53–69.

28. McGuire DB. The perception and experience of pain. *Semin Oncol Nurs.* 1985;1(2):83–86.

29. Holm K, Cohen F, Dudas S, Medema PG, Allen BL. Effects of personal pain experience on pain assessment. *Image.* 1989;21(2):72–75.

30. Cohen FL. Postsurgical pain relief: patients' status and nurses; medication choices. *Pain.* 1980;9(2):265–274.

31. Kolcaba KY. Holistic comfort: operationalizing the construct as a nurse-sensitive outcome. *ANS.* 1992;15(1):1–10.

32. Updike P. Music therapy results for ICU patients. *Dimens Crit Care Nurs.* 1990;9(1):39–45.

33. Frank JM. The effects of music therapy and guided visual imagery on chemotherapy induced nausea and vomiting. *Oncol Nurs Forum.* 1985;12(5):47–52.

34. Cook JD. Music as an intervention in the oncology setting. *Cancer Nurs.* 1986;9(1):23–28.

35. Smith CA, Morris LW. Effects of stimulative and sedative music on cognitive and emotional components of anxiety. *Psychol Rep.* 1976;38:1187–1193.

36. Peretti PO, Zweifel J. Effect of musical preference on anxiety as determined by physiological skin responses. *Acta Psychiatr Belg.* 1983;83:437–442.

37. Moss VA. The effect of music on anxiety in the surgical patient. *Perioperative Nurse Q.* 1987;3(1):9–16.

38. Davis-Rollans C, Cunningham S. Physiologic responses of coronary care patients to selected music. *Heart Lung.* 1987;16:370–378.

39. Melzack R. The McGill pain questionnaire: major properties and scoring methods. *Pain.* 1975;1:277–299.

40. McDonald SF. The relationship between visible lightwaves and the experience of pain. In: Malinski VM, ed. *Explorations on Martha Rogers' Science of Unitary Human Beings.* Norwalk, Conn: Appleton-Century-Crofts; 1986.

41. Capra F. *The Tao of Physics.* Boulder, Colo: Shambhala; 1983.

42. Ference HM. The theory of motion. *Nursing Science Institutes Monograph.* Carmel, Calif: Nightingale Society; 1988.

43. Ference HM. *Human Field Motion Tool Word Form.* Pebble Beach, Calif: HM Ference Co; 1988.

An Introduction to Music Therapy: Helping the Oncology Patient in the ICU

Kelly Johnston, MSN, RN, CCRN
Staff Nurse
Department of Nursing
Ann Arbor Veterans Administration Hospital
Ann Arbor, Michigan

Jacqueline Rohaly-Davis, MS, RN, OCN
Staff Nurse
Edward J. Hines Jr. Veterans Administration
  Hospital
Hines, Illinois

Intensive care units (ICUs) are probably the most frightening and threatening environment in the hospital to patients and families.[1] Some of the common components of an ICU that may cause fear or anxiety in an individual include: sensory overload in terms of sounds and number of individuals attending to the patient, sensory monotony in terms of repetitious sights and sounds, absence of familiar individuals, and lack of day–night sequence. Other components include the physical and emotional discomfort of the illness, lack of privacy, medications interfering with cognitive processes, and illness and death of other patients.[2] Music therapy is a noninvasive intervention that offers a means of creating familiarity and a source of comfort for the ICU patient. It is an intervention that ICU nurses can initiate to support a holistic approach in caring for the critically ill.[3] The purpose of this article is to introduce the ICU nurse to music therapy as an alternative therapy for the critically ill patient.

Music therapy has been around for centuries. Music and medicine have been linked throughout history. According to Greek mythology, Orpheus was given a lyre by Apollo (the god of music) and was taught how to use it by the muses: hence the word music. Apollo's son Aesculapius was the god of healing and medicine. The Greeks believed that music had the power to heal the body and soul.[4]

Source: Reprinted from K. Johnston and J. Rohaly-Davis, *Critical Care Nursing Quarterly,* Vol. 18, No. 4, pp. 54–60, © 1996, Aspen Publishers, Inc.

Throughout history, music therapy has been used in a variety of clinical settings as a noninvasive therapeutic modality to promote relaxation and pain control. It was first used in World War II to help the recovery of shell-shocked soldiers.[5] Some of the clinical settings in which music has been used include: coronary care, surgery, postanesthesia recovery, and neonatal intensive care units.[6] It has also been used as soothing background music in hospital waiting areas, dentist and physician's offices, nursing homes, delivery suites, psychiatric settings, occupational and physical therapy, oncology units, and operating rooms.[5,7]

DEFINITION OF MUSIC THERAPY

Music therapy is defined as the "controlled use of music and its influence on the human being in physiologic, psychologic, and emotional integration of the individual during treatment of an illness or disability."[5(p37)] Music therapy is also defined as a "behavioral science that is concerned with the use of specific kinds of music and its ability to produce changes in behavior, emotions, and physiology."[7(p610)]

REVIEW OF LITERATURE

Historically, the use of music has been well documented, and scientific studies have shown physiologic benefits, as well as psychologic benefits, both invaluable in an intensive care environment.[8] Music has been a successful intervention in the oncology setting in ameliorating chemotherapy-induced nausea and vomiting.[9] There are several studies looking at the effects of music therapy, but there is limited information specific to the critical care population. Several authors noted the beneficial effects of music therapy in patients with acute pain. Munro and Mount[10] demonstrated in their study of chronic pain that music was useful in palliative care to break the vicious cycles of pain exacerbations. They found an overall decrease in intensity of the pain experience. This study supports the beneficial effect music may have on the psychologic dimension of the cancer pain experience.[10]

Moss[11] in her study of seventeen 1-day surgery patients reported a significant decrease in postoperative anxiety among adults who received music therapy. The subjects were assigned to an experimental or control group. They chose music from four selections. Music was started after the preoperative injection, played throughout surgery, and discontinued when they reached the postanesthesia care unit. Many of the participants commented positively on the experience.

Several studies demonstrated a reduction of heart rate and blood pressure with sedative music.[3,10,12,13] Stone et al[14] investigated the physiologic and psychologic effects of music therapy on critically ill patients in the ICU (11 males and 11 females). Patient music preferences that were utilized for the study included jazz, popular, classical, new age, gospel, soft rock, and country western. Their study indicated that music therapy positively affects the critically ill patient by reducing heart rate, systolic blood pressure, pain, and anxiety.

Herth,[16] a nursing coordinator of a 40-bed medical–surgical unit, did a 6-month study on music therapy. Her unit staff utilized a random case study protocol. They did a music history on admission, then played music 5 minutes prior to painful activities (ie, getting out of bed after surgery and exercising). They found a 30% decrease in the use of pain medication by those patients who listened to music when experiencing pain. Guzetta's study[7] consisted of 80 cardiac care unit patients in three eastern United States hospitals admitted with a presumptive diagnosis of anterior myocardial infarction. The subjects were randomly selected to one of three groups: music therapy group, relaxation group, or control group. The relaxation group received a relaxation technique 20 minutes twice a day for a total of 3 sessions over a 2-day period. The music therapy group received music following the same schedule. She found that patients had fewer cardiac complications than expected when exposed to music.

Guzetta[7] found in her study that 92.5% of the participants found music to be extremely helpful, and 94.3% said music would be extremely helpful for future patients. Participants (77.4%) said they would continue with the music after they went to a non-ICU setting/step-down unit or home. Most of the participants said they enjoyed the music therapy and that it helped them to relax during their coronary care unit admission.

Downey and Flood[17] completed studies highlighting myocardial infarction patients using music in an intensive care setting. They reported that an intensive care patient may benefit from mental diversion using intermittent background music. They also noted a reduction of mortality rate from 20% to 8% to 12% after music was introduced into the intensive care setting.

The literature frequently identifies pain and anxiety as common concerns of all patients as well as of medical staff. Pain is defined as a complex subjective phenomenon that has interacting physiologic, psychologic, social, cultural, and spiritual components. Meinhart and McCafferty define pain as "whatever the experiencing person says it is, exiting whenever he says it does."[18(p377)] An anxiety state is defined in terms of the intensity of subjective feelings of tension, apprehension, nervousness, and worry experienced by an individual at a particular moment and by heightened activity of the autonomic nervous system that accompanies the feelings.[19]

Music Therapy Plan of Care

Alteration in comfort: anxiety	The patient will demonstrate positive psychologic outcomes in response to music therapy: decreased anxiety/depression, decreased restlessness/agitation, increase in motivation.
Nursing intervention	1. Assess patient's level of anxiety, restlessness, agitation, and motivation. 2. Assess patient's interest in music. 3. Assess patient's music preference. 4. Provide a quiet milieu; dim lights; close drapes; assist patient to a comfortable position. 5. Avoid interruptions for a designated period. 6. Play music for 20–30 minute intervals BID. 7. Evaluate patient's subjective and objective responses to music.
Alterations in comfort: pain	The patient will demonstrate decrease in pain: verbalize improvement in pain using a 0–5 scale; use less pain medication.
Nursing interventions	1. Assess patient's pain using a 0–5 scale in which 0 is no pain and 5 is severe pain. 2. Medicate as prescribed. 3. Assess patient's interest in music therapy. 4. Assess patient's music preferences. 5. Provide a quiet milieu; dim lights; close drapes; assist patient to a comfortable position. 6. Avoid interruptions for a designated amount of time. 7. Play music for 20–30 minute intervals BID. 8. Evaluate patient's subjective and objective responses to music.

Totas,[20] in her study observing anxiety levels in preoperative patients, found that high preoperative anxiety levels increase the cardiac work load and diminish cardiac reserve. Therefore, it is imperative that anxiety levels be reduced to prevent adverse physiologic and psychologic outcomes. Cassem and Hackett[21] identified anxiety as a major management problem among the critical care population. Factors that have been identified to contribute to anxiety levels in patients include the admission/transfer to the ICU, the nature of the illness, the environment, and the interaction with the staff. Other contributing factors are visiting hours, interrupted sleep, use of the bedpan/urinal, and noise in the unit.[22] It is believed by these authors that reducing anxiety will decrease the potentially

Suggested Music Selections

Popular
Cat Stevens—Morning Is Broken
Big Bands—Smoke Rings
Nat King Cole—Red Sails
Anderson—Trumpeter's Lullaby
John Denver—It's Up To You

Movie Sound Track
Born Free
Chariots of Fire
The Sound of Music

Country-Western
Willie Nelson
—Star Dust
—Sweet Memories
—Moonlight in Vermont

Guitar
Will Ackerman—Childhood and
  Memories
Passage

Symphonic
Kitaro—Silk Road Suite

Piano
George Winston
—Autumn
—December
—Winter into Spring

Religious
Mormon Tabernacle Choir—The
  Old Beloved Songs
—The Lord Is My Shepherd

Classical
Bach—Air for G String
Beethoven—Moonlight Sonata
Bizet—Intermezzo from Carmen
  Suite
Brahms—Lullaby
Chopin—Nocturne in G
Canteloube—Songs of the
  Auvergne Brezairola
Debussy—Clair de Lune
Dvorak—Serenade for Strings
  Larghetto
Haydn—Minuet from Berenice
Liszt—Liebestraum
Marcello—Oboe Concerto in
  Dm Adagio

Classical
Mascagni—Cavalleria
  Rusticana Intermezzo
Massenet—Scenes
Alsaciennes—Sous let Tilleuls
Mendelssohn—A Midsummer
  Night's Dream
Pachelbel—Canon in D
Respighi
—Pines of Rome
—The Pines of Giancolo
Saint-Saens—The Swan
Tchaikovsky—Panorama from
  Sleeping Beauty
Vaughn-Williams—Fantasia on
  Greensleeves
Villa Lobos—Brasileiras #5
Vivaldi—Concerto in B Flat M
  Andante

Source: Dated from Bonny H, Savary L. *Music and Your Mind.* New York: Harper & Row; 1978; Bolwerk CA. Effects of relaxing music on state anxiety in myocardial infarction patients. *Crit Care Nurs Q.* 1990;13:65–72; Heitz L, Symreng T, Scamman FL. Effect of music therapy in the postanesthesia care unit: a nursing intervention. *J Postanesthesia Nurs.* 1992;7:22–31; and O'Sullivan RJ. A musical road to recovery: music in intensive care. *Intens Care Nurs.* 1991;7:160–163.

harmful physiologic outcomes. One such method to decrease anxiety will be implementation of music therapy.

GOALS

The goal of music therapy is the reduction of psychophysiologic stress, pain, anxiety, and isolation.[7] This can be achieved by diverting the person's attention away from pain and refocusing on something more pleasant.[12,23,24]

The effects of music therapy on hospitalized surgical, obstetric, oncology, and pediatric patients have been well documented in nursing literature. However, there are limited publications on the effects of music therapy in the critically ill patient population.[14] The literature identifies a variety of advantages that music therapy offers to patients. Alvin[25] noted that music can be used as a means of nonverbal communication when oral communication is limited because of mental, physical, or emotional challenges (ie, endotracheal tubes).

Music has long been recognized as a nonthreatening form of communication. Music is often referred to as the universal language because of its ability to break down cultural, educational, linguistic, and emotional barriers. Music can reduce feelings of loneliness by producing familiar, comforting stimulation reminiscent of family, homeland, or past experiences.[26]

Music is an effective means of providing recreational and social diversion from the monotony and isolation of hospitalization and may play a role in meeting the patients' physiologic and emotional needs.[27] It is also a method to filter unpleasant and unfamiliar sounds associated with hospitalization. Music can offer a means to reduce self-preoccupation, thereby limiting the need for excessive medication, minimizing side effects of medication, and facilitating shorter recovery.[28]

RECOMMENDATIONS

To start a music therapy program in an ICU, the ICU nurse needs to consider the era, tempo, volume, and tone of the music. Choosing the correct music is critical in developing music therapy as an effective intervention.[5]

Tempo is the major cause of physiologic response to music. Beats of 70 to 80 per minute, approximately the same as the heart rate, are considered soothing, whereas faster beats may create tension. High pitch creates or increases tension, and low pitch causes relaxation. Loud volume (ie, greater than 130 decibels, such as a jumbo jet landing) causes pain. Music appropriate for reduction of anxiety should have a slow steady rhythm, low-frequency tones, orchestral effects, and relaxing melodies.[29] "Sedative music is defined as having regular rhythm, predictable dynamics, harmonic consonance, and recognizable vocal and instrumental timbre."[9(p40)] On the other hand, Halpern and Savary[30] suggested that musical selections not have words because the patient may focus on the words and their meanings rather than allowing themselves to flow with the music. Music should not be played continuously, otherwise it is a nuisance rather than a pleasure.[29] Zimmerman et al[31] suggested 30-minute intervals that have been shown to be effective in reduction of cancer pain.[31]

Two nursing diagnoses for cancer patients in the ICU include, but are not limited to, alteration in comfort related to pain and/or anxiety. The intensive care nurse can develop a plan of care with music therapy (see box "Music Therapy Plan of Care"). The ICU nurse must first assess the level of pain or anxiety. This is most often done using a simple scale, such as for pain 0–5, where 0 is no pain and 5 is severe pain. The next step in assessment would be a music history to determine patient preference or interest. The ICU nurse should then establish a music schedule for the patient in which a quiet milieu can be provided to enhance the positive effects of music therapy. This schedule should be repeated at least twice a day. Certain musical compositions have been identified that promote a relaxed response (ie, reduction in heart rate, regular deep breathing, muscular relaxation, and sleep) (see box "Suggested Music Selections"). It is essential for the ICU nurse to evaluate the subjective and objective responses of the patient to the music intervention.

• • •

In summary, music can be a valuable, noninvasive therapeutic nursing intervention. Music is the universal language that can be used in the critical care setting to assist patients through their intensive care experience. Music has several positive benefits (eg, it decreases anxiety/stress, heart rate, systolic blood pressure, and pain and is a diversional activity) that are essential to the critical care population. Music therapy may bridge the gap of this frightening experience for the patient in the ICU.

REFERENCES

1. Kimball CP. Reactions to illness: the acute phase. 1979;2:307–319.
2. Bonny HL. Music listening for intensive care units: a pilot project. *Music Ther*. 1983;3:4–16.
3. Coughlan A. Music therapy in ICU. *Nurs Times*. 1994;90:35.
4. Dossey BM, Keegan L, Guzzetta CE, Kolkoneier LG. *Holistic Nursing: A Handbook for Practice*. 2nd ed. Gaithersburg, Md: Aspen Publishers; 1995.
5. Biley F. Using music therapy in hospital settings. *Nurs Standard*. 1992;6:37–39.
6. Collins SK, Kuck K. Music therapy in the neonatal intensive care unit. *Neonatal Network*. 1991;9:23–26.
7. Guzzetta CE. Effects of relaxation and music therapy on patients in a coronary care unit with presumptive acute myocardial infarction. *Heart Lung*. 1989;18:609–616.
8. Bonny H, Savary L. *Music and Your Mind*. New York: Harper & Row; 1978.
9. Updike P. Music therapy results for ICU patients. *Dimens Crit Care*. 1990;9:39–45.
10. Munro S, Mount B. Music therapy in palliative care. *Can Med Assoc J*. 1978;119:1029–1034.
11. Moss VA. Music and the surgical patient: the effect of music on anxiety. *AORN*. 1988;48(1):64–69.
12. Owens KM, Ehrenreich D. Literature review of non-pharmacologic methods for the treatment of chronic pain. *Holistic Nurs Practice*. 1991;6:24–31.
13. Bonny HL. *The Role of Taped Music Program in the Guided Imagery of Music (GIM) Process*. Baltimore, Md: ICM Press; 1978.
14. Stone SK, Rusk F, Chambers A, Chafin S. The effects of music therapy on critically ill patients in the intensive care. Presented at the sixteenth annual National Teaching Institute, held by the American Association of Critical Care Nurses in Atlanta, Ga. *Heart Lung*. 1989;18:291.
15. Steelman VM. Intraoperative music therapy. *AORN J*. 1990;52:1026–1034.
16. Herth K. The therapeutic use of music. *Nurs Supervisor*. October 1978;22–23.
17. Downey G, Flood S. In this ICU, the downbeat helps the heartbeat. *Modern Hosp*. 1972;118:91.
18. Meinhart N, McCafferty M. *Pain: A Nursing Approach and Analysis*. East Norwalk, Conn: Appleton-Century Crofts; 1983.
19. Bolwerk CA. Effects of relaxing music on state anxiety in myocardial infarction patients. *Crit Care Nurs Q*. 1990;13:63–72.
20. Totas ML. The emotional stress of the preoperative patient. *J Am Assoc Nurse Anesth*. February 1978;27–30.
21. Cassem NH, Hackett TP. Psychological aspects of myocardial infarction. *Med Clin North Am*. 1977;61:711–721.
22. Davis MZ. Socioemotional component of coronary care. *J Nurs*. 1972;72:704.
23. Doody SB, Smith C, Webb J. Nonpharmacological interventions for pain management. *Crit Care Clin North Am*. 1991;3:69–75.
24. Heitz L, Symreng T, Scamman FL. Effect of music therapy in the postanesthesia care unit: a nursing intervention. *J Postanesthesia Nurs*. 1992;7:22–31.
25. Alvin J. Principles of music therapy. *Physiotherapy*. 1978;64:77–79.
26. Cook JD. Music as an intervention in the oncology setting. *Cancer Nurs*. 1986;9:23–28.
27. Goloff MS. The response of hospitalized medical patients to music therapy. *Music Ther*. 1981;1:51–56.
28. Bonny HL, McCarron N. Music as an adjunct to anesthesia in operative procedures. *Amer Assoc Nurse Anesth*. 1984;52:55–57.
29. O'Sullivan RJ. A musical road to recovery: music in intensive care. *Intens Care Nurs*. 1991;7:160–163.
30. Halpern S, Savary L. *Sound Health: Music and Sounds That Make Us Whole*. San Francisco, Calif: Harper & Row; 1985.
31. Zimmerman L, Pozehl B, Duncan K , Schmitz R. Effects of music in patients who had chronic pain. *West J Nurs Res*. 1989;11:298–309.

Therapeutic Touch: A Healing Modality

Steffanie S. Mulloney, MS, RN
Brigham and Women's Hospital
Newborn Intensive Care Unit

Carol L. Wells-Federman, MEd, RN
Division of Behavioral Medicine
New England Deaconess Hospital
Boston, Massachusetts

For more than two decades, nursing has pioneered inquiry about healing through the human energy field. A substantial body of literature exists on the energetic healing modality known as therapeutic touch (TT). As an extension of professional skills, TT is practiced around the world by an estimated 20,000–30,000 health care professionals in hospitals, hospices, and community health settings. In addition, it is being taught in numerous universities and health care institutions around the country.

TT is a contemporary interpretation of several ancient healing practices, including the laying on of hands. Dolores Krieger, a nurse and professor emeritus at New York University and Dora Kunz, a gifted healer, developed this nursing intervention in the late 1960s and early 1970s after extensive study of well-known healers.

DEFINITION

TT is a consciously directed process of energy modulation during which the practitioner uses the hands as a focus to facilitate healing. The technique involves simultaneously centering awareness, directing compassionate intention, and modulating the flow of human energy using the hands. TT may include physical contact, but it is not a requirement for assessment and treatment.

Although derived from the laying on of hands, TT differs in several ways. TT is not typically done within a religious context, and its effectiveness is not contingent on the patient's belief in

Source: Reprinted from S.S. Mulloney and C. Wells-Federman, *The Journal of Cardiovascular Nursing,* Vol. 10, No. 3, pp. 27–49, © 1996, Aspen Publishers, Inc.

the intervention. Developed as a nursing intervention, TT has a specific, standardized procedure and continues to be scientifically tested. The ability to practice TT is not a special talent for healing bestowed on a few gifted individuals. Rather, TT can be practiced by anyone with the desire, discipline, and educational resources to learn it.

HEALING

Healing or restoring wholeness, is an intrinsic process of living and is derived from the Anglo-Saxon word *haelan*, which means to make or become whole. The healing process is the innate ability to integrate and balance body, mind, and spirit. Healing is described by Estby and colleagues as "not predictable in terms of time frame, cause, or outcome" because of the "many variables that influence it."[1(p408)]

Healing is not something the nurse does for the patient; rather, the nurse facilitates the healing process through knowledgeable caregiving. As Nightingale stated, "Nature alone cures . . . and what nursing has to do . . . is to put the patient in the best condition for nature to act upon him."[2(p133)] The nurse, through assessment, therapeutic intervention, and compassionate caregiving, facilitates the healing process.

Healing can become blocked in times of stress such as illness or hospitalization because of the dynamic interaction of mind and body. The stress response is triggered when a person perceives a situation to be a threat to physical or psychological well-being and that he or she is unable to cope effectively with the demand.[3] This interpretation generates a cascade of biochemical events initiated by the central nervous system that affect the body. Most specifically, the autonomic nervous system via the sympathetic branch produces a generalized arousal of the body including increased heart rate and blood pressure, heightened awareness of the environment, the shifting of blood from the visceral organs to the large muscle groups, increased muscle tension, altered lipid metabolism, increased platelet aggregability, and in-

creased respiration. This basic adaptive response to physical stress was named the "fight or flight" response by Cannon in the early 1900s.

In response to stress, the psychoneuroendocrine system (hypothalamic-pituitary-adrenal axis) is also affected, causing the adrenal cortex to secrete glucocorticoids. Glucocorticoids are responsible for increased blood sugars, sodium retention, alterations in lipid metabolism, increased anti-inflammatory response, and with time, a decrease in immune function. Similarly, other hormones regulated by the psychoneuroendocrine system such as reproductive and growth hormones as well as endorphins and encephalins can be affected by the stress response.

In its acute phase, the stress response may cause or exacerbate symptoms such as anxiety, angina, cardiac dysrhythmias, pain, tension headaches, insomnia, and gastrointestinal complaints. With repeated or prolonged exposure to physical or psychological stress, this response can exacerbate symptoms of diseases that are influenced by central nervous system stimulation, precipitating arousal of the musculoskeletal system, autonomic nervous system, or the psychoneuroendocrine system.[4] There is, however, an innate ability to counter this response and, therefore, promote healing. This innate ability is known as the relaxation response.

The *relaxation response* is the antithesis of the stress response. It is an integrated physiologic response originating in the hypothalamus that leads to a generalized decrease in central nervous system arousal.[5] To the extent that stress causes or exacerbates a symptom or illness, eliciting the relaxation response can break the stress–symptom cycle. The immediate physiologic effects are a decrease in heart rate, blood pressure, respiratory rate, and muscle tension. The long-term physiologic effect is a decrease in central nervous system arousal with its concomitant decrease in musculoskeletal system, sympathetic nervous system, and psychoneuroendocrine system arousal.

Research and practice literature suggest that through TT patients can experience a relaxation response.[6–8] In addition to eliciting the relaxation response, another research finding has been the reduction of anxiety.[6,9] Eliciting the relaxation response, reducing anxiety, and interrupting the stress–symptom cycle through TT can enhance the body's natural healing process, facilitate recovery from illness or injury, promote health, and prevent further complications.

THEORETICAL FRAMEWORK

Krieger drew from a philosophy common to many Eastern cultures to support the view of TT as an energy field interaction. This philosophy holds that a universal, unitary life force, or vitality, flows through all living systems. A healthy individual has an abundance of vitality and therefore can consciously sense and direct this energy through the hands to facilitate healing in others.[6] It is important to note that to date there is no empirical evidence to support the existence of universal life force or a personal energy field. However, this view is still used as a working hypothesis and serves as a guidepost for researchers and practitioners. As with many other valuable therapies such as hundreds of medications, biofeedback, relaxation techniques, and therapeutic use of presence, the mechanism of action in TT is still unknown. However, outcome-based studies that demonstrate its effectiveness, all without adverse effects, help guide practice and further research.

As a nursing intervention, TT is best described from Martha Rogers' science of unitary human beings.[10,11] Her theory provides conceptual support for the clinical practice and research of TT. Rogers' model is developed from the quantum field theory of contemporary physics and von Bertalnaffy's[12] general system theory. Its primary assumptions are that (1) a person is a unified whole rather than the sum of his or her parts; (2) a person is characterized as a complex human energy field; (3) a person and the environment are open systems that are continually, simultaneously, and mutually in process with each other; and (4) the identity and integrity of the human energy field is maintained through patterning and organization. Macrae eloquently summarizes these assumptions of Rogers'[11] field model:

Body, mind, and spirit . . . are not separate substances or categories, but rather different energy frequencies that are continually interacting. A human being is a complex, multidimensional energy system. From this point of view, health or wholeness implies an inner balance among these different levels or dimensions of energy as well as an open harmonious interchange between the individual and the environment.[13(p18)]

Research on the science of unitary human beings reinforces the belief that health and healing evolve within the context of the mutual human–environment field process. Rogers' framework views professional nursing practice as seeking to "strengthen the coherence and integrity of the human and environmental fields, and to knowingly participate in patterning of the human and environmental fields for realization of maximum well-being."[14(p74)]

Integrating this framework, Meehan describes a TT treatment as a "purposeful patterning of the mutual energy field process in which the nurse uses his/her hands to meditate patterning of the patient–environmental energy field process."[14(p74)] Any change in a patient's energy field facilitated by TT occurs in the human–environmental energy field. This change proceeds as the nurse enters a focused moment-to-moment awareness, uses compassionate intent to potentiate the patient's capacity for self-healing, and consciously modulates the flow of the human energy field.

Rogers and others[15,16] propose that to the trained sense of touch, the human energy field can be perceived. Through training, one develops skills that facilitate perception and modulation of the human energy field. There is a normal pattern to the human energy field that varies from person to person. Disease, injury, pain, and negative affective states such as anxiety affect this pattern.[15,17] These negative states can create disturbances in the human energy field such as areas of energy depletion, blockages in the flow of energy, accumulations or congestion of energy around areas of the body, or dysrhythmic pulsations.

The five phases of TT intervention are centering, assessment and scanning, unruffling or clearing, treatment, and evaluation. These are briefly described in the box, "The Five Phases of Therapeutic Touch Process." Further elaboration of the process of TT can be found in Macrae's[13] book and the National League for Nursing instructional video by Quinn.[18]

RESEARCH FINDINGS

The evaluation and testing of TT was based on research on the laying on of hands by Grad,[19,20] Grad et al.,[21] and Smith.[22] Nonhuman subjects were selected in these investigations because they were not amenable to suggestion or faith, thus eliminating this artifact from the results. These studies found increases in the rate of wound healing in mice,[21] an increase in activity of the enzyme trypsin in vitro,[22] and increases in rate of germination and height in barley seedlings.[20]

Based on the above observations, Krieger developed a model for investigating TT within a hospital setting. In 1975 Krieger[23] published her investigation of the effect of TT on hemoglobin values on hospitalized patients. Although methodologic problems preclude scientific support for the positive outcome, the observation indicated a di-

---

The Five Phases of Therapeutic Touch Process

1. *Centering*
   Centering is the most critical phase of therapeutic touch and occurs throughout the treatment. It is a moment-to-moment awareness and an ability to be fully present. Sustaining a centered state of awareness during a TT treatment is why some refer to it as a "meditation in motion" or the "yoga of healing."

2. *Assessment*
   This involves scanning the field by moving the hands in a rhythmical, symmetrical manner about 2 to 6 inches from the head to the feet. The practitioner perceives the quality of the flow of energy looking for changes in sensory cues. In a state of health, the field is open and symmetrical and may be perceived as having a soft warmth, smoothness, or gentle vibration. Conversely, subtle changes in sensory cues associated with imbalance are perceived as feelings of congestion, pressure, warmth, coolness, blockage, pulling or drawing, static or tingling.

3. *Unruffling/Clearing*
   This is a technique that is usually the first step in treatment although some sources have it preceding the treatment phase of TT. Unruffling facilitates the symmetrical, rhythmical flow of energy through the field. The practitioner uses long downward strokes through the field over the entire body, from head to toe.

4. *Treatment*
   The fourth phase is directing and modulating energy to reestablish order. It is also known as balancing, rebalancing, and intervention. Treatment is the least structured phase as it is determined by the needs of the patient. During this phase, practitioners use hands both on and off the body to facilitate energy flow. Imagery often helps the practitioner conceptualize areas of imbalance and direct the flow of energy.

5. *Evaluation*
   This phase involves the reassessment of the field as changes often occur spontaneously and new areas of congestion can occur. At the end of a treatment, ideally the field will feel symmetrical and energy will be flowing in a more open manner.

rection for future research and provided a meaningful foundation for the investigation of a new and evolving intervention.

Since Krieger's initial study, research has clustered around the investigation of TT's effects on stress, anxiety, pain, psychoimmunity, and wound healing. Qualitative research has examined the experience of both the recipient of TT as well as the practitioner.

There are a wide range of methodologic problems researchers confront when studying TT, the most important of which is the differentiation between TT and the placebo effect. To control for this, most quantitative studies reported after 1983 included control groups that received a mimic TT intervention developed and validated by Quinn.[24]

Mimic TT was designed to control for the intent of the practitioner, the effects of the presence of a helping person, and the placebo effect. In mimic TT a practitioner with no prior knowledge of the process mimics the movements of the hands off the body with no attempt to center, no intention to assist the subject, no attuning to the condition of the subject, and no direction of energy. Practitioners are asked to count backward from 100 by sevens while moving the hands over the body to distract them from focusing their intention on assisting the subjects.

In addition to the published qualitative and quantitative research, numerous doctoral dissertations and masters' theses have focused on TT. This article, however, focuses only on those studies that have been published. Table 1 is limited to quantitative, nonmethodologic studies. For clarity, the qualitative studies are described within the body of the paper.

Stress studies

Four research studies explore the relationship between TT and physiologic measures of stress reduction.[7,8,25,26] Krieger, Peper, and Ancoli[8] conducted a pilot study that sought evidence of physiologic change during TT in both the healer and the recipients of TT. Three subjects, all having specific physical complaints, received TT administered by Krieger on 2 consecutive days.

Data on Krieger were recorded with an electroencephalograph (EEG), electromyograph (EMG), and electrooculograph (EOG) while she administered TT and while she meditated alone. The subjects were monitored with EEG, EMG, and EOG, and recordings of galvanic skin response (GSR), hand temperature, and heart rate were made as well.

The observation suggested that TT could promote a relaxation response. Krieger's EEG showed rapid, rhythmical beta waves and her EOG was without movement, which indicated a stable state of deep concentration. This type of beta EEG activity has been observed in advanced meditators.[8] Most of the subjects' data were not significantly changed during TT except that they were relaxed as indicated by alpha states in both eyes-open and eyes-closed conditions. Alpha states of consciousness are rarely present in the eyes-open condition and is an indicator of a state of deep relaxation. Subjects' self-reports confirmed that they felt feelings of relaxation and well-being during TT treatments. Subjects also reported improvement in their physical conditions; however, the placebo effect may have been responsible for this subjective report of improvement.

Limitations of this study are its small sample size and lack of control subjects. Absent from the report are the pretreatment and posttreatment physiologic data. The presence of alpha brain waves was the only correlation between subjects' comments of having experienced relaxation and the physiologic data.

Randolph[25] studied the effect of TT on physiologic responsiveness to experimentally induced stress in healthy female college students. Subjects in the experimental group watched a distressing film that had been validated as a stress-producing stimulus while receiving TT. Data analysis revealed no significant difference between experimental and control groups on any of the three indices of physiologic stress response (skin temperature, muscle tension, and skin conductance). One possible explanation for the failure of the study to demonstrate a therapeutic effect from TT is that a substantial deviation in the

Table 1. Quantitative therapeutic touch research: 1975–1994

Author	Year	Outcomes variables	Population	Intervention	Min/Rx	Instruments	N	Significance
Krieger	1975	Hgb	Hospitalized pts.	TT, routine care	7	Hgb monitor	64	$P<.001$
Heidt	1981	Anxiety	Hospitalized CV pts.	TT, CT, NT	5	STAI	90	$P<.001$TT; TT vs. NT $P<.01$; TT vs CT $P<.01$
Quinn	1984	Anxiety	Hospitalized CV pts.	TT, MTT	5	STAI	60	$P<.0005$
Randolph	1984	Stress response	College students	TT, MTT	13	GSR, EMG, temp	60	NS
Keller & Bzdek	1986	Tension headache	Adults	TT, MTT	5	3 scales MMPQ	60	$P<.005$; $P<.002$; $P<.0001$
Quinn (NIH)	1989	Anxiety, SBP, HR	Hospitalized preop. CV pts.	TT, MTT, NT	5	STAI, SBP, DBP, HR	153	DBP $P<.02$ NT vs TT; NS-STAI, SBP, HR
Meehan et al (NIH)	1990	Pain & meds	Postop. pts.	Narcotic & TT, narcotic & MTT, narcotic alone	5	Med Ct; time, VAS	159	<meds; > wait, NS - VAS
Wirth	1990	Punch wound (60 mm²)	University students	TT, no Rx	5	Digitalizing line-area meter	44	$P<.001$
Olson et al	1992	Anxiety	Hurricane survivors	TT	7.8–11.8	Skin temp, HR, BP, RR, VAS for ST anxiety	23	Anxiety $P<.05$; NS - skin temp, HR, BP, RR
Meehan	1993	Pain & meds	Postop. pts.	TT, MTT, narcotic analgesics	5	VAS; time	108	$.05>P<.06$; $.05>$ >wait
Quinn & Strelkauskas	1993	Anxiety, affect, immune function	RNs & bereaved subjects	TT	Varied	STAI, ABS, blood samples	2 RN 2S	S < anxiety; S + RN > affect; S + RN < OKT8
Simington & Laing	1993	Anxiety	Institutionalized elders	TT with back rub, back rub alone	3	STAI	105	$P<.001$
Wirth et al.	1993	Punch wound	Adults	TT, no Rx	5	Physician assessment	24	$P<.005$
Wirth & Cram	1993	ANS & CNS arousal	Adults	TT, MTT	5–7	EMG, temp, HR, $ETCO_2$	12	< energy; < arousal
Gagne & Toye	1994	Anxiety	Psychiatric inpatients	TT, RT, MTT	15 min = TT & MTT 25–30 min = RT	STAI	31	TT $P<.001$; RT $P<.01$; MTT $P>.05$

ABS = Affect Balance Scale; ANS = autonomic nervous system; BP = blood pressure; CT = casual touch; CNS = central nervous system; CV = cardiovascular; DBP = dystolic blood pressure; EMG = electromyography; $ETCO_2$ = end-tidal CO_2; GSR = galvanic skin response; Hgb = hemoglobin; HR = heart rate; Med ct = medication count; MMPQ = McGill Melzack Pain Questionnaire; MTT = mimic TT; NS = no significance; NT = no touch; OKT8 = a suppressor T cell; Postop. = postoperative; RN = registered nurse; RT = relaxation therapy; Rx = treatment; S = subjects; SBP = systolic blood pressure; STAI = State Trait Anxiety Inventory; temp = temperature; TT = therapeutic touch; VAS = Visual Analog Scale.

administration of TT had occurred. TT was administered by centering then placing hands on the lower abdomen and back of the recipient and without the phases of assessment, clearing, or evaluation. Another possible explanation for the study's results is that Randolph used healthy college students as subjects. Previous research used subjects who were ill or injured.[19,22,23] Grad[19] empirically validated the assumption that little change occurs in a healthy subject receiving the laying on of hands, and studies generally use populations that have some degree of illness.

Quinn[27] relates another possible explanation for Randolph's findings. TT is helpful in eliciting relaxation in nonemergent situations in which external threats are not present. Quinn sees TT being used to support and enhance health rather than to "suppress appropriate physiologic responses to external stressors."[27(p39)]

Olson and colleagues'[26] descriptive study investigated the effectiveness of TT in reducing stress in 23 adults following the natural disaster Hurricane Hugo. Outcome measures were collected in a repeated-session design. The subjects received TT during the first two sessions, and the third session served as a control with the practitioner and subject sitting quietly for 20 minutes. Measures of physiologic and psychologic stress were collected before, during, and after each session. Physiologic measures included heart rate, skin temperature, blood pressure, and respiratory rate; psychologic measures used two visual analog scales, one each for state and trait anxiety.

Data analysis showed significant decreases in state anxiety comparing pre- and post-TT intervention and TT intervention with the control session at the 0.05 level of significance. Physiologic outcomes of TT reflected relaxation trends but showed no significant differences between treatment and control groups. Typically, stress research has lacked correlation between self-report and physiologic measures of stress.[28]

This study was constrained by the conditions in the community following the hurricane that affected participation. Of the 23 subjects, only 18 returned for a second session and 8 for the third control session. In addition, environmental conditions such as room temperature were difficult to control because the heating and cooling systems in the room used to collect data had been damaged by the hurricane. This lack of controlled room temperature may have confounded physiologic measures such as skin temperature. These results underscore the importance of environmental conditions as a critical element in research examining physiologic effects of TT.

Wirth and Cram[7] studied the objective, quantifiable effect of TT on physiology. The study used a randomized ABAC methodologic design to investigate the effect of TT on autonomic and central nervous system parameters. The 12 subjects were blinded to the true nature of the experimental protocol to control for placebo and expectation effects. All meditators, they were told that the study was designed to examine the effect of meditation on a variety of electrophysiologic potentials. Each subject was monitored for one evaluation session. The session was divided into the following four segments: (1) Baseline, (2) mimic or TT, (3) baseline, and (4) mimic or TT. The subjects were randomly assigned to receive mimic or TT during segment 2. If mimic was received in segment 2, TT was received in segment 4. Conversely, if TT was received in segment 2, mimic was received in segment 4. Each segment lasted for 5 to 7 minutes with a total session time per subject of 20 to 28 minutes. Both the TT and mimic segments were performed from behind the subject by an independent TT practitioner (eight of the subjects) or by the first author (four of the subjects).

The impact of TT was assessed by multisite surface electromyographic recordings. Autonomic indicators of physiologic activity were also monitored and included hand and head temperature, heart rate, and end-tidal CO_2 levels. The results demonstrated that all of the autonomic indicators showed a general trend toward lowered levels of arousal over time. In a majority of cases (eight), the subjects' respiratory rates during the TT segment were reduced by half. Previous studies have also demonstrated that a reduced respiratory rate and increased hand temperature are indicative of an increase in relaxation.[29-31] The EMG readings for three of the four muscle regions monitored—C4, T6, and L3—indicated a significant reduction in energy during and following the TT treatment for the majority of subjects. For example, the cervical region demonstrated a significant relaxation effect at the $P<.009$ level, and the T = 6 paraspinals and the lumbosacral region showed significance at the $P<.004$ and $P<.005$ levels, respectively.

These findings are confounded by some methodologic issues. The standardized practice of TT was altered in that the practitioners assessed and treated subjects from behind only. Second, the findings must be considered preliminary because this was an exploratory study that used a specialized subject population, namely, meditators. Therefore, the results of the experiment may not be generalizable to other subject populations. Further research is needed either to confirm or repudiate the hypothesis that TT has a normalized effect on the central nervous system. To date, scientific support for the view that TT decreases stress is equivocal. Further replication and extension of these studies are needed.

Anxiety studies

Studies by Heidt,[9] Quinn,[24,32] Simington and Laing,[33] and Gagne and Toye[34] investigated effects of TT on anxiety. Anxiety is an index of psychologic distress and considered incompatible with physical relaxation. These studies test whether TT can influence the subjective psychologic experience of anxiety. The strength of this segment of TT research is that it builds on theoretical and clinical knowledge through replication and extension. Populations include adult patients awaiting cardiac surgery, older medical patients, and psychiatric inpatients.

Heidt's[9] study of 90 hospitalized cardiovascular patients had three groups. One group received a 5-minute TT treatment by the principal investigator; the second group received casual touch that consisted of the nurse taking apical, radial, and pedal pulses for a total of 5 minutes; and the third received no touch (ie, a brief verbal interaction). Anxiety state was evaluated before and after the interventions with the Spielberger State–Trait Anxiety Scale (STAI),[35] a self-evaluation tool that was normalized with neuropsychiatric and medical–surgical patients.

Heidt found that subjects who received TT had a significant decrease in anxiety ($P<.001$). There were no significant decreases in anxiety in either the casual touch or no touch groups. There was a significant reduction in anxiety with the TT group compared with both the casual touch ($P<.01$) and the no touch groups ($P<.01$).

Quinn[24] replicated Heidt's study on the same cardiovascular unit with several differences in study design. She investigated the theory of energy exchange as a basis for TT as it relates to actual contact or lack of touch in TT. Quinn theorized that energy exchange can occur and bring about change without direct physical contact. The experimental group received TT without any direct contact. This intervention, known as noncontact TT, was administered by nurses who had been taught TT by Krieger and who had a minimum of 4 years of experience. The control group received mimic TT. Results replicated Heidt's findings and revealed that the experimental group's anxiety scores decreased more following TT than the control group's scores following the mimic treatment ($P<.0005$).

Quinn[32] replicated and extended her previous research in an investigation that was the first TT study funded by the National Institutes of Health. This study examined the effects of TT on anxiety in 153 patients who were awaiting cardiovascular surgery. Blood pressure and heart rate were the physiologic indices of anxiety, and Spielberger's STAI was the instrument used to measure state anxiety. The TT and mimic TT treatments varied from Quinn's previous study in that they were administered by the principal investigator and the subjects were asked to assume a side-lying position, with their backs to the nurse. This change in subjects' position was an attempt to further test the energy exchange theory by ruling out some subtle communication that may occur through eye contact or facial expression.

Analysis revealed that there were no significant differences among the groups in any of the measures except for a decrease in diastolic blood pressure in the group receiving TT compared with the no touch control group (P<.02). Quinn suggests that the lack of support for TT decreasing anxiety is most likely a result of the investigator delivering both TT and the mimic treatment and the confounding presence of cardiovascular medications. Eye contact may also be necessary with regard to the intervention's effectiveness.

Simington and Laing[33] studied the effects of TT on state anxiety of 105 institutionalized older patients. A three-group experimental design was used. State anxiety was measured using the Spielberger STAI. The anxiety level of subjects who received TT combined with a 3-minute back rub was found to be significantly lower than the anxiety level of subjects who received a 3-minute back rub without TT (P<.001). This study varied in its approach in that TT was exclusively performed in the context of a back rub. The authors state that the control group's back rubs were performed by a nurse having no previous experience in TT. The experimental group received a back rub from nurses who were experienced in TT and centered during the procedure and who frequently removed their hands in order to balance and direct the energy flow.

Gagne and Toye[34] examined the effects of TT and relaxation therapy on the anxiety of 31 inpatients at a Veterans Administration psychiatric facility. The study compared three groups that received two sessions within 24 hours of TT, relaxation therapy (RT) as described by Benson,[5] or mimic TT with psychiatric inpatients suffering moderate to severe anxiety. TT and mimic TT treatments each lasted 15 minutes, and the RT treatments lasted 25–30 minutes. A female nurse or nursing assistant dressed in street clothes administered TT, a female nurse dressed in standard nursing attire administered mimic TT, and a male chaplain dressed in clerical garments administered RT.

Anxiety was measured pre- and postintervention using the Spielberger STAI. Additionally, subjects were rated on an unnamed instrument for the amount of their motor activity during rest pre- and postintervention. Because RT was regularly used in the hospital and TT was new, the researchers considered the possibility of positive expectation effects having an impact on treatment outcome. An attempt was made to analyze expectancy effects with the use of a questionnaire labeled "Final Summary." However, expectancy did not correlate with outcome. This result created statistical problems and prevented further analysis of this effect.

Anxiety reduction was realized in all groups following intervention. Both TT and RT groups showed significant reductions in anxiety scores on STAI immediately after treatment, with the TT group demonstrating the greater reduction (P<.001) and the RT group demonstrating a lesser effect (P<.01). The mimic TT group showed a small but nonsignificant change (P >.05).

The only group to show a change in motor behavior after treatment was the RT group (P<.001). This change may have been caused by the intentional focus of RT on decreasing muscular tension and activity. Oddly, the mimic TT control group had a lower motor activity score before treatment than the other groups, suggesting that the groups were not comparable on this variable.

Questions arise around the methodology used in this study. Specifically, the significant differences in treatment length between the TT and mimic TT groups and the RT group could conceivably have statistical impact. Standardizing treatment length for all interventions would clarify this point. It is unknown whether the mimic TT practitioner recited multiplication tables aloud or silently. If they were recited aloud, this would have been a significant deviation from the standard administration of mimic TT and could have disturbed the subject and skewed the results. Differences in role, gender, and dress among the professionals administering the interventions disturbed the constancy of conditions, which may also have altered the results.

This disturbance could have been minimized by using multiple therapists to decrease therapist-specific effects. The years of experience of the TT practitioners also is unknown. The instruments for expectancy and motor activity lack information on reliability and validity, which weakens their usefulness.

Still, the results are promising. There is preliminary support for the use of TT for the relief of subjective anxiety, and it appears at least as effective as RT as a clinical strategy for anxiety reduction in psychiatric inpatients. TT are tested in a new population, which represents an extension of previous research. Gagne and Toye[34] noted that many methods of anxiety reduction were ineffective in psychiatric inpatients. Passive anxiety reduction techniques such as TT were valuable for many of these patients whose degree of anxiety interferes with their cognitive ability to engage in mental focusing or visual imagery techniques.

Constructive replication and extension of research of TT's effect on anxiety is needed. To date, scientific support for the view that TT decreases anxiety beyond the placebo effect is equivocal.

Pain studies

Inasmuch as anxiety influences the pain experience through increases in muscle tension, it could be assumed that TT would have an effect on decreasing pain by affecting anxiety. Three studies investigated the effect of TT on pain, one on tension headache pain[37] and two on postoperative pain.[38,39] Keller and Bzdek[36] investigated the effect of TT on tension headache pain in a group of 60 college students. The experimental group received a 5-minute TT treatment and the control group received a 5-minute mimic TT treatment; both treatments were administered by Keller.

The McGill-Melzack Pain Questionnaire,[39] a subjective instrument that evaluates the experience of pain, was given before, 5 minutes after, and 4 hours after treatment. Data analysis revealed that TT significantly reduced tension headache pain immediately following the intervention and relief continued for up to 4 hours later ($P<.005$) compared with the control group. Pain scores decreased an average of 70% in the TT group and 37% in the control group ($P<.005$). This research supports the claim that TT may be an effective modality for pain relief above and beyond the placebo response.

Meehan[38] examined the effect of TT on acute abdominal or pelvic pain. Hospitalized postoperative patients (108) were randomly assigned into three groups. The experimental group received a 5-minute TT treatment for pain with the option for further medication; the placebo group received a 5-minute mimic TT treatment, again with the same option for medication; and the control group received the usual postoperative narcotic analgesics medications for pain.

The Pain Visual Analog Scale[40] was administered to measure pain before all interventions. Posttest measures were obtained 1 hour after the interventions. Subjects from either the TT or mimic TT group who asked for pain medication before 1 hour after intervention received it, and a posttest score was recorded as equal to their pretest score.

Data analysis revealed that narcotic analgesia was more effective in reducing postoperative pain than either TT or mimic TT. There were no significant differences between the TT and mimic TT posttest scores, although subjects receiving TT had pain scores that approached significance ($.05<P<.06$). The lack of significant findings may be related to comparing the analgesic effects of TT with the narcotic analgesia of meperidine injections rather than measuring its effectiveness as an adjunct for acute pain relief. A more realistic comparison may be with a milder, oral analgesic such as acetaminophen.

Another explanation for the lack of significance is the brevity of the treatment. Treatment time was restricted to 5 minutes to be consistent with previous research; however, Meehan[38] suggested that 5 minutes was not enough time for an analgesic effect. Given that a significant effect was almost achieved in 5 minutes, it is reasonable to assume that a longer treatment would have had a greater effect. Meehan recommended that the study be replicated, lengthening the time allotted for TT treatment.

Meehan and colleagues[39] investigated the effects of TT on postoperative pain in 159 subjects who underwent abdominal or pelvic surgery. Subjects were randomly assigned to one of three groups; an experimental group receiving TT, a single-blind control group receiving mimic TT, or a standard control group receiving standard nursing care. Subjects received the assigned treatment the evening before surgery and seven times during the postoperative period. The number of doses and amount of analgesic medication received over the postoperative period were calculated. Pain was measured before and at four intervals following each treatment administered with as-needed analgesics on the first postoperative day. The study used a Visual Analog Scale to measure pain. The time lapse before receiving the next analgesic medication was also calculated.

The authors reported that subjects who received TT with an as-needed narcotic analgesic waited a substantially longer time before requesting further medication ($P<.01$). No significant difference was found in pain intensity scores over the initial 3-hour posttreatment period. Subjects who received TT requested fewer doses of analgesics and received less analgesic medication over the entire postoperative period than the control groups, but this decrease was not significant ($P >.05$). The analgesic effect was significantly greater in women than men.

The authors concluded that TT in conjunction with narcotic analgesic medication can reduce the need for further analgesic medication. This finding replicates Meehan's first study,[38] suggesting that TT may have potential beyond the placebo effect in the treatment of postoperative pain.

A critical discussion of certain aspects of this study is limited (eg, treatment length), because information was extracted from a research abstract. Nevertheless, because of its significant findings this study is important to mention in a review of the research literature.

Methodologic limitations confounded some findings in these studies on pain. The principal investigator administered the intervention in Keller and Bzdek's study,[36] and patients required analgesic medication before the completion of the 1-hour postintervention time in Meehan's[37] study. Replication and extension of these findings are needed to include patients with other types of mild pain such as low back pain along with studying the use of TT with other medical interventions such as nonnarcotic analgesics.

Wound healing studies

Two studies have been conducted on the effect of TT on wound healing beyond Grad and colleagues'[19,21] investigations on the effect of the laying on of hands in mice. Using a randomized, placebo-controlled protocol, Wirth,[41] and Wirth et al[42] studied the effect of TT on the healing rate of full-thickness dermal wounds in human subjects.

In Wirth's[41] initial study, a physician using local anesthesia and a skin punch biopsy instrument incised full-thickness dermal wounds in the lateral deltoid region of the arm of healthy male subjects. The 44 university students who volunteered were randomly assigned to either an experimental group that received a 5-minute TT treatment from an experienced practitioner or a control group in which no treatment was given and the subject merely sat for 5 minutes. The TT practitioner was hidden behind a specially modified door. Subjects in both groups placed their wounded arms through an opening in this modified door. Once through the door, subjects rested their arms on a platform and positioned themselves comfortably for the 5-minute period. Subjects were unable to see the other side of the door or know whether anyone was present on the other side.

To control for placebo and the potentially confounding effects of belief, caring, and compassion, subjects and the physician were kept blind to both group assignment and to the nature of the treatment modality. In fact, both were unaware that healing was the experimental focus until the conclusion of the study.

Data analysis revealed that subjects treated with TT experienced a substantial acceleration in the rate of wound healing compared with the nontreated subjects at the 0.001 level of significance. Complete healing occurred in 13 of 23 treated subjects versus 0 of the 21 control subjects by day 16.

A methodologic issue that confounds these findings was in the administration of TT only to the subject's arm. This treatment varied substantially from the standardized method described by Krieger.[15] Missing from Wirth's discussion[41] of his research were a detailed description of the TT intervention and evidence of a review by a human subjects committee or external reviewer relating to the protection of human subjects. At the same time, this randomized, placebo-controlled study demonstrated a rigor that is unequaled in previous TT research. Wirth's study effectively eliminated the placebo effects and any suggestion or expectation of healing that most often confounds healing research. This elimination was accomplished by isolating subjects from the TT practitioner, blinding them to the nature of the intervention during the study, and using an independent experimenter who was also blinded to the nature of the intervention. This study's findings indicate that TT is an effective healing modality for full-thickness human dermal wounds.

Wirth and colleagues[42] replicated this study in 1993 and again found a significant acceleration in the rate of healing in subjects treated with TT compared with those in the control group. The observations of four physicians blind to the procedure showed that the treated subjects experienced a significant acceleration in the rate of wound healing compared with the control subjects ($P<0.005$). Again the method used varied from standard TT procedure in that patients were treated behind a one-way mirror. The results suggest that TT has the potential to be an effective noninvasive treatment modality for full-thickness human dermal wounds.

Psychoimmunologic study

A pilot study published by Quinn and Strelkauskas[43] in 1993 investigated the effect of TT on anxiety, mood, and immune function of practitioners (N = 2) and recently bereaved recipients (N = 4) using a descriptive study design. One purpose of the study was to address the more recent conceptualization that the TT practitioner, knowingly participating in the mutual human–environment process by shifting consciousness into a state that may be thought of as a "healing meditation," facilitates repatterning of the recipient's energy field, rather than "energy exchange or transfer."[44] At the center of the TT practice is the intent of the practitioner to focus with compassion on the well-being of the recipient. Recent research suggests that positive emotions can have a beneficial effect on the health of the individual. As demonstrated by McClelland,[45] feelings of compassion and unconditional love may increase the effectiveness of the immune system in the experiencer. If this hypothesis is correct, the practice of TT should enhance or support the immune system of the practitioner.

Recently bereaved subjects were selected for this study because bereavement is known to depress immune function temporarily. The authors proposed that this situational shift might be expected to respond favorably to TT treatment because it is assumed to accelerate the natural healing process.

Practitioners had been trained by Krieger and Kunz and had practiced the modality for more than 5 years. Unlike other TT research where practitioners were only allowed to treat control and experimental subjects for 5 minutes, practitioners in this descriptive study were allowed to administer treatments for the length of time that they deemed appropriate. This freedom allowed for the study of the phenomenon as practiced clinically rather than adherence to a specific protocol.

All subjects (practitioners and recipients) completed questionnaires designed to measure baseline anxiety and affect. Blood was drawn for baseline immunologic analysis. These measures were repeated on recipients after treatment and on practitioners after completion of all the day's treatments. Anxiety scores for practitioners were on or near zero both pre- and posttreatment. For recipients, however, state anxiety was 29%

lower posttreatment. Scores of affective mood improved for all recipients. Posttreatment serum analysis revealed no consistent variation in subsets identified by the markers Leu-16, OKT11, OKT3, and OKT4 across recipients. However, there was a consistent decrease in the percentage of OKT8 cells (suppressor T cell) from the initial baseline blood sample to terminal sample in all four recipients (21%, 10%, 20%, and 17%, respectively).

Both practitioners in the study, interestingly, were lower in percentage of OKT8 cells at the beginning than were the recipients. The more experienced practitioner was 47% lower than the highest bereaved recipient and 35% lower than the lowest bereaved recipient. These large differences continued throughout the study, even though the recipients experienced a decrease in OTK8 percentages. The second practitioner began the study 30% lower than the highest recipient and 13% lower than the lowest recipient. By the end of the first treatment, however, she was virtually identical to the more experienced practitioner and remained that way throughout the study. At the end of the study, the more experienced practitioner had a 16% decrease in OKT8 cells, and the second practitioner had a 23% decrease.

No statistical tests and P values were used in this pilot study because of the small sample size. Percentages do not necessarily indicate statistical significance or difference from chance. The authors suggested that the data seem to indicate that something about the treatment (ie, the actual TT, the environment, and so forth) influenced lymphocyte subset composition. An explanation of what this means, why this subset should respond differentially to TT, and what the impact of the response is in terms of the rest of the immune system and health status will need to be investigated in future research. One potential hypothesis derived from this study is that TT enhances immunologic functioning by the inhibition of immune suppression. One major focus of the pilot study was the relationship between the practitioner and the recipient of TT because the nature of the TT interaction is unitary. Some of the most interesting findings involved the comparison of these data and helped to establish a direction for future research of the phenomenon.

Continued replication and extension of quantitative research is needed. To date, quantitative findings suggest that TT may have the potential to reduce anxiety in hospitalized cardiovascular patients, institutionalized older patients, people exposed to natural disasters, and psychiatric inpatients. TT may reduce autonomic and central nervous system arousal and the pain of tension headache and decrease the need for as-needed analgesic medication. Data suggest that TT is a safe and effective intervention for healing full-thickness dermal wounds, and preliminary findings point to the importance of further investigation into the effects of TT on the immune system.

Qualitative studies

Heidt[46] explored the lived experience of TT from the perspective of seven pairs of practitioners and patients. Data were collected from interviews before and after TT treatments and from continuous notes that were made of all verbal and nonverbal expressions, interactions, and body movements of each nurse and patient before, during, and after treatment.

Data analyzed using the grounded theory method developed by Glaser and Strauss[47] focused most heavily on the experience of the practitioner. The primary experience reported by nurses was that of "opening to the flow of universal life energy."[47(p180)]

Interestingly, and consistent with the theory of repatterning, the accounts of nurses and patients frequently paralleled each other. When the nurse reported an inner experience of wholeness, the patient also reflected the same feeling. Similarly, when nurses quieted themselves and projected a sense of inner calm to the patient, the patients relaxed and focused on the healing process. Heidt's investigation of the lived experience of TT lays the groundwork for future exploration into this phenomenon.

Samarel[48] explored the lived experience of TT from the recipient's perspective. Data were obtained by interviewing 20 volunteer subjects with varied diagnoses that included depression, osteoarthritis, multiple sclerosis, cancer, and acquired immune deficiency syndrome. Each participant was interviewed twice, the first being an open-ended interview and the second interview serving to clarify information from the first.

The data were subject to content analysis using Parse's[49] adaptation of Giorgi's[51] operations of phenomenologic analysis. Results indicate that TT is a "dynamic multidimensional experience of developing awareness that facilitates personal change leading to a resonating fulfillment."[48(p655)] Samarel explains that TT is multidimensional because it encompasses all dimensions of living; it reflects developing awareness because of the deepening consciousness of self and of others over time; and it "resonates fulfillment because it is described as intensifying and prolonging feelings of satisfaction, peace, and serenity."[48(p655)]

Despite an admittedly biased sample (ie, subjects were seeking treatment at a TT conference), this study elucidates the patient's experience. Further qualitative investigation into the simultaneously occurring physiologic, emotional, and spiritual experiences described by patients receiving TT is necessary.

France[52] studied the child's lived experience of the TT process. Data were collected from a series of videotaped interviews, drawings by 11 children, and the diaries of parents and the investigator. Each child drew pictures depicting his or her experience before and during TT treatments administered by the investigator. Each child then described the pictures to France. This was repeated over four to six sessions. Usually at about the third to fifth session, the child was asked whether he or she could feel the energy around someone else and selected the energy field of a parent, a sibling, the investigator, or a pet to feel. This exploration was followed by picture drawing and explanation, as was the final session in which the child felt the energy around another child in the study.

The phenomenologic methodology of Husserl[53] guided the generation and analysis of data. The children described kinesthetic, visual, and affective experiences of receiving TT sometimes using analogy and metaphor. Their body language while receiving TT reflected the elicitation of the relaxation response, suggesting that children respond similarly as adults to TT. Each child indicated that he or she could feel the energy of others and distinguish energetic differences in various parts of the body. Many of the parents reported events in which their child was spontaneously "feeling the energy" of others with a purpose or with the intention to help. This supports the assumption that TT is an innate human potential. France[52] identified "being with," "taking in the world to know more," and "struggling to make sense of it" as the essential structures that emerged during data analysis.

Although the investigation of a child's lived experience of receiving TT may be a phenomenon of interest, what this study offers to the advancement of clinical practice is unclear. The subjects in France's sample were healthy children. Both qualitative and quantitative investigation of TT as a nursing intervention focusing on its efficacy in health restoration, health promotion, and illness prevention is recommended.

Carefully designed quantitative studies with more rigorous methodologies and a wide range of subjects and health problems are clearly necessary to corroborate the above findings. Clinically, TT continues to be experienced as an intervention that can promote relaxation, reduce anxiety, increase wound healing time, and reduce pain. The research outcomes thus far are compatible with an energy field process. In other words, there is some kind of correspondence between human beings and the universe in which they live. Perhaps "energy" is not the best word to describe this phenomenon; others suggest communication, information, or correspondence.[54–57] Further discussion, articulation, and research on the subject will help to define and describe the process. One avenue of inquiry may be to compare TT with other caring modalities (eg, presence, empathy, and the therapeutic use of self), which may help address the hypothesis of energy field process.

Although modulation and transfer of energy continue to be used as the working hypothesis, there is no empirical evidence to date to support this theory. In theory development, both quantitative and qualitative approaches should be used. Research endeavors must continue to postulate and test competing explanations for the phenomenon.

This is an enormous area for research and may best be approached through an interdisciplinary effort. Other professionals researching subtle energy and energy medicine are striving to articulate and test a comprehensive paradigm that can account for the phenomena of healing through the human energy field. Although other disciplines are involved in the research, nurse researchers can make a significant contribution because of their substantial experiential expertise and expertise in the design and conduct of clinical research.

CLINICAL APPLICATIONS

Nurses' interest in the clinical application of TT has been described in an expanding body of literature. TT has been used and recommended in the management of pain[37,58–60] including childbirth.[61–63] Braun and colleagues[64] and Dall[65] reported its effectiveness in promoting sleep and Heidt[66] in helping patients to rest. It has been found to be helpful in managing symptoms of persons with acquired immune deficiency syndrome,[67] facilitating physical rehabilitation[68] and a peaceful death in those who are terminally ill.[69,70] TT has been reported to comfort and calm hospitalized infants,[71–73] provide support and allay fears during the perioperative experience,[74] and relieve anxiety[34] and depression in older nursing home residents.[75]

Anecdotal reports of D. Kunz and D. Kreiger (annual workshops, 1972–1995) and of other TT practitioners suggest that it is useful in accelerating the healing of traumatic injuries (eg, sprains, burns, fractures, and wounds);[76,77] managing suicidality; relieving respiratory distress during acute asthma attacks;[76,77] alleviating emotional and spiritual distress;[78] easing chemotherapy-induced nausea and vomiting; and facilitating recovery from incest and abuse.[79]

As with any nursing intervention that includes touch, assessment should include the patient's spiritual or religious beliefs as they pertain to touch as well as other related beliefs and values. Assessment should consist of past experience with touch therapies and the possibility of detecting overt pathology that might require referral for further evaluation.[79] Also, caution is advised in administering TT to patients who have psychiatric disorders or who have been physically abused. These patients are extremely sensitive to human interaction, may misunderstand the intent of the treatment, and may feel threatened and upset by it.[80] Patients who are sensitive to repatterning of the energy field include premature infants and newborns; children; pregnant women; older or debilitated people; or those who are in critical, labile conditions such as burn patients or those with head injuries. Administering TT with these patients must be done with discernment, drawing on clinical judgment and skill.

Simple principles of TT such as centering, intention, and unruffling can be taught to patients and their families as a means of encouraging their participation and partnership in health and healing. It is important to educate patients that TT is a complementary approach, not a substitute for medically effective treatments.

IMPLICATIONS FOR SELF-CARE

Nurses who are involved in the practice of TT report a natural transformation in their lives, lifestyles, and self-perceptions.[81,82] Krieger[61] calls this process "living the Therapeutic Touch" in her book by that title and describes the process that occurs when commitment to healing becomes a lifestyle. Nurses report experiencing increased vigor, confidence, commitment, and satisfaction with their work and an increased overall sense of well-being.

During the experience of TT, nurses report an expansion of consciousness as they assume and maintain a meditative state. With this comes an attitude of nonjudgmental awareness. Meehan[80] asserts that the simple form of meditation that informs TT practice promotes a process of self-healing in the nurse. This self-healing is congruent with Newman's[83] framework, in which the expansion of consciousness is equivalent to health and healing. Future research investigating the psychophysiologic effects of TT on the healer will help elucidate this process of self-healing.

GUIDELINES FOR PRACTICE

For more than 20 years, there has been a growing body of literature on TT reflecting the interest and growing acceptance of it as a nursing intervention. TT policy and procedure guidelines for health professionals are published by Nurse Healers-Professional Associates, Inc. (NH-PA), the professional association that promotes TT. That organization encourages nurses to use TT in clinical settings. These guidelines include documentation of TT treatments in patient records. Recorded data can include objective changes and patient comments and should be recorded in the patient's chart and the personal journal of the practitioner. A journal of TT experiences is a valuable tool for skill development.

Recommendations for practice have been suggested by Meehan[80] for the introduction of TT into acute care settings and can be modified for use in other settings. They are intended for nurses who have at least 6 months' experience in an acute care setting. Meehan's recommendations include being mentored by a nurse with at least 2 years' experience with TT and, preferably, a master's degree and receiving at least 30 hours of instruction covering the theory and practice of TT in a nursing or continuing education program, along with 30 hours of supervised practice with relatively healthy individuals.[80(p14–15)] Being well-versed in the TT literature will help in communicating to physicians, nursing administrators, and colleagues what this nursing intervention can offer patients.

In 1994, the North American Nursing Diagnosis Association (NANDA) accepted a new nursing diagnosis that relates to the human energy field. It is known as *energy field disturbance* and is defined as "a disruption of the flow of energy surrounding a person's being which results in disharmony of the body, mind, and/or spirit." Its defining characteristics include "temperature change (warmth/coolness); visual changes (image/color); disruption of the field (vacant/hole/spike/bulge); movement (wave/spike/tingling/dense/flowing); sounds (tone/words).)[84(p37)] TT is one intervention that is recognized by NANDA for use in the treatment of energy field disturbance. A bonafide nursing diagnosis related to energy field processes brings a new level of recognition to nurses who practice TT. The value of this nursing diagnosis is that it can serve as a vehicle to increase visibility of the healing role of the nurse. It also grounds TT documentation in standardized nursing nomenclature, which may facilitate reimbursement for TT treatment.

CURRENT ISSUES IN HEALTH CARE

A recent national survey by Eisenberg and colleagues[85] reported a significantly higher prevalence of consumer utilization of unconventional medical practices than what had previously been reported. The authors describe unconventional or alternative practices as those that are not commonly taught in medical schools or used in hospitals in the United States. These practices include acupuncture, chiropractic, massage therapy, and homeopathy. Thirty-four percent of their sample of 1,539 adults used at least one unconventional therapy in the past year, and a third of these saw a provider for unconventional therapy. Of those who saw a provider for unconventional therapy, 32% saw a provider for energy healing. This result indicates a greater acquaintance with energy healing modalities such as TT than expected.

In 1992, the National Institutes of Health (NIH) established the Office for Alternative Medicine (OAM) when the Senate Appropriations Committee mandated $2 million of NIH's 1992 budget for the purpose of investigating the efficacy and safety of complementary health practices. Since then, the OAM budget has grown substantially with the 1995 budget set at $5.4 million.

TT was recognized by the OAM as the most evolved of energetic healing modalities because of its body of published research. Nursing was also recognized for its leadership in the development, research, and practice of complementary practices such as TT.[86] In 1994, the OAM awarded a grant to nurse researcher Melodie Olson for a study investigating the effect of TT on the immune system's response during stress. Future plans at the OAM include investigating the possibility of funding a Center for Subtle Energies.[87] Such a center could provide unequaled opportunities for the advancement of knowledge related to healing through human energy fields.

The increasing use of complementary health care practices supports nursing's leadership role in the understanding and application of adjunctive healing modalities. Krieger[88] describes the body of knowledge pertaining to the healing act as being ". . . derived from logical deduction, formal and clinical research findings, the compendium of world literature concerning the therapeutic use of human energies, and deep experiential knowledge that grows into a personal knowing."[(p13)] The challenge of illuminating the nature of health and healing calls for nursing to develop a comprehensive paradigm and to advance clinical practice and research.

In addition to courses offered at the graduate and undergraduate level, TT instruction is currently available at conferences and workshops by the organizations listed in the box entitled "Recommended Resources for TT." Support groups worldwide are designed for members to share their experiences and to continue developing their abilities.

Certification in TT is not currently available, although it is a controversial topic within the organizations that support TT practice. Proponents suggest that certification can promote standards of practice, empower nurses in practice settings, contribute to TT's credibility within the health care community, and facilitate consumer acceptance and the likelihood of reimbursement.[89] Quinn views certification as an exclusionary process that is based on a patriarchal model of fear and control that buys into the dominant medical paradigm.[90] At present, there are no plans to establish certification for TT practitioners or educators. However, standards of practice are being developed and disseminated by Nurse Healers-Professional Associates, Inc.

•   •   •

The practice of TT is intrinsic to the holistic nature of professional nursing. For many nurses, TT embodies the spirit of nursing practice, but others question its effectiveness.[91–93] Both quantitative and qualitative research must continue to build a scientific basis for the practice of TT.

Recommended Resources For Therapeutic Touch

Nurse Healers-Professional Associates, Inc.*
P.O. Box 444
Allison, Park, PA 15101-0444
(412)355-8476
   *Information available on Therapeutic Touch Satellite Chapters, updated bibliographies, newsletters, upcoming workshops, and a directory of TT practitioners throughout the world.

International Society for the Study of Subtle Energies & Energy Medicine
356 Coldco Circle
Golden, CO 80403
(303)278-2228

Pumpkin Hollow Farm
1184 Route 11
Craryville, NY 12521
(518)325-3583

With new opportunities for TT and subtle energy research, collaboration can make the best use of talent and resources.

In this age of cost containment and emphasis on sophisticated technology, one of nursing's most important challenges will be to create a healing environment for each patient within the health care system. Therapeutic touch is one nursing intervention that has been shown to provide nurses with a way to expand their caregiving skills for the health and well-being of their patients and themselves.

REFERENCES

1. Estby SN, Friel MI, Hart LK, Reese JL, Clow TJ. A delphi study of the basic principles and corresponding care goals of holistic nursing practice. *J Holist Nurs.* 1994;12(4):401–413.

2. Nightingale F. *Notes on Nursing: What It is and What It Is Not.* New York, NY: Dover Press; 1859/1969.

3. Wells-Federman C, Stuart E, Deckro J, Mandle CL, Baim M, Medich C. The mind/body connection: the psychophysiology of many traditional nursing interventions. *Clin Nurse Spec.* 1995;9:30–37.

4. Benson H, Stuart EM. *The Wellness Book: The Comprehensive Guide to Maintaining Health and Treating Stress-Related Illness.* New York, NY: Birch Lane Press; 1992.

5. Benson H. *The Relaxation Response.* New York, NY: William Morrow; 1975.

6. Jurgens A, Meehan MTC, Wilson HL. Therapeutic touch as nursing intervention. *Holist Nurs Pract.* 1987;2(1):1–13.

7. Wirth DP, Cram JR. Multi-site electromyographic analysis of non-contact therapeutic touch. *Int J Psychosom.* 1993;40(1–4):47–55.

8. Krieger D, Peper E, Ancoli S. Physiologic indices of therapeutic touch. *Am J Nurs.* 1979;79(4):660–662.

9. Heidt P. Effect of therapeutic touch on anxiety level of hospitalized patients. *Nurs Res.* 1981;30:32–37.

10. Rogers ME. *An Introduction to the Theoretical Basis of Nursing.* Philadelphia, Pa: FA Davis; 1970.

11. Rogers ME. Nursing: science of unitary, irreducible human beings: update 1990. In: Barrett EAM, ed. *Visions of Rogers' Science-Based Nursing.* New York, NY: National League for Nursing; 1990. NLN Publication 15-2286.

12. von Bertalnaffy L. *General Systems Theory.* New York, NY: George Braziller; 1968.

13. Macrae J. *Therapeutic Touch: A Practical Guide.* New York, NY: Knopf; 1987.

14. Meehan MTC. Science of unitary human beings and theory-based practice: therapeutic touch. In: Barrett EAM, ed. *Visions of Rogers' Science-Based Nursing.* New York, NY: National League for Nursing; 1990. NLN Publication 15-2286.

15. Krieger D. *The Therapeutic Touch: How to Use Your Hands to Help or Heal.* Englewood Cliffs, NJ: Prentice Hall; 1979.

16. Malinski VM, ed. *Explorations on Martha Rogers' Science of Unitary Human Beings.* Norwalk, Conn: Appleton-Century-Crofts. 1986.

17. Kunz D, Peper E. Fields and their clinical implications. In: Kunz D, ed. *Spiritual Aspects of the Healing Arts.* Wheaton, Ill: Theosophical Publishing House; 1984.

18. Quinn JF. *Therapeutic Touch: Healing through Human Energy Fields* [videotape series]. New York, NY: NLN; 1992. Publication 42-2485, 42-2486, 42-2487.

19. Grad B. A telekinetic effect on plant growth. *Int J Parapsychol.* 1963;5(2):117–131.

20. Grad B. A telekinetic effect on plant growth: experiments involving treatment of saline in stoppered bottles. *Int J Parapsychol.* 1964;(94):473–494.

21. Grad B, Cadoret RJ, Paul GI. An unorthodox method of wound healing in mice. *Int J Parapsychol.* 1961;3:5–24.

22. Smith MJ. Enzymes are activated by laying-on of hands. *Hum Dimens.* 1972;2:46–48.

23. Krieger D. Therapeutic touch: the imprimatur of nursing. *Am J Nurs.* 1975;75:784–787.

24. Quinn JF. Therapeutic touch as energy exchange: testing the theory. *Adv Nurs Sci.* 1984;6(2):42–49.

25. Randolph GL. Therapeutic touch and physical touch: physiological response to stressful stimuli. *Nurs Res.* 1984;33(1):33–36.

26. Olson M, Sneed N, Bonadonna R, Ratliff J, Dias J. Therapeutic touch and post–Hurricane Hugo stress. *J Holist Nurs.* 1992;10(2):120–136.

27. Quinn JF. Building a body of knowledge: research on therapeutic touch 1974–1986. *J Holist Nurs.* 1988;6(1):37–45.

28. Fagin CM. Stress: implications for nursing research. *Image.* 1987;19(1):38–41.

29. Kesterson J, Clinch NF. Metabolic rate, respiratory exchange ratio, and apneas during meditation. *Am J Physiol.* 1989; 256:632–638.

30. Fried R. Relaxation with biofeedback-assisted guided imagery: the importance of breathing rate as an index of hypoarousal. *Biofeedback Self Regul.* 1987;12:273–279.

31. Fuller GO. *Biofeedback Methods and Procedures in Clinical Practice*. San Francisco, Calif: Biofeedback Press; 1977.

32. Quinn JF. Therapeutic touch as energy exchange: replication and extension. *Nurs Sci Q.* 1989a;2(2):79–87.

33. Simmington JA, Laing GP. Effects of therapeutic touch on anxiety in the institutionalized elderly. *Clin Nurs Res.* 1993;2(4):438–450.

34. Gagne D, Toye RC. The effects of therapeutic touch and relaxation therapy in reducing anxiety. *Arch Psychiatr Nurs.* 1994;8(3):184–189.

35. Spielberger CS, Gorsuch RL, Lushene RE. *STAI Manual for the State Trait Anxiety Inventory*. Palo Alto, Calif: Consulting Psychologists Press; 1970.

36. Keller E, Bzdek VM. Effects of therapeutic touch on headache pain. *Nurs Res.* 1986;35:101–105.

37. Meehan MTC. Therapeutic touch and postoperative pain: a Rogerian research study. *Nurs Sci Q.* 1993;6(2):69–77.

38. Meehan MTC, Mersmann CA, Wiseman ME, Wolff BB, Malgady RG. Therapeutic touch and surgical patients' stress reactions, abstracted. *J Pain.* 1990;5(suppl):149.

39. Melzack R. The McGill Pain Questionnaire: major properties and scoring methods. *Pain.* 1975;1:227–299.

40. Husklsson EC. Measurement of pain. *Lancet.* 1974;9:1,127–1,131.

41. Wirth DP. The effect of non-contact therapeutic touch on the healing rate of full thickness dermal wounds. *Subtle Energies.* 1990;1(1):1–20.

42. Wirth DP, Richardson JT, Eidelman WS, O'Malley AC. Full thickness dermal wounds treated with non-contact therapeutic touch: a replication and extension. *Compl Ther Med.* 1993;1:127–132.

43. Quinn J, Strelkauskas AJ. Psychoimmunologic effects of therapeutic touch on practitioners and recently bereaved recipients: a pilot study. *Nurs Sci Q.* 1993;6(2):13–26.

44. Malinski VM. Therapeutic touch: the view from Rogerian nursing science. *Visions.* 1993;1(1):45–54.

45. McClelland DC. Cited by: Borysenko J. Healing motives: an interview with David C. McClelland. *Advances.* 1985;2(2):29–41.

46. Heidt P. Openness: a qualitative analysis of nurses' and patients' experiences of therapeutic touch. *Image.* 1990;22(3):180–186.

47. Glaser B, Strauss A. *The Discovery of Grounded Theory*. Chicago, Ill: Aldine Press; 1967.

48. Samarel N. The experience of receiving therapeutic touch. *J Adv Nurs.* 1992;17(6):651–657.

49. Parse RR. The phenomenological method. In: Parse RR, Coyne AB, Smith MJ, eds. *Nursing Research: Qualitative Methods*. Bowie, Md: Brady Communications; 1985.

50. Giorgi A. Convergence and divergence of qualitative methods in psychology. In: Giorgi A, Fisher CL, Murray EL, eds. *Duquesne Studies in Phenomenological Psychology*. Vol 2. Pittsburgh, Pa: Duquesne University Press; 1975.

51. Giorgi A. *Psychology as a Human Science: A Phenomenologically Based Approach*. New York, NY: Harper & Row; 1970.

52. France N. The child's perception of the human energy field using therapeutic touch. *J Holist Nurs.* 1993;11(4):319–331.

53. Husserl E. *Logical Investigations*. New York, NY: Humanities Press; 1970.

54. Dossey L. But is it energy? reflections on consciousness, healing and the new paradigm. *Subtle Energies.* 1992;3(3):69–82.

55. LeShan L. Language in the human development movement. In: *Proceedings of the 6th International Conference on the Psychology of Health, Immunity, & Disease*. Mansfield Center, Conn: National Institute for the Clinical Applications of Behavioral Medicine;1994:262–268.

56. Rubik B. Energy medicine and the unifying concept of information. *Alt Therap in Health & Medicine.* 1995;1(1):34–39.

57. Straneva JE. Therapeutic touch: placebo effect or energetic form of communication. *J Holist Nurs.* 1991;9(2):41–61.

58. Boguslawski M. Therapeutic touch: a facilitator of pain relief. *Top Clin Nurs.* 1980;2(1):27–37.

59. Owens MK, Ehrenreich D. Application of nonpharmacologic methods of managing chronic pain. *Holist Nurs Pract.* 1991;6(1):32–40.

60. Wright SM. The use of therapeutic touch in the management of pain. *Nurs Clin N Am.* 1987;22(3):704–715.

61. Krieger D. *Living the Therapeutic Touch: Healing as a Lifestyle*. New York, NY: Dodd, Mead; 1987.

62. Wolfson IS. Therapeutic touch and midwifery. In: Brown CC, ed. *The Many Facets of Touch*. Skillman, NJ: Johnson & Johnson; 1984.

63. Lothian JA. Therapeutic touch. In: Nichols F, Humenick S, eds. *Childbirth Education: Practice, Research, and Theory*. Philadelphia: Pa: WB Saunders; 1988.

64. Braun C, Layton J, Braun J. Therapeutic touch improves resident's sleep. *Am Health Care Assoc J.* 1986;12(1):48–49.

65. Dall JV. Promoting sleep with therapeutic touch. *Addict Nurs Network.* 1993;5(1):23–24.

66. Heidt P. Helping patients to rest: clinical studies in therapeutic touch. *Holist Nurs Pract.* 1991;5(4):57–66.

67. Newshan G. Therapeutic touch for symptom control in persons with AIDS. *Holist Nurs Pract.* 1989;3(4):45–51.

68. Payne MB. The use of therapeutic touch with rehabilitation clients. *Rehabil Nurs*. 1989;15(2):69–72.

69. Fanslow CA. Therapeutic touch: a healing modality throughout life. *Top Clin Nurs*. 1983;5(2):72–79.

70. Messenger T, Roberts KT. The terminally ill: serenity nursing interventions for hospice clients. *J Gerontol Nurs*. 1994;29(11):17–22.

71. Leduc E. Using therapeutic touch on babies. *Neonatal Netw*. 1987;5(6):46–47. Letter to the editor.

72. Leduc E. The healing touch. *Matern Child Nurs J*. 1989; 14(1):41–43.

73. Macrae J. Therapeutic touch in practice. *Am J Nurs*. 1979;79(4):664–665.

74. Jonasen AM. Therapeutic touch: a holistic approach to perioperative nursing. *Today's OR Nurse*. 1994;16(1): 7–12.

75. Rowlands D. Therapeutic touch: its effects on the depressed elderly. *Aust Nurs J*. 1984;13(11):45–46,52.

76. Wytias CA. Therapeutic touch in primary care. *Nurse Pract Forum*. 1994;5(2):91–96.

77. Mackey RB. Discover the healing power of therapeutic touch. *Am J Nurs*. 1995;95(4):25–33.

78. Bright MA. Energetic imbalances rooted in physical and emotional abuse. *Cooperative Connection*. 1993;14(4): 1,4.

79. Keegan, L. Touch: connecting with the healing power. In: Dossey BM, Keegan L, Guzzetta CE, Kolkmeier, LG. *Holistic Nursing: A Handbook for Practice*. Gaithersburg, Md: Aspen Publishers; 1995.

80. Meehan MTC. Therapeutic touch. In: Bulecheck GM, McCloskey JC, eds. *Nursing Interventions: Essential Nursing Treatments*. 2nd ed. Philadelphia, Pa: WB Saunders; 1992.

81. Quinn JF. One nurse's evolution as a healer. *Am J Nurs*. 1979;79(4):662–664.

82. Woods-Smith D. Therapeutic touch: a healing experience. *Maine Nurse*. 1988; 74(2):3,7.

83. Newman M. *Health as Expanding Consciousness*. St Louis, Mo: Mosby; 1986.

84. North American Nursing Diagnosis Association (NANDA). *NANDA Nursing Diagnosis: Definitions and Classifications 1995–1996*. Philadelphia, Pa: NANDA; 1994.

85. Eisenberg DM, Kessler RC, Foster C, Norlock FE, Colkins DR, Delbanco TL. Unconventional medicine in the United States: prevalence, costs, and patterns of use. *N Engl J Med*. 1993;328(4):246–252.

86. Samarel N. Report to the membership and board of the National Institutes of Health office of unconventional medical practices workshop. *Cooperative Connection*. 1993;14(1):1,3–5.

87. Holzman D. Advisory council meeting: NIH Office of Alternative Medicine Program. *Alternat Compl Therapies*. 1995;1(2):109.

88. Krieger D. *Accepting Your Power to Heal: The Personal Practice of Therapeutic Touch*. Santa Fe, NM: Bear & Co; 1993.

89. Weber S, Coppa DF. An open letter to the board of trustees and the membership. *Cooperative Connection*. 1993;14(1):10.

90. Quinn JF. An open letter to the board of trustees and the membership. *Cooperative Connection*. 1992;13(4):12–13.

91. Clark PE, Clark MJ. Therapeutic touch: is there a scientific basis for the practice? *Nurs Res*. 1984;33(1):37–41.

92. Jaroff L. A no-touch therapy. *Time*. November 21, 1994:88–89.

93. Oberst MT. Our naked emperor, editorial. *Res Nurs Health*. 1995;18:1–2.

Nursing Grand Rounds

Cynthia M. Steckel, RN, MSN, CCRN
Director, ICU/SDU/Telemetry
Scripps Memorial Hospital-La Jolla and Green
Hospital of Scripps Clinic

Rauni Prittinen King, RN, BSN, CCRN
Staff Nurse, Intensive Care Unit
Scripps Memorial Hospital
La Jolla, California

Source: Reprinted from C.M. Steckel, R.P. King, *The Journal of Cardiovascular Nursing,* Vol. 10, No. 3, pp. 50–54, © 1996, Aspen Publishers, Inc.

THERAPEUTIC TOUCH IN THE CORONARY CARE UNIT

The Scripps Memorial Hospital coronary care unit (CCU) became involved with therapeutic touch (TT) through a persistent colleague who felt that there was great potential for the healing arts in the CCU. Ultimately, the staff decided that if this was a new heart pump they would want to be on the cutting edge of learning about it and incorporating it into their practice. In this spirit, eight practitioners attended a weekend-long class in November 1993. Although skeptical, all were curious and motivated by a vision of walking into an agitated patient's room, performing TT, and rapidly creating calm. Today, the experiences of the staff suggest there may be benefits from adding TT into the patient's current medical treatment as a noninvasive, potentially healing nursing practice. Twenty nurses in the CCU have completed TT training through the level I healing touch class. In August 1994, the hospital began to offer the level I healing touch classes on site and has trained more than 100 employees throughout the hospital system.

Healing Touch is the name given to a national program presented by the American Holistic Nurses' Association that includes a collection of various energy-based interventions. There are many classes available throughout the United States. TT is one of the techniques taught in this class. TT is the most well-researched technique and the one with which the authors have had the most experience. It is supported by the National League for Nursing (NLN) and has been taught in more than 70 countries. This article, therefore, focuses on clinical experiences using TT. The current practice of TT was developed in 1974 by Dolores Krieger,[1] and a noted healer, Dora Kunz. It has its basis in the nursing conceptual model of Martha Rogers,[2] a pioneer in developing the theoretical view of human energy fields as they relate to nursing practice.[2]

CLINICAL EXPERIENCES WITH TT

Over the past year, Scripps' staff has performed TT many times in the CCU. Anecdotally, a reduction of pain in arthritic joints, headaches, and backaches and a decrease in anxiety have been observed. Practitioners do not attest to miracle cures or sudden reversals but have achieved positive changes. Following open heart surgery, one extremely anxious patient in the CCU required a bronchoscopy after extubation. Low blood pressure and hypoxia made him a poor candidate for sedation. Using TT, however, the staff was able to successfully complete the bronchoscopy procedure.

After cardiac surgery, decreased sedation is essential to enable early extubation. The authors found TT to be of assistance in helping patients awaken calmly from anesthesia, in some cases reducing the need for sedation. In one case, a patient, the victim of a self-inflicted stab wound to the heart, was too agitated postoperatively to be extubated. Staff did not want to continue heavy sedation because this would delay extubation. TT was successfully applied in this situation to help calm the patient and he was subsequently extubated.

One patient was admitted after a myocardial infarction (MI) in massive pulmonary edema requiring intubation for more than 1 week. He repeatedly suffered periods of anxiety and agitation and required increased oxygenation, frequent suctioning, and almost daily bronchoscopy. The staff decided to add daily TT to his treatment plan. After implementing TT as part of the plan, the patient began requiring less sedation and became more compliant. In fact, the patient looked forward to his TT treatments. He eventually went on to have a mitral valve replacement and was extubated without complications the day after his surgery.

The authors documented the course of one particularly striking case involving a patient on the intraaortic balloon pump (IABP). At one point in his course the patient had a systolic blood pressure in the 70s, a cardiac index (CI) of 1.46, and systemic vascular resistance (SVR) of 2,427 dyne/sec/cm⁵. These measurements were taken when he was on vasodilator drips. His ST segments were rising despite intravenous nitroglycerin, morphine, and oxygen. His nurse, having exhausted the options available in the treatment plan for improving his cardiovascular status, elected to add TT with a subsequent drop in his ST segment despite no other changes in treatment. The patient's SVR dropped to 1,498 and CI rose to 2.06. It is not known which specific factor at that moment caused the ST elevation to resolve. It is known, however, that in the presence of elevated ST segments being treated with vasodilators, an IABP, and pain medication, the addition of TT coincided with the resolution of symptoms. Was it serendipity or design? No one knows for sure, but it is an interesting observation that bears repeating.

The best similar example the authors have noted was in a newly injured quadriplegic patient acting out loudly and refusing medication to help settle him. After many unsuccessful attempts at soothing the agitated patient by talking to him, the patient was offered TT and the staff was able to calm the patient enough for him to accept the necessary medication; he slept for more than 1 hour. Again, TT was not the complete treatment. Rather, as a valuable adjunct to traditional approaches, it actually put the patient in the best condition for nature and the medical regimen to act.

TT—WHAT IT IS

Florence Nightingale presented one of the most practical descriptions of nursing in use today. "Nature alone cures. And what nursing has to do . . . is put the patient in the best condition for nature to act upon him."[3(p133)] This description may be applicable as well to TT, the goal of which has been stated as restoring harmony and balance in the energy system to help the patient self-heal. TT is based on the assumption that each person has a physical body and a subtle body comprised of many layers or fields of energy. The earth has an energy field of gravity that becomes more intense around a planet. Similarly, people have a human energy field that is more concentrated around their bodies. Originally known as the "aura," this energy field is now understood as an electromagnetic field found throughout nature. An energy field can be experienced any time a person outside the visual field quietly enters a room and you "feel" his or her presence. This energy field has been described in many ancient cultures.

A congestion or disturbance of flow in these energy layers is one of the first signs of illness in the physical body. The practitioner works in these energy fields to restore balance, smooth out disturbances or blocks, and help the person to self-heal. The mechanism of action among energy fields, health, and illness is not well understood. However, many careful studies describing the phenomenon of interaction have been done. TT is not meant as a substitute for medical treatment but as an adjunct to assist medical treatment—another tool in a nurse's repertoire. It requires no particular spiritual belief system in either the practitioner or the patient. While physicians have become increasingly specialized, nurses have traditionally maintained their focus on the whole being, even expanding into the family and social environment to assist the patient's healing. TT may be a natural step in this progression, moving from the visible physical body into the energy field of the body to treat the whole person.

THE PROCESS OF TT

The process of TT contains five steps[1]:

1. The first step is for the practitioner to become centered. This is the state of bringing the body, mind, and emotions to a quiet, focused state of awareness.

2. The second step is to assess the energy field. The practitioner uses his or her hands to assess the nature of the energy field. This assessment is done by holding the hands in a relaxed, cupped position several inches from the body and moving them symmetrically from head to feet. Descriptions such as "tingling," "vibrating," "cold," and "heat" may be noted in various areas of the body.

3. The third step is to unruffle the field. The practitioner uses a similar movement as in assessing but in a brushing, more vigorous manner. This unruffling smooths out disturbances in the field.

4. The fourth step is the modulation of energy to problem areas. Energy is directed locally to an area by resting the hands over it to bring fullness to the energy field in that location.

5. The final step is to reassess for changes and conclude the treatment.

The TT treatment takes approximately 15 minutes to complete and does not deplete energy from the practitioner. To the contrary, many practitioners feel invigorated after a patient treatment. It can be done on anyone at any time, unrestricted by the equipment attached to the patient or patient instability. TT follows a process consistent with the nursing process. Experience is necessary for skill acquisition. When learning to discern heart sounds, it is only with practice and experience that the nurse begins to differentiate split sounds from extra heart sounds. Likewise, it is only with repeated practice of TT that the practitioner becomes increasingly sensitive to the subtle changes in the energy field.

EFFECT OF TT ON PRACTITIONER AND FAMILIES

Some of the most interesting results are the relaxing and calming effect the practice of TT has on the practitioner. Whether it be the time concentrated on one task that temporarily shuts out the stress of the CCU atmosphere, the effect of the practitioner centering, or the TT itself, the authors have themselves been refreshed following a treatment given to their patients. Family members have commented that they have felt their loved one to be in caring hands because the nurse practiced TT. Some families that are aware of TT as a treatment modality have requested the intervention for a family member. They have expressed pleasant surprise to find TT practiced in such a "high tech" traditional hospital setting. Patients themselves have become accepting of the treatment. Rather than being reluctant to accept TT, most patients who receive TT request it again.

A patient admitted after a cardiac arrest following an MI had a long CCU course with multiple setbacks and was eventually determined not to be a candidate for open heart surgery. His wife was anxious, stemming from her husband's long hospitalization and poor prognosis. She approached the staff to ask whether anyone in the hospital performed TT because she had just seen it on television the night before. TT treatments were begun on both the patient and his wife who provided much positive feedback about how it helped them through the hospitalization.

The authors have been successful using TT on fellow colleagues. One of the pulmonary physicians, after completing a procedure in the CCU, said he had pulled his back and was in acute pain. He planned to take pain medication for his back spasm and go home. The authors offered TT as an option for treating his back pain and he accepted. After TT was performed on his back, he stood up claiming he was able to walk without pain. This physician not only stayed at work, but also kept returning to the CCU throughout the day to comment on how amazed he was that his back felt well. In addition, staff members have successfully performed TT on each other to help relieve headaches and backaches as well as promote general relaxation after a stressful shift.

FUTURE DIRECTIONS

TT is a healing modality that may have met its moment in time. Patients and families have been open to its use, and practitioners in health care are beginning to accept the relationships between mind and body and between emotion and organic response. When the subject of TT arises in the hospital, the number of physicians and practitioners who will come forward to support such a venture is surprising. In the authors' experience, some of the strongest supporters have been surgeons and cardiologists with traditional approaches to medical care. In general, these physicians have expressed the belief that whatever helps the patient and is noninvasive is worth trying. The authors have elected to continue pursuing the use of TT because their experiences have shown some value in helping to stabilize patients, relieve pain, decrease anxiety, and possibly accelerate wound healing. The fact that it can be taught to families helps them get involved in a hands-on manner. The authors would encourage further research on TT to help determine its mechanism of action and place in nursing practice, and they want to participate in this line of inquiry.

REFERENCES

1. Krieger D. *The Therapeutic Touch: How to Use Your Hands to Help or to Heal.* Englewood Cliffs, NJ: Prentice Hall; 1979.
2. Rogers M. *The Theoretical Basis of Nursing.* Philadelphia, Pa: FA Davis; 1970.
3. Nightingale F. *Notes on Nursing: What It Is, and What It Is Not.* New York, NY: Dover Publications; 1969.

Psychoimmunologic Effects of Therapeutic Touch on Practitioners and Recently Bereaved Recipients: A Pilot Study

Janet F. Quinn, PhD, RN, FAAN
Associate Professor and Senior Scholar
Center for Human Caring
University of Colorado School of Nursing
Denver, Colorado

Anthony J. Strelkauskas, PhD
Associate Professor
Microbiology and Immunobiology
Medical University of South Carolina
Charleston, South Carolina

Therapeutic Touch (TT) is a modern approach to healing that derives from the ancient practice of the laying on of hands. Research on TT is built on the work by Bernard Grad, Sister Justa Smith, and Dolores Krieger. These researchers studied the phenomenon of laying on of hands and found that it could increase the rate of wound healing in mice,[1,2] the rate of growth in plants,[2-4] the rate of activity of the enzyme trypsin,[5] and the level of human hemoglobin.[6,7] Outcome studies to date indicate that TT can increase human hemoglobin level,[8,9] induce physiologic relaxation,[10] decrease state anxiety,[11,12] decrease pain,[13,14] decrease diastolic blood pressure,[15] reduce stress in hospitalized children,[16] and accelerate wound healing.[17]

THEORETICAL FRAMEWORK AND PURPOSE

The Rogerian conceptual system has provided the foundation for most of the TT studies that followed Krieger's initial work drawing on the insights of Eastern philosophic thought. Rogers defines people as irreducible, indivisible, multidimensional energy fields integral with the environmental energy field.[18] In earlier conceptualizations of TT, the idea that there was an "energy transfer or exchange" between the practitioner and the recipient was a primary explanatory

Source: Reprinted from J.F. Quinn, A.J. Strelkauskas, *Advances in Nursing Science,* Vol. 15, No. 4, pp. 13–26, © 1993, Aspen Publishers, Inc.

This study was funded by the Institute of Noetic Sciences, Sausalito, California.

theory,[11,12,15] deriving from Rogers' conceptual system and consistent with theoretical explanations offered by earlier researchers.[1-6] More recently, it has been postulated that the TT practitioner, knowingly participating in the mutual human/environment process by shifting consciousness into a state that may be thought of as a "healing meditation," facilitates repatterning of the recipient's energy field through a process of resonance, rather than "energy exchange or transfer."[10,19,20]

In spite of these conceptualizations that the practitioner and the recipient of TT are not separate but are interconnected and integral with the total universal energy field, outcome studies have continued to focus on the effects of TT treatment on recipients and have ignored the effects of treatment on the practitioner. This focus has been and will continue to be helpful in expanding our database of research-demonstrated outcomes of TT—a process that has stimulated the introduction of TT into many nursing schools and hospitals nationally and internationally. Yet these research studies are not wholly consistent with our conceptual framework. We have conducted our research studies from particulate–deterministic and interactive–integrative perspectives, yet TT is clearly an example of a phenomenon belonging to the unitary–transformative perspective.[21]

The purposes of this descriptive pilot study were to address this conceptual inconsistency and several other methodologic problems identified in earlier TT research,[15] while also providing direction for future TT studies by attempting to determine the appropriateness and suitability of a combination of psychologic and immunologic measures in the ongoing empiric evaluation of TT. The following understandings informed the decision-making process about which outcome variables to explore within this unitary context.

At the core of the TT process is the intent of the practitioner to help the recipient; that is, the practitioner attempts to focus completely on the well-being of the recipient in an act of unconditional love and compassion. For this reason TT has been called a "healing meditation."[10] Recent research suggests that positive emotions can have a beneficial effect on the health of the individual. McClelland[22] has demonstrated that feelings of compassion and unconditional love may increase the effectiveness of the immune system in the experiencer. If McClelland's hypothesis is correct, the practice of TT should be enhancing of or supportive to the practitioner's immune system. Anecdotally, TT practitioners claim that they are sick less often and that when they do become ill they consistently recover more quickly than others or themselves prior to becoming TT practitioners. Research on the practice of TT could thus reasonably ask about the effects of administering TT on the practitioners' immune systems. In seeking a population of recipients for such an investigation, recently bereaved individuals were chosen because they often have a temporarily suppressed immune system[23-25] in the absence of other immunologic problems. These situational shifts might be expected to respond favorably to treatment by TT, which is assumed to accelerate natural healing processes. These considerations led to the framing of the following questions for study, explored using a descriptive study design.

RESEARCH QUESTIONS

1. Are there differences from baseline in the immunologic profile of recipients and practitioners immediately after and following a series of treatments with TT?

2. Are there patterns among or relationships between recipient's and practitioner's immunologic profile before, immediately after, and following a series of treatments with TT?

3. Are there differences from baseline in selected psychologic measures in recipients and practitioners immediately after and following a series of treatments with TT?

4. Are there patterns among or relationships between recipient's and practitioner's psychologic measures before, immediately after, and following a series of treatments with TT?

5. Are there patterns among or relationships between immunologic and psychologic measures in the recipients and practitioners immediately after and following a series of TT treatments?

6. Are there patterns among or relationships between the perceptions of effectiveness of treatments and psychoimmunologic outcomes of recipients and practitioners immediately after and following TT treatments?

7. Are there patterns among or relationships between the time experiences, perceptions of effectiveness, and psychoimmunologic outcomes of recipients and practitioners immediately after and following a series of TT treatments?

METHODOLOGY

Subjects

The subjects were two TT practitioners (SB and GA) and four recently bereaved individuals who received TT treatments (CB, VD, MG, and GS). Demographic data on the subjects appear in Table 1. The TT practitioners had been trained by Krieger and Kunz and had been practicing TT for more than 5 years. TT practitioners were recruited through collegial contacts of the investigator. Two bereaved subjects were recruited through a newspaper ad, one responded to a request through a church bulletin, and one was referred by a colleague of the investigator. Bereaved individuals were told that we were interested in studying the potential benefits of

Table 1. Demographic characteristics of the subjects

	TT recipients				TT practitioners	
Subject	CB	VD	MG	GS	GA	SB
Sex	F	M	M	F	F	F
Age (years)	61	47	72	62	46	57
Deceased relative	Husband	Mother	Wife	Husband	—	—
Length of bereavement	8 wks	24 wks	7 wks	15 wks	—	—
Religion	Pres*	RC*	RC*	RC*	RC*	Epis*
Occupation	Housewife	MD	Retired	Retired	RN, professor	Nurse
Highest grade	14	MD	GED*	AS*	EdD	AD*
Health problems	None	Gastritis; CAD*; hypercholesterolemia	Seizure disorder	Anxiety; depression; ASHD*	Obesity	Food allergies; Candida
Medication	Vitamins	None regularly	Dilantin	Persantine; Limbitrol	None	Nizoral; estrogen
Regular exercise	No	Runs	No	No	Walks	No
Meditation/relaxation	No	No	No	No	Daily	Daily

*Pres = Presbyterian; RC = Roman Catholic; Epis = Episcopalian; GED = General Education Certificate; AS = Associate of Science Degree; AD = Associate Degree; CAD = coronary artery disease; ASHD = arteriosclerotic heart disease.

TT for bereaved people like themselves. All subjects signed written informed consent, which included the instruction (also verbally given) that they may exit from the study at any time and for any reason.

Definition of terms and measures

TT is an intervention that is a derivative of laying on of hands, during which it is assumed that the practitioner knowingly participates in the repatterning of the recipient's energy field for the purpose of helping or healing the person.[20] In treating a person with TT, the practitioner

- makes the intention mentally to assist the subject therapeutically
- moves the hands over the body of the subject from head to feet, attuning to the condition of the subject by becoming aware of changes in sensory cues in the hands
- redirects areas of accumulated tension in the subject's energy field by movement of the hands; and
- focuses attention on the specific direction of energies to the subject using the hands as focal points[11,12]

Psychologic measures

A psychologic profile was obtained on both recipients and practitioners. The profile included the following measures, among others: anxiety as measured by the State-Trait Anxiety Inventory (STAI)[26] and mood as measured by the Affect Balance Scale (ABS).[27] Reliability and validity of the STAI are well established, while there are no reliability and validity data available for the ABS.

Unitary measures

Included in this category are two experiential measures that might traditionally be considered within the psychologic dimension. Yet within a human energy field model, they may be better conceptualized as reflections of shifts in field pattern.

Effectiveness of treatment

Perception of the effectiveness of the treatment was measured by the Effectiveness of Therapeutic Touch [visual analogue] Scale (ETTS).[28] There is no established reliability or validity for this scale.

Time perception

Altered states of consciousness are known to be associated with distortions in time perception, and TT is assumed to involve an altered state of consciousness. Time perception was measured as a way of beginning to examine the nature of the change in consciousness that accompanies both the administration and receipt of TT and also to see if there might be any relationship between the time perception of the recipients and that of the practitioners as an index of their interconnectedness and mutual process.[21] Each recipient and practitioner was asked to write down, out of view of each other, an estimate of the length of time that had elapsed during the treatment that had just ended.

Immunologic measures and methods

A profile of immune functions was developed for each practitioner and recipient, consisting of the following four measures:

1. lymphocyte subset composition as determined by cytofluorographic analysis
2. responsiveness toward foreign cells as shown by mixed lymphocyte reactivity (MLC) and cell-mediated toxicity (CML)
3. lymphocyte stimulation using phytohemagglutinin (PHA), concanavalin A (Con A), and pokeweed mitogen (PWM); and
4. natural killer cell (NK) assays

Lymphocyte types were determined by utilizing commercially available fluorescence conjugated monoclonal antibodies, with cells being identified on a coulter cytofluorograph. Each sample was tested for percentage of T and B cells as well as for specific T4 (helper) and T8 (suppressor) T-cell subsets. This type of evaluation is becoming routine, and the percentages of these cells are becoming increasingly important for the delineation of immune potential.[29]

MLC and CML were obtained by utilizing standard radiolabeled assays with tritiated thymidine uptake indicating MSL reactivity and chromium release from target cells used to identify CML. These assays provide information on the ability of the subject's immune system to react to a foreign cell type. These functions represent a fundamental part of the immune response, with mixed lymphocyte responses being an indicator of recognition and cell-mediated lympholysis an indicator of the cytotoxic capability of sensitized lymphocytes.

Lymphocyte stimulations were performed using standard procedures for inducing lymphocyte division. These divisions were quantitated by the uptake of tritiated thymidine. The lymphocyte stimulation assay is a standard means to identify the reactivity of lymphocytes.[30] Mitogens such as PHA, Con A, and pokeweed have been used for many years to induce lymphocyte division. Most of the studies that seek to evaluate psychoneuroimmunologic changes have employed lymphocyte stimulation studies.[23–25]

NK assays were performed using a transformed cell line K562. Unlike the CML response, natural killing is a lymphocyte function that does not require the killer cells to be previously sensitized to their targets. It is thought that the natural killing event is directed predominantly toward tumor cells. Radioactive assays to determine NK activity are routine.[31]

Testing procedures: Each blood sample was approximately 50 cc of heparinized blood and was divided into 2 aliquots. Whole blood was used for lymphocyte profiles, while the majority of the blood was fractionated over ficoll Hypaque gradients to purify the lymphocytes. Isolated lymphocytes were then split into two aliquots and frozen in liquid nitrogen until the time of testing. One of the frozen samples was used for CML and MLR. All of the samples were tested for CML and MLR on the same day to prevent interassay variability. The second aliquot of cells was used for the NK assays, again doing all testing on the same day to prevent variability.

Protocols

On day one all subjects completed baseline questionnaires and baseline bloods (B1) were drawn before TT treatments were administered. Repeat questionnaires were administered and repeat bloods (B2) were drawn on recipients following their first TT treatment. Questionnaires were administered and repeat bloods were drawn on practitioners after all of their treatments for that day were completed.

Treatment consisted of the practitioner administering TT in the manner in which it has been taught, that is, using the sequential steps as specified in the definition. Beyond this general guideline, the practitioners were permitted to administer TT as they usually did and for the length of time that they deemed appropriate. The length of time of the procedure was monitored by the research assistant. This is a shift from previous studies, critiqued by Quinn,[15] that have prescribed the exact length of treatment—a protocol that works well in the context of experimental design but does not allow for study of the phenomenon as practiced clinically.

Final questionnaires were administered and final bloods were drawn pretreatment (B3) and posttreatment (B4) on the last day of participation for each subject. The trial was for 4 treatments for CB; 7 for VD, MG, and GS; 18 given by SB, and 14 given by GA. The numbers of treatments given reflects treatments given to an additional nonbereaved subject, for which data are not reported herein.

DATA ANALYSIS AND RESULTS

A research assistant administered and scored all psychologic tools and collected the time estimates after each session. Immunologic data was compiled and examined for clinical significance by the cellular immunologist (AS) on the project. The data were examined for patterns and trends using simple descriptive statistics. Only the most important findings will be summarized in the following discussion. A full report of this study is available from the first author.

Psychologic measures

Table 2 summarizes the changes that occurred in STAI, and Table 3 presents changes in ABS over the course of the study period in both recipients and practitioners.

State and trait anxiety

Recipients

State anxiety was measured before and after the first and the last TT treatments, providing two change scores for each subject. These scores were averaged for each subject and are presented in Table 2. There was an average decrease in state anxiety, following treatment by TT, of 29% in recipients. This average percent change is considerably larger than that obtained in any of the TT studies to date, the largest percent change being 17% found by Quinn in 1984. Many possible explanations exist for this finding; however, it seems that a very likely one involves the method of administering the TT treatments. In former studies, these treatments have been operationally defined quite specifically, particularly in terms of length of treatment (5 minutes) and the use of touch or nontouch. The TT practitioners in these earlier studies were instructed to follow the protocols exactly. In this study, the TT protocol was not specified; that is, practitio-

ners were permitted to administer the treatment as they determined and for as long as they determined. This may have contributed to the larger effect on state anxiety. There was a decrease in trait anxiety score from first to last TT treatments in two recipients and an increase in two recipients. No obvious explanation exists for this finding.

Practitioners

State and trait anxiety scores for practitioners both before and after administering TT were at or close to zero and so percent changes in their scores reflect very little real change. Their low anxiety may be a reflection of TT practice, meditation practice, or the unique setting of the study.

Patterns/relationships

Examination of these data does not reveal any obvious relationships between scores of recipients and scores of practitioners on state or trait anxiety. Further, there does not appear to be a pattern of response variability between the recipients treated by SB and those treated by GA.

Affect Balance Scale

Table 3 reveals that there was a dramatic increase in virtually all of the dimensions of positive affect (joy, vigor, contentment, and affection) and in the positive total in all TT recipients and a dramatic decrease in virtually all of the negative affect (anxiety, guilt, hostility, and depression) dimensions and the negative total in all TT recipients. The Affect Balance Index (relationship between positive and negative ex-

Table 2. Percent changes from first to last measure on State-Trait Anxiety Inventory

Measure	Recipients		Nurse	Recipients		Nurse
	CB	*VD*	*SB*	*MG*	*GS*	*GA*
Pretest state anxiety	+56	−32	−38	−39	−14	+27
Mean percent change pretest to posttest state anxiety	−26	−32	−23	−34	−25	+8
Trait anxiety	+32	−21	0	−15	+19	−24

Table 3. Percent changes from first to last measure on Affect Balance Scale

Measure	Recipients		Nurse	Recipients		Nurse
	CB	VD	SB	MG	GS	GA
Joy	+38	+38	−9	+4	+38	+10
Contentment	+43	+47	0	+100	+11	+8
Vigor	+60	+56	0	+25	+18	+8
Affection	+79	+54	0	−7	+56	+6
Positive total	+67	+76	−9	+32	+42	+8
Anxiety	−33	−27	−25	−20	−18	−44
Depression	−25	−45	0	−33	−17	0
Guilt	0	−39	0	+64	−18	0
Hostility	+33	−43	−17	0	0	0
Negative total	−14	−43	−14	+3	−16	−23
Affect balance	+50	+152	−3	+29	+36	+8

pressed in standardized score—the higher, the more positive) increased across all recipients. The pattern of results in the practitioners was similar to that of the recipients.

There are much larger increases in the positive total and much larger decreases in the negative total in SB's recipients than in GA's recipients. There is an average of 48% difference between the two groups in positive total, 77% in negative total, and 68% in Affect Balance Scale.

Unitary measures

Effectiveness of Therapeutic Touch Scale

Following each TT treatment, both recipients and practitioners placed a mark on a visual analogue ETTS. These marks were scored as a number between 0 and 10, with 10 representing the maximum positive rating. Recipients treated by SB rated the effectiveness of their treatments 54% higher than did recipients treated by GA. Practitioners tended to rate their treatments similarly, although there was less variability in the ratings of SB. There was greater congruence between the ratings of SB and those of her recipients than between the ratings of GA and her recipients.

The congruence observed in SB and her recipient's ratings is quite interesting, well beyond the simple question of whether or not the treatment was perceived as helpful. There were many differences in outcomes between subjects treated by SB and those treated by GA. Perhaps the congruence we see in the effectiveness ratings is an index of the degree to which this practitioner was able to "get inside" of or "get into sync" with the recipients she was treating. Additional evidence that this may indeed by so appeared when examining the perception of time experience.

Time estimation

As noted earlier, this measure was included as an initial attempt to see if the shift in consciousness that is assumed to occur during TT and that has also been observed in recipients of TT might in some way be reflected in a subject's experience of time. Each practitioner and recipient estimated the amount of time that had elapsed during treatment. The actual time elapsed was also recorded, and the difference between the two measures was labeled as "time distortion." A full presentation of this data appears elsewhere.[20] For the purpose of this article, a brief summary of this data will now be presented with emphasis on the relationship of these findings to the other measures in the study and on implications of the findings for future TT research.

Subjects treated by SB and those treated by GA again differed. SB's recipients experienced a distortion in time that was about three times that of the recipients treated by GA. Similar observations were made about the practitioners. SB experienced time distortion that was about four times greater than that experienced by GA. Actual length of treatment did not appear to relate to the amount of distortion on a case by case basis in either recipients or practitioners.

When examining how practitioner–recipient pairs experienced time, there was not any observable relationship in the *magnitude* of time distortion in these pairs—ie, in the actual number of minutes that were over- or underestimated. However, there was a very clear relationship in terms of the *direction* of time distortion. In all of SB's sessions, the direction of time distortion (ie, over- or underestimations) was the same for both her and her recipients, and this estimation varied each day with the same recipient. On some days they both overestimated, and on some they both underestimated. In GA's two recipients, there were two different patterns. With MG there was 100% congruence in direction of time distortion, and with GS there was 50% congruence. Interestingly, when SB treated GS, there was an inverse relationship in the direction of their time distortion as well. One possible explanatory note seems important here. GS, treated by GA, also had the least magnitude of time distortion, and her effectiveness ratings were also the lowest. It is possible that the ability of her system to shift into an altered state of consciousness, and thus to experience the time distortion, was influenced by her antidepressant medication. Further, it may be that the degree to which consciousness shifts in TT recipients influences how "effective" they perceive the intervention to be. Future study may shed light on this possibility.

There are many questions for future investigation raised by this set of findings. Are we seeing the emergence of an index of practitioner–re-cipient resonance? To date, no such index exists. If altered states of consciousness are correlates of alternative healing modalities, and if time perception/distortion is an index of consciousness, then perhaps we are. Can this index be used to determine if a given practitioner is able to enter the "healing state of consciousness?" Is this variable, time distortion, correlated with outcomes? The data in this study suggest such a possibility. Recall that we have seen what appears to be evidence of a connection, a resonance, between SB and her recipients, reflected in the congruence of their effectiveness scores and that, of the two recipients treated by GA, the more positively responsive one was in fact MG, with whom GA had 100% congruence on the distortion measure. Recall also that the two recipients treated by SB had the greatest positive changes in the ABS. Finally, we shall see that in some of the immunologic parameters the responses of SB's two subjects are again very similar.

Immunologic profile

Lymphocyte subset composition as determined by cytofluorographic analysis

Recipients

Table 4 presents the changes in lymphocyte subset populations from the first blood drawing to the last for all study participants. There are no consistent variations in subsets identified by the markers Leu-16, OKT11, OKT3, and OKT4 across recipients. However, examination of the OKT8 (suppressor T cell) subset presents a different pattern. Here there is a consistent change across all of the recipients, namely a diminution of the percentage of suppressor T cells. The percentage of OKT8 cells at B4 is lower in all four recipients, with a difference of over 20% in the case of CB. Such a change, particularly in light of the random pattern appearing in all other subsets, seems highly unlikely to be due to chance.

Table 4. Lymphocyte profile percent change from B1 to B4*

Marker/cell type	Recipients				Practitioners	
	CB	VD	MG	GS	SB	GA
Leu-16/B cells	+37	−26	−57	+11	+8	−29
OKT3/T cells	−5	−10	+15	+9	+2	+18
OKT11/T cells	−8	−9	+4	+0.3	−6	+8
OKT4a/helper T cells	−1	−0.2	+13	+9	+6	−5
OKT8/suppressor T cells	−21	−10	−20	−17	−16	−23

*B1 = initial baseline blood sample; B4 = terminal sample.

Practitioners

Table 5 reveals that SB has a disproportionately low percentage of T8 cells across all testing times, and very little fluctuation is seen between B1, B2, B3, and B4. GA began the study with a lower percentage of T8 cells than the recipients but a higher percentage than the other practitioner. Her pattern then resembled the initial drop in T8 cells seen in the recipients, such that her percentage of suppressor T cells became virtually identical with SB's percentage, with little fluctuation thereafter.

Patterns/relationships

It is particularly interesting to note the substantial difference between the recipients and the practitioners on the parameter of OKT8. As noted, both practitioners are lower in percentage of T8 cells than the recipients at the initial measurement. SB is 47% lower than the highest bereaved recipient (CB at 31.4) and 35% lower than the lowest bereaved recipient (VD at 25.4). These large differences between SB and the bereaved recipients continue throughout the study, even though the recipients experience a decrease in T8 percentages. GA begins the study 30% lower than CB and 13% lower than VD. She is 34% higher than SB. By the end of the first treatment (B2), however, she is virtually identical to SB and essentially remains that way throughout the rest of the study. It is interesting to note that

SB is the more experienced of the two practitioners. She engages in TT practice on a daily basis and administers TT approximately 50 to 60 times per month. GA is an experienced practitioner who does not practice TT daily, administering an average of 10 TT treatments per month. While there is obviously no conclusive interpretation of this data that can appropriately be made, there are important questions raised for future study. For example, is there some relationship between frequent practice of TT and the findings related to the T8 population? Is a low percentage, a diminution, of suppressor T cells a marker in TT practitioners? Note that GA's percentage quickly came into line with SB's when she began treating people.

Table 5. OKT8—suppressor T cell subset percentage of total lymphocytes at B1 through B4*

	B1	B2	B3	B4
Recipients				
CB	31.4	30.8	26.4	24.7
VD	25.4	23.7	23.8	22.9
MG	30.3	26.6	21.9	24.1
GS	30.7	28.4	35.5	25.6
Practitioners				
SB	16.4	15.1	15.2	13.7
GA	22.0	16.4	15.3	17.0

*B1 = initial baseline blood sample; B4 = terminal sample.

Summary

These data seem to indicate that something about the treatment (ie, the actual TT, the environment, etc) impacts on lymphocyte subset composition. The magnitude of the changes and the consistency of the pattern of diminution in T8 cells across both recipients and practitioners is unequivocal. Explanation of what this means, why this subset should respond differentially to TT, and what the impact of the response is in terms of the rest of the immune system and health status will have to wait for future investigations. One potential hypothesis deriving from this finding is that TT enhances immunologic functioning by the suppression of suppression, which, immunologically, is the equivalent of increasing helping.

Lymphocyte stimulation using PHA, Con A, and PWM

Recipients

Several patterns may be observed in these data, presented in Table 6. First, there are clear and substantial changes in the values across testings in all recipients, particularly in Con A and PHA. The percent changes from B1 to B4 clearly identify the magnitude of the change. Second, the direction of the change is not consistent across recipients. Both CB and VD have a diminution of response to the mitogens from B1 to B4, while MG and GS have very large increases.

Practitioners

We have an incomplete dataset here due to an inadequate number of cells at several of the testings. The data that are available reveal several patterns. First, both SB and GA demonstrate a dramatic decrease in lymphocyte response to mitogen stimulation by PHA. SB's response to Con A is increased by B4 while response to PWM is small and unlikely to be significant.

Patterns/relationships

There are unequivocal changes in both the recipients' and the practitioners' lymphocyte response to mitogen stimulation. In addition, there are patterns of response across testings that are easily identified and are shared by SB's recipients CB and VD, who have been similar on many measures thus far. Why this should be and what this means in terms of TT and health, remain to be determined through further study.

MLC, CML, and NK assays

Inadequate numbers of cells were available for analysis of MLC and CML in practitioner GA. In SB and in recipients, there was a pattern of response that indicated an adequate recognition response (to foreign cell types) and a diminution of killing response. There does not appear to be any consistent effect of the TT treatment on NK in either recipients or practitioners. As noted, these findings are discussed in detail in the full report.

Table 6. Percent change from B1 to B4* in lymphocyte response to mitogen stimulation

Mitogen	Recipients				Practitioners	
	CB	VD	MG	GS	SB	GA
Con A*	−19	−71	+140	+105	+17	—
PHA*	+5	−38	+59	+218	−50	−97
PWM*	−41	−61	+82	+596	+10	—

*B1 = initial baseline blood sample; B4 = terminal sample; Con A = Concanavalin A; PHA = phytohemagglutinin; PWM = pokeweed mitogen.

SUMMARY

A major focus for this pilot study was the relationship between the practitioner and the recipient of TT. Specifically, it was postulated that, since the nature of the TT interaction is unitary, it would be meaningful to study both sides of that relationship rather than one in isolation. The findings of this pilot study provide affirmation of that perspective. Some of the most interesting and theoretically significant findings of the study involve the comparison of practitioner and recipient data. In summary, it is clear that several changes occurred in both practitioners and recipients following the series of treatments with TT. There is no way to know which one or combination of factors discussed best explains the results; and there are many possible intervening variables, all of which will need to be explored in further study. This pilot has served to demonstrate that further study of the effects of TT on immune systems of both practitioners and recipients is appropriate and that future studies should concentrate on the lymphocyte response to mitogenic stimulation, the modulation of subsets as a result of treatment, and perhaps most importantly, the immunologic differences between practitioners and nonpractitioners. Further, an entirely new area of study has emerged relative to the time experience of both practitioners and recipients of TT, which has theoretical implications beyond those concerned with TT.

DIRECTIONS FOR FUTURE RESEARCH

The following are recommendations for future research on TT within a unitary framework based on this pilot study.

This study should be replicated with larger samples of both practitioners and recipients. However, the design should allow for a longitudinal approach rather than the 2-week time frame we used. The recruitment of the bereaved population is not without difficulty; and to get an adequate sample, the study will need to go on over time with flexible entry and exit points for the bereaved subjects.

The design for the above replication should remain descriptive. This approach will allow the development of a much needed baseline of data that demonstrates the "best case" possibilities for this treatment prior to development of controlled intervention trials. However, even in controlled investigations, the TT treatment itself should not be manipulated. A control group of some sort could be added, but the TT treatment practitioners should be permitted to do the treatments as they determine.

Time estimation seems to have great descriptive and predictive potential in our attempts to understand healing and the practitioner–recipient mutual process. This variable should be measured in a more precise way. Computerized measurement would be ideal.

The ideal study would include computerized videotaping of the treatments with analysis of the videotapes for time, amount of physical contact, body closeness, the position of the eyes (ie, open or closed) the amount of movement of both practitioners and recipients, etc. Methodologies for such analysis exist and are used in anthropologic and sociologic studies.

A descriptive psychoimmunologic study of TT practitioners should be done. This could be done simultaneously with a study of TT treatments (ie, with recipients), or it could be done in its own right. The goal would be to determine whether the pattern in the suppressor T cell subset and the poor mitogen stimulation responses that we observed are uniform in TT practitioners or were unique to SB and GA. The methodology for such a study would be fairly straightforward using a descriptive correlational design and both TT practitioners and matched controls. Information about experience with TT, frequency of meditation, retrospective and prospective information on frequency of illness, and other psychophysiologic data could be collected and the results correlated with the immune profiles.

REFERENCES

1. Grad B, Cadoret RJ, Paul GI. An unorthodox method of wound healing in mice. *Int J Parapsychol.* 1961;3:5–24.

2. Grad B. Some biological effects of the laying-on of hands: review of experiments with animals and plants. *J Am Soc Psychical Res.* 1965;59:95–127.

3. Grad B. A telekinetic effect on plant growth. *Int J Parapsychol.* 1963;5:117–133.

4. Grad B. A telekinetic effect on plant growth, II. *Int J Parapsychol.* 1964;6:473–485.

5. Smith MJ. Paranormal effects on enzyme activity. *Human Dimens.* 1972;1:12–15.

6. Krieger D. The response of in-vivo human hemoglobin to an active healing therapy by direct laying-on of hands. *Human Dimens.* 1972;1:12–15.

7. Krieger D. Healing by the laying-on of hands as a facilitator of bioenergetic change: the response of in-vivo human hemoglobin. *Psychoenergetic Systems.* 1974;1: 121–129.

8. Krieger D. The relationship of touch, with the intent to help or heal, to subjects' in-vivo hemoglobin values: a study in personalized interaction. In: *Proceedings of the Ninth American Nurses' Association Research Conference.* New York, NY: American Nurses' Association; 1973.

9. Krieger D. Therapeutic Touch: the imprimatur of nursing. *Am J Nurs.* 1975;5:784–787.

10. Krieger D, Peper E, Ancoli S. Physiologic indices of therapeutic touch. *Am J Nurs.* 1979;4:660–662.

11. Heidt P. Effect of therapeutic touch on anxiety level of hospitalized patients. *Nurs Res.* 1981;30:32–37.

12. Quinn JF. Therapeutic touch as energy exchange: testing the theory. *ANS.* 1984;6:42–49.

13. Keller E, Bzdek VM. Effects of therapeutic touch on tension headache pain. *Nurs Res.* 1986;35(2):101–106.

14. Meehan TC. The effect of therapeutic touch on the experience of acute pain in postoperative patients. *Dissertation Abs Int.* 46, 795B. (University Microfilms No. 8510765), 1985.

15. Quinn JF. Therapeutic touch as energy exchange: replication and extension. *Nurs Sci Q.* 1989;2(2):79–87.

16. Kramer NA. Comparison of therapeutic touch and casual touch in stress reduction of hospitalized children. *Pediatr Nurs.* 1990;16(5):483–485.

17. Wirth D. The effects of non-contact Therapeutic Touch on the healing rate of full thickness dermal wounds. *Subtle Energies.* 1990;1(1):1–20.

18. Rogers ME. Nursing: science of unitary, irreducible, human beings: update 1990. In: Barrett EAM, ed. *Visions of Rogers' Science-Based Nursing.* New York, NY: National League for Nursing; 1990.

19. Cowling RW. A template for unitary pattern-based nursing practice. In: Barrett EAM, ed. *Visions of Rogers' Science-Based Nursing.* New York, NY: National League for Nursing; 1990.

20. Quinn JF. Holding sacred space: the nurse as healing environment. *Holistic Nurs Prac.* 1992;6(4):26–35.

21. Newman M, Sime AM, Corcoran-Perry SA. The focus of the discipline of nursing. *ANS.* 1991;14(1):1–6.

22. Borysenko J. Healing motives: an interview with David C. McClelland. *Advances.* 1985;2(2):29–41.

23. Clayton PJ. The sequelae and nonsequelae of conjugal bereavement. *Am J Psychiatry.* 1979;136:1530–1534.

24. Bartrop R, Luckhurst E, Lazarus L, Kiloh LG, Penny R. Depressed lymphocyte function after bereavement. *Lancet.* 1977;1:834–836.

25. Schleifer SJ, Keller SE, Camerino M, et al. Suppression of lymphocyte stimulation following bereavement. *JAMA.* 1983;250(3):374–377.

26. Spielberger CD, Gorsuch RL, Lushene RE. *STAI Manual for the State-Trait Inventory.* Palo Alto, Calif: Consulting Psychologists Press, Inc.; 1983.

27. Derogatis LR. *The Affect Balance Scale.* Baltimore, Md: Clinical Psychometrics Research; 1975.

28. Ferguson C. *Subjective Experience of Therapeutic Touch—Psychometric Examination of an Instrument.* Austin, Tex: University of Texas at Austin; 1986. Dissertation.

29. Georgi J. Lymphocyte subset measurements: significance in clinical medicine. In: Rose NR, Friedman H, Fahey JL, eds. *Manual of Clinical Laboratory Immunology.* Washington, DC: American Society for Microbiology; 1986.

30. Maluish A, Strong D. Lymphocyte proliferation. In: Rose NR, Friedman H, Fahey JL, eds. *Manual of Clinical Laboratory Immunology.* Washington, DC: American Society for Microbiology; 1986.

31. Herberman R, Ortaldo J. Natural killer cells: their role in defenses against disease. In: Rose NR, Friedman H, Fahey JL, eds. *Manual of Clinical Laboratory Immunology.* Washington, DC: American Society for Microbiology; 1986.

The Power of Touch: Massage for Infants

Elaine Fogel Schneider, PhD, CCC-SLP, ADTR, CIMI
Founder and Executive Director
Baby Steps/Antelope Valley Infant
    Development
First Touch
Lancaster, California

Ancient civilizations believed that one way to promote health and prevent disease was by rubbing, stroking, and kneading of the body. Massage can be found in Eastern as well as Western histories, being traced to China 3,000 years before the birth of Christ. The Indian books of the Ayur Veda, written about 1800 BC, refer to massage as shampooing and rubbing the body, which they recommend to help the body heal itself. In literature of other civilizations, Egyptian, Persian, and Japanese physicians made references to the benefits and usefulness of massage. The Romans and the Greeks also believed in massage. The word *massage* comes from the Greek word *messein,* "to knead."[1] Those who praised massage included Homer, Hippocrates, Plato, and Socrates, among others. Massage was used to rub down war heroes, preserve health, and cure disease, and was applied for specific illness. A way of healing the sick, as written in the Bible, was with "laying on of hands." It was at

I would like to acknowledge Vimala McClure, Founder of the International Association of Infant Massage (IAIM), and Kalena Babeshoff, President of IAIM, for awakening the infant within me and bringing me the message of massage; Drs. Deepak Chopra and David Simon, and Mark Lamm (BioSync), for enlivening the mind/body/spirit connection; Dr. Marion Taylor Baer for supporting and encouraging this work; all the infants/toddlers and families that I have been privileged to serve; and Jack and Karli Schneider for their patience, love, and understanding.

Source: Reprinted from E.F. Schneider, *Infants and Young Children,* Vol. 8, No. 3, pp. 40–55, © 1996, Aspen Publishers, Inc.

the time of the Middle Ages that massage lost ground in the medical community, as the general attitude was of the spirit and not of the flesh. Christianity placed an importance on the spiritual self. The Renaissance brought back an interest in the body and health of the physical structure. In the 1500s, physicians began to integrate massage into their practices. Then in the 1780s, a Swede, Per Henrik Ling, returned from China to assemble the technique of The Swedish Movement Treatment. This form of massage is widely used as is the Japanese method of massage known as Shiatsu.[2-7] (See Table 1.) Each one of us, young or old, at risk for delay or not, houses within our bodies our own pharmacologic warehouse of natural wonders—hormones, enzymes, neuropeptides, amino acids, and the like. Current clinical studies are trying to

Table 1. Historical overview of massage

Period	Area	Description
3000 BC	China	Rubbing, stroking, and kneading of the body was to promote health and prevent diseases.
2300 BC	Egypt	Physicians made references to the benefits and usefulness of massage.
1800 BC	India	Ayur Vedic practices with herbs and aromatic oils being rubbed into skin with two massage therapists simultaneously.
101–44 BC	Rome	Pliney, naturalist, was rubbed to relieve asthma.
2nd C	Rome	Roman Emperor's physician, Galen, wrote 16 books relating to massage. Julius Caesar was pinched to ease headaches and neuralgia.
5th C	Greece	Hippocrates studied massage for use with sprains and constipation, named massage *anatripsis*. "The physician must be experienced in many things, but assuredly in rubbing. . . . For rubbing can bind a joint that is too loose, and loosen a joint that is too rigid."
5th–15th C (Middle Ages)	Europe	Massage not applied now, as spirit is valued more than the body.
11th C	Arabia	Avicenna, physician, massaged to disperse wastes in muscles not expelled by exercise.
16th C (Renaissance)	France	Ambroise Pare revived massage, became physician to 4 kings.
	Italy	Mercurialis, physician, wrote a treatise on massage and gymnastics.
17th–18th C	Tahiti	Capt Cook, 1779, recovered from painful sciatica via massage therapy.
17th–18th C	Sweden	Per Henrik Ling (1776–1839) developed scientific system of massage based on principles of anatomy and physiology. Swedish College established for massage, 1813. Swedish Institute opened in London, 1838. Society of Physiotherapy established.
19th C	Sweden	Swedish Institute opened in Russia, America, and France.
20th C	United States	Massage used for nerve injury and shell shock for World War II. Massage reawakened in Esalen, California, by the Esalen Institute. Scientific studies exploring the benefits of massage.

determine if these chemicals are released, stimulated, or reduced during the massage process. For example, during massage, are endorphins released to reduce pain naturally; does serotonin facilitate the production of killer cells; and does vagal activity induce greater digestion, slowing the heart and stimulating the gastrointestinal tract?[8]

Scientists, physicians, and educators have raised questions about the importance of touch in infant development and for older children and adolescents.[9–27] The attention massage is receiving is an indication of the increasing interest in the sense of touch. This article is a review of the literature on the power of touch; the role of the skin; the relationship between touch, attachment, and bonding; and the influence of massage on the growth and development of at-risk infants/toddlers and their caregivers. Recommendations for further research topics will also be explored. In order to discover if massage is important to health, growth, and development, the role of touch and the skin must first be examined.

THE ROLE OF THE SKIN

The skin is made from the same cells as is the brain. Neurology shows us that the size of an organ is related to the multiplicity of functions it performs, and the skin is the largest organ in the body, weighing from 8 to 10 lbs in an adult and covering nearly 20 sq ft if laid end to end.[28] A piece of skin the size of a quarter contains more than 3 million cells, 100 to 340 sweat glands, 50 nerve endings, and 3 ft of blood vessels.[9] The skin has an expansive representation in the brain.

The sensory feedback that the brain receives from the skin is continuous, even when the body is sleeping. Montagu stated that "next to the brain, the skin is the most important of all our organ systems. A human being can spend his life blind and deaf and completely lacking the senses of smell and taste, but he cannot survive at all without the functions performed by the skin."[9(p8)] Current studies are attempting to determine the effect of skin stimulation on the immune and nervous systems, release of hormones, and the effect on glandular activity and behavior.

Montagu suggested that we get to know the skin intimately because it has great powers and abilities that are not yet fully explored.

THE ROLE OF TOUCH

Touch is the most general of the bodily senses, diffused through all parts of the skin. No other sense plays such a vital role in our survival than does the touch sense.[9] At birth, the rooting reflex (the instinctive reflex of an infant to turn to suckle when the skin around the mouth is stimulated) occurs and is critical for survival. In the first month, the sensation of touch is an important source of emotional satisfaction. "Touching is the first communication a baby receives and the first language of its development is through the skin."[9(p126)]

Scientific research looking at the relationship of touch and development first took place in laboratories using animals. An animal study performed by Hammett explored the role of touch in the development of physical and behavioral functions.[9,29–30] This study showed that when rats were gentled and petted after undergoing removal of thyroid and parathyroid glands, they survived longer than those rats who underwent the surgery but only received cage cleaning and feeding. The latter rats were apprehensive, high strung, tense, resistant, and timid and exhibited fear and rage by biting. The rats who were gentled and petted were more relaxed and yielding. They were not easily frightened and felt secure in the hands of whoever held them. When the parathyroid and thyroid of 304 animals from both groups were removed, within 48 hours of the operation, 79% of the irritable rats died, and only 13% of the gentled rats died; when the parathyroid was removed alone, then 76% of the irritable rats died, and only 13% of the gentled rats died. The critical elements of this 1922 study were that gentle touching of rats made the difference between life and death; gentling produced gentle, unexcitable animals; and lack of gentling resulted in excitable and fearful animals. Harlow's animal experiments with infant monkeys showed that given the choice between an artificial mother made of wire offering liquid nourishment and a soft, cuddly artificial mother with no nourishment, the infant monkeys chose the latter, demonstrating that contact comfort was more important than nursing comfort.[31] Schanberg and associates of Duke University investigated deprivation of tactile stimulation to rat pups and discovered that the pups produced fewer growth hormones when briefly deprived of tactile stimulation. Postmaternal stimulation normalized when researchers "licked" pups systematically with a paintbrush. Also, touch-deprived rat pups possessed lesser amounts of a specific growth gene.[32] Other animal studies have been performed that suggest to be held, fondled, and touched with warmth and gentleness conveys meanings beyond the feeling state, as physiological states are also enhanced.[9] (See Table 2.)

Observing human infant studies, Leboyer revealed that "Being touched and caressed, being massaged, is food for the infant. Food as necessary as minerals, vitamins, and proteins."[33(p1)] Infants with failure to thrive can have all the food they need but continue to deteriorate without intervention that includes emotional nurturing, care, and contact comfort.[33] Research studies throughout the last two decades have explored the importance of touch in infant development[9-26] for infants of low birth weight and prematurity,[34-69] drug exposure,[70-77] acquired immune deficiency syndrome (AIDS),[78-79] motoric disturbances,[80] low incidence and/or developmental disorders,[81-83] and mental health difficulties.[84-87]

Whereas scientists and physicians at one time thought that infants were not processing any information until 1 or 2 months postbirth, current research shows that infants are participating in their worlds, not only at the time of birth, but in utero.[17] Challenging us to rethink how infants learn, many scientists and researchers continue to examine the importance of touch: Dr. Tiffany Field, director of the Touch Research Institute (TRI) in Miami, Florida, (which opened in May 1992 with grants from private industry and the National Institutes of Health)[88] and colleagues are engaged in over 30 studies relating to touch. Areas of study include newborns (cocaine, human immunodeficiency virus [HIV]-exposed,

and preterm); infants (cancer, colic, depression, food texture, sleep disorders, and toy textures); children (abuse, asthma, autism, burn, diabetes, neglect, pediatric skin disorders, preschool, etc); adolescents (depression among teen mothers, eating disorders); adults (chronic fatigue syndrome, HIV, job performance/stress, etc); and the elderly (volunteer foster grandparents providing vs receiving massage). In Sweden, Uvnas-Mosberg reported that stimulating the inside of the mouth of the newborn and the breast of the mother led to the increased release of gastrointestinal food absorption hormones such as gastrin and insulin, suggesting that massage on different body parts could also lead to the release of hormones.[89]

Barnard and Brazelton, editors of *Touch the Foundation of Experience,* provide an overview of issues and outcomes in the field of touch research,[90] and Ackerman, author of *The Natural History of the Senses,* addresses the importance of sensory input.[91] Klaus and Kennell found that an extra 16 hours of contact in the first 3 days of life appeared to have affected maternal behavior for 2 years. Mothers were more affectionate prior to the hospital discharge and more affectionate when the baby cried.[25] Ringler et al[92] found that mothers who had extra contact with their infants talked to their infants differently. Ainsworth[93] found that mothers whose responsiveness was low in the first 3 months of the infant's life had infants whose feedings were characterized as unhappy throughout the first year. Infants who were securely attached by 12 months of age had mothers who were sensitive to the infants' signals during the first 3 months.

THE ROLE OF TOUCH ON ATTACHMENT AND BONDING

To understand the infancy period and the role of touch, you must first appreciate the nature of infant survival. Bowlby formulated the attachment theory in 1958, combining psychoanalytic insights into early childhood development with findings from the field of ethology, the science of animal behavior.[14-15] Freudian theory views

Table 2. Sampling of touch studies using animals

Study year	Chief researcher	Animals used & application	Results
1920s	Hammett[29]	Albino rats—removal of thyroid glands. One colony was petted and held. The second group was given routine feeding and cage cleaning. Second series investigated mortality rate in para-thyroidectomized Norway rats.	Rats petted and gentled: • did not die after thyroid and parathyroid removals; • were gentler, friendlier; • lacked muscular tension. Rats not petted: • died, • were more angry, • died within 48 hours (90%).
1950s	Harlow[31]	Four monkeys given choice of wire mother substitute with food, or comfy cloth mother substitute with no food.	Monkeys went to the cloth mother, even when the wire mother had food. Contact comfort more important than nursing comfort.
1950s	Benjamin[137]	Twenty rats given same kinds and amounts of food in similar living conditions. One group was cuddled and caressed, other group was not.	Cuddled rats: • learned faster, • grew faster, • stimulation from the external world enhanced the growth factor for the cuddled group.
1960s	Rosenblatt & Lehrman[138]	During 15-minute observations, maternal rats licked their newborn pups for an average of 2 minutes, 10 seconds, in an anogenital region and lower abdomen, and 12 seconds on back of head.	Results sustaining bodily systems, stimulating and improving functional responses of organ systems.
1980s	Schanberg et al[32,139]	Rat pups deprived of tactile stimulation.	Rat pups produced fewer growth hormones when briefly deprived of tactile stimulation. Host maternal stimulation normalized when researchers "licked" pups systematically with a paintbrush. Touch-deprived rat pups possessed lesser amount of specific growth gene ornithine decarboxylase (ODL).

the infants' attachment to the mother related to her role in feeding and provision of gratification.[94] Learning theorists see that attachment is developed from stimulation and reinforcement occurring between a mother and her infant.[94] Some indicators of attachment include cuddling, kissing, fondling, prolonged gazing, and physical touch. The direction of attachment from mother to infant that can occur in the first 3 days of life and after includes simultaneous interactions of touch, eye-to-eye contact, high-pitched voice, entrainment, time giver T and B lymphocytes macrophages, bacteria flora, odor, and heat. The simultaneous interactions that occur from the infant to the mother include eye-to-eye contact, cry, oxytocin (stimulates contraction of the uterus), prolactin (stimulates lactation in the mother), odor, and entrainment.[25,33] It is vital for the development of attachment behavior and early social development of the young child that both the infant and caregiver (mother and/or father) have the capacity to elicit and respond to behaviors in mutually pleasurable ways.[95]

The infant–mother attachment in most cases is an infant's first real social experience and is the beginning of social and emotional development.[14] The physical and social stimulation infants receive as a result of the mother–child attachment is necessary for continued normal physical and social development[94] and is crucial to the survival and development of the infant. The role of the father is also important as noted by Parke and others.[96–98] Parke demonstrated that when fathers are given the opportunity to spend time alone with their newborn, they spend almost the same amount of time as mothers in holding, touching, and gazing at them.[96] "Early emotional development is a function of complex reciprocal interaction of behaviors between infants and caregivers."[80(p61)] The infant's motor and sensory abilities evoke responses from the parent/caregiver and begin the communication that is helpful for the attachment to begin. The interdependency of rhythms seems to be the root of their attachment as well as their communications.[99–100]

Research about the role of touch on attachment/bonding has entered the field from a vast variety of disciplines, including anthropology, ethology, ethics, nursing, obstetrics, pediatrics, psychology, psychiatry, and sociology.[25] Klaus and Kennell coined the word *bonding* not only as an adhesive property but as the process that occurs between people, developing a "unique relationship between two people that is specific and endures time."[25(p2)] Klaus and Kennell suggest that there "is a sensitive period"[25(p38)] in the first minutes and hours of life and afterward where it is necessary that the mother and father have close contact with their neonate. In this bi-

directional interaction of bonding, the parents give, and the newborns signal back, thus the relationship continues "from the embryonic state, infant gestating inside of its mother, to the outside, where the infant is totally dependent on the caregivers for survival, until the individual separates and lives on his/her own."[25(p3)] This original infant–parent tie is so important for all infants and society because it is from this original attachment and bonding that all subsequent attachments will follow. It is also this infant–parent tie that is the formative relationship in the course of which the child develops a sense of self.[1]

THE ROLE OF MASSAGE

Massage is generally a manipulation of the body that combines tactile (touch) and kinesthetic (perception of movement) stimulation performed in a purposeful, sequential application. Vimala McClure, founder of the International Association of Infant Massage, states that the massage technique for infants is not manipulative, but rather a gentle, warm communication.[33] It is a technique that allows the parents to engage and relax their child in a mutually pleasurable interaction.[21] "As baby grows stronger, so should your touch. All of your strokes should be long, slow, and rhythmic, with just enough pressure to be comfortable but stimulating."[33(p65)] With healthy infants, massage can be started as soon as parents desire, beginning with a daily massage for the first 6 or 7 months, using unscented natural oil, in a warm environment. As the child becomes more active, through crawling or walking, the massage may be reduced to once or twice a week, as desired. A toddler may enjoy a rubdown before bedtime every night or after bathtime. Massage provides a model for becoming more sensitive to the subtle cues of the infant and techniques for eliciting positive reactions from the child. Skin-to-skin contact may not be the "massage touch" of first choice for parents/caregivers of severely medically fragile premature infants. Direct touch may be disruptive and unbearable to the sensitivity of that infant. Each infant's unique needs must be addressed.

WHY MASSAGE INFANTS

Many studies have been performed on the effects of massage for premature infants. Few studies looked at massage for full-term healthy infants. Of performed studies, a connection between massage and physical, emotional, and intellectual development is suggested.[9] According to Montagu, "the early development of the nervous system of the infant is to a major extent dependent upon the kind of cutaneous (skin) stimulation it receives. There can be no doubt that tactile stimulation is necessary for its healthy development."[9(p215)] The need for peripheral skin stimulation and contact exists throughout life, but it appears to be most intense and crucial in the early phase of reflex attachment.[100] As mentioned previously, learning theorists see that attachment is developed from stimulation and that this interaction between parent and child is crucial for the infant's survival and development. Also, two conditions that have been found to enhance development of bonding are the ability of the caregiver to be sensitive in understanding and responding to his or her infant's cues and the amount and nature of the interactions between them.[14] It is through nurturing touch that forming attachments (and furthering of bonding) may be deepened.

"Babies by their very nature are social creatures, and much of what they learn comes from their interactions with people."[101(p205)] Social interaction is significant for the caregivers' well-being, essential for the child's development during the first 3 years of life, and paramount thereafter.[102–104] Expanding children's repertoires of interactive behaviors can assist them to influence their world and deepen their quality of life and the lives of their parents/caregivers.[105] During the first 1 or 2 years of life (the sensory stage according to Erikson) infants rely on others in their social environment for their needs. If children receive a good quality of care and nurturing during this period, they will learn to trust and rely on their caregivers to feel secure.[106] One such strategy to improve parent–child interaction is early meaningful stimulation. Stroking an infant is the first form of communication an infant experiences. It is a giving and taking, a sharing of information, thoughts, and feelings. Synchronous with communication are infants' movements.[92]

According to Ramsey, when you engage an infant in massage, you begin to listen to the infant. You listen to his or her sounds, and you watch his or her movements.[17] Even though infants cannot speak, they communicate through their bodies. In the infant massage process, described by McClure,[33] communication plays an active part, as the caregiver talks to the infant, asks permission to start the massage, questions the infant, and facilitates dialogue.

Infant massage is a "dance" between parent/caregiver reading cues of the infant and the infant being understood, listened to, and responded to in a fashion that resembles social reciprocity.[107] This ongoing interactive process between infants and their primary caregiver is a mutual one. The infant provides signals and cues (engagement or disengagement) to a parent/caregiver, who interprets these cues and responds to them. The parent gives signals that the infant gradually understands. Examples of engagement cues are stilling, smiling, looking at the caregiver's face, reaching out, raising the head, and so forth. Examples of disengagement cues are pulling away, crying and being fussy, having hiccups, frowning, turning head away, and so forth.[108] The actual bonding process is more stimulation than chain-like.[25] The mutual give and take, understanding, and responding to each other's cues influences the child's development.[26] (See Table 3 and Figure 1.) If touch is a child's first language, and if touch fosters attachment and bonding, then infant massage, including tactile and kinesthetic stimulation, may also be a way to foster bonding and attachment.

THE IMPLICATIONS OF MASSAGE FOR SPECIAL NEEDS INFANTS

When an infant is born with a special need, anxieties about the well-being of the infant may result in long-lasting concerns that adversely

Table 3. Reported benefits of infant massage based on research studies and observations

Benefit type	For the infant	For the parents/caregivers
Psychosocial	Bonding Body/mind connection Increased self-esteem Enhanced sense of love Enhanced sense of acceptance Enhanced sense of respect Enhanced sense of trust Enhanced communication	Improved ability to read infant cues Improved synchrony between parent and infants Bonding Increased confidence Promoted intimacy Increased communication Developed trust Developed respect
Physiological/physical growth	Improved body awareness Stimulated circulation Increased digestion, which can lead to weight gain Reduced colic symptoms Muscle tone coordination Body/mind connection Calmed nervous system leading to more restful sleep Increased elimination Increased respiration Touch relaxation Increased vagal activity Reduced stress Increased hormonal function (ie, stimulates endorphins, serotonins, somatotropins, gastrin, oxytocin, and insulin) Stimulated lymphatic circulation Improved sleep patterns	Improved sense of well-being Reduced blood pressure Relaxation Increased prolactin Promoted health Reduced stress

shape the development of the child.[25] Social reciprocity may be of great issue with infants who are disabled. Studies by Klaus and Kennell[25] and Levy-Shiff[109] revealed that mothers of mentally disabled children initiated fewer interactions and were less likely to respond favorably to their children than mothers of nondisabled children, and, conversely, children who were mentally disabled were less responsive to their parents.[110–117] They smiled, laughed, socialized, and vocalized less than their nondisabled counterparts. The reciprocal nature of interaction can also be compromised if the child with severe motor problems is unable to react

positively when being cuddled by the parent or to form their body into their parent's arms.[118] The child with a disability who does not respond to the parent's touch may inhibit the development of interactive behaviors, since many typical reinforcers may not be present. Comparing mothers of preterm and full-term infants, Rossetti found, too, that even if the length of time of interaction was similar to that for the full-term infants, the quality of the interaction differed.[119]

Minde found "that mothers of ill infants touched and smiled at their infants significantly less during all nursery observations, and at home they not only touched and smiled less but also

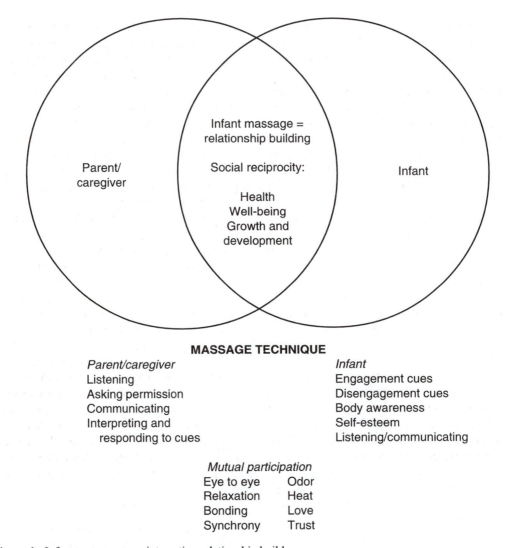

MASSAGE TECHNIQUE

Parent/caregiver
Listening
Asking permission
Communicating
Interpreting and
   responding to cues

Infant
Engagement cues
Disengagement cues
Body awareness
Self-esteem
Listening/communicating

Mutual participation

Eye to eye	Odor
Relaxation	Heat
Bonding	Love
Synchrony	Trust

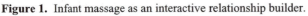

Figure 1. Infant massage as an interactive relationship builder.

looked at their infants less, and vocalized to them less than did the mothers of the well infants."[120(p83)] Also, the mothers' actual behavior correlated more with their perceptions of how ill their infant was, rather than the infant's actual degree of illness. The quality of interaction for a full-term and a premature infant, over the first year of life, was observed to differ.[119] Rossetti tells us that "observations of human mothers separated from their infants consistently show that attachment, bonding, and inter-

action patterns do differ between the mothers of healthy and high-risk newborns."[119(p83)] Parents of premature infants undergo additional stress. When the time to prepare for birth is lost, failure to produce a full-term infant can result in grief and depression. Taylor and Hall[121] pointed out that parents can feel guilty, depressed, angry, and preoccupied with the infant, along with fearing the death of the infant or severely handicapping conditions. Furthermore, additional losses replace expectations. Mothers of high-risk infants face an exceptional emotional trauma at the birth of their child. They may feel extreme loneliness or an inability to do anything of significance for the frail infant.

Increasingly, neonatologists and other health care professionals are concerned about separating the high-risk infant from the mother in the newborn period. Early maternal–infant separation leads to deviant caretaking behavior that may develop into patterns of abuse and neglect later in infancy.[122–129] Barnett and colleagues showed that mothers who were separated from their infants displayed differences in three areas over mothers who did not have disturbance to their bonding: (1) commitment to the infant, (2) self-confidence in the ability to mother the infant, and (3) other nurturing behavior such as stimulating the infant.[130]

The sensitive period when bonding can take place may not be adequately realized when an infant is born with special needs, setting in motion disruption of growth and development.[119] This dysfunctional social reciprocity may lead to a sense of inadequacy; dysfunctional infant and parent self-images; disordered communication; and decreased self-esteem, intimacy, love, and trust. This sensitive period for bonding may be interrupted as well if the parents are fearful that their child may not survive. Also, if the child is in the neonatal intensive care unit (NICU), there is limited contact, and the sensitive period may pass without the amount of necessary touch and contact. Touch and eye-to-eye contact may not be available to the premature infant in an incubator. However, the need for touching and being with a fragile infant is now acceptable, whereas 40 years ago it was not.[25,119] The mother may not be able to look at her infant or touch her or him should the newborn not match the portrait she had of her infant when he or she was in utero. An infant born blind may never develop the longed for eye-to-eye contact with its mother, and yet eye-to-eye contact is expressed as a need for both preterm and full-term infants.[131]

In recent years, there is an increased interest in helping parents attach and bond with their high-risk infants. Parents are encouraged to be close to and have regular contact with their in-

fants.[25] To achieve the aim of serving infants through strengthening families, we must look toward therapeutic interventions that engage the infant and the family. Themes of intervention strategies emerge from the work of Brazelton and others in the field of child development, and researchers are attempting to define strategies to enhance parent–child interaction.[26] One such strategy that improves parent–child interaction and overall growth and development is early meaningful stimulation.[103] Research in the field of early child development shows that such stimulation enhances physical, emotional, and intellectual development.[26,101–102]

Hanson and Lynch tell us that "early intervention efforts are aimed at assisting the child to become more competent and develop more normally."[101(p205)] Since this effort may take more time to occur, and some may never gain these skills, another goal of intervention is to assist parents/caregivers to modify their interactional patterns and understand and read their infants' cues. Massage is being viewed as a way to develop this closeness with high-risk infants in a family-focused, family-interactive process.[132] The mother is helped to begin building a close, affectionate tie to her infant, developing mutual interaction so that she will be attuned to her infant's special needs as the infant grows.[119] The infant massage process may enliven the five aspects of early intervention skill development:

1. *communication*—engages prespeech components and emerging speech (ie, direct eye gaze, listening, turn taking, etc)
2. *motor*—may reduce or tone muscles, increase body awareness, etc
3. *socialization*—infant and caregiver engage one another, infant usually in quiet, alert state
4. *self-help*—may stimulate oral motor musculature awareness, lip closure, relaxation of tension needed for swallowing, etc; and
5. *cognition*—overall awareness of self and body boundaries, cause and effect, etc.

The field of early intervention offers a nurturing, rich environment to study the effects of infant massage on child/family relations (including parent competency in caring for a handicapped infant); child growth and development (including communication, cognition, gross- and fine-motor movements, socialization, self-help, bonding, trust, intimacy, and self-esteem development); and infant and caregiver well-being.[132]

RESEARCH FINDINGS

In a meta-analysis of 19 studies of stimulation, researchers estimate that 72% of infants receiving some form of tactile stimulation were positively affected.[22] Although studies from the TRI revealed that tactile and kinesthetic stimula-

Table 4. Science focuses on premature infants: sampling of research studies

Study year	Chief researcher	Application	Results
1976	Rice[50]	Premature babies were massaged and control group was not.	Massaged premies were ahead in • weight gain • neurological development. Found that massage does not medically compromise oxygen tension in the preterm neonate during stressful procedures.
1986	Field et al[48]	Studied the effects of stroking and passively manipulating newborns for 15 minutes, three times daily, for a 10-day period.	The massaged premies • gained 47% more weight than did the premies in the nonmassaged control group • scored better on the Brazelton scale • were more alert and active • stayed 6 fewer days in the hospital for a per-infant hospital cost savings of $3,000 • continued into their first year to receive relatively higher scores than the nonmassaged group on testing
1987	White-Traut and Nelson[63]	Premature infants were massaged, rocked, and talked to, and control group was not.	Premies who were massaged, rocked, and talked to • gained weight • left the hospital in 19 days • thrived on extra cuddling
1990	Scafidi et al[68]	Added physiological and biochemical measures to their first study (1986).	This study confirmed their earlier study that stimulated infants • showed a 21% greater daily weight gain • were discharged 5 days earlier from the hospital, showing superior performance on the Brazelton Habituation items • showed less stress behaviors • catecholamines (norepinephrine, epinephrine) had increased across the situation period, which is desirable in the neonatal period
1993	Acolot et al[140]	Mean gestational age was 29 weeks and median postnatal age 20 days. Blood samples drawn 45 minutes before massage and 1 hour after massage.	Cortisol concentrations decreased. Catecholamines did not decrease.

tion of the skin produced different immediate effects on behavior (tactile stimulation had an activating effect that resulted in more episodes of active sleep and greater motor activity; kinesthetic stimulation had a quieting effect), these findings are in contrast to Hasselmeyer's studies of the 1960s and 1970s, which reported that handled infants were less active than control infants.[59] Barnard[134] also found no differences in the amount of waking activity between the control and the experimental infant groups. It would seem logical that increased activity would result in increased energy, resulting in a lesser weight gain. However, in at least three studies that showed increased weight gain, activity levels were also greater. Studies involving weight gain for premature infants who received massage also revealed mixed findings.[67,79,135] The studies of Hasselmeyer[59] and Barnard[134,136] revealed no differences in weight gain for massaged premature infants. However, more recent studies performed by Field and colleagues did reveal greater weight gains and earlier hospital discharge for massaged premature infants. These studies also suggest the massaged infants experienced a reduction in stress, increased circulation, respiration, and elimination as well as better sleep patterns

and greater relaxation.[45,48,57–58,62,68] The caregiver administering the massage also experienced benefits through increased self-esteem and competency, lower anxiety levels, reduced blood pressure, and greater relaxation.[135] The discrepancy in findings may be due to the variability in the infant's activity levels or to the different stroking qualities that were used.

Suggestions for future ongoing massage research include assessing the differential and cumulative effects of the tactile and kinesthetic types of stimulation, determining the most appropriate time for executing infant massage with special needs populations, and reviewing family competencies for infants/toddlers with special needs. Longitudinal studies using larger sample sizes and comparative research designs need to be conducted before definitive conclusions are drawn.

Table 4 and Table 5 highlight massage studies and results that apply to infants born with gastrointestinal illness, cocaine addiction in utero, and motor disturbances.

• • •

The power of touch and the benefits of infant massage for those being massaged and those giving the massage is being widely studied to-

Table 5. Science focuses on other at-risk conditions

Study year	Chief researcher	Application	Results
		Gastrointestinally Ill Infants	
1989	Unvas-Mosberg[89]	Stimulating the inside of the mouth of the newborn (and the breast of the mother)	The increased release of gastrointestinal food absorption hormones such as gastrin and insulin
		Infants Drug Exposed In Utero	
1990	Field et al[89]	Touch therapy to infants exposed to cocaine in utero	Massaged cocaine babies gained weight Scored better on the Brazelton scale
		Infants with Motor Problems	
1980s	Hansen and Ulrey[80]	Mothers massaged infants with motor problems over time.	Parents and their babies had more positive interaction Compatible positive interactions Parents' expectations and behavior toward their children changed, enhancing parent–infant interactions

day. If current research continues to demonstrate a connection between touching through massage, increased bonding, and enhanced growth and development for infants, as well as benefits for those giving the massage, these new findings may become a cornerstone in the delivery of early intervention services to special needs infants and their families.

REFERENCES

1. *Webster's Dictionary of the English Language.* New York, NY: Lexicon Publications; 1988.

2. West OMT. *The Magic of Massage.* 3rd printing. Mamaroneck, NY: Hastings House; 1990.

3. Lidell L, Thomas S, Beresford C, Porter A. *The Book of Massage: The Complete Step by Step Guide to Eastern and Western Techniques.* New York, NY: Simon & Schuster; 1984.

4. Hudson CM. *Complete Book of Massage.* New York, NY: Random House; 1988.

5. Zerinsky S. *Introduction to Pathology for the Massage Practitioner.* New York, NY: Swedish Institute, Inc; 1987.

6. Feltman EJ. *Hands on Healing.* Emmaus, Pa: Rodale Press; 1989.

7. Juhan D. *A Handbook for Body Work.* Barrytown, NY: Station Hill Press; 1987.

8. Gerwirtz D, ed. Scientists outline the many benefits of touch. *Touchpoints.* 1993;1(1):3–5.

9. Montagu A. *Touching: The Significance of the Skin.* New York, NY: Harper & Row; 1986.

10. Gottfried A, et al. Touch as an organizer for learning and development. In: Brown C, ed. *The Many Facets of Touch.* Elsevier, NY: Johnson and Johnson; 1980; 10.

11. Brazelton TB. Behavioral competence of the newborn infant. *Semin Perinatol.* 1979;3:35–44.

12. Ayres AJ. *Sensory Integration and the Child.* Los Angeles, Calif: Western Psychological Services; 1985.

13. Bender M, Baglin CA. *Infants and Toddlers: A Resource Guide for Practitioners.* San Diego, Calif: Singular Publications; 1992.

14. Bowlby J. *Attachment and Loss.* New York, NY: Basic Books; 1969.

15. Bowlby J. *The Making and Breaking of Affectional Bonds.* London, England: Tavistock Publications; 1979.

16. Piaget J. *The Origins of Intelligence in Children.* New York, NY: Norton; 1952.

17. Ramsey TK. *Baby's First Massage.* International Association of Infant Massage; 1992.

18. Brazelton TB, Cramer BG. *The Earliest Relationship: Parents, Infants and the Drama of Early Attachment.* Reading, Mass: Addison-Wesley; 1990.

19. Samuels M, Samuels N. *The Well Baby Book.* New York, NY: Simon & Schuster; 1979.

20. Walker P. *The Book of Baby Massage.* New York, NY: Simon & Schuster; 1988.

21. Leboyer F. *Loving Hands.* Paris, France: Collins; 1977.

22. Ottenbacher KJ, Muller L, Heintzelman A, Hojem P, Sharpe P. The effectiveness of tactile stimulation as a form of early intervention: a quantitative evaluation. *J Dev Behav Pediatr.* 1987;8:68–76.

23. Gunzenhauser N, ed. *Advances in Touch.* Elsevier, NY: Johnson & Johnson; 1990.

24. Horowitz FD. Infant stimulation efforts: theoretical challenges for research and intervention. In: *Infant Stimulation: For Whom, What Kind, When, and How Much?* Elsevier, NY: Johnson and Johnson; 1987; 13.

25. Klaus M, Kennell JH. *Parent-Infant Bonding.* 2nd ed. Springfield, Mo: Mosby; 1982.

26. Brazelton TB, Koslowski B, Main M. The origins of reciprocity: the early mother–infant interaction. In: Lewis M, Rosenblum L, eds. *The Effect of the Infant on its Caregiver.* New York, NY: Wiley; 1974.

27. Field T, Morrow C, Valderon C, Larson S, Kuhn C, Schanberg S. Massage reduces depression and anxiety in child and adolescent psychiatric patients. *Journal of the American Academy of Adolescent Psychiatry.* 1992;31:125–131.

28. Weiss S. Communication-touch. *UCSF Magazine.* February 1992:31–35.

29. Hammett FS. Studies of the thyroid apparatus. *Endocrinology.* 1922;6:221–229.

30. Hammett FS. Studies in the thyroid apparatus. *Am J Physiol.* 1921;56:196–204.

31. Harlow HF. The nature of love. *Am Psychol.* 1958;13:673–685.

32. Schanberg S, Field T. Sensory deprivation stress and supplemental stimulation in the rat population and the pre-term human neonate. *Child Dev.* 1987;58:1,431–1,447.

33. McClure V. *Infant Massage: A Handbook for Loving Parents.* 2nd edition. New York, NY: Bantam Books; 1985.

34. Klaus MH. Bach, Beethoven, or rock and how much? *J Pediatr.* 1976;88:300.

35. Rose S. Pre-term responses to passive, active, and social touch. In: Brown C, ed. *The Many Facets of Touch.* Elsevier, NY: Johnson and Johnson; 1980; 10.

36. Field T, Dempsey J, Shuman HH. 5 year follow up of preterm respiratory distress syndromes and post term maturity syndrome infants. In: Field T, Sostek A, eds. *Infants Born at Risk: Physiological Perceptual and Cognitive Processes.* New York, NY: Grune & Stratton; 1984.

37. Barnard B. Paradigms for intervention: infant state modulation. In: *Infant Stimulation: For Whom, What Kind, When, and How Much?* Elsevier, NY: Johnson and Johnson; 1987; 13.

38. Field T. Alleviating stress in ICU neonates. In: *Infant Stimulation: For Whom, What Kind, When, and How Much?* Elsevier, NY: Johnson and Johnson; 1987; 13.

39. Brazelton TB. Early intervention: what does it mean? In: *Infant Stimulation: For Whom, What Kind, When, and How Much?* Elsevier, NY: Johnson and Johnson; 1987; 13.

40. Bernbaum J, Perreira GR, Watkins JB, Peckkman J. Non-nutritive sucking during gavage feeding enhances growth and maturation in preterm infants. *Pediatrics.* 1983;71:41–45.

41. Burns KA, Deddish RB, Burns WJ, Hatcher RP. Use of oscillating waterbeds and rhythmic sounds for premature infant stimulation. *Developmental Psychology.* 1982;19:746–751.

42. Long JG, Alistair GS, Philip MB, Lucey JF. Excessive handling as a cause of hypoxemia. *Pediatrics.* 1980; 65:203–207.

43. Masi W. Supplemental stimulation of the premature infant. In: Field T, Sostek A, Goldberg S, Shuman HH, eds. *Infants Born at Risk.* New York, NY: Spectrum; 1979.

44. Rausch P. A tactile and kinesthetic stimulation program for premature infants. In: Brown C, ed. *The Many Facets of Touch.* Elsevier, NY: Johnson and Johnson; 1984; 10.

45. Field T, Dempsey J, Schanberg S, et al. Tactile/kinesthetic effects on preterm neonates. *Pediatrics,* 1986;77:654–658.

46. Goldson E. The neonatal intensive care unit: premature infants and parents. *Inf Young Children.* 1992;4(3):31–42.

47. Hughes M, McCollom J, Sheftal D, Sanchez G. How parents cope with the experience of neonatal intensive care. *Children's Health Care.* 1994;27:1–14.

48. Field T, Scafidi F, Schanberg S. Massage of pre-term newborns to improve growth and development. *Pediatric Nursing.* 1987;3:385–387.

49. Rausch PB. Effects of tactile and kinesthetic stimulation on premature infants. *Journal of Obstet and Gynecol.* 1981;10:34.

50. Rice R. Neurophysiological development in premature infants following stimulation. *Developmental Psychology.* 1977;13:69–76.

51. White J, La Barbara R. The effects of tactile and kinesthetic stimulation on neonatal development in the premature infant. *Developmental Psychology.* 1976;9:569.

52. Kuhn C, Schanberg S, Field T. Tactile/kinesthetic stimulation effects on sympathetic and adrenocortical function in premature infants. *J Pediatr.* September 1991;434–440.

53. Solko N, Matuszak D. Tactile stimulation and behavioral development among low birthweight infants. *Child Psychiatry Hum Dev.* 1975;6:33–37.

54. Estabrooks CA. Touch: a nursing strategy in the intensive care unit. *Heart Lung.* 1989;18:392–401.

55. Affonson D, Bosque E, Wahlberg V, Brady J. Reconciliation and healing for mothers through skin-to-skin contact provided in an American tertiary level intensive care nursery. *Neonatal Network.* 1993;12:25–32.

56. Cornell EH, Gottfried AW. Intervention with premature human infants. *Child Dev.* 1976;47:32–39.

57. Field T. Supplemental stimulation of preterm neonates. *Early Hum Dev.* 1980;4:301–314.

58. Field T, Ignatoff E, Stringer S, et al. Tactile/kinesthetic stimulation effects on preterm neonates. *Pediatrics.* 1986;77:654–658.

59. Hasselmeyer EG. The premature neonate's response to handling. *American Nurses' Journal.* 1964;1:15–24.

60. Barb SA, Lemons PK. The premature infant: toward improving neuro development outcome. *Neonatal Network.* 1989;7:7–15.

61. Sinclair M. A look at massage for children of the United States. *Massage Therapy Journal.* Spring 1991;52–58.

62. Field T, Schanberg SM, Scafidi F, et al. Tactile/kinesthetic stimulation effects on pre-term neonates. *Pediatrics.* 1977;654–658.

63. White-Traut R, Nelson M. Maternally administered tactile and visual vestibular stimulation: relationships to later interactions between mothers and premature infants. *Res Nurs Health.* 1986;1:31–39.

64. Field T. Alleviating stress in the NICU. *Neonatal Journal of the American Osteopathic Association.* 1987;87:646–650.

65. Richmond J. Low birth weight infants: can we enhance their development? *JAMA.* 1990;263(2):3,069. Editorial.

66. Gross R, Spiker D, Constantine N, et al. Enhancing the outcomes of low-birth weight premature infants. A multi-site randomized trial. *JAMA.* 1990;263(22):3,035–3,042.

67. Scafidi FA, Field T, Schanberg SM, et al. Effects of tactile kinesthetic stimulation on the clinical course

and sleep/wake behaviors of pre-term neonates. *Infant Behavior and Development.* 1986;9:91–105.

68. Scafidi FA, et al. Massage stimulates growth in pre-term infants. A replication. *Infant Behavior and Development.* 1990;13:167–188.

69. Brooks FD. Skin to skin contact in the NICU. *Kangaroo Care.* 1993;18:250–253.

70. Knaster M. Premature infants grow with massage. *Clearinghouse for Drug Exposed Children Newsletter.* Summer 1991:50–51.

71. Gregory R. Infant massage makes the difference. *Clearinghouse for Drug Exposed Children Newsletter.* Summer 1991:3.

72. Gerwitz D, ed. *Touchpoints.* Touch Research Institute; Fall 1993:1–6.

73. Weber K. Massage for drug exposed infants. *Massage Therapy Journal.* Summer 1991:62–64.

74. D'Apolito K. What is an organized infant? *Neonatal Network.* 1991;10(1):27–29.

75. Myers B, et al. Cocaine exposed infants: myths and misunderstanding. *Zero to Three.* 1992;13(1):1–5.

76. Griffith DR. Comforting techniques for your baby. *Northwestern Memorial Hospital/The Perinatal Center for Chemical Dependence.* Chicago, Ill; 1988.

77. Russell FF, Free TA. Early intervention for infants and toddlers with prenatal drug exposure. *Inf Young Children.* 1991;3:78–85.

78. Falloon J, et al. Human immunodeficiency virus infection in children. *J Pediatr.* 1989;114:1–30.

79. Scott GB, et al. Mothers of infants with acquired immunodeficiency syndrome. *JAMA.* 1985;253(3):363–366.

80. Hansen R, Ulrey G. Motorically impaired infants: impact of a massage procedure on caregiver–infant interaction. *Journal of Multihandicapped Persons.* 1988;1:61–68.

81. Warren D. *Blindness and early childhood development.* New York, NY: American Foundation for the Blind; 1984.

82. Bigelow A. The development of reaching in blind infants. *British Journal of Developmental Psychology.* 1988;4.

83. Sinclair M. *Massage for Healthier Children.* Oakland, Calif: Wingbow Press; 1992.

84. Welch M. Toward prevention of developmental disabilities. *Pre and Perinatal Psychology.* 1989;3:319–326.

85. Field T. Neonatal stress and coping in intensive care. *Infant Mental Health Journal.* 1990;2(1):57–65.

86. Bonkowski SE, Yanoss JH. Infant mental health: an expanding field of social work. *National Association of Social Workers.* 1992;37(2):144–148.

87. Paulsen M. Strategies for building resilience in infants and young children at-risk. *Inf Young Children.* 1993;6(2):29–40.

88. Villano D. Just the right touch. *Miami Magazine.* Fall 1992;31–35.

89. Field T. Infant massage therapy. *Touchpoints.* Benjamin Y, ed. Touch Research Institute. Fall 1994;1(4):1.

90. Barnard K, Brazelton TB, eds. *Touch the Foundation of Experience.* Madison, Conn: International Universities Press; 1990.

91. Ackerman D. *The Natural History of the Senses.* New York, NY: Random House; 1990.

92. Ringler NM, Kennell JH, Jarvella R, Navojosky BJ, Klaus MH. Mother to child speech at two year effects of early postnatal contact. *J Pediatr.* 1975;86:141–144.

93. Ainsworth M. Early caregiving and later attachment problems. In: Klaus M, ed. *Birth-Interaction and Attachment.* Elsevier, NY: Johnson and Johnson; 1982; 6.

94. McCandless BR, Trotter RJ. Children's behavior and development. New York, NY: Holt, Rinehart & Winston; 1977.

95. Emde RN, Harmon RJ, eds. The development of attachment and affiliative systems. New York, NY: Plenum; 1982.

96. Parke RD. Perception of father–infant interaction. In: O Soloky JD, ed. *Handbook of Infant Development.* New York, NY: Wiley; 1979.

97. Tuttman. The father's role in the child's development of the capacity to cope with separation and loss. *J Am Acad Psychoanal.* July 1986.

98. Parke RD. Father–infant interaction. In: *Maternal Attachment and Mothering Disorders.* Elsevier, NY: Johnson and Johnson; 1978.

99. Condon W, Sander L. Neonate movement is synchronized and adult speech: interactional participation and language acquisition. *Science.* 1974;183:99–101.

100. Clay VS. *The Effect of Culture on Mother–Child Tactile Communication.* New York, NY: Teachers College, Columbia University; 1966. Dissertation.

101. Hanson MJ, Lynch EW. *Early Intervention Implementing Child and Family Services for Infants and Toddlers Who Are At-risk or Disabled.* Austin, Tex: Pro Ed; 1989.

102. Rosenburg SA, Robinson CC. Interactions of parents with their young handicapped children. In: Odom SL, Karnes MB, eds. *Early Intervention for Infants and Children with Handicaps: An Empirical Base.* Baltimore, Md: Paul H. Brookes; 1988.

103. Barrera M, Rosenbaum P. The transactional model of early home intervention. *Infant Mental Health Journal.* 1986;7:112–131.

104. Calhoun ML, Rose TL, Prenergast DE. *Charlotte Circle Intervention Guide for Parent–Child Interactions.* Tucson, Ariz: Communication Skill Builders; 1991.

105. Babeshoff K. *Personal communication.* October 1994.

106. Erikson EH. *Childhood and Society.* New York, NY: Norton; 1950.

107. Bromvich R. *Working with Parents and Infants: An Interactional Approach.* Baltimore, Md: University Park Press; Austin, Tex: PRO ED; 1981.

108. *Nursing Child Assessment Satellite Training (NCAST): A Parent's Guide to Learning How Babies Behave: Booklet 3: Infant Cues.* Seattle, Wash: University of Washington; 1990.

109. Levy-Shiff R. Mother–father–child interactions with a mentally retarded young child. *Am J Ment Defic.* 1982;91:141–149.

110. Tyler N, Kogan K. Turner P. Interpersonal components of therapy with young cerebral palsied children. *Am J Occup Ther.* 1974;28:395–400.

111. Ramey CT, Farran D, Campbell F, Finkelstein N. Observations of mother–father interactions: implications for development. In: Minifie F, Lloyd L, eds. *Communicative and Cognitive Abilities: Early Behavioral Assessment.* Baltimore, Md: University Park Press; 1978.

112. Burkhalt J, Rutherford R, Goldberg K. Verbal and non-verbal interaction of mothers with their Down's syndrome and non-retarded infants. *Am J Ment Defic.* 1978;82:337–343.

113. Cunningham CE, Reubal E, Blackwell J, Jr, Deck J. Behavioral and linguistic development in the interactions of normal and retarded children with their mothers. *Child Dev.* 1981;52:62–70.

114. Eheart B. Mother–child interactions with non-retarded, mentally retarded preschoolers. *Am J Ment Defic.* 1982;87:20–25.

115. Brookes-Gunn J, Lewis B. Temperament and affective interaction in handicapped infants. *Journal of the Division for Early Childhood.* 1982;5:31–41.

116. Crawley SB, Spiker D. Mother–child interactions involving two year olds with Down's syndrome. A look at individual differences. *Child Dev.* 1983;54:1,312–1,323.

117. Hanzlik J, Stevenson M. Interaction of mothers with their infants who are mentally retarded with cerebral palsy or non-retarded. *Am J Ment Defic.* 1982;90:513–520.

118. Langley M. *The Teachable Moment of the Handicapped Infant.* Washington, DC: National Institute of Education; 1980. ERIC Document Reproduced. Service No. ED 191254.

119. Rossetti L. *High-Risk Infants, Ideas, Assessment and Intervention.* Boston, Mass: Little, Brown; 1986.

120. Minde K. Low birth weight infants: a psychosocial perspective. In: Parron D, Eisenberg L, eds. *Infants at Risk for Developmental Dysfunction. Health and Behavior: A Research Agenda Interim Report.* Washington, DC: National Academy Press; 4.

121. Taylor PM, Hall BL. Parent–infant bonding: problems and opportunities in a prenatal center. *Semin Perinatol.* 1979;3:73–84.

122. Jeffcoate J, Humphreys M, Lloyd J. Disturbance in parent–child relationship following preterm delivery. *Dev Med Child Neurol.* 1979;21:344–352.

123. Klaus MH, Kennell JM. *Maternal Infant Bonding.* St. Louis, Mo: Mosby; 1976.

124. Klein M, Stern L. Low birth weight and the battered child syndrome. *Am J Dis Child.* 1971;122:122.

125. Elmer and Gregg. Developmental characteristics of abused children. *Pediatrics.* 1967;40:596–602.

126. Weston J. The pathology of child abuse. In: Helfer R, Kempe C, eds. *The Battered Child.* Chicago, Ill: University of Chicago Press; 1968.

127. Fomufod A, Sinkford SM, Lovy VT. Mother–child separation at birth. A contributing factor in child abuse. *Lancet.* 1975;2:549–550.

128. Ackerman D. The magic touch. *American Health.* October 1993:70–71.

129. Leiderman P. Human mother to infant social bonding. Is there a critical phase? In: Barlow G, Maine M, Petrinovich L, eds. *Behavioral Development: An Interdisciplinary Approach.* Cambridge: Cambridge University Press; 1980.

130. Barnett C, Leiderman H, Grolisteir R, Klaus M. Neonatal separation: the maternal side of the interactional deprivation. *Pediatrics.* 1970;45:2.

131. Robinson K. The role of eye-to-eye contact in maternal–infant attachment. *J Child Psychol Psychiatry.* 1967:8–13.

132. Schneider EF. The role of infant massage in early intervention. Presented at the Infant Development Association Conference; February 1995; San Jose, Calif.

133. Field T. Reduced blood pressure, and greater relaxation. Volunteer grandparents benefit more from massaging others than from receiving massage. *Touchpoints.* Benjamin Y, ed. Touch Research Institute, 1994;1(3):1–4.

134. Barnard KE. The effect of stimulation on the sleep behavior of the premature infant. *Communicating Nursing Research.* 1973;6:12–40.

135. Solkof N, Yaffe S, Weintraub D, Blase B. Effects of handling on the subsequent development of premature infants. *Developmental Psychology.* 1969;1:765–768.

136. Freedman DB, Boverman H, Freedman N. Effects of kinesthetic stimulation on weight-gain and smiling in premature infants. Presented at the American Orthopsychiatric Association; San Francisco, Calif; 1966.

137. Gray GW. Human growth. *Sci Am.* 1953;189:65–67.

138. Rosenblatt JS, Lehrman DS. Maternal behavior of the laboratory rat. In: *Material Behavior in Mammals,* HL Rheingold, ed. New York: Wiley; 1963.

139. Gerwitz D. Scientists outline the many benefits of touch. *Touchpoints.* Fall 1993:3.

140. Acolot D, et al. Changes in plasma cortisol and catecholamine concentrations in response to massage in preterm infants. *Arch Dis Child.* 1993;68:29–31.

Unit VI

Exemplars of Holistic Nursing Practice

The articles in this unit represent exemplars in holistic nursing practice. The authors share with us a special gift—their wisdom and experience in providing holistic nursing care. Perhaps even more important, these authors have taken the quantum leap in translating theoretical concepts of holism and healing into tangible, down-to-earth examples of what it means to deliver holistic care to a select group of clients. Although most nurses ascribe to a holistic philosophy of nursing, many struggle when trying to apply such concepts in their daily practice. Holistic philosophy and concepts frequently are not easily understood and often are filled with abstract terminology and impractical ideas. It is from such exemplars, however, that the rest of us can visualize the process and begin the journey of transforming theory into practice. These exemplars give us specific ideas, creative suggestions, practical recommendations, basic behaviors, and details of implementation that can be replicated, altered, or adapted within our own practice.

Applying holistic care to neonates (Modrcin-McCarthy and colleagues) is illustrated using a STRESS tool (really a mnemonic for practice developed from Roy's Adaptation Model rather than a tool) for assessing and intervening with preterm infants. Likewise, holistic care of children undergoing surgery (Rundio and colleagues) is fully described in terms of the development of a program that spans preoperative teaching, the pediatric holding area, anesthetic induction, the wake-up room, and postoperative recovery. Specific details are outlined to create a holistic and healing experience for the child including the use of distraction, role rehearsal, educational preparation, therapeutic play activities, relaxation skills, imagery, and a child-friendly environment.

An innovative approach to providing holistic care to patients with cardiac illness was developed from the results of a qualitative research study (Medich and colleagues). From this research, the framework of Healing through Integration was developed as a guide to assess and implement relevant body-mind-spirit interventions to promote wellness and recovery following a cardiac crisis. A detailed case study is used to describe and illustrate fully each step of the framework.

The Trauma Bereavement Program for families of trauma victims (Buchanan) delineates the components of another concrete approach in delivering holistic care. The article is filled with rich examples and case studies, specific responses that nurses can use when confronted with difficult family questions, tangible methods of providing family reassurance, actual support letters written to families during the holidays and death anniversary, and many supplementary details that could be replicated in other settings. The article also includes the support that is provided for the trauma staff who are an integral part of these difficult patient deaths.

349

Nurses who wish to integrate holistic nursing in nursing homes (Drugay) should be aware of the institutional barriers and problem solving approaches encountered in this practice setting. Details of implementing holistic strategies, establishing support groups, using touch, prayer, and imagery as well as movement and music therapy and stress-management strategies to enhance health outcomes are shared.

What is impressive about several of these exemplars is the multidisciplinary character of the programs. Many of the programs were conceived, developed, and implemented by the collaborative efforts of various professional disciplines (e.g., nurses, physicians, chaplains, social workers, child life specialists, and pharmacists, as well as respiratory, physical, and occupational therapists) whose primary goals are to meet the body-mind-spirit needs of their clients and families. Too often in nursing, we assume the role of providing holistic care in isolation of our colleagues. Collaborative, multidisciplinary holistic practice is necessary for true healing and wholeness to occur in our clients.

One can read the details of these exemplars and intuitively know that such programs help clients. To demonstrate scientifically that they do make a difference, however, elevates their value and justifies their existence. The effectiveness of providing holistic care could be evaluated for each of these exemplars by using a number of psychophysiologic, educational, behavioral, financial, and satisfaction endpoints. For example, it would be possible to evaluate the effects of the STRESS tool in guiding practice (Modrcin-McCarthy and colleagues) by developing an instrument that scored the autonomic, motor, and state behavioral signs of stress in preterm infants (Table 1 of the article) before and after implementing the TRESS (of STRESS) interventions described in the article.

As we approach the 21st century, we will continue to be challenged to demonstrate that the results of our nursing care are effective in enhancing client outcomes. If holistic health care programs have the potential to make a difference in the lives of our clients and families, then it is critical that we investigate and document such outcomes.

Preterm Infants and STRESS: A Tool for the Neonatal Nurse

Mary Anne Modrcin-McCarthy, PhD, RN
Director and Associate Professor
Undergraduate Program
College of Nursing

Susan McCue, MSN, RN, PNP
Former Graduate Student

Julie Walker, MSN, RN, PNP
Former Graduate Student
College of Nursing
University of Tennessee
Knoxville, Tennessee

Infants born prematurely are not physiologically or developmentally prepared for life outside the supportive environment of the mother's womb. Their response to stimuli is usually immature or disorganized. This article examines actual and potential stressors of premature infants; describes specific autonomic, motor, and state behavioral responses; and proposes a clinical tool (the STRESS tool: *s*igns of stress, *t*ouch interventions, *r*eduction of pain, *e*nvironmental considerations, *s*tate, and *s*tability) that nurses can use to prioritize interventions when caring for fragile preterm infants. The Roy Adaptation Model is used to provide a conceptual framework for the discussion.

THE ROY ADAPTATION MODEL AND THE PRETERM INFANT

The Roy Adaptation Model is one of the most commonly implemented conceptual models in nursing today. The model uses a systems theory approach with the person (defined as a biopsychosocial entity) as the core of an adaptive system. The scientific assumptions are based on both systems and adaptation theories. The philosophical assumptions about the adapting person in society are founded on humanistic values and the principle of veritivity. Roy's theory of the person as an adapting system was

Source: Reprinted from M.A. Modrcin-McCarthy, S. McCue, and J. Walker, *Journal of Perinatal and Neonatal Nursing,* Vol. 10, No. 4, pp. 62–71, © 1997, Aspen Publishers, Inc.

Submitted for publication: August 8, 1996
Accepted for publication: November 6, 1996

developed from the Roy Adaptation Model. Input to the system in the form of stimuli—focal (immediate), factor contextual (contributing factors), and residual (innate, unknown factors)—determines the person's adaptation level and adaptive response.

According to Roy and Andrews,[1] coping mechanisms assist the person in adapting to environmental changes. These coping mechanisms can be innate (genetically determined and automatically processed) or acquired (a deliberate, learned response). These mechanisms are further categorized into regulator and cognator subsystems. Roy and Andrews posited that the regulator subsystem is a "basic type of adaptive process" and "responds automatically through neural, chemical and endocrine coping processes."[1(p14)] The cognator subsystem coping process "responds through four cognitive-emotive channels: perceptual/information processing, learning, judgment and emotion."[1(p14)] Additionally, neurologic function is essential to regulator and cognator processing and thus is important to a person's adaptation.[1] The cognator and regulator coping processes act to maintain adaptation in the four adaptive modes: physiologic, self-concept, role function, and interdependence.

Roy states that an infant is born with two adaptive modes, physiologic and interdependence: "out of the interactions that are primarily affectional or nurturing in nature arises the beginning self-concept (self-concept mode), and finally roles (role function mode) are learned."[2(p310)] The firm establishment of the physiologic and interdependence modes is pivotal for the overall growth, development, and general well-being of the infant. Additionally, because of the holistic nature of the person, Roy and Andrews[1] posit that the adaptive modes are interrelated and affect the other modes. Adaptive or ineffective responses may be characteristic of more than one mode. Specifically, the physiologic mode is concerned with how the infant responds physically to stimuli. The interdependence mode involves the infant's bonding process and the developing ability to give and receive love.

The idea of adaptation must be examined within the context of the infant in the neonatal intensive care unit (NICU). The infant is viewed as a system that has the capacity to adapt positively to stimuli. The model suggests that positive adaptation depends on several factors: the stimuli, the adaptation level of the infant, and the coping mechanisms available to the infant. To understand the infant in the context of Roy's theory of an adapting person, one need only observe the infant as a simple heelstick is done. The painful penetration of the skin is the focal stimulus. The ambient noise and bright lights are two of the contextual stimuli. The residual stimuli may include the memory of previous heelsticks. These stimuli combine with the infant's internal conditions to determine the infant's adaptation level.

Finally, the coping mechanisms are innate and acquired abilities to respond to stimuli. Innate coping mechanisms are those with which the infant is born, such as reflex withdrawal from the painful stimulus of the heelstick. This is an example of a function of the regulator subsystem. Acquired coping mechanisms are those that the infant develops through experience with various stimuli, such as bringing a hand to the mouth for self-comfort. In this, the infant demonstrates functioning of the cognator subsystem. It is readily apparent that the premature infant will have immature innate coping mechanisms and limited acquired coping mechanisms. Thus the vulnerable preterm infant is likely to demonstrate ineffective responses to stimuli that are commonly recognized as signs of stress.

CLARIFICATION OF TERMS

To apply Roy's theory of an adapting person to the care of the preterm infant, one must grasp Roy's definition of stress and how it differs from the common understanding of the concept. The *Oxford English Dictionary* defines stress as "a condition or adverse circumstance that disturbs, or is likely to disturb, the normal physiological or psychological functioning of the individual." In Roy and Andrews' work, stress is defined as "the transaction between the environmental demands requiring adaptation and the individual's cognator and regulator coping mechanisms."[1(p238)] Although similar, these definitions differ in that Roy and Andrews' definition considers the actual connection between the demands of the environment and the response of the infant to those demands; it further requires that caregivers be mindful of the particular regulator and cognator coping mechanisms available to the infant.

Although rarely clearly defined in the literature in relation to preterm infants, the concept of stress is discussed extensively. Events and conditions that are assumed to produce stress in preterm infants include environmental noise,[3,4] bright lighting,[4,5] nursing interventions,[6] certain types of infant handling,[4,5] and so-called painful procedures such as suctioning, intubation, and heelsticks.[7,8]

A review of the literature reveals that stress responses observed in preterm infants are generally divided into two categories: physiologic and behavioral. It is understood, however, that these are not truly separate categories; rather, they represent points on a continuum of behavior. This is revealed through examination of the *Oxford English Dictionary* definition of behavior: "an observable pattern of actions; a response to a stimulus." Roy and Andrews define behavior as "internal or external actions and reactions under specified circumstances."[1(p4)] Regardless of which definition is accepted, it is clear that the term *behavior* includes physiologic/autonomic, measurable responses, such as heart rate and oxygen saturation, as well as those responses that are traditionally viewed as motor and state behaviors, such as crying, sleeping, and limb movement. For the purposes of this article, signs of stress in preterm infants are discussed in terms of autonomic, motor, and state behaviors.

AUTONOMIC, MOTOR, AND STATE BEHAVIORAL SIGNS OF STRESS

It is known that during the third trimester of pregnancy the fetal brain, especially the autonomic nervous system, undergoes rapid development. Layering and organization of cortical neurons, expansion of dendrites and axons, development of synapses, and differentiation occur.[5] Although this development continues after birth, the premature infant lacks the initial maturation that normally occurs in utero, where the environment is warm, dark, and isolated and sounds are buffered.[5] The infant enters the extrauterine world of the NICU with immature neurologic and physiologic systems,[4] which makes it difficult for the infant to develop, interact, and adapt in the NICU environment. Infants may be bombarded with environmental stimuli, such as bright lights, loud noises, frequent nursing interventions, and painful procedures. These extrauterine conditions and events may lead to hypoxic episodes, which often result in damage to brain tissue and the formation of idiopathic neuron connections.[5] Until the autonomic system reaches a more organized, integrated, mature level, premature infants react to their environment with disorganized, ineffective responses.[9]

Autonomic responses to stress are summarized in Table 1.[4,9–18] It is thought that many of these responses are due to withdrawal of parasympathetic tone.[19] The majority of the literature focuses on three specific physiologic reactions: heart rate, respiratory rate, and oxygen saturation. Some investigators discuss blood pressure instability[10] and hormonal reactions to stress, including increased serum cortisol levels[11] and decreased serum growth hormone concentration.[12]

It is well known that oxygen is necessary for body functions, brain development, and tissue growth. During stressful events in preterm infants, a decrease in transcutaneous oxygen levels has been documented.[7,14] A decrease in alveolar ventilation and thus decreased oxygenation occur when an infant is crying.[3,20] When infants experience hypoxia, they are at risk for neurologic damage. It is currently unknown what length of hypoxia results in brain damage.[7] With repeated stressful events, the infant may experience prolonged hypoxemia and have more difficulty recovering from the episodes.[4,5] This places the infant at an even greater risk for long-term sequelae.

Table 1. Autonomic, motor, and state behavioral signs of stress in preterm infants

Autonomic	Motor	State
Decreased transcutaneous oxygen levels	Frantic body movements	Inadequate state modulation
Increased heart rate	Jitteriness	Sudden changes of state
Increased respiratory rate	Tremors	Prolongation of alert state
Increased intracranial pressure	Startles	Fussiness
Fluctuations in systolic blood pressure	Flaccidity	Crying
Increased cortisol secretion	Hyperextension of legs, arms, trunk	Inconsolability
Decreased serum growth hormone levels	Finger splays	Panicked or worried alertness
Skin color changes	Facial grimacing	Staring
Increased stooling	Tongue extension	Eye floating
Decreased tolerance of feedings	Hand to face movement	
Hiccoughs	Fisting	
Sneezing	Limited use of self-comforting behaviors such as hand/finger sucking, hand clasping, rooting, sucking	
Gagging		
Yawning		
Seizures		
Twitching		
Sighing		
Coughing		

Sources: References 4, 9–18.

Increased heart rates and respiratory patterns are documented as physiologic signs of stress. An increase in these rates leads to greater energy requirements, resulting in higher oxygen demand and calorie consumption. Unnecessary energy expenditure leaves less oxygen available for body functions and tissue growth and fewer calories for growth and healing. If the stressful event is prolonged, the infant may become apneic and bradycardic.[4,5,21] Energy depletion may even lead to exhaustion and death.[22]

Intraventricular hemorrhage is a significant contributor to neurologic sequelae and death in preterm infants.[20] Increases in intracranial pressure, blood pressure fluctuations, and hypoxia can lead to intraventricular hemorrhage.[23,24] Brown[10] found a statistically significant alteration in systolic blood pressure both during and after a painful stimulus, and Stevens and colleagues[24] noted changes in intracranial pressure. Carefully selected nursing interventions may de-

crease episodes of hypoxia, thereby minimizing the occurrence and sequelae of intraventricular hemorrhage in neonates.[20]

Tissue healing, growth, and recovery can be affected by alterations in hormone levels during stress. Investigators have reported an increase in cortisol, adrenaline, and catecholamines.[11,23,25,26] Increases in glucocorticoids can lead to hyperglycemia and metabolic acidosis in preterm infants. Schanberg and Field[12] found that serum growth hormones are decreased in stressed infants.

Ineffective adaptation may be manifested in the preterm infant in ways other than the measurable autonomic/physiologic responses described above. Motor and state behaviors also provide insight into the adaptation level of the infant. Motor behaviors, such as frantic body movements, jitteriness, and decreases in muscle tone to flaccidity or limpness, are among the many motor indicators of ineffective responses to stimuli.[9] State behavior refers to the sleep and wake states, which are further divided into quiet sleep, active sleep, drowsy, awake alert, active awake, and crying states.[27] Behaviors that indicate immature, ineffective responses related to state regulation include inability to modulate state, sudden state changes, prolonged alert state, and limited use of self-quieting behaviors, such as hand-to-mouth movement[9] (Table 1). An infant who exhibits disorganized motor and state activity is compromised as a result of the futile expenditure of available oxygen, nutrients, and energy, which leaves these precious resources unavailable for healing, growth, and development.

The concept of state organization is central to our understanding of the stress response in preterm infants and our interpretation of their related behavioral cues. State organization refers to the frequency of transition from one sleep/wake state to another. Infants who are disorganized exhibit frequent and rapid changes in their state. Organized infants have the capacity to modulate responses to stimuli, including the transitional state periods. Murphy suggests that "the range and variety of states, and the amount of time spent in each state have a great influence on the physiological and emotional well-being of high risk infants."[28(p369)]

Gorski and coworkers provide a list of behavioral responses that represent evidence of a high level of organization:

> 1) the capacity to respond reliably and selectively in a social interaction with a nurturing adult or with attractive auditory or visual stimuli, 2) the capacity to regulate [the] state of consciousness in order to be available for positive stimulation and to defend [the self] from negative stimulation, 3) the capacity to maintain adequate tone, to control motor behavior, and to perform integrated motor activities such as hand-to-mouth maneuvers, and 4) the capacity to maintain physiologic homeostasis.[13(p62)]

These behavioral responses are built one on another, beginning with physiologic homeostasis and ultimately developing into the capacity to respond positively to social stimuli as the infant matures.

Als and Brazelton[29] and Murphy[28] suggest that physiologic stability is the foundation for higher levels of organization, including motor control and state regulation, leading ultimately to the capability for successful social interaction. "Until the infants have established homeostasis there is little progress through higher levels of maturation. Until immature infants are sufficiently organized with some motor control they cannot attend to or be alert for long enough to make social contact."[28(p368)] In terms of the Roy Adaptation Model, adaptive responses in the physiologic mode are a prerequisite to adaptive functioning in the interdependence mode.

THE STRESS TOOL

It is extremely important that caregivers be knowledgeable of autonomic, motor, and state behavioral signs of stress in preterm infants. Repeated stressful events can lead to serious consequences, including increased morbidity and mortality. In fact, it has been suggested that high-intensity stimulation correlates with lower levels of cognitive development.[3] For these reasons, it is necessary to intervene on behalf of the premature infant, who is unable to respond effectively or adapt to stressful situations that are encountered.

The STRESS tool was developed to assist the neonatal nurse in recognizing and reducing stress in preterm infants (see the box titled "Summary of the STRESS Tool"). As mentioned previously, STRESS stands for signs of stress, touch interventions, reduction of pain, environmental considerations, state, and stability. Remembering the word *stress* and the related key phrases may facilitate nurses in assessing, diagnosing, planning, implementing, and evaluating care of the stressed preterm infant. Selected nursing diagnoses approved by the North American Nursing Diagnosis Association (NANDA) that may be actual or potential concerns for the stressed preterm infant are listed in

Summary of the STRESS Tool

Signs of stress: caregivers must be knowledgeable of the signs of stress in preterm infants

Touch interventions: touch interventions such as gentle human touch may be appropriate, and thus utilized, to promote physiologic and interdependence adaptation

Reduction of pain: actions may need to be taken to reduce painful events experienced by preterm infants in the NICU

Environmental considerations: environmental factors such as ambient temperature, noise level, and lighting must be controlled appropriately

State: interventions should be tailored with regard to the infant's autonomic, motor, and state behaviors

Stability: the nurse needs to monitor the stability of the preterm infant continuously and modify care as warranted

the box titled "NANDA Nursing Diagnoses for the Preterm Infant."[30] Once the nurse has determined the nursing diagnoses, appropriate interventions can be implemented.

Signs of stress

It is important for the nurse to monitor the preterm infant continually for signs of stress. As discussed earlier, stress can have adverse effects on the health of the preterm infant. Table 1 gives a compiled list of autonomic, motor, and state behavioral signs of stress.

Nursing interventions include the following:

- Educate self and other caregivers in identification of autonomic, motor, and state behavioral signs of stress in preterm infants.[3,4]
- Assist parents in recognizing and interpreting their infant's behavioral stress cues. Teach them how to provide the support their infant needs.[3,22]

- Include stress identification and intervention education when training new employees of the NICU.[22]

Touch interventions

Appropriate touch interventions, such as gentle human touch, can be used to promote physiologic and interdependence adaptation. Gentle human touch is a form of continuous touch; the individual places his or her hands gently on the infant's body, usually one hand on the head and the other hand on the arm or back and holds that position for a designated amount of time.[31,32]

Nursing interventions are as follows:

- Gentle human touch may be an appropriate nursing/parental intervention for preterm infants.[31,32]
- Stroking, massage, tactile/kinesthetic, and kangaroo care types of touch may be appropriate,[23,33,34] but the nurse needs to know that stroking, massage, and tactile/kines-

NANDA Nursing Diagnoses for the Preterm Infant

Activity intolerance
Anxiety
Ineffective breathing pattern
Altered comfort
Impaired communication
Ineffective individual coping
Fatigue
Impaired gas exchange
Altered growth and development
High risk for infection
Ineffective infant feeding pattern
Altered nutrition: less than body requirements
Pain
Altered protection
Relocation stress syndrome
Sensory perceptual alterations
Sleep pattern disturbance

thetic touch may be inappropriate or too much stimulation for some fragile infants.
- Monitor oxygen saturation, heart rate, and motor and state behaviors during touch if there is any concern that the touching may overstimulate and thus stress the preterm infant.
- Interventions should be altered or stopped if the infant manifests signs of stress.
- Eliminate routine and unnecessary procedures on the unstable infant.[4]
- Implement appropriate touch into the care plan.[4,31]
- Cluster nursing care.[4,5,14,33]

Reduction of pain

Pain is an obvious but sometimes unavoidable stressor to the preterm infant. The following nursing interventions, however, may mitigate the pain associated with the many necessary procedures:

- Consider kinesthesia, soothing music, or touch to reduce the sensation of pain.[10]
- Use containment or facilitated tucking during painful procedures to lessen the stress responses.[35,36]
- Use spring-loaded lances for heelsticks.[8]
- Provide opioid[6] or other analgesics during stressful procedures.
- Consider nonnutritive sucking (pacifier) during painful procedures.[19]

Environmental considerations

The infant in the NICU is often bombarded with sensory stimuli. There has been much discussion about the possibility that the inappropriateness of this stimuli in the NICU is stressful to the preterm infant. Evaluation and modification of the NICU environment may be warranted.

Nursing interventions are as follows:

- Be aware of sound levels at all times in the NICU[4,5] (eg, doors slamming, objects being dropped on the floor, loud conversations).
- When purchasing new equipment for the NICU, consider machine noise and alarms.[4,5]

- Physician and nurse rounds should be conducted away from the infant's bedside.[4,14]
- Implement quiet times in the NICU during shifts.[23]
- Place the most fragile and vulnerable infants in an incubator[23] if resources are limited.
- Educate nursing staff, parents, and ancillary staff about noise reduction.[3]
- Monitor and evaluate sound levels in the NICU.[3]
- Close incubator doors carefully and quietly.[14,33]
- If radios are used, keep them at a low volume.[14]
- Respond promptly to alarms.
- Keep all ventilation tubing free from excess water.[14]
- Place a blanket over incubators and oxygen hoods periodically to reduce lighting and also absorb noise.[14]
- If the infant is on an open warmer, create a tentlike covering over the infant's head for light and noise reduction.[4,14,33]
- Implement periods of darkness or reduced lighting to simulate diurnal rhythm.[4,5]
- Shield the infant's eyes from bright lighting when holding the infant outside the incubator.[14]

State

The immature status of the preterm infant is often demonstrated by disorganization and state instability, such as a decreased amount of time in quiet sleep and more time in the other sleep/wake states. It is important that caregivers be sensitive to and respectful of the state of these infants to promote their well-being.

Nursing interventions for state include the following:

- Cluster nursing care.[4,5,14,33]
- Provide for rest periods.[4,14,33]
- Promote smooth transitions from one state to another by awakening infants slowly before performing nursing procedures.

- Provide support, such as nonnutritive sucking, swaddling, and gentle touch, during periods of disorganization.[14,19,23]
- Avoid inappropriate stimulation, such as initiation of social interaction, before the infant demonstrates physiologic organization.[14,28]

Stability

The nurse needs to monitor the stability of the preterm infant continuously and modify care as warranted. This can be best accomplished by discriminately selecting and evaluating nursing interventions, individualizing care, and providing continuity of caregivers for the preterm infant.

The following are nursing interventions for stability:

- Be choosy about nursing interventions (just because it worked for Baby Smith doesn't mean it's right for Baby Jones).[14]
- Get to know the infants in your care and respect their individuality (do not refer to the infant as "it").

- Organize nursing shifts and rotations so that infants receive care from the same few nurses throughout their stay in the NICU.
- Encourage parents to be with their preterm infant as soon and as often as possible.
- Evaluation and reevaluation are key to achieving stability in the preterm infant.

•   •   •

This article has examined the idea of adaptation, which is so central to the Roy Adaptation Model, in the context of the preterm infant in the NICU. The vulnerable preterm infant is likely to demonstrate immature and disorganized responses to stimuli that are commonly recognized as signs of stress. These ineffective responses present themselves through the physiologic and interdependence modes via autonomic, motor, and state behavioral signs seen in the fragile preterm infant. Neonatal nurses can utilize the STRESS tool when caring for fragile preterm infants.

REFERENCES

1. Roy C, Andrews HA. *The Roy Adaptation Model: The Definitive Statement.* Norwalk, Conn: Appleton & Lange; 1991.
2. Roy C. *An Adaptation Model: Introduction to Nursing.* 2nd ed. Englewood Cliffs, NJ: Prentice Hall; 1984.
3. DePaul D, Chambers SE. Environmental noise in the neonatal intensive care unit: Implications for nursing practice. *J Perinat Neonat Nurs.* 1995;8:71–76.
4. Catlett AT, Holditch-Davis D. Environmental stimulation of the acutely ill premature infant: Physiological effects and nursing implications. *Neonat Network.* 1990;8:19–26.
5. Allen A. Stressors to neonates in the neonatal unit. *Midwives.* 1995;108:139–140.
6. Pokela M. Pain relief can reduce hypoxemia in distressed neonates during routine procedures. *Pediatrics.* 1994;93:379–384.
7. Norris S, Campbell LA, Brenkert S. Nursing procedures and alterations in the transcutaneous oxygen tension in premature infants. *Nurs Res.* 1982;31:1330–1336.
8. McIntosh N, vanVeen L, Brameyer H. Alleviation of the pain of heel prick in preterm infants. *Arch Dis Child.* 1994;70:F177–F181.

9. D'Apolito K. What is an organized infant? *Neonat Network.* 1991;10:23–29.
10. Brown L. Physiologic responses to cutaneous pain in neonates. *Neonat Network.* 1987;5:18–22.
11. Economou G, Andronikou S, Chella A, Cholevas V, Lapatsanis PD. Cortisol secretion in stressed babies during the neonatal period. *Horm Res.* 1993;40:217–221.
12. Schanberg S, Field T. Sensory deprivation, stress and supplemental stimulation in the rat pup and the human neonate. *Child Dev.* 1987;58:1431–1447.
13. Gorski PA, Davison MF, Brazelton TB. Stages of behavioral organization in the high-risk neonate: Theoretical and clinical considerations. *Semin Perinatol.* 1979;3:61–72.
14. Lawhon G. Management of stress in premature infants. In: Angelinini DJ, Whelan Knapp CM, Gibes RM, eds. *Perinatal/Neonatal Nursing: A Clinical Handbook.* Boston, Mass: Blackwell Scientific; 1986.
15. Stevens BJ, Johnston C. Physiological responses of premature infants to a painful stimulus. *Nurs Res.* 1994;43:226–231.
16. Als H, Lester BM, Tronick EZ, Brazelton TY. Toward a research instrument for the assessment of preterm in-

fants' behavior. In: Fitzgerald ME, Lester BM, Togman MW, eds. *Theory and Research in Behavioral Pediatrics.* New York, NY: Plenum; 1982;1.

17. Cole JG. Infant stimulation reexamined: An environmental and behavioral-based approach. *Neonat Network.* 1985;3:24–31.

18. Vanderberg KA. Revising the traditional model: An individualized approach to developmental interventions in the intensive care nursery. *Neonat Network.* 1986;3:32–38.

19. DiPietro JA, Cusson RM, O'Brien-Caughy M, Fox NA. Behavioral and physiologic effects of nonnutritive sucking during gavage feeding in preterm infants. *Pediatr Res.* 1994;36:207–214.

20. Beaver PK. Premature infants' response to touch and pain: Can nurses make a difference? *Neonat Network.* 1987;6:13–17.

21. Tribotti S. Admission to the neonatal intensive care unit: Reducing the risks. *Neonat Network.* 1990;8:17–22.

22. Gunderson LP, Kenner C. Neonatal stress: Physiologic adaptation and nursing implications. *Neonat Network.* 1987;6:37–42.

23. Glass P. The vulnerable neonate and the neonatal intensive care environment. In: Avery GB, Fletcher MA, McDonald MG, eds. *Neonatology: Pathophysiology and Management of the Newborn.* 4th ed. Philadelphia, Pa: Lippincott; 1994.

24. Stevens BJ, Johnston CC, Horton L. Multidimensional pain assessment in premature neonates: A pilot study. *J Obstet Gynecol Neonat Nurs.* 1993;22:531–541.

25. Bozzette M. Observation of pain behavior in the NICU: An exploratory study. *J Perinat Neonat Nurs.* 1993; 7:76–87.

26. Gunnar MR, Isensee J, Fust S. Adrenocortical activity and the Brazelton Neonatal Assessment Scale: Moderating effects of the newborn's biobehavioral status. *Child Dev.* 1987;58:1448–1458.

27. Brazelton TB. *Neonatal Behavioral Assessment Scale.* 2nd ed. Philadelphia, Pa: Lippincott; 1984.

28. Murphy F. The high-risk infant. *Physiotherapy.* 1991;77:367–371.

29. Als H, Brazelton TB. A new model of assessing the behavioral organization of preterm and fullterm infants. *J Am Acad Child Psychiatry.* 1981;20:239–263.

30. North American Nursing Diagnosis Association (NANDA). *Nursing Diagnoses: Definitions and Classification.* Philadelphia, Pa: NANDA; 1995.

31. Modrcin-McCarthy MA. *The Physiological and Behavioral Effects of a Gentle Human Touch Nursing Intervention on Preterm Infants.* Knoxville, Tenn: University of Tennessee at Knoxville; 1992. Thesis.

32. Harrison LL, Groër M, Modrcin-McCarthy MA, Wilkerson J. Effects of gentle human touch on preterm infants: Results from a pilot study. *Infant Behav Dev.* 1992;15:12.

33. Langer VS. Minimal handling protocol for the intensive care nursery. *Neonat Network.* 1990;9:23–27.

34. Field TM, Schanberg SM, Scafidi F, et al. Tactile/kinesthetic stimulation effects on preterm neonates. *Pediatrics.* 1986;77: 654–658.

35. Corff KE. An effective comfort measure for minor pain and stress in preterm infants: Facilitated tucking. *Neonat Network.* 1993;12:74.

36. Taquino L, Blackburn S. The effects of containment during suctioning and heelstick on physiological and behavioral responses of preterm infants. *Neonat Network.* 1994;13:55.

Children's Experience of Surgery: Creating a Holistic Environment

Albert A. Rundio, Jr, PhD, MSN, RN, CNAA
Vice President for Nursing Services

Marion E. Rudek, MSN, RNC, CRNP
Maternal Child Health Nurse Practitioner

Maria Spear, BS
Child Life Specialist

Patricia LaCarrubba, RN
Pediatric Sedation Nurse

Betty Halpern, RN, CPAN
Postanesthesia Care Unit Staff Nurse
Shore Memorial Hospital
Somers Point, New Jersey

Shore Memorial Hospital's Pediatric Perioperative Program represents a combination of developmental approaches to the child's and family's experience of surgery. Each phase of perioperative care has surfaced throughout the decades of pediatric technology and has developed a progression of overall identified needs within the following areas: preoperative teaching, the operating room (OR) and anesthesia experience, and recovery room care. Subcomponents of these phases have addressed the issues of pain management and parental presence and reunitement with the child. Shore Memorial has strived to combine the most progressive components of these phases for a program focused on the specific physical and emotional needs of children and families who experience surgery as a change to their normal daily environment.

REVIEW OF THE LITERATURE

Attention to the developmental needs of children has an origin in the research of responses to hospitalization.[1] A comprehensive review of 20 years of theories and psychological response data was conducted to support the importance of prepa-

The authors thank the members of the Shore Memorial Hospital Pediatric Perioperative Program, especially David Azar, MD, and Nabil Younan, MD. Also, we appreciate the support of Mr. Richard Pitman, CEO, the Board, and the contributions of Dianne S. Charsha, RNC, MSN.

Source: Reprinted from A. Rundio, M. Rudek, M. Spear, P. LaCarrubba, and B. Halpern, *Holistic Nursing Practice,* Vol. 6, No. 4, pp. 44–52, © 1992, Aspen Publishers, Inc.

ratory teaching with children. Medical, nursing, psychiatric, and psychological literature continued to define methodologies for supportive care procedures to minimize stress reactions.

Data collection in the area of pediatric surgical preparation revealed two significant intervention styles that would serve as a cornerstone to preoperative preparation with children. These approaches remain integral to modern preoperative teaching and were defined as social interaction theory and stress-point preparation.

Mahaffy[2] and Skipper and colleagues[3] placed emphasis on the supportive efforts for the mothers rather than the child undergoing surgery. Social interaction theory was incorporated into the data collection. The results of these two studies indicated a reduction in the mother's emotional stress when information was provided about hospital routines, medical and nursing procedures, and the role of the parent in caring for the child.[2,3]

Stress-point preparation expanded on the original single-session approach and extended information across the total surgery experience for improved assimilation by both parent and child.[4] An experimental design with random assignment of control versus intervention included 84 children between the ages of 3 to 12 years and their families for the conditions of elective short-term surgery such as tonsillectomy and/or adenoidectomy, myringotomy, and ear tube placement. The intervention group of 21 children and their parents were provided information, instruction, rehearsal, and support from a single nurse at critical time periods. Intervention was interspersed at admission, shortly before blood tests, late in the afternoon the day before surgery, shortly prior to administration of preoperative medications, prior to transport into the OR suite, and on return from the recovery room. These critical intervention periods were events found to be typically stressful for children and integrated both parent and child needs.[4] Key elements of stress-point intervention utilized today incorporate parental information, sensory expectations, role support, and rehearsal through play activities.

An emotionally supportive environment soon expanded the focus to OR and anesthesia detail. Throughout the early 1980s, preoperative injections and the induction of anesthesia were invasive procedures for children because the child often experienced this portion of care without the benefit of parental support.[5] Attention to the waiting room areas, preoperative procedures including "shots" (still utilized at that time), transfer to the OR suite, activities of the staff in the OR, and the induction phase placed pediatric care within a developmental framework. Sensory detail was geared to tailoring the surgery experience through the eyes and ears of a child. Lighting, manipulation of equipment (ie, face mask, monitor electrodes, blood pressure cuff), terminology with simple comparisons, and assurance of parental reunitement were measures to provide a less stressful perception of surgery as well as a calm child.

The postanesthesia care unit (PACU) became the next area of examination of issues aimed at relieving parent-child separation anxiety. Editorials[6] and unpublished data that were later documented[7] surfaced as a direct challenge to the controversial textbook discussions of whether parents should be present in the recovery room. A study comprised of unit-specific comparisons that examined the child's behavior after surgery was able to support parental presence in the recovery room.[8] The intervention sequence included preoperative preparation (tour and teaching session) for both units; therefore, a *t*-test was performed to identify the most significant intervention for the child's stress reduction. There were 25 children surveyed on each of the two units for a total of 50 children in the sample. Parental presence was found to reduce stress symptoms to a "virtually nonexistent level" independent of preoperative teaching. Significant emotional behavior problems found in the nonintervention group of children (lack of parent presence in PACU) included nightmares; bedwetting; clinging; thumb sucking; decreased interest in activities, eating, and talking; and overconcern with body parts. Children's ages spanned 2 to 12 years with a mean of 7 years.

Advances in medical procedures such as elimination of preoperative intramuscular injections and/or the use of the alternate route of nasal medications,[9] and increased awareness of pediatric pain management in the recovery room[10] complete the cycle of perioperative care for the child. Individual assessment, developmental considerations, and family participation now have the potential to join together for a continuum of pediatric care rather than separate areas for the common goal of stress and anxiety reduction. Maximal coping skills are encouraged throughout preadmission, the day of surgery, in the recovery room, and during postoperative follow-up as the thrust of pediatric surgical care in the 1990s.

INTEGRATION AND DEVELOPMENT OF A PEDIATRIC PERIOPERATIVE PROGRAM

Shore Memorial Hospital's Pediatric Perioperative Program spans a 6-year history for establishment in the present form, and mirrors a pattern of progressive expansion and meshing of surgery phases. Stress-point intervention and family-centered care are central themes to the physical and emotional environment of the service.

The role of the child life specialist became integrated into Shore Memorial Hospital as an initial step to developmentally appropriate and supportive care for all pediatric patients. By 1985, the preadmission testing area incorporated the child life specialist for preoperative teaching. Provision of equipment manipulation and play activities was extended to the same-day surgery area with presence of the child life specialist the day of surgery.

PACU nurse interest in the pediatric specialty led to the establishment of toys and activities for children as well as family visitation by 1988. Children and their families were receiving significant procedural support at two critical time periods during the surgery process.

Progressive anesthesia practice invoked an interest in newer routes of sedative administration. OR personnel and clinical nurse specialist input

for safety and parental support combined for a search of functional space to house a pediatric holding area. November 1990 brought completion of former storage space to a room with oxygen outlet and equipment capacity for preanesthesia care.

The clinical nurse specialist role for the area of maternal-child health modeled the function of the pediatric sedation nurse for a trial period of 6 months from January to June 1991. Pediatric staff and two key recovery room nurses were targeted for workshop educational instruction of the pediatric sedation process. An independent pediatric sedation nurse role was conceived. The pediatric sedation nurse has become an essential member to the multidisciplinary team of pediatric, OR, anesthesia, and recovery or PACU personnel.

DESCRIPTION OF THE ENVIRONMENT

Preadmission testing is the initial introductory area for all children who will experience same-day surgery. The activities and teaching comprise the pediatric atmosphere at this phase rather than a physical space. Progressive phases of the program expose the child and family to the pediatric-specific areas of PACU.

A child's and family's experience the day of surgery spans the OR areas and recovery. The pediatric holding area hosts a friendly forest theme with large animal decals on the walls, including a sleeping bunny, a raccoon jumping rope, and a mama bear holding a baby bear. Room size accommodates two stretchers at once with a curtain divider for privacy. Supportive items include a videocassette recorder (VCR) with short features and cartoons, dimmer light switch, developmentally appropriate toys (Mr. Potatohead, Legos, bubble solution), chairbed for patient(s), and emergency equipment.

Mock respiratory arrests are conducted quarterly involving same-day surgery ancillary staff, child life specialist, pediatric sedation nurse, and PACU nurses. Review of emergency equipment includes bag-valve-mask apparatus bags (infant/child/adult), suction apparatus, oxygen, intravenous line equipment, pulse oximetry, and drug supply from the PACU emergency cart. This emergency component provides an essential safety aspect to the pediatric holding area.

Transport of the child to the OR area is facilitated by either the child being carried or placed on a stretcher. One OR suite is currently decorated with the same friendly forest theme. The wake-up room hosts similar diversional activities as the pediatric holding area, and provides rockers for parents to comfort their child.

The wake-up room is a six-bed unit with cardiac monitors, oxygen, suction, and an automatic blood pressure machine. Emergency drugs are available. This room also houses two televisions and two shelves filled with toys, games, and books. Posters of airplanes; soccer, basketball, and football sports players; and cats, dogs, and bears occupy the visual space around the wake-up room.

Postoperative care is either completed within the wake-up room prior to discharge, or facilitated on the pediatric unit for overnight stay situations. The entire continuum of care targets child-specific sensory information, and child-friendly environments for optimal transition through the surgery process.

PREOPERATIVE PREPARATION

Preparation for elective surgery begins at the time of preadmission testing, which takes place several days before surgery. At this time, the child life specialist meets with the child and family to begin, or in many cases, to continue the preparation process. Preparation is geared to the child's developmental level, and a variety of techniques are utilized. The goals of preparation are as follows:

- Determine the child's understanding of what will be done and why surgery is necessary.
- Provide accurate, developmentally appropriate information regarding the sequence of events. This information should include both procedural and sensory information.
- Provide the child an opportunity to see and handle related medical equipment.

- Introduce appropriate coping skills as needed.
- Provide emotional support to the family.
- Allow the child an opportunity to establish a relationship with one person who will represent surrogate support when parents cannot be present.
- Provide child and family with information and materials to continue the preparation process at home.

Preparation for infants and toddlers is primarily focused to the parents. While the child life specialist is talking with the parents, hospital equipment is available for infants and toddlers to handle. Parents are given information about how the day will proceed so that they can feel more relaxed. Suggestions regarding items to bring with their child are given. This time is usually spent in emotional support of the family and discussion of fears. Our belief is that a calm parent contributes to a calmer process for the child. The parents are then given an OR mask to take home for peek-a-boo play the night before surgery.

Preschool and school-age children benefit greatly from in-depth preparation. Initial discussions with use of body outlines or anatomically correct dolls involve determination of the child's understanding of where and why surgery will happen. A photo book then assists the child in seeing the sequence of events and sights of the day of surgery. The use of equipment is demonstrated using the dolls, and the child is given an opportunity to handle all equipment. A large portion of preparation time for this age group is spent practicing use of the face mask. All children are given a choice of scents that can be placed inside the mask. Children are instructed to take deep breaths when they smell the sweet air and to blow away any air they don't like. When necessary, deep breathing or mental imagery are introduced at this time. At the end of the session, children are given some play time while further instructions are given to the parents. Before going home, the child is given a hospital bag that includes a doctor/nurse hat, mask and gloves, a same-day surgery coloring book, a box of crayons, and a hospital sticker.

Adolescents are prepared using similar methods but with less play. However, adolescents are given an opportunity to see and handle hospital equipment. The reason for surgery and the various rooms during the phases of surgery are discussed. The need for an intravenous (IV) and how it will be inserted is explained. Appropriate relaxation skills are introduced at this time. Throughout the session, adolescents are encouraged to ask questions and share their feelings regarding their surgery.

THE DAY OF SURGERY

Transition to the pediatric holding area

Parents and the child are greeted by the pediatric sedation nurse. The parents receive a gown, shoe covers, and hat. Parents accompany their child to the pediatric holding area where a curtain is drawn for privacy so that the child can be assisted into "OR pajamas."

Initial moments within the pediatric holding area are spent adjusting to the new environment. Photographs of the child and his or her family are taken. The child is given the photograph in order to encourage discussion of the day at home and at school.

Nursing measures

Procedural readiness for the child and family is facilitated by the pediatric sedation nurse. The nurse must pay specific attention to the psychosocial needs of the child. The OR staff are integrated as a vital part of procedural care. The overall goals of the pediatric holding area are emphasized:

- Acquire a database on the child's physical and psychological status prior to anesthesia.
- Provide a nonthreatening environment with a familiar face (child life specialist).
- Administer sedation/amnesia drugs to soften the initial moments of OR anesthesia (referred to as induction).

- Involve and support parents' participation in comforting their child.

The pediatric sedation nurse briefly describes the anticipated procedures to parents and child (if developmentally appropriate). These procedures assist the rapid collection of baseline data:

- vital signs
- brief body system review
- preoperative checklists
- ongoing emotional assessment

Physical parameters and nursing assessment are essential to ensuring safe transit through surgery. The nurse's findings assist first-line confirmation that the surgery can be initiated. Essential elements include vital signs within acceptable limits for that child's medical condition, uncongested lung fields, clearance of any prior anesthesia problems including adverse familial history, assurance of empty stomach and urination, laboratory values within acceptable limits for the child's medical condition, complete history of drug or food allergies, identification of loose or "wiggly" teeth, and formal completion of the preoperative checklist for legal documentation of consent and knowledge base.[11]

During this assessment phase, the nurse pays attention to the family member who shows objective signs of anxiety or increased concern. While the nurse is assessing the child, appropriate diversional activities are provided to help reduce the child's and family's anxiety. Once the assessment is completed, the events that will occur in the OR are reviewed with the child.

Ongoing emotional support is a team responsibility and priority inclusive of the pediatric sedation nurse and the child life specialist, anesthesia, OR, and PACU staffs.

Sedation phase

Sedation is performed for children ages 10 months and older. Dosages are calculated according to the child's body weight obtained in preadmission and consideration for the length of surgical procedure. A frequent route involves instillation of nose drops, although other routes may be utilized based on the anesthesiologist's preference. The family and child receive intense emotional support, detailed explanation of the sedation process, and safety instructions. Environmental elements emphasize a calm, quiet atmosphere. Once sedation is given, the lights in the room are dimmed and a soothing videotape is placed in the VCR.

Nursing measures during the sedation phase also concentrate on reassessment of vital signs, respiratory effort, and general physical status. Before transfer to the OR, the OR nurse and anesthesia staff introduce themselves to the child and family, and answer any last-minute questions.

Transition to the operating room

The child is then transferred to the OR suite while the parents remain in the pediatric holding area. OR and anesthesia staff provide simple, developmentally appropriate explanations while attaching the necessary monitoring equipment (ie, "house for your finger," seat belt, Band-Aid/stickers).

Parental orientation to postoperative care

Parents are initially given the opportunity to adjust to the actual separation from their child. The pediatric holding area remains the physical space for this phase of care.

A critical element of postoperative care is explanation of the child's physical appearance and anticipated equipment and procedures within the "wake-up room" (PACU). Parents are prepared to visually experience a pale child who is connected to a cardiac monitor and oxygen assistance. Children emerging from anesthesia often exhibit restlessness and "fretful" disorientation.[10,12] Parents are cautioned that they may hear their child's awakening cry on entrance to the wake-up room as part of the initial arousal period.

A nursing database is then obtained for children who will require admission to the Pediatric

Unit. A brief orientation to the Pediatric Unit is provided. Parents are physically escorted to the same-day surgery waiting area. Space within the pediatric holding area can support two families awaiting the surgery process at one time.

Wake-up room (PACU)

All pediatric patients are recovered in the same-day surgery "wake-up room" because this recovery room allows visitors. Early visitation of the child by the significant family member(s) supports literature findings of reduced stress surrounding the surgery experience.[8,10] Both the child and the parents experience abandonment until reunion in the recovery area. Parents need to see with their own eyes that the child "has made it through surgery and is okay." This early visitation would not be possible without prior preparation. The monitoring equipment, IV, and oxygen are familiar to the child and family when they arrive in the wake-up room. Goals to be achieved in the wake-up room include the following:

- Involve and assist parents in comforting their child.
- Keep child safe.
- Keep child as free from pain as possible.

Once the child is able to respond verbally or open his or her eyes, the parent or guardian is allowed to stay at the child's bedside. Parents are encouraged to touch and talk to the child. Once the child becomes reactive to the room and staff, the parents may hold the child while seated in a chair or rocker. During this awakening phase or emergence from anesthesia the child may cry, kick, hit, and not recognize his or her family. Families are prepared for this behavior and state they would prefer to be present in the wake-up room as a source of comfort. In addition to continuing postoperative teaching, parents are responsive to the comfort, attention, and supportive care administered to their child.

The actual emergence phase lasts a brief period until the disorientation resolves. Parents may become faint on a very rare occasion. Visitors receive a close observation for pallor, upon which a brief break from the immediate recovery area is provided inclusive of cold beverage and the opportunity to lie down in a lounge area. These measures allow a more sensitive visitor to return to the bedside.

The use of pain management during the OR procedure and during the recovery phase has also contributed to establishing an almost tearless environment for the child. Common pain relief drugs are as simple as acetaminophen (Tylenol), possibly with codeine. Nurses must observe the child for signs of pain, such as crying beyond emergence, irritability, clenched fists, or curling of the toes. A short-acting class drug called sublimaze (Fentanyl) is useful for pediatric pain management and may be administered in the OR suite.

Once the disorientation, delirium, and trashing behaviors cease, the child is allowed to express anger at being in a situation out of his or her control. Recognition of the painful separation from family and daily routine is expressed. Diversional activities continue when the child is interested. Toys, television, puzzles, bubbles, or very often the interest established in the pediatric holding area are offered. Bravery stickers are given with the child's name as a reward for maintenance of IV lines and participation in procedures. Physical care includes establishing oral intake such as popsicles and other fluids. The child's choice of popsicle flavor is often much anticipated, only second to the request for "Mom"!

Education of the family continues as does all prior detail of nursing assessment from head to toe, with particular attention to the level of arousal. The child usually plays and smiles after pain and disorientation have resolved. Average watchful time in the wake-up room is approximately 1½ hours with assurance of retained fluids and lack of nausea. All same-day surgery patients who return home after recovery discharge receive a follow-up call the next day. Children who remain in-house for an overnight hospital stay are discharged to their room on the Pediatric Unit within 1 hour. The pediatric sedation nurse provides either immediate or next-day follow-up care by actual visitation to the child's hospital room.

•   •   •

Shore Memorial Hospital has devised a pediatric perioperative program that contains the philosophy of family-centered care and the intervention approach of stress-point preparation. Each phase of pediatric surgery care is integrated to provide continuity in specially designed physical and emotional environments. Preoperative teaching, the pediatric holding area, OR induction, wake-up room, and postoperative components comprise a flow of the most advanced and developmentally supportive approaches for children. One parent's perspective best summarizes Shore Memorial Hospital's efforts:

> For too long the medical community has attended solely to the physical well-being of the patient. Thank you for stepping out of the "dark ages" and focusing on emotional support and preparation and parental involvement. We credit your program and those talented and dedicated folks for implementing it and transforming a potentially scary, painful, and lonely experience to one of informed calm, with friendly, familiar faces. We will continue to brag about this wonderful program and hope for its continual support and expansion.

REFERENCES

1. Vernon DTA, Foley JM, Sipowicz RR, Schulman JL. *The Psychological Responses of Children to Hospitalization and Illness.* Springfield, Ill: Charles C Thomas; 1965.

2. Mahaffy PR. The effects of hospitalization on children admitted for tonsillectomy and adenoidectomy. *Nursing Research.* 1965;14:12.

3. Skipper JK, Leonard RC, Rhymes J. Child hospitalization and social interaction: An experimental study of mother's feelings of stress, adaptation and satisfaction. *Medical Care*. 1968;6:496.

4. Visintainer MA, Wolfer JA. Psychological preparation for surgical pediatric patients: The effect on children's and parent's stress responses and adjustment. *Pediatrics*. 1975;56:187–202.

5. Gatch G. Caring for children needing anesthesia. *Association of Operating Room Nurses Journal*. 1982;35:219–226.

6. Mayhew JF. Parents in the recovery room. (Editorial). *Anesthesia Analogs*. 1983;62(1):124.

7. Dew TA, Bushong ME, Crumrine RS. Parents in pediatric RR. *Association of Operating Room Nurses Journal*. 1977;26:266–273.

8. Diniaco MJ, Ingoldsby BB. Parental presence in the recovery room. *Association of Operating Room Nurses Journal*. 1983;38:685–693.

9. Berry FA, ed. Unique challenges in pediatric anesthesia. *Anesthesia Management of Difficult and Routine Pediatric Patients*. New York, NY: Churchill Livingstone; 1990.

10. Kline J. Recovery room care for the child in pain. *American Journal of Maternal-Child Nursing*. 1984;9:261–264.

11. Cote CJ, Todres ID, Ryan JF. The preoperative evaluation of pediatric patients. In: Ryan JF, et al, eds. *A Practice of Anesthesia for Infants and Children*. New York, NY: Grune & Stratton; 1986.

12. Drain CB, Shipley SB. *The Recovery Room*. Philadelphia, Pa: WB Saunders; 1979.

SELECTED READINGS

Bates TA, Broome M. Preparation of children for hospitalization and surgery: A review of the literature. *Journal of Pediatric Nursing*. 1986;(4):230–239.

Byers ML. Same day surgery: A pre-schooler's experience. *Maternal-Child Nursing Journal*. 1987;16(3):277–282.

Crocker E. Preparation for elective surgery: Does it make a difference? *Journal for the Association for the Care of Children's Health*. 1980;9(1):3–11.

Ferguson BF. Preparing young children for hospitalization: A comparison of two methods. *Pediatrics*. 1979;65:656–664.

Korsch BM. The child and the operating room. *Anesthesiology*. 1975;43:251–257.

McClintic J. Preoperative care of the pediatric patient. *Today's OR Nurse*. 1980;2:7–10.

Niall CTW, Leigh J, Rosen DR, Pandit UA. Preanesthetic sedation of preschool children using intranasal midazolam. *Anesthesiology*. 1988;69:972–975.

Perin G, Frase D. Development of a program using general anesthesia for invasive procedures in a pediatric outpatient setting. *Journal of the Association of Pediatric Oncological Nurses*. 1985;2(4):8–10.

Petrillo M, Sanger S. *Emotional Care of the Hospitalized Child*. Philadelphia, Pa: Lippincott; 1980.

Healing Through Integration: Promoting Wellness in Cardiac Rehabilitation

Cynthia Jean Medich, PhD, RN
Clinical Director
Affiliate Programs
Faculty and Scientist
The Mind/Body Medical Institute
Beth Israel Deaconess Medical Center and
*   Harvard Medical School*

Eileen Stuart, MS, RN, C
Project Director, CAD Reversal Project
The Mind/Body Medical Institute
Beth Israel Deaconess Medical Center and
*   Harvard Medical School*
Boston, Massachusetts

Susan K. Chase, EdD, RN
Assistant Professor
Boston College
Graduate School of Nursing
Chestnut Hill, Massachusetts

Clinical trials have demonstrated that aggressive risk factor reduction through behavioral and lifestyle change, with and without lipid-lowering medications, can result in the regression of atherosclerotic lesions.[1–7] However, efforts to sustain needed lifestyle changes remain a challenge.[8] Risk factor reduction programs are limited by poor patient adherence to dietary modifications including cholesterol and weight control management,[9] hypertension management,[10] physical activity regimens,[11–13] and smoking cessation.[14,15]

Motivational models have provided a structure for clinicians and researchers to observe and predict biopsychosocial and behavioral determinates of health-related behavioral change.[16–25] These models have failed, however, to advance understanding of the processes inherent in sustained behavioral change or the personal meaning of health behavior change to the individual.[8,26,27] Thus, models of care may not adequately support those processes through which recovery and repatterning of behavior occur following diagnosed coronary artery disease (CAD).

Brownell,[9,28] Lincoln and Guba,[29] and Sandelowski[30] suggest that the best way to learn about the synergistic influences of all aspects of the person and the natural environment on behavioral change

The authors thank Dorothy A. Jones, PhD, RN, Carol L. Mandle, PhD, RN, Aggie Casey, MS, RN, Jim Huddleston, MS, PT, Judy Palken, MS, RD, and Jane Hayward, BA (graphic artist) for their support.

Source: Reprinted from C.J. Medich, E. Stuart, S. Chase, *The Journal of Cardiovascular Nursing,* Vol. 11, No. 3, pp. 66–79, © 1997, Aspen Publishers, Inc.

efforts is through a qualitative approach, where the experiences and perspectives of the patients themselves form the understanding. Thus, the acknowledgment of individual motivational responses that influence the repatterning of health behavior throughout the recovery process may enable the development of rehabilitative interventions that increase motivation toward and participation in cardiovascular risk-reduction efforts.[31]

This article provides a synopsis of the lived experience of one woman with diagnosed CAD who participated in an innovative program of cardiac rehabilitation. The data presented are part of a larger study that was designed to explore and describe the basic life processes, transitions, and meanings of adult patients with CAD who were participating in an outpatient cardiac rehabilitation program.[32]

METHODS

Phenomenologic methods were used to explore and describe the basic life processes, transitions, and meanings experienced by 16 adult patients with diagnosed CAD who participated in an innovative outpatient program of cardiac rehabilitation.[32] Data gathering and analysis were accomplished using the steps outlined by Spiegelberg[33,34] and van Manen.[35] Standards of rigor were upheld using four major criteria outlined by Lincoln and Guba:[29] truth value, applicability, consistency, and neutrality.

As described in this case study, Mary was interviewed 65 days after discharge from the formal, monitored cardiac rehabilitation program. Listed below are some of the questions that were asked by this investigator during a 1-hour audiotaped interview:

- Describe for me what it has been like for you to live with the diagnosis of CAD.
- Have you had to change any of your behaviors?
- What has affected your ability or inability to make lifestyle change(s)?
- Describe what healing means to you.
- Was there anything in the cardiac rehabilitation program that affected your healing?

The case study presented provides a synopsis of the lived experience of one study participant and is used to illustrate the process of healing through integration. Detailed descriptions of the concepts and the relationships among concepts that make up the structure are provided.

MARY'S STORY: A MODEL CASE OF THE PROCESS OF HEALING THROUGH INTEGRATION

Clinical history

Mary's history was obtained from her medical record so the nature of her cardiac health status and functional capacity could be understood from the perspective of both the health care team and the patient. Mary, a 65-year-old white female with a history of silent myocardial infarction (MI) noted on routine electrocardiography (ECG), arrived at the emergency department on July 11 with sudden onset of stabbing left chest pain radiating to the left scapular area. Chest pain was associated with nausea, diaphoresis, and weakness that lasted 20 minutes.

Mary sustained an anteroseptal MI and was treated with a thrombolytic agent. One hour after tissue plasminogen activator (TPA) infusion, she exhibited accelerated idioventricular rhythm but remained hemodynamically stable. No evidence was found of early reperfusion. A cardiac catheterization on July 14 revealed a 90% proximal left anterior descending (LAD) artery stenosis, 80% first obtuse marginal stenosis, and 90% nondominant right coronary artery stenosis. Comorbidities included diabetes, retinopathy, thalassemia B anemia, and a history of hiatal hernia and cholelithiasis.

Mary's hospital course was complicated by episodic chest pain treated successfully with percutaneous transluminal coronary angioplasty (PTCA) of the LAD on July 16. An echocardiogram demonstrated a decreased left ventricular ejection fraction of 35% to 45%. Mary expressed an interest in participating in cardiac rehabilitation for support. She was discharged on July 20 with a friend, a registered nurse, who initially stayed with her.

Personal motivation and goals for cardiac rehabilitation

Mary enrolled in cardiac rehabilitation approximately 4 weeks after hospital discharge with the goal "to heal and return to a normal healthy lifestyle." According to Mary, her motivation for participating in cardiac rehabilitation was to regain her heart health, schedule an exercise regimen, and learn to cope with loss. Mary completed the full course of cardiac rehabilitation and embraced the concepts of modifying her lifestyle and behaviors. At the time of her discharge from cardiac rehabilitation, Mary adhered to the following lifestyle behaviors:

- Eating a low-fat (25 fat grams/day), no added-salt, low-sugar, reduced-caffeine diet.
- Walking and/or biking four times per week for 30 minutes to 1 hour.
- Eliciting the relaxation response daily through meditation.
- Performing "mini" relaxation exercises several times per day to relieve mind and body tension, and
- Using cognitive therapy to reframe thought-generating stressors and control her actions.

HEALING THROUGH INTEGRATION

A central theme, integration, emerged from the data to explain healing and engagement in behaviors that promote recovery after diagnosed CAD. Healing reflects "movement toward wholeness or to make whole on all levels—physical, mental, emotional, social, and spiritual."[36] Through healing individuals may negotiate personal transitions and move toward new levels of self-organization and personal growth after a cardiac event.[31,32,37]

Integration reflects the process of bringing together some complex internal and external human responses with past and present biologic, psychologic, social, spiritual, and behavioral experiences for the individual to achieve new life meaning, growth, and development. This process includes an assimilation of the experience

of living with CAD into a meaningful personal perspective and requires a clarification of one's relationship to self, others, and the environment. Integration manifests itself as the essential factor for healing and engagement in behaviors that promote well-being and recovery. Figure 1 illustrates the critical attributes of the central theme of integration: the experience of vulnerability, awareness, and responding, as well as context within which integration occurs. The process of integration is enhanced by eliciting the relaxation response, healing awareness, and social support. Although the process includes movement in stages, integration is not conceptualized as a linear progression. Rather, integration reflects a process of individual questioning, patterning, feedback, and repatterning that creates personal transformation, strength, and balance over time.[31,32,37]

THE CONTEXT FOR HEALING THROUGH INTEGRATION

The context within which integration occurs determines its essential properties. A context for recovery includes personal experiences that occur both before and after a cardiac health crisis and determine the meaning of the event. For Mary the context for healing through integration included her unique history and the experience of a cardiac health crisis.

Unique history

A *unique history* includes past and present biologic, psychologic, social, spiritual, and behavioral experiences that reflect underlying life patterns. These experiences occur within the context of ongoing person–environment interactions and play a role in determining one's relationship to self, others, and the environment. This relationship in turn influences the meaning given to a cardiac health crisis and directions for repatterning. A unique history is illustrated in Figure 1 by an inner and outer circle depicting continuous person–environment interactions. For Mary, a unique

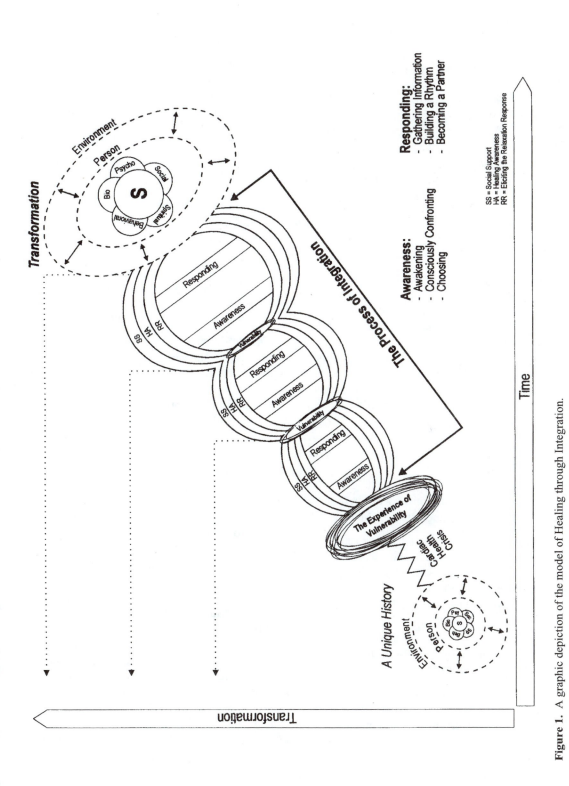

Figure 1. A graphic depiction of the model of Healing through Integration.

history included an enormous amount of stress and strain. She stated:

> At the time of the attack I was actually helping two brothers who unfortunately died within 6 months' time and I had to run the family business which I did not like. I had too much stress. I had the heart attack on July 11th and Joseph died on the 12th and I was in the hospital for 10 days. When I came out, it was business as usual 'cause I still had a daily business to take care of.

Cardiac health crisis

The *cardiac health crisis* represents a multifaceted disruption of the parts of oneself as whole, healthy, and predictable. This crisis is a crucial time and/or event where there is a perceived decline in one's cardiac health status. Thus, a cardiac health crisis forces a person to confront basic assumptions and beliefs about the self and the possibility of death. Old patterns and behaviors are no longer adequate and lead to disorder and degrees of dysfunction in the biologic, psychologic, social, spiritual, and behavioral domains. A cardiac health crisis is graphically represented as a jagged line in Figure 1.

The cardiac health crisis came as little surprise to Mary, given her family history of CAD and a series of stressful life circumstances. Mary stated:

> We were in the gourmet fruit basket business and in 3 weeks you send out 10,000 baskets. So it's not even manageable. So I had the business to contend with and he [her brother] was in a hospital that was about 30 minutes away. I knew something had to break. I didn't think about what it was going to be but I knew something would break.

Mary's state of mind at the time of her heart attack also influenced the meaning she gave to the event. She had lost two brothers and assumed leadership of a stressful family business that she viewed with some ambivalence. This situation

contributed to her sense of relief and acceptance when the heart attack occurred. Mary stated:

> When it happened and I was going to the hospital, took us only 15 minutes to get here . . . the thought came through my mind that, you know Mary, you've been a loner all your life and here you are having a heart attack and you're having it alone but what crossed my mind was . . . well I'm 64 going to be 65. I had three careers. I've outlived two husbands and two doctors. You know, if it had to happen, this was a fine time. You know even if it was the end, I wasn't frightened. I had done everything. And I think I personally was exhausted because of all the illnesses in the family and all the stress I had to go through.

During the initial crisis of the cardiac event, Mary resigned herself to the possibility of death. Once it became apparent that she was going to survive, her energy for life began to rekindle. She stated, "I've learned to look forward to living, not that I was anxious to die, but I was at an acceptance stage."

THE EXPERIENCE OF VULNERABILITY

The experience of vulnerability is a human response to the cardiac health crisis and events associated with the illness experience. Feeling vulnerable is unique for each person, with varying degrees of perceived threat to physical, intra- and/or interpersonal well-being. Vulnerability is both a process and a state of being in which an individual perceives a threat to self-definition and feels unable to cope with the threat. When the degree of threat is sufficient to stimulate the need or desire to change, an opportunity is created to facilitate individual growth and development. Vulnerability is illustrated by the chaotic spheres along the spiral of integration in Figure 1. The experience of vulnerability for Mary was marked by information specifying the nature of her cardiac event. She was shocked by the extent of heart damage and stated:

> I think she [the clinical nurse specialist] saved my life because I felt good when I got out of the hospital and I was under the impression I'd had a mild heart attack, very, very mild heart attack. And when she gave me the facts of life it was a shocker but that's when I knew I had to do something about it.

Some degree of perceived vulnerability is an essential condition for integration to occur. Because vulnerability creates a disruption in one's reality, it forces one to find meaning in the illness experience and to repattern behavior. Becoming aware of the reality of what happened left Mary feeling uncertain about her prognosis and her physical limits and boundaries. This uncertainty contributed to Mary's perception of physical vulnerability. She remarked, "Up until a particular time after a heart attack it feels as though you're walking on eggs. You don't know what's going to happen so you're very cautious about everything." She went on to say, "It's the uncertainty you know. . . . Am I going to have another heart attack? See, I had ischemia which had no warnings, so that could happen again."

Mary also experienced intrapersonal vulnerability because of a perceived loss of control and a decreased ability to cope with the threat of the cardiac event. Mary experienced a change in how she viewed herself, her identity, and her role within relationships as a result of her CAD diagnosis. Mary spoke of this vulnerability when she said; "I guess when you have a heart attack, your self-confidence is a bit shattered because you don't have the control for yourself that's been built up."

THE PROCESS OF HEALING THROUGH INTEGRATION: AWARENESS AND RESPONDING

The process of healing through integration is conceptualized as a human response to the cardiac health crisis and the concomitant experience of vulnerability. Through integration, a greater sense of control, order, and harmony is restored within the biologic, psychologic, social, spiritual and behavioral domains, and human potential may be enhanced. The process of integration includes the components of awareness and responding. Integration components are depicted by the bars within the ascending and expanding spiral of integration in Figure 1 and indicate achievement of deeper levels of integration.

Awareness

Awareness reflects a conscious awakening to the nature of the cardiac event and is characterized by a search for meaning and choice of direction for the repatterning of lifestyle. When creating new meaning, individuals begin to explore and redefine their relationship to self, others, and the environment.

Mary's awareness of her cardiac illness began in response to perceived physical and intrapersonal vulnerability. Not only had she awakened to "what is," but she also consciously confronted the nature of her illness by questioning "what does it mean to me?" and chose to alter her lifestyle. Mary stated:

> When I had the heart attack I questioned whether I could use the same philosophy . . . can the heart attack live my way of life? And I had to say, no it couldn't because I was always on the fast track. So I knew I had to adjust to heal. And at that point I guess it's not that I didn't want to live before. I was accepting death but now I guess I felt, well, gee, maybe I have a few more good years left. Maybe I'd better make the best of it. So I was very careful in everything I did.

Mary's ability to accept the implications of her illness on her work status involved clarifying values. Mary became in touch with her most basic values by clarifying them. These values included the need to make a contribution and to be happy. In this context she realized that she needed to focus more on caring for herself; business and professional accomplishments were recognized as secondary to her basic core values. Mary stated:

> Well I've always done for others. I've always worked very diligently for my own companies. And I said to myself, maybe it's time to put Mary first . . . and I never did in my life. Maybe there is something to this retirement, traveling, and things of that sort. I did all of my traveling when I was much younger. So, I was kind of looking forward to doing something different.

By letting go of the burden and responsibility associated with her past life, particularly the stress associated with working, Mary moved toward an increased sense of wellness early in her recovery. She commented, "I guess I changed my thinking about retirement and said, well, I'll go and play like other people."

By awakening to the reality of her health status and consciously confronting the meaning of the illness experience, Mary recognized the need to change her life. As she clarified her basic values, she redefined retirement as a continuation of life with changes. She stated:

> I had to slow down. I never thought I would use the word retire but I will be turning 65 now. I'll be 65 in February and I'm seriously thinking toward the retirement area, but I never did before because I think that's when your brain gets idle. But I'm having second thoughts.

Through awareness Mary created a lifestyle that supported health and healing. Mary resumed certain health-enhancing behaviors such as meditating daily and altering unhealthy behaviors. As patients awaken to "what happened," and begin to understand the implications of the cardiac health crisis, they begin to feel more in control of the uncertainties surrounding their illness. Deeper levels of awakening to "what is" unfold as meaning is assigned and patients strengthen their ability to make consistent, self-directed behavioral choices for disease management and risk modification. As Mary continued to gain awareness about the nature of her illness, her understanding of what a healthy lifestyle meant with CAD became more clear.

Responding

Responding involves the acquisition, refinement, and mastery of biologic, psychologic, social, spiritual, and behavioral skills needed for self-management of illness and recovery. Responding includes gathering information, building a rhythm of new behaviors into one's life, and becoming an active participant in recovery.

For Mary, responding involved gathering information about certain relevant behaviors and specific skills needed to manage her illness. Information was gathered to understand what is needed to modify risk factors and build skill in behavioral change. Mary said:

> If I had not come here I probably would have been afraid to do the exercise because to me if you had a heart attack and then you exercise, are you promoting another heart attack? When in fact now I know you're opening up your arteries and you're helping your heart.

Building a rhythm of new behaviors into life involves a difficult process of forming habits and integrating new behaviors into a daily routine. Health care providers help in building new behaviors by assisting patients to acquire new skills and form habits. Mary stated:

> I guess she [the clinical nurse specialist] made the biggest impression on me. She got us to go on diets, to exercise, to write down everything we did during the day, to keep a chart of our nutrition . . . that was hard for business to find the time to do, but I never saw anyone neglect that. And after twelve weeks, you become in the habit of doing that.

Mary referred to the importance of being exposed to the health-enhancing behaviors in a consistent, integrated fashion to build new behaviors into her lifestyle. She stated, "I think it is because it's a whole structure that takes in everything you need—your nutrition, your exercise, your meditation—and it becomes part of your life. It's an integral part of your life like eating and sleeping. You just do it."

Building a rhythm of new behaviors included testing the limits and boundaries of the new behaviors by allowing for flexibility in carrying out the behavior. Although Mary had integrated certain behaviors into her lifestyle, she recognized that she may lapse or intentionally engage in old behavioral patterns. She said, "I know with having been diabetic for so long that you can't be good all the time, I mean it's not humanly possible."

To prevent relapse Mary allowed for some behavioral flexibility in her diet by building lapses into her routine. This flexibility let her test the limits and boundaries of the new behaviors in a more controlled manner. She said, "I know that if I wanted to go out every night and eat out and live the high life that we do when we're in business, I'd be just asking for trouble. So I allow myself maybe one dinner out a week."

The negative feedback experienced with relapse provided important information and helped reestablish intended goals for self-management. Mary said,"You do get off track once in a while but then you don't feel good so you go right back on if you want to stay well."

Finding ease, confidence, or pleasure in new behaviors consistently supported the new habits in Mary's life. She stated:

> I had been on a fat-free diet anyway but when I came here to cardiac rehab, they reinforced the fat-free, low-fat diet, they reinforced the exercise. I had done transcendental meditation maybe for 25 years but unfortunately didn't think to do it when I needed it the most during the stressful time, so I got back in the habit of doing my meditation. So I

found it all easy enough to do because it wasn't new to me.

Becoming an active partner in care required mastering self-regulation in the management of CAD. As self-regulation is mastered, a gradual decrease is seen in the need for instrumental support from others; patients begin to function more independently in initiating behavioral change. Mary stated, "Well, I think they made such a lasting impression on me that I do it automatically."

ENHANCERS OF THE PROCESS OF HEALING THROUGH INTEGRATION

Three experiences were found to enhance or support the process of integration: social support, healing awareness, and eliciting the relaxation response. These concepts are indicated by the three circles encasing each section of the spiral integration in Figure 1.

Social support

Mary's process of integration was enhanced by the *social support* received during rehabilitation. Social support is the experience of giving and/or receiving information, feedback, and encouragement; and/or demonstrations of caring by family, friends, or health care professionals. Through this support, Mary confronted and managed her illness while maintaining her commitment toward risk modification and recovery. This support promoted a sense of certainty about her prognosis and helped foster a sense of personal balance. Mary said, "You don't know what's going to happen. I use that expression, you're walking on eggs . . . you could have a heart attack at any time. They gave me the confidence that . . . do your exercise, stay on your diet, get all your tests back to normal, that you have a good chance."

By sharing personal issues surrounding the nature of her illness with other participants in rehabilitation, Mary reached out and connected with others for the first time. She considered this important for her healing as well as for the healing of others in the program. Mary stated:

> I never tell anyone about my problems, so to speak. Always been a leader. But even with the heart attack, I didn't tell anyone. The only ones I allowed in the hospital were my brother, my accountant, my lawyer. It [the cardiac rehab program] is probably the first time that I talked about personal things to other people.

She continued, "I just felt it was part of the healing process. I think we all learned something from each one [other]."

Healing awareness

Healing awareness was described as the recognition of improvement in biologic, psychologic, social, spiritual, and behavioral domains. Healing awareness helped Mary to awaken and consciously confront the events surrounding her cardiac event that helped her to cope more effectively with the fear and threat associated with a CAD diagnosis. Choosing to respond differently to life through behavioral and lifestyle changes was enhanced through healing awareness by allowing Mary to acknowledge improvement in physical and psychologic well-being over time. Mary said, "I wasn't lethargic or tired all the time. The pulling sensation over my heart was going away. I was beginning to enjoy life more. I could see the progress . . . I can honestly say, I could feel the heart healing process all the way through the program."

Eliciting the relaxation response

The relaxation response is a physiologic state of deep rest that results in quieting of the mind and body. The relaxation enhances one's ability to reflect in an open, objective manner, and opens the mind and heart to the possibilities in recovery. According to Mary,"I think it [relaxation response] awakens reality and

gives you more creative ideas." She went on to say; "It's [relaxation response] kept me in a good disposition. It's strange to say but I think it's empowered my mind to clearer thinking and better decisions."

As Mary incorporated meditation back into her life, she became realigned with a core philosophy of living that included a growing spirituality. According to Mary, "I've experienced out-of-body type of meditation, complete relaxation. I used to use the expression, when I was on top of the mountain, that was the closest I'd ever get to heaven, but in the meditation you do feel very close to, I'd like to say a deity."

TRANSFORMATION: THE OUTCOME OF THE PROCESS OF HEALING THROUGH INTEGRATION

Transformation occurs as part of the context of healing through integration and reflects a new state of being that transcends the preillness state across some or all of the biologic, psychologic, social, spiritual, and/or behavioral domains. Transformation is the primary outcome of the process of integration and represents an expansion of consciousness with new ways of seeing, being, and responding. Transformation also reflects personal balance or a greater sense of control, order, and harmony within one's life as perceptions of vulnerability decrease. Transformation is represented on a continuum as shown in the vertical axis in Figure 1. Dotted lines connect the integration spiral to the vertical axis and represent low to high levels of transformation.

The most visible feature of transformation in Mary's recovery was her positive, upbeat attitude. She also acknowledged the influence of a lifelong attitude about the interaction of mind and body and their role in guiding recovery when she said, "I've always felt that the mind could heal the body and I always knew that a positive attitude could heal the body also." Mary's ability to integrate past and present strengths consciously with the nature of her current illness allowed her to transform her life toward a newfound sense of wholeness. This expansion of consciousness with a movement toward being instead of doing was evident when Mary stated:

> It may seem strange after being off in the fast lane . . . I enjoy getting up late. I have breakfast at 9, watch the birds, listen to my music, read the paper. It's 2 hours. I never had that time in my life to do the simple things: take a walk in the woods, all these things that are very pleasurable, but when you're a working person you're up and out at 7 in the morning. It's dark when you get home . . . You don't do these little things. So I find that very pleasurable.

Although Mary had always been self-directed, she was now able to accept direction from others to find new ways to make decisions that were self-authorizing in an effort to bring about better health. Mary stated, "I've never taken orders before. This was a very new experience for me. I've always given orders. I figured I was coming to the course, I had to play the game according to their rules. And I said, 12 weeks . . . if it's going to help me, that's great."

• • •

This case illustrates the processes, transitions, and meanings that Mary experienced as she recovered from her cardiac health crisis and learned to live with diagnosed CAD from a newfound place of wellness. The case presented proposes a view of recovery after a cardiac health crisis that incorporates the potential for healing, growth and change. The data generated support for the findings of Johnson and Morse,[38] Keller,[39] Bartz,[40] and Fleury,[31,37] that emphasize individual recovery after a cardiac event as a process that incorporates struggle through vulnerability, personal loss, the repatterning of valued activities, and the rediscovery of personal strength.

Healing through integration occurred for Mary as an emerging process that included personal movement toward biologic, psychologic, social, and spiritual wholeness. Through healing, Mary negotiated personal transitions and moved toward new levels of personal growth after the cardiac event.[31,32,37] This process includes assimilating the experience of living with CAD into a meaningful, personal perspective and requires clarification of one's relationship to self, others, and the environment.

Nursing's way of understanding a patient has traditionally come from assessment approaches that do not necessarily reflect holistic understandings. Instead, assessment tools and the nature of history taking create a view of individuals as body systems and assume that the whole is understood. Although an assessment tool may guide the cardiovascular clinician in eliciting more specific and thorough information, the questions asked and the way that data are interpreted are structured by the clinician's perspective rather than the patient's. A limited view of the person may result, with an incomplete understanding of the life patterns, realities, values, and meanings that contribute to current definitions of self that ultimately guide repatterning efforts after a cardiac event.

The conceptualization of healing through integration proposed in this case provides a basis for cardiovascular nursing assessment and the implementation of relevant mind, body, social, spiritual, and behavioral interventions designed to promote wellness. Cardiovascular nurses working with individuals seeking to initiate and sustain lifestyle changes have a unique role in facilitating repatterning and healing.

Findings from this case study emphasize the need for clinicians to include narrative descriptions of the patient's illness experience as part of setting rehabilitation goals and strategies for recovery. The potential to understand the life processes, meanings, and transitions inherent in human responses to a cardiac health crisis may be increased by asking the patient questions during the cardiac rehabilitation intake evaluation such as, "Describe for me what it has been like for you to live with the diagnosis of CAD." Through listening to individuals' stories, cardiovascular nurses can learn what resources are needed—physically, intrapersonally, and environmentally—so that a realistic basis for mutual problem solving can be established.[41]

Patient's perception that a worsening in cardiac health status has occurred. In this way, patients' perceptions hold value in determining changes in health status and are a valid indicator of overall health and adaptation. An assessment of perceived vulnerability at points along the illness trajectory may become a guide for clinical intervention. Because vulnerability creates a disruption in one's reality, it forces one to search for meaning in the illness experience and to evaluate the worth of previous behavior patterns.[31,32,37] If degrees of vulnerability are too low or too high after a cardiac health crisis, the clinician may provide information about CAD and its implications or encourage effective coping mechanisms to facilitate integration.

Throughout integration, Mary clarified her core values, grieved losses, assigned meaning to her illness experience, and chose a direction for repatterning that was consistent with what was important and meaningful to her. This process influenced her commitment to goals and motivated her to learn and sustain those behavioral skills needed for self-management of CAD. Interventions that empower behavioral change may include imparting information necessary for change and self-monitoring of symptoms and progress in achieving behavioral change. Self-monitoring of physical and psychologic symptoms and behavioral change efforts via patient logs is essential in recognizing patterns and the factors that may worsen or improve such patterns. Self-management of symptoms or psychophysiologic self-regulation supports the goal of self-care. Consistent feedback from family, friends, and health care providers that recognizes positive changes can strengthen patients' recognition of the benefits of change and healing awareness. Having access to needed resources such as other patients, social services, psychiatry and psychology, pastoral care, vocational rehabilitation, pharmacy, and dietary counseling is important in an integrative model of cardiac rehabilitation.

Healing and self-management of CAD require an integrated mind, body, social, spiritual, and behavioral model of care with state-of-the-art biomedical therapies. This approach views illness and suffering as a powerful catalyst for changing not only behaviors such as diet and exercise, but also for helping to transform more fundamental determinants of wellness such as values, meanings, and relationships.

REFERENCES

1. Blankenhorn DH, Nessim SA, Johnson RL, et al. Beneficial effects of combined colestipol-niacin therapy on coronary atherosclerosis and coronary venous bypass grafts. *JAMA*. 1987;257:3,233–3,240.

2. Brown GB, Lin TJ, Schaefer SM, et al. Niacin or lovastatin, combined with colestipol, regress coronary atherosclerosis and prevent clinical events in men with elevated apoliprotein B. *Circulation*. 1989;80:II–266.

3. Hambrecht R, Niebauer J, Marburger C. Various intensities of leisure time physical activity in patients with coronary artery disease: effects on cardiorespiratory fitness and progression of coronary atherosclerotic lesions. *J Am Coll Cardiol*. 1993;22:468–477.

4. Haskell W, Alderman E, Fair J. Effects of intensive multiple risk factor reduction on coronary atherosclerosis and clinical cardiac events in men and women with coronary artery disease: the Stanford Coronary Risk Intervention Project (SCRIP). *Circulation*. 1994;89:975–990.

5. Ornish D. Can lifestyle changes reverse coronary heart disease? *Lancet*. 1990; 336:129–132.

6. Schuler G, Hambrecht R, Schierf G. Myocardial perfusion and regression of coronary artery disease in patients on a regimen of intensive physical exercise and low-fat diet. *J Am Coll Cardiol*. 1992;19:34–42.

7. The Simvastin Trial. Effect of simvastatin on coronary atheroma: the Multicentre Anti–Atheroma Study (MAAS). *Lancet*. 1994;344:633–638.

8. Fleury J. The application of motivational theory to cardiovascular risk reduction. *Image*. 1992;24(3):229–239.

9. Brownell KD, Marlatt GA, Lichenstein E, Wilson GT. Understanding and preventing relapse. *Am Psychol*. 1986;41(7):765–782.

10. Kinsey MG, Fletcher BJ, Rice CR, et al. Coronary risk factor modification followed by home-monitored exercise in coronary bypass surgery patients: a four year follow-up study. *J Cardiopulm Rehabil.* 1989; 9:207–212.

11. Ice R. Long-term compliance. *Phys Ther.* 1985;65(12): 1,832–1,840.

12. Oldridge NB, Spencer J. Exercise habits and perceptions before and after graduating or dropout from supervised cardiac rehabilitation. *J Cardiopulm Rehabil.* 1985; 5(7):313–320.

13. Fontana AF, Kearns RD, Rosenberg RL, et al. Exercise training for cardiac patients: adherence, fitness and benefits. *J Cardiopulm Rehabil.* 1986;6:334–357.

14. Godin G. The effectiveness of interventions in modifying behavioral risk factors of individuals with coronary heart disease. *J Cardiopulm Rehabil.* 1989;9:223–236.

15. Curry S, Marlatt GA, Gordon JR. Abstinence violation effect: validation of an attributional construct with smoking cessation. *J Consult Clin Psychol.* 1987; 55(2): 145–149.

16. Lewin K. *Dynamic Theory of Personality.* New York, NY: McGraw-Hill; 1944.

17. Maimen LA, Becker MH. The health belief model: origins and correlates in psychological theory. In: Becker MH, ed. *The Health Belief Model and Personal Health Behavior.* Thorofare, NY: Slack; 1974:9–26.

18. Rosenstock IM. The health belief model and preventive health behavior. *Health Educ Monogr.* 1974;2:354–383.

19. Pender NJ. *Health Promotion in Nursing Practice.* 3rd ed. Norwalk, Conn: Appleton & Lange; 1996.

20. Ajzen I, Timko C. *Attitudes, Perceived Control, and the Prediction of Health Behavior.* Worcester, Mass: University of Massachusetts; 1983.

21. Ajzen I. From intentions to actions: a theory of planned behavior. In: Kuhl J, Beckman J, eds. *Action-Control: From Cognition to Behavior.* Heidelberg, Germany: Springer; 1985:11–39.

22. Wallston KA, Wallston BS, DeVellis BM. Development of the multidimensional health locus of control (MHLC) scales. *Health Educ Monogr.* 1978;6(2):160–170.

23. Bandura A. *Social Foundations of Thought and Action: A Social Cognitive Theory.* Englewood Cliffs, NJ: Prentice-Hall; 1986.

24. Cox CL. An interaction model of client health behavior: theoretical prescription for nursing. *Adv Nurs Sci.* 1982;5:41–56.

25. Prochaska JO, DiClemente CC. Stages and processes of self-change of smoking: toward an integrative model of change. *J Consult Clin Psychol.* 1983;51:390–395.

26. Hilgenberg C, Crowley C. Changes in family patterns after myocardial infarction. *Home Health Nurs.* 1987;5(3):26–35.

27. Parse RR. Man-living-health theory in nursing. In: Parse RR, ed. *Nursing Science: Major Paradigms, Theories and Critiques.* Philadelphia, Pa: WB Saunders; 1987: 159–180.

28. Brownell KD & Wadden T. Etiology and treatment of obesity: understanding a serious, prevalent and refractory disorder. *J Consult Clin Psychol.* 1992;60:505–517.

29. Lincoln Y, Guba E. *Naturalistic Inquiry.* Beverly Hills, Calif: Sage Publications; 1985.

30. Sandelowski M. The problem of rigor in qualitative research. *Adv Nurs Sci.* 1986;8:27–37.

31. Fleury J, Kimbrell C, Kruszewski MA. Life after a cardiac event: women's experience in healing. *Heart Lung.* 1995;24:474–482.

32. Medich CJ. *Healing Through Integration: The Lived Experience of Cardiac Rehabilitation.* Ann Arbor, Mich: UMI Dissertation Information Service; 1995.

33. Spiegelberg H. *The Phenomenological Movement: A Historical Introduction.* The Hague, Netherlands: Martinius Nijhoff; 1975.

34. Spiegelberg H. *The Phenomenological Movement: A Historical Introduction.* 3rd ed. The Hague, Netherlands: Martinius Nijhoff; 1982.

35. van Manen M. *Researching Lived Experience: Human Science for an Action Sensitive Pedagogy.* Canada: Althous Press; 1990.

36. Dossey BM, Keegan L, Guzzetta C, Kolkmeier L. *Holistic Nursing: A Handbook for Practice.* 2nd ed. Rockville, Md: Aspen Publishers; 1995.

37. Fleury J. Empowering potential: a theory of wellness motivation. *Nurs Res.* 1991; 40:286–291.

38. Johnson JL, Morse JM. Regaining control: the process of adjustment after myocardial infarction. *Heart Lung.* 1990;19:126–135.

39. Keller C. Seeking normalcy: the experience of coronary artery bypass surgery. *Res Nurs Health.* 1991;14:173–178.

40. Bartz C. An exploratory study of the coronary artery bypass graft surgery experience. *Heart Lung.* 1988;17: 179–183.

41. Stuart EM. *Regression Project Manual.* Boston: Division of Behavioral Medicine, Beth Israel Deaconess Medical Center; 1995.

Trauma Bereavement Program: Review of Development and Implementation

Harriette L.K. Buchanan, MS, Ed, MS
Counseling
Former Full-Time Volunteer
Trauma Unit
Codeveloper and Past Coordinator
Allegheny General Hospital Trauma
Bereavement Program

Marie D. Geubtner, RN, CCRN
Staff Nurse
Trauma Unit
Coordinator
Allegheny General Hospital Trauma
Bereavement Program

Carolyn Kay Snyder, MSW, LSW
Clinical Social Worker
Trauma Unit
Codeveloper and Supervisor
Allegheny General Hospital Trauma
Bereavement Program
Allegheny General Hospital
Pittsburgh, Pennsylvania

Source: Reprinted from H.L.K. Buchanan, M.D. Geubtner, and C.K. Snyder, *Critical Care Nursing Quarterly,* Vol. 19, No. 1, pp. 35–45, © 1996, Aspen Publishers, Inc.

"I just walked in the door. I was at the cemetery. It was the first time that I have been to my brother's grave." These were the first words that John, age 22, spoke during a telephone consultation made by the trauma bereavement coordinator. John's younger brother, Ron, age 20, died 3 months earlier in the trauma unit while receiving treatment for injuries sustained in a motor vehicle accident. (Patient remarks in this article are taken from the journal of the Trauma Bereavement Program.)

As John continued to talk that day, his pain was still fresh and raw. He said that one of his jobs had been to care for the graves at the cemetery where his brother was buried, but he had given up the job temporarily because he was unable to go there. John felt guilty because he was not with Ron in the automobile accident that claimed Ron's life. He thought he might have saved his brother's life had he been with him. As sons of a single mother, John, as the older brother, had assumed the reponsibility of taking care of Ron throughout their childhood and adolescence. Without denying his guilt or pain, the bereavement coordinator gently suggested to John that realistically he could not always be with his brother. Ron, at the age of 20, was an adult and responsible for his own care, and John stated that he had been trying to encourage that independence. John was experiencing overwhelming grief in response to Ron's death.

When he visited his brother's grave John had taken one small step toward acceptance and healing. The bereavement coordinator's suggestion that he might take another step forward by returning to his job at the cemetery and to continue his love and care for Ron by tending his grave seemed comforting to John. More important, perhaps, was a timely telephone call to Ron's family from a person with listening and grief therapy skills. The call was not serendipitous, but rather, one of many calls made by the trauma bereavement coordinator at Allegheny General Hospital, a Level 1 trauma center. These calls are part of a comprehensive bereavement program.

Ron was just one of the 119,886 people nationwide who died as a result of traumatic injuries, including homicides and suicide, in 1992.[1] In 1994, Allegheny General Hospital treated 2,578 trauma patients, 114 of whom died of their injuries and/or complications (Allegheny General Hospital Trauma Registry, 1994).

From the time a person learns of a traumatic injury or death as a result of such an injury, there is a barrage of reactions, particularly total shock and disbelief. The person is often thrust into a position of rushing to a hospital not knowing whether the loved one is dead or alive. The uncertainty and dread of what will be found is overwhelming. A person usually arrives in a totally distraught and disoriented state. A survivor's reaction after arrival will vary according to the situation and the individual. However, all of these variants and circumstances must be considered by bereavement coordinators as they individualize and personalize the follow-up contacts.

The deaths of trauma patients may be shockingly sudden or may occur after days or weeks in which a family's emotions vacillate between hope and despair. More than one person has described this experience as being on an awful, emotional roller coaster. Unlike a death that occurs after a lingering and debilitating illness, sudden traumatic injury and subsequent death does not allow surviving family members or loved ones to grieve and resolve issues over time. The grieving process is condensed into hours, days, or weeks of intense, unrelenting emotional pain. The dynamics of such an experience have great significance for eventual healing and recovery by surviving family members and loved ones. The Allegheny General Hospital Trauma Bereavement Program is designed to assist families in this process.

PROGRAM DEVELOPMENT

The Allegheny General Hospital Trauma staff has long recognized the need for a follow-up bereavement program for a number of reasons. For example, a family that leaves a trauma unit after a death often feels overwhelmed with the feelings that accompany the loss and the circumstances surrounding the loss. If the survivor's support system is not activated, or if one does not exist, the bereaved person will feel isolated and abandoned. The bereavement program, therefore, was established to continue the support that the staff had provided to the family during the patient's hospitalization and to extend that support to the family during the year following the death.

After several planning sessions involving representatives from the administration, nursing, social work services, and volunteer services departments, the Allegheny General Hospital Trauma Bereavement Program was established in January 1991. Social work has been an integral part of the medical staff since the inception of the trauma unit. Social workers educated at the master's level meet with each family, prepare an in-depth patient and family assessment, and use crisis intervention skills to focus on stabilizing the family. In addition, volunteer services have been an integral part of Allegheny General since the hospital's founding in 1886. The volunteer administrator has recruited and trained volunteers to serve in every hospital department, including the emergency department and the critical care units. Both social work and volunteer services provided valuable components to the development of the program.

From its inception, the administrators of the Allegheny General Hospital Trauma Unit embraced the concept of the project, as proposed by the social worker. Although most facilities are able to provide patients' medical care, the administrators understood that the total care of the patient and family requires much more effort. The trauma unit administrator, in particular, believed in the need for extended bereavement assistance for a family. This administrator was a key figure in the development of the program and also approved the financial support for the program's implementation.

It became apparent that a family, after leaving the trauma unit following the death of a loved one, had not had a sufficient closure. Many families would call the social worker following the death to talk about the patient, to ask questions, and to receive reassurance that everything was done to save the patient's life. On several occasions a family would ask to return to the deceased patient's room in an attempt to relive the death, reexperience the grief, and begin to develop some understanding and resolution of the event. In remembering the event, a family found that many details and facts had been forgotten as a result of the crisis state. Often, a family had forgotten to ask the physician specific questions or could not remember descriptions of procedures or other medical explanations. Some families returned to resolve simpler issues, such as where the patient's room was located, the view from the window, the position of the bed in the room, or what the medical equipment monitored. For some families, to revisit the trauma unit and talk with the trauma staff at a less stressful time provided a measure of closure for the hospital experience.

The concept of the trauma bereavement program originated because the social worker recognized the need for finalization. Using the hospice model, the social worker designed the program to accommodate the grief experience following a sudden, traumatic death. The program had to address the issues of unexpected, ill-prepared-for death, rather than the hospice program, which addresses expected, inevitable death.

The need for extended bereavement services was recognized by the nursing staff. Bonds develop as the staff intellectually, medically, and emotionally care for patients and their families.

Whether holding the hands of family members who are receiving bad news or watching silently as they cry at a patient's bedside and say their final good-bye, staff members often witness the most intimate moments of any human's life. The difficulty in saying good-bye to these devastated families at times was overwhelming to staff members. The insightful ideas and suggestions from nursing assisted the social worker and volunteer as they addressed specific issues. The trauma bereavement program now gives staff members an opportunity to extend their caring as families leaves, and it encourages closure with a feeling of completeness in each case. Staff members also are better prepared for the next difficult trauma death, and possibly, the next loss they may face in their own lives.

Valuable suggestions from the volunteer administrator and volunteers, as well as adaptations of various volunteer models, were incorporated into the present bereavement program. The hospice bereavement coordinator, specifically, provided insight about the use of volunteers in a bereavement program. A volunteer is carefully placed and supervised in the trauma setting to maximize specific and individual experiences and skills. Use of volunteers has proven to be a valuable asset in the waiting room where families are greeted and made as comfortable as possible. Families often need directions to different hospital departments, to the cafeteria, and to other hospital facilities. Some simple comfort measures such as water, coffee, pillows, and blankets can be provided by the volunteer. A volunteer with appropriate credentials and experience may be trained to actively assist the bereavement coordinator with some program aspects, such as researching literature, compiling resource material, and record keeping. Other duties might be assigned as appropriate.

For the first 2½ years of the program, a full-time volunteer with a master's degree in counseling and prior work experience in the mental health field and grief counseling served as the bereavement coordinator and was supervised by the trauma social worker. The current trauma bereavement coordinator is a trauma staff nurse with CCRN certification and 15 years of varied experience in trauma nursing. She has specific crisis intervention and grief training and has worked closely with bereaved families in both professional and volunteer capacities.

PROGRAM IMPLEMENTATION

The Allegheny General Hospital Trauma Bereavement Program is designed to accomplish the following eight goals:

1. Provide immediate and sympathetic acknowledgement of the death and the family's pain.
2. Make personal contact so a family has opportunities to deal with grief issues and unanswered questions.
3. Demonstrate the staff's ongoing concern for the survivors.
4. Assess the grief process through a family member's words and the behavior described and follow immediately with specific interventions.

5. Provide information, referrals, and suggested literature that might be helpful.
6. Give assurance that the staff will continue to be available for them.
7. Acknowledge and support anticipated difficulties with holidays, birthdays, anniversaries, and so forth.
8. Bring closure to staff involvement 1 year after the death, even though an open invitation is extended to the family to remain in contact with the Trauma Bereavement Program as long as desirable.

To achieve these goals the bereavement coordinator follows specific steps for each death. The Program's components are outlined in the Box. Following the death of a patient, the family enters the Trauma Bereavement Program. Specific details concerning the patient's injuries, hospitalization, and family dynamics are recorded by the bereavement coordinator. Within 2 weeks of the death a sympathy card is sent to the family. The card includes a note of condolence, which often refers to something personal

---

Allegheny General Hospital Trauma Bereavement Program

1. Day 1	Date of patient's death.
2. Week 1	A sympathy card is sent to the family from the trauma unit with messages and signatures from appropriate staff members.
3. 2–4 months	A telephone call is made to family members dealing with grief issues, support systems, and appropriate referrals. At least two or up to three phone calls are made. If contact is not made, a personal handwritten note is sent advising the family of the attempt to reach them by phone and inviting them to call if they would like, or need, to talk.
4. Week following telephone call	If it is determined necessary or desirable during the phone call, selected follow-up material is sent.
5. 2–4 weeks before Thanksgiving	A holiday letter is mailed to help the family be aware of and deal with emotions and memories during the winter holiday season (Fig 1).
6. Between Thanksgiving and the winter holidays	A modified holiday letter is sent to families of patients who died between Thanksgiving and the winter holidays.
7. 3–4 weeks before the first anniversary of death	An anniversary letter is mailed to the family addressing issues significant to the anniversary (Fig 2).
8. Record keeping	Accurate records are maintained for each step of the program.

that occurred at the hospital. These notes are written with much thought and empathy for each particular family. Cards also include notes and signatures from the staff members who cared for the patient. The family often recognizes the names of the nurses who provided the final care and concern that their loved one and they themselves received at the hospital.

Although it is believed that each step of the program has value and provides opportunities for healing and recovery to begin, perhaps the most helpful, and certainly the most poignant, contact is the personal telephone call to surviving family members. The telephone call addresses many of the goals of the program. At this point the bereavement coordinator can assess the family's support system, express the continuing concern and availability of the staff members to the family, and refer family members to resources in the hospital or resources in their own community. Nurses and physicians are available to answer nagging medical questions. Social workers with experience in family counseling and knowledge of community agencies consult with the coordinator about various family needs. A medical library is an on-site resource for the coordinator. Clergy from the pastoral care department are available 24 hours a day to speak with those in crisis. A bimonthly memorial service for hospitalwide deaths is also offered by the pastoral care department.

Crucial to the success of the telephone call are the bereavement coordinator's skills in listening, interpersonal relationships, and grief therapy. A call is made 2 to 4 months after a death occurs. Very often during this period, support for the family diminishes and reality and loneliness intensify. A survivor is sometimes expected to be getting over a death, when in fact healing and recovery may take many months or years.[2]

The call may range in length from a few minutes to several hours. The conversation can be heartbreaking or heartening and is often a mixture of both. The issues and comments that families bring to these conversations are as varied as the situations and as the individuals. There are, however, some common themes expressed as

families struggle with loss and grief. Guilt, the "if onlys," anger, and feelings of emptiness and despair almost always surface in some way. Underlying the emotions are usually some feelings of lethargy, depression, and a sense of being overwhelmed or going crazy. All of these feelings often contribute to a sense of hopelessness and helplessness. Families need to hear that these feelings are normal and that there is no right or wrong way to grieve.

Responding appropriately to whatever is said is critical to the success of the contact. A mother who was grieving the death of a 17-year-old son said, "I feel so guilty when I laugh because Craig will never laugh again." In this case the response was, "You have told me many extraordinary things about Craig, and how he loved life and loved to laugh. What a wonderful way for you to honor Craig by your being able to laugh again." This thought appeared helpful to her as her guilt was reframed as a positive affirmation of her son. As this mother learns to laugh again, even brief moments of joy may rekindle hope and promise for her own life.

Another mother, that of a 41-year-old son, expressed her grief most graphically. She talked for several minutes about her six other children, several grandchildren, and three great-grandchildren. Then she said, "I am the shepherd with 99 sheep in the fold and one lost one, and I can't rest until the lost one is found." Understanding and accepting this statement was so important to her. How damaging it would have been to deny her loss or try to make her feel better by suggesting that all of the others could make up for her lost one. Sometimes, the compulsion to make things better is so great that inappropriate things are said. One must remember that nothing can change what happened. Appropriate interventions that provide understanding and continuing support may enable a grieving survivor or loved one to find and build on positive elements in his or her life.

The father of a 29-year-old, divorced daughter who died and whose 6-year-old daughter was then placed in the custody of her father expressed his pain, "Not only did we lose our own daughter, but in reality we lost her daughter, too. Every day of my life I live with this terrible, sad, empty, feeling." These particular parents had heard about the Compassionate Friends Organization, a worldwide bereavement organization that provides assistance after the death of a child and, with encouragement, were able to contact the organization. This family has now begun the long road to recovery.

Parents' expressions of grief reflect the pain of a child's death regardless of the child's age. It is out of the normal life cycle for parents to outlive their children. It is expected that parents will die before their children. When the opposite happens, parents feel betrayed and that they have not only lost their present but also their future.

During the telephone conversations, concern is expressed for other family members. Young children are of special concern as a family copes with the death of a parent or sibling. Parent save encouraged to listen to a child's words, to observe behavioral changes, to express their own sadness and loss, and to be honest in answering questions. Assuring a child that he or she is not responsible for a death is most important. Providing love and security during this time of loss and grief is also critical to acceptance and recovery.

No loss to traumatic death can be minimized. The loss of a spouse can be acute at any age or at any time. A young married couple has not had time to realize dreams or to establish family traditions that might provide some comfort and solace while grieving the loss of a mate. A young widow wrote, "I received your holiday letters and the letter regarding the anniversary of my husband's death. I want you to know how much I appreciate your remembrance and your words of caring. Jim's mother and I are still very much grieving our loss." An older couple may have looked forward to retirement and years of enjoyment without other family pressures, only to have those dreams destroyed in an instant. An older widow wrote, "Thank you for your lovely card . . . it helped me in my great loss of my beloved Henry."

A common fear expressed by spouses when a mate has collapsed suddenly is that the patient may have suffered before being found. A surviving spouse often expresses guilt and seeks answers to questions about the time between loss of consciousness and receipt of medical attention. Reassurance is given that physicians describe the loss of consciousness after falls or head injuries as instantaneous and that it is believed that the patient did not suffer. This explanation usually relieves this concern. However, with this issue or other troubling, unanswered questions, everyone is encouraged to call the attending physician to discuss any concerns and to find acceptable answers to all questions.

One frequently misunderstood or misinterpreted issue is that of brain death. A family served by the Traumatic Death Bereavement Program may never even have heard this term until it pertains to a loved one. During a call to a woman whose 56-year-old husband had been pronounced brain dead, she said "I will have to hide the secret that I let them take John off the ventilator because his sister and our daughter would never understand." Relief was clearly heard in her voice after it was explained that, following the determination of brain death, it is a medical decision that life support be terminated and that she was not responsible for her husband's death. She had no secret to hide. It is sometimes even difficult for staff members to understand and to become comfortable with brain death and its criteria. It is much more difficult for lay persons to understand this issue, particularly when they are in a crisis state.

The previous comments and anecdotes are but a few of those heard from loved ones. The immediate feedback from the majority of families indicates that the program has been helpful. Many express surprise and appreciation that a hospital provides such a caring and empathetic service. There are times, however, when such deep despair is expressed, or family dysfunction is noted, that members staff are also left with feelings of helplessness and ineffectiveness. Accepting one's own limitations and possible failures are realities that must be faced.

Although the program's primary goal is to provide support to trauma families, it also provides support for the trauma staff members who must be a part of these difficult deaths. Nurses are often the first contact for family members when they arrive at the hospital and the last contact as the family leaves the trauma unit. After saying good-bye to a family, a nurse usually returns to other patients where her nursing skills are in immediate demand. At the same time, the nurse feels a bond for the departing family and may have strong, emotional feelings that have to be postponed. To address these needs of nurses and other trauma staff members, debriefing sessions led by the social worker are held at appropriate intervals. These sessions provide ways for trauma staff members to deal with issues that arose and feelings they experienced while caring for a patient and family members. Nurses will often express feelings of helplessness, anger, and despair when their patients die. Nurses, too, can feel isolated in their grief if there is no opportunity to share these feelings. The debriefing sessions enable them to receive support from their peers who have had similar experiences and feelings. Led by an experienced social worker, the sessions help nurses learn how to cope with their feelings and where to seek professional counseling if necessary.

Although this article has focused largely on the personal telephone contact, other aspects of the program recognize grief issues and provide suggestions for a family to comfort and support each other as some specific steps are taken toward healing. Specifically, the follow-up letters address issues related to coping with holidays and the anniversary of the death. Although the letters (Figures 1 and 2) are standard in form, a family name is used and appropriate pronouns are selected to reflect the particular individual. The letters are personally signed by the trauma bereavement team, which includes two social workers, the trauma bereavement coordinator, and trauma nurses. Although these may seem like small details, this personalization reinforces the staff's care for the bereaved family.

•   •   •

The Trauma Bereavement Program assisted 347 families during the period of January 1, 1991, through December 31, 1994. All of the families received the personalized sympathy card. Telephone contacts were made to 202 families; 107 handwritten notes were sent when telephone attempts were unsuccessful, and 580

The winter holidays are rapidly approaching. Normally, Thanksgiving, Chanukkah and Christmas are days of celebration and of sharing time with those people we love. However, because of your loss this past year, these holidays may be times of sadness and may, in fact, only emphasize the absence of the one you loved.

We of the Allegheny Hospital Trauma Unit recognize some of the difficulties you may experience this year, and we would like to encourage you to consider the following thoughts which we believe might be helpful to you in the days ahead.

- Recognize that these holidays may be very strenuous for you. Try to pay attention to activities that will help you. Try not to overextend yourself or over commit.
- Eliminate the unnecessary chores and help reduce holiday pressures on yourself and others.
- Your family members may also be grieving in different ways. Discuss your feelings with each other and how you want to handle the holidays. While keeping some old traditions, it may also be helpful to establish some new ones this year.
- You may feel uncomfortable when someone says to you: "Happy Holidays." A simple reply of "Thank You," or "Best Wishes to You," are graceful responses.

In conclusion, be kind to yourself and allow yourself to grieve. If there is any way that we can be helpful to you, please feel free to call us.

Figure 1. Holiday letter, Allegheny General Hospital Trauma Bereavement Program. *Source:* Reprinted with permission from Allegheny General Hospital Trauma Unit.

As the first anniversary of _____ death approaches, we of the Trauma Team want you to know that _____ has not been forgotten.

While we cannot really understand the depth of your pain and loss, we do remember _____, and we want to be available for you and your family as your recover. We do not believe that time alone heals unless it is accompanied with people who care, and with ways to enable healing.

At this time you may be surprised at the feelings you have, and with the intensity of them. You may expect to feel sadness and despair, but may be surprised to feel guilt, anger, or even relief as you relive the death over and over. Remembering and reliving the event can sometimes cause these feelings to seem overwhelming or frightening. We want to assure you that this is normal, and that there is no right and wrong way to grieve. We hope that as you relive the event that resulted in the loss of your loved one, that you will be kind to yourselves; that you will be able to rejoice in your good memories which honor _____; that you will seek help from those who love and care for you; that you will forgive yourselves for any thoughts or feelings of neglect or guilt which you might have; and that you will use this time to move toward acceptance of this tragedy in ways which could help you move forward with your own lives. We in the Trauma Unit are available to assist you in your effort. Please call at any time in the future if we can help in any way.

Figure 2. Anniversary letter, Allegheny General Hospital Trauma Bereavement Program. *Source:* Reprinted with permission from Allegheny General Hospital Trauma Unit.

anniversary and holiday letters were sent. Approximately 40 calls and 60 cards and letters were received by the trauma unit or bereavement coordinator in response to the program. Although these numbers do not measure the worth of the program, they do reflect the commitment that the trauma team has made to grieving family members. The feedback suggests that a family that has a support system available and that receives assistance in the grieving process is more likely to experience healthy, normal grieving and avoid prolonged, pathologic grieving. A plan for a formal evaluation of the program's first 4 years is underway.

The need for closure and finality when death occurs in the acute care setting is evident. The Allegheny General Hospital Trauma Bereavement Program provides for this closure and assists the family as it begins to establish some hope, order, and promise for its recovery. Additionally, it is hoped that readers of this article will be encouraged to develop and implement bereavement programs for families of patients who die in their critical care units. Although resources will vary in different hospitals, with the support and commitment of administration, nursing, social services, and volunteer services as described in this article the authors believe that this program can be successfully modified or replicated. They are available to discuss further this program and to assist in the establishment of meaningful bereavement programs in other hospital settings.

REFERENCES

1. Itasca IL. *Accident Facts.* Chicago, Ill: National Safety Council; 1993.

2. Brown JT. Grief response in trauma patients and their families. *Adv Psychosom Med.* 1986;16:93–114.

SUGGESTED READING

Brothers J. *Widowed.* New York, NY: Simon & Schuster; 1990.

Brown JT, Stoudemire. Normal and pathological grief. *J Am Med Assoc.* 1983;250:378–382.

Dubin W. Sudden unexpected death: intervention with the survivors. *Am J Emerg Med.* 1986;15:54–57.

Donnelley NH. *I Never Know What to Say.* New York, NY: Ballantine Books; 1987.

Fitzgerald H. *The Grieving Child: A Parent's Guide.* New York, NY: Simon & Schuster; 1992.

Gravelle K. *Teenagers Face to Face with Bereavement.* Englewood Cliffs, NJ: J. Messner; 1989.

Lindemann E. *Beyond Grief, Studies in Crisis Intervention.* New York, NY: Jason Aronson; 1979.

Lukas C. *Silent Grief: Living in the Wake of Suicide.* New York, NY: Scribner's; 1987.

Raphael B. *The Anatomy of Bereavement.* New York, NY: Basic Books; 1983.

Rosof D. *The Worst Loss: How Families Heal from the Death of a Child.* 1st ed. New York, NY: Holt; 1994.

Schiff HS. *Living Through Mourning: Finding Comfort and Hope When a Loved One Has Died.* New York, NY: Penguin Books; 1987.

Schiff HS. *The Bereaved Parent.* New York, NY: Penguin Books; 1978.

Shaw E. *What to do When a Loved One Dies: a Practical Guide to Dealing with Death on Life's Terms.* Irvine, Calif: Dickens Press; 1994.

Tatelbaum J. *The Courage to Grieve: Creative Living, Recovery, and Growth Through Grief.* New York, NY: Lippincott & Crowell, 1980.

Worden J. *Grief Counseling and Grief Therapy—A Handbook for the Mental Health Practitioner.* New York, NY: Springer; 1982.

Influencing Holistic Nursing Practice in Long-Term Care

Marge Drugay, MS, RN, C
Consultant
Drugay & Associates
Glenview, Illinois
Associate Faculty
Rush University
Department of Gerontological Nursing
Chicago, Illinois

Nursing homes can present formidable barriers to the practice of holistic nursing, or they can be fertile ground for the development of expanded practice. The critical issue may be how a particular nurse or institution defines holistic nursing, and what implications this has for practice.

DEVELOPMENT OF THE CONCEPT OF HOLISM

In a recent article, Johnson[1] reported a research study that attempted to identify the concepts and activities that represent the holistic paradigm of health in nursing, and the manner in which this information is being communicated within the profession. She stated:

> In recent years a new paradigm has come forward, a holistic viewpoint that has captured the attention of many researchers and practitioners. Its definitions of the nature of disease and the healing arts have resulted in major changes in the practice of health professionals and unanticipated results among the client population. This new paradigm, labeled by many as the holistic paradigm of health, is a major innovation in today's rapidly changing health care system.[1(p129)]

According to Johnson, since 1966 some of the key words found and indexed in nursing literature to express holism/holistic nursing include well-

Source: Reprinted from M. Drugay, *Holistic Nursing Practice,* Vol. 7, No. 1, pp. 46–52, © 1992, Aspen Publishers, Inc.

ness, lifestyle, holistic health, self-care, consciousness, caring, and Therapeutic Touch. Between 1966 and 1987, a total of 924 articles relating to the holistic paradigm were published in nursing journals, the majority of those in practice areas as opposed to areas of research, education, or administration. The author concludes that "the increase in the number of articles on holism supports the argument that a holistic perspective is being diffused in the nursing literature."[1(p137)]

HOLISTIC PRACTICE IN LONG-TERM CARE

Whether we agree with Johnson's conclusions or not, the concept of holism has a seductive appeal in gerontological nursing, particularly in a long-term care facility. Kastenbaum[2] posited that care of the institutionalized aged should incorporate a philosophy of care. Accepting Barnum's[3] definition that holism is a philosophy facilitates the practice of holistic care in any nursing interaction. If innovative care and a paradigm change are indeed occurring in nursing, then long-term care/gerontology is a practice area in which these new behaviors and activities may be viewed longitudinally.

The nursing home is often the final home that the older person may know, and many health professionals are not always sensitive to the fact that this is truly "home" for these residents. It is easy to focus on the process and procedures of the institutional reality, rather than the reality of the resident, yet it is one environment where holism should be assiduously practiced because of the very nature of long-term relationships that can develop between residents and staff. Cognitive impairment in residents may alter the process and procedures in the relationships, but it has no effect on the need for a holistic nursing perspective.

Relocation to a nursing home represents a significant life passage for many older adults. Often-quoted statistics indicate that 5% of all older adults, and 25% of those older than 85 reside in nursing homes. This transition is often caused by a change in functional and/or cognitive status, and individual response to this type of move var-

ies greatly. Chenitz,[4] Rosswrum,[5] and Dimond and associates[6] have studied the effect of relocation on residents, and their adjustment over time, and have described some of the difficulties people encounter.

Assuming the validity of the observations that relocation represents a major transition in the life experience of older adults, we need to examine how nurses can assist these people in the adjustment processes to enrich and enhance the quality of their life. A holistic nursing perspective has multiple benefits to this end, for both the residents and the nurse, and provides a means to evaluate the cultural and societal support necessary at this time.

FACTORS AFFECTING THE PRACTICE OF HOLISTIC NURSING IN THE NURSING HOME SETTING

Barriers to the practice of holistic nursing, that is, nursing care that takes into consideration the interconnectedness of the whole individual—mind, body, and spirit—may be related to three factors:

1. External factors such as federal and state rules and regulations, which govern overall policies and procedures of the institution;
2. Internal factors such as a shortage of registered nurses and assistive personnel; the strict adherence to a medical model of care; or the presence of specific institutional policies; and
3. Personal factors such as lack of knowledge about how to incorporate holistic practice; issues of control or territoriality of practice; and fear of the unknown concept of holism.

External factors

Federal and state rules and regulations were designed with the intent to protect the individual resident. Standardization of factors within the physical plant to provide appropriate space, light, heat, safety, so forth, and regulations governing the physical care of the individual while protecting their civil rights have developed to prevent substandard care and abuse of any nature. In the process, however, regulations and their required documentation have frequently interfered with the ability to provide high-quality care.

The adherence to "paper compliance" has crippled institutions because of the number and qualifications of personnel required to document compliance. This concern for minutiae may prevent nurses from spending appropriate time with residents, and may restrict their ability to develop meaningful therapeutic relationships. The Omnibus Reconciliation Act of 1987, was designed to allow registered nurses to assess the individual residents more completely, thereby being able to plan more accurately for their needs. If an institution's administration views this as a restrictive regulation, and has insufficient staff to comply with the required documentation, that segment of nursing control and involvement may be lost or redistributed to other disciplines.

Internal factors

According to an American Nurses Association report in 1991, the nursing shortage in long-term care was 18.9%.[7] This represents a significant inability to provide appropriate assessment and evaluation of critical older adult needs. If there are insufficient registered nurses to provide adequate care, it is inevitable that the general quality of care will suffer, and so too will those nursing home residents.

Institutional routines can also adversely affect the practice of holistic nursing. To tailor daily routine to the needs of the individuals is almost impossible in any institutional setting if there are not built-in supports for that behavior. For example, the older adult who has always stayed up late in the evening and slept later in the morning will challenge the system; so also will the individual who prefers meals at any time other than the established hours. Regardless of the individual nurse's willingness to "bend the rules," institutional policy usually dominates. Changing institutional policy is not routinely tackled by an overburdened nurse.

Certain institutional policies may contribute to the fragmentation of the role of the professional nurse, so that other disciplines are providing care or services that should appropriately be nursing responsibilities. In some institutions, the nurse may have duties that rightly belong within other disciplines, and the need for role-appropriate responsibilities is a critical one.[8]

Personal factors

These may be the largest hurdles that the nurse wishing to incorporate a holistic philosophic approach may face. As previously discussed, holism has assumed various definitions, not all of which are readily accepted in traditional nursing circles. The association of the term holistic with alternative and nontraditional therapies creates an impression of the use of "voodoo" or nonscientific methods in care. The lack of knowledge regarding the scope of activities in holistic nursing, personal issues of control or territoriality of nursing practice, or fear of the unknown concept of holism can obstruct the best intentions of the nurse hoping to incorporate this approach.

SUPPORT FOR HOLISTIC NURSING PRACTICE IN THE NURSING HOME

In these same institutions there may be a multitude of resources and supports available to promote a more holistic approach to care. If part of the process of positive adaptation to the transition of relocation is to retain a sense of control of one's personal environment, then it is imperative for nurses to assist the resident with defining those areas of control and autonomy. Residents' civil rights are built-in guidelines for viewing the whole person. Techniques in holistic nursing include but are not limited to such modalities as the use of imagery (guided or otherwise), Therapeutic Touch, biofeedback, breathing techniques, use of prayer and spirituality, movement, dance and art therapies, massage, humor, music, reminiscence, acupressure, and pet therapy.[1,9–12,13–16,19–22]

These techniques have been used by nurses, nursing assistants, physical therapists, occupational therapists, social workers, physicians, ministers, and activity program personnel in many long-term care institutions, usually as isolated entities, not as part of an intentional holistic focus. Establishing a coalition of these interested individuals is one method of identifying organizational supports, and may be one of the most effective means of "diffusing the paradigm of holistic health"[1(p129)] as Johnson claims.

Another area where nurses can capitalize on the potential for a supportive atmosphere is in collaborating with nurses in advanced practice roles. If the nursing home is fortunate to have a geriatric nurse practitioner or clinical nurse specialist, or if the nursing home has linkages with a college or university affiliations, such as the Teaching Nursing Home Programs,[17] the home may already be an arena more responsive to change in practice.

If the nursing home has a progressive and open-minded administration, acceptance of a creative nursing plan may be dependent only on its being proposed. A recent innovation in this respect is creation of restraint-free, or restraint-appropriate facilities. It was believed that this could never be done, but nursing homes across the country are learning not only that it *can* be done, but also that there are observable benefits for residents and staff.

IMPLICATIONS FOR PRACTICE IN THE NURSING HOME SETTING

A nursing home can present formidable barriers to the practice of holistic nursing practice, or provide fertile ground for development of expanded practice. Activities and strategies can be implemented to expand nursing practice within a holistic philosophical framework. The following suggestions may be used in isolation, or as part of a globally integrated plan to promote high-level wellness with a holistic perspective.

Use of support groups

Long-term care settings are ideal arenas for support groups designed for residents, families, or staff.[18] An Alzheimer's disease support group

can provide education on the disease itself, management of common problems, and multigenerational issues. Groups for coping with functional limitations such as arthritis, or impaired vision or hearing, are logical choices for many nursing home residents.

Taylor and Ferszt[13] feel that support groups with a spiritual focus can be especially helpful for those staff members who work with death and dying on a regular basis. Not only does this allow for the expression of grief at the loss of a resident, but it may also provide staff with an opportunity for closure of the relationship, which might not otherwise occur.

If the nursing home is part of a larger retirement community or continuum of care, issues that relate to coping with actual or impending losses, aging itself, relocation, living with an ill spouse, or "surviving cancer" support groups may also be welcomed. Those groups that focus on maintaining wellness throughout aging can have a positive impact on the health and well-being of residents as well. In each of these areas, the mind–body–spirit interaction should be emphasized, and can provide the focus for improved self-care behaviors at all levels.

Use of touch as communication

The value of touch, as distinguished from the modality of Therapeutic Touch, as a tool of nonverbal communication is often underestimated or neglected in our increasingly technically oriented health care society. The acute care setting was often defined as high tech, low touch, and long-term care was seen as the opposite. In today's world of long-term care, high tech consumes an ever-widening portion of the care that is provided. In long-term care, however, we often have the advantage of establishing longer-term relationships that encourage a more frequent use of touch as an expression of friendship and caring, beyond the clinical task-oriented touch, which occurs with bathing, dressing, and physical assessment.

The need for human touch is a separate issue from sexuality in aging. Only a very small minority of nursing home residents are currently married or have access to an appropriate sexual partner. Institutional policy often inhibits intimacy of any type, including expressions of sexuality.

Kass[14] noted that nursing home residents felt a lack of sexual attractiveness, and a restriction in their sexual expression because of a lack of privacy. According to Allen,[15] in a study reported in 1984, Portonova and associates[16] discovered that in the elderly women they studied the "subjects' attitudes were more positive toward married sexually active older adults and widowed sexually active older adults living in an apartment than widowed sexually active older adults residing in a nursing home."[15(p78)]

The need for security, love, and social belonging does not disappear with lack of an acceptable partner. Thus nonsexual touch may fulfill some of the needs of the nursing home resident for relating to other human beings. It is important to consider the needs of the resident who constantly reaches out physically to staff members, as a plea to meet the desire for warm human contact.

Use of prayer

Participation in prayer with a resident is often overlooked in the day-to-day nurse–resident relationship, which routinely centers on functional tasks, voluminous paperwork, and time schedules. Too frequently praying is a function relegated to the chaplain, minister, priest, rabbi, or volunteer when they visit with the resident. But prayer can be a powerful presence in the lives of older adults, and should not be left to happenstance. "More things are wrought by prayer than this world dreams of."[23(p569)] Tennyson's words echo a deep spiritual belief that fuels the existence of many older adults. Prayer can provide a refuge, solace, strength, comfort, and guidance. Losses that occur with relocation to a nursing home can include a disruption in the previous pattern of prayer or religious worship, and nurses interested in holistic care must be aware of the effect this may have on residents.

Spiritual needs may be assessed when a resident enters a nursing home, but neglected in the days, months, and years to follow. Providing an atmosphere that supports and acknowledges the resi-

dents' desire for prayer or other religious activity should be a role of the nurse advocate. Taking a few moments to join in prayer with a resident who desires it may mean the difference in the resident's ability to cope with frustrations and problems encountered on a daily basis, or may provide serenity in the face of illness and stress.

Use of other noninvasive techniques

Movement therapy is a term used to describe a variety of techniques that incorporate the development of a conscious awareness of body movements. This constellation of modalities is a natural product of holism, with the mind–body–spirit connection clearly outlined. Snyder[19] discusses several of the activities included under the rubric of movement therapy, with familiar ones such as creative dance, social dance, relaxation exercises, yoga, Tai Chi, and rhythmic games. She identifies some of the positive outcomes to be reduction of stress and pain, improvement in mobility and interactions, increased self-esteem, and decreased confusion. The author reviews two specific forms of movement therapy, and suggests a variety of ways in which they can be introduced. In addition, she has also referenced two additional studies related to use of movement therapy with the elderly as a specific group.[20,21]

Guzzetta[22] described a study comparing the effects of relaxation technique and music therapy in a coronary care unit. This author noted that music appeared to have more effect on that population, but both modalities showed positive physiologic outcomes as opposed to the lack of change in the control group. Humor has also been used as a therapeutic approach, primarily with a pediatric population, and research needs to be expanded to include information about effects with older adults.

Use of research findings and diffusion of the paradigm of holistic health

It is incumbent on the nurse interested in holistic care of the older adult to have the ability to articulate what holistic care *is*, and what it means for his or her practice. Sharing this perspective with other nurses and health care professionals validates the existence of the resident as a "whole person." As an all-encompassing philosophical framework for assessing and recognizing the mind–body–spirit interaction, holistic nursing offers a tempting approach to caring for older adults. In Johnson's words:

> Spirituality, consciousness, self-concept, life style and well-being are important dimensions of this person that need to be considered within the practice of nursing . . . the relationship between the client and the nurse is a reciprocal one in which each benefits

from the interactions and each grows in self-awareness.[1(p137)]

• • •

The use of simple techniques, such as touch, imagery, art and music therapy, prayer, and stress-management strategies may produce positive health outcomes if they are consciously and consistently applied as one means of therapeutic intervention. Overcoming barriers in the practice setting and diffusing this holistic innovation may open up a new vision of holistic nursing practice for future generations of nurses in long-term care.

REFERENCES

1. Johnson MB. The holistic paradigm in nursing: the diffusion of an innovation. *Research in Nursing and Health.* 1990;13:129–139.

2. Kastenbaum RJ, Barber TX, Wilson SC, Ryder BL, Hathaway LB. *Old, Sick, and Helpless: Where Therapy Begins.* Cambridge, Mass: Ballinger; 1981.

3. Barnum BJ. Holistic nursing and nursing process. *Holistic Nursing Practice.* 1987;1(3):27–35.

4. Chenitz WC. Entry into a nursing home as status passage: theory to guide nursing practice. *Geriatric Nursing.* 1983;4(2):92–97.

5. Rosswrum MA. Relocation and the elderly. *Journal of Gerontological Nursing.* 1983;9:632–637.

6. Dimond M, McCance K, King K. Forced residential relocation: its impact on the well-being of older adults. *Western Journal of Nursing Research.* 1987;9:445–464.

7. American Nurses Association. *The Nursing Shortage and the 1990s: Realities and Remedies.* Kansas City, Mo: American Nurses Association; 1991.

8. Drugay M. Solutions to nurse shortage include "role-appropriate" responsibilities. *Provider.* 1991;17(1):66–68.

9. Levine ME. Holistic nursing. *Nursing Clinics of North America.* 1971;6:253–264.

10. Rogers ME. *An Introduction to the Theoretical Basis of Nursing.* Philadelphia, Pa: F.A. Davis; 1970.

11. Sarkis JM, Skoner MM. An analysis of the concept of holism in nursing literature. *Holistic Nursing Practice.* 1987;2(1):61–69.

12. Brallier LW. Biofeedback and holism in clinical practice. *Holistic Nursing Practice.* 1988;2(3):26–33.

13. Taylor PB, Ferszt GG. Spiritual healing. *Holistic Nursing Practice.* 1990;4(4):32–38.

14. Kass MJ. Sexual expression of the elderly in nursing homes. *The Gerontologist.* 1978;18(4):372–378.

15. Allen ME. A holistic view of sexuality and the aged. *Holistic Nursing Practice.* 1987;1(4):76–83.

16. Portonova M, Young E, Newman MA. Elderly women's attitudes toward sexual activity among their peers. *Health Care for Women International.* 1984;5:289–298.

17. Mezey MD, Lynaugh JE. The teaching nursing home program. *Nursing Clinics of North America.* 1989; 24(3):769–775.

18. Barker E. Support groups: holistic nursing. *Journal of Neuroscience Nursing.* 1987;19(3):121–122.

19. Snyder M. Movement therapy. *Journal of Neuroscience Nursing.* 1988;20(6):373–376.

20. Goldberg WG, Fitzpatrick JJ. Movement therapy with the aged. *Nursing Research.* 1980;29:339–346.

21. Lindner EC. Dance as a therapeutic intervention for the elderly. *Educational Gerontology.* 1982;8:167–174.

22. Guzzetta CE. Effects of relaxation and music therapy on patients in a coronary care unit with presumptive acute myocardial infarction. *Heart and Lung.* 1989;18(6):609–616.

23. Tennyson A. *The Passage of Arthur.* In: Pfordresher J, Veidemanis GV, McDonnell H, eds. *England in Literature.* Glenview, Ill: Scott Foresman; 1989.

Index

C